Principles of
PHARMACOLOGY
for DENTAL STUDENTS
Third Edition

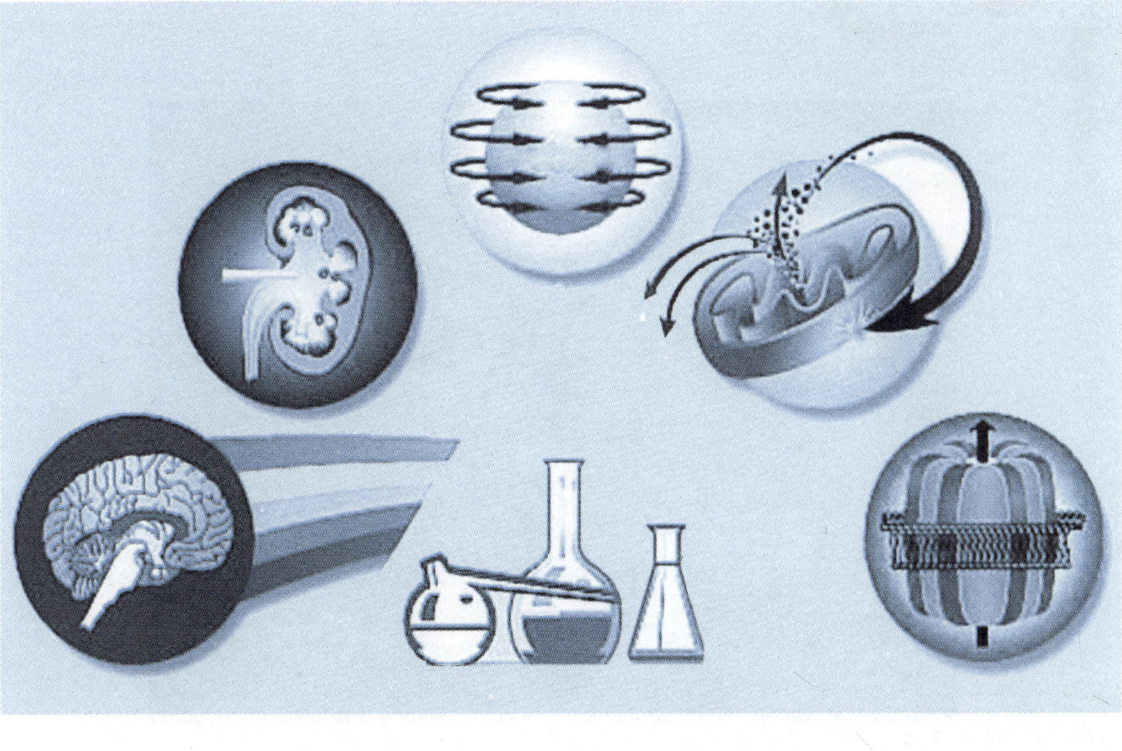

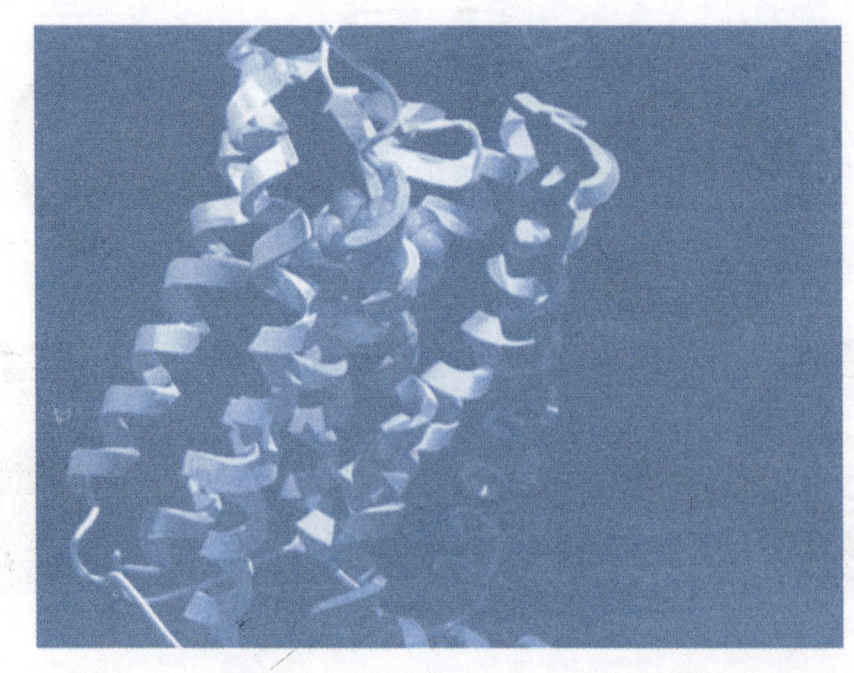

Principles of

PHARMACOLOGY

for DENTAL STUDENTS

Third Edition

Naresh Kumar Khanna

MBBS, MSc (Med.), MD, FIMSA, MNAMS

Professor and Head
Department of Pharmacology
Jaipur Dental College, Jaipur

Formerly

Senior Professor and Head
Department of Pharmacology
SMS Medical College, Jaipur, and MGNIMS, Jaipur

Director, Maharishi Arvind College of Pharmacy, Jaipur

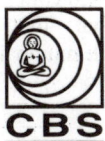

CBS

CBS Publishers & Distributors Pvt. Ltd.

New Delhi • Bengaluru • Chennai • Kochi • Kolkata • Mumbai
Hyderabad • Nagpur • Patna • Pune • Vijayawada

ISBN: 978-81-239-1858-7

First Edition: 1999
Second Edition: 2005
Third Edition: 2010
Reprint: 2016

Published by:
Satish Kumar Jain for CBS Publishers & Distributors Pvt. Ltd.,
4819/XI Prahlad Street, 24 Ansari Road, Daryaganj, New Delhi - 110002
delhi@cbspd.com, cbspubs@airtelmail.in • www.cbspd.com
Ph.: 23289259, 23266861, 23266867 • Fax: 011-23243014

Corporate Office: 204 FIE, Industrial Area, Patparganj, Delhi - 110 092
Ph: 49344934 • Fax: 011-49344935
E-mail: publishing@cbspd.com • publicity@cbspd.com

Branches:
• *Bengaluru:* 2975, 17th Cross, K.R. Road, Bansankari 2nd Stage,
  Bengaluru - 70 • Ph: +91-80-26771678/79 • Fax: +91-80-26771680
  E-mail: cbsbng@gmail.com, bangalore@cbspd.com
• *Chennai:* No. 7, Subbaraya Street, Shenoy Nagar, Chennai - 600030
  Ph: +91-44-26681266, 26680620 • Fax: +91-44-42032115
  E-mail: chennai@cbspd.com
• *Kochi:* Ashana House, 39/1904, A.M. Thomas Road, Valanjambalam,
  Ernakulum, Kochi • Ph: +91-484-4059061-65
  Fax: +91-484-4059065 • E-mail: cochin@cbspd.com
• *Kolkata:* 6-B, Ground Floor, Rameshwar Shaw Road, Kolkata - 700014
  Ph: +91-33-22891126/7/8 • E-mail: kolkata@cbspd.com
• *Mumbai:* 83-C, Dr. E. Moses Road, Worli, Mumbai - 400018
  Ph: +91-9833017933, 022-24902340/41 • E-mail: mumbai@cbspd.com

Representatives:

• Hyderabad: 0-9885175004	• Nagpur: 0-9021734563
• Patna: 0-9334159340	• Pune: 0-9623451994
• Vijayawada: 0-9000660880	

Printed at:
India Binding House, Noida (UP)

to

_____

my wife and daughter

and

my students

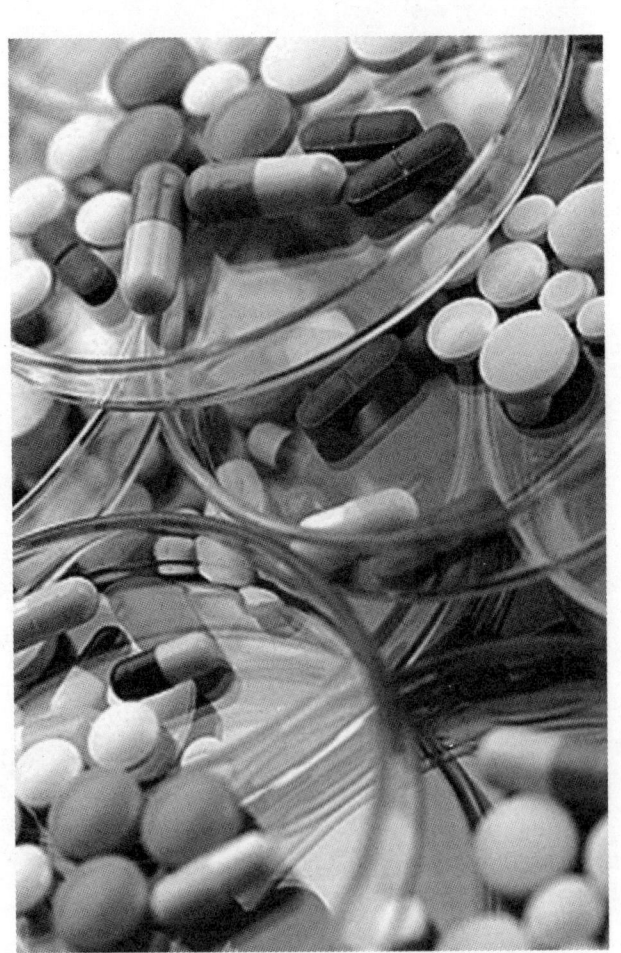

Preface to the Third Edition

The Dental Council of India (DCI) has recently revised the syllabus in pharmacology for BDS students. Keeping that in mind the book has been revised. Points for dental students are given at the end of each chapter to cover the implications of drugs in dental practice as desired by the DCI. Treatment of common dental problems has also been included in the portion of dental pharmacology. Further, all the chapters have been updated and meticulously revised. I have also tried to include the new drugs as for as possible. As usual, I am sure dental students will find the text precise and reader-friendly. This will enable them to acquire the basic knowledge of drugs for their rational use in dental practice.

I am thankful to my colleague, Dr HL Sharma, for his valuable suggestions. I am sure to receive constructive comments and suggestions from my fellow colleagues, students, and other readers in future also. This will help me to revise the book in future.

I thankfully acknowledge the meticulous work of the staff of CBS Publishers & Distributors, and the cooperation of my wife.

Naresh Kumar Khanna

Preface to the First Edition

Students of BDS course are supposed to attend about forty lectures in pharmacology as per syllabus. On the other hand, the students of MBBS course are required to attend 100–110 lectures as per recommendations of Medical Council of India. At present the major object of teaching pharmacology to the students of BDS is to provide rational basis for choosing and using drugs skillfully in dental practice. It is highly desirable that they should be educated to develop a critical outlook towards various drugs as per syllabus. So they are supposed to know the basic principles of whole of the pharmacology with particular stress on certain groups of drugs used routinely in dental practice. Since there are no suitable books available for them, they have to read the same books of pharmacology meant for MBBS students.

It is time consuming as they have to prepare their own notes in concise form. Further this fact is still more important as these students have many other subjects to go through which are equally important and advanced. Keeping this in mind I have attempted to write this book which is not unduly voluminous or too concise. I hope it should provide adequate, balanced and up-to-date information on the subject for these students. For the benefit of these students a section on dental pharmacology and therapeutics has also been written.

Although the book is written mainly for BDS students, it will also prove useful to undergraduate MBBS, Diploma in Pharmacy and B Pharmacy students for quick revision as well as to practising doctors as pharmacotherapeutic reference book.

I welcome comments, criticism and suggestions from my colleagues and students.

Naresh Kumar Khanna

Contents

Section 11: HORMONES AND RELATED DRUGS

Section 12: CHEMOTHERAPY

Section 13: DENTAL PHARMACOLOGY AND THERAPEUTICS

Section 14: MISCELLANEOUS TOPICS

Appendix

Section 1

General Pharmacology

1. Definitions, Sources of Drugs and Routes of Drug Administration

2. Pharmacokinetics

3. Pharmacodynamics

4. Adverse Drug Reactions, Prescription Writing and Drug Interactions

Chapter 1

Definitions, Sources of Drugs and Routes of Drug Administration

DEFINITIONS

1. **Pharmacology** (Greek: *Pharmacon*—drug; *logos*—discourse in) is the science of drugs. Its two main divisions are pharmacodynamics and pharmacokinetics.

2. **Pharmacodynamics** deals with physiological and biochemical effects of drugs and their mechanism of action at macromolecular/subcellular/organ/system level.

3. **Pharmacokinetics** deals with absorption, distribution, binding, localization, storage, biotransformation and excretion of drugs.

4. **Drug** (French: *Drogue*—a dry herb) is any substance or product that is used or intended to be used to modify physiological system or pathological states for the benefit of recipient.

   Some other pharmacological aspects of importance are:

5. **Pharmacotherapeutics** means use of a drug for prevention, mitigation or cure of the disease.

6. **Clinical pharmacology** deals with the scientific study of drugs in man (healthy volunteers and patients). It is carried out for evaluation of efficacy and safety of drugs, and provides data for optimum use of drugs in human beings.

7. **Chemotherapy deals** with treatment of systemic infection/malignancy with specific drugs. Usually these drugs have selective toxicity for the infecting organisms/malignant cell with no/minimal effects on the host cells. Thus drugs can be divided into:
   i. *Pharmacodynamic agents:* These are designed to have pharmacodynamic effects in the recipient.
   ii. *Chemotherapeutic agents:* These are used to inhibit/kill invading parasite/malignant cell. These have been designed to have no/minimal pharmacodynamic effects in the recipients.

8. **Pharmacy** is a branch of pharmacology. It deals with collection, identification, purification, isolation, synthesis, standardization, compounding and dispensing of a drug. Large scale manufacture of drugs is called pharmaceutics. It is primarily a technological science.

9. **Toxicology** is the study of poisonous effects of drugs and other chemicals. It deals with detection, prevention and treatment of poisoning.

10. **Pharmacovigilance** is defined as the pharmacological science which deals with the detection, assessment, understanding and prevention of adverse effects, particularly long-term and short-term adverse effects of medicines. It is an important and integral part of clinical research. Both clinical trials safety and postmarketing pharmacovigilance are critical throughout the product life cycle.

SOURCES OF DRUGS

Drugs can be obtained from various sources such as:

1. **Animal,** e.g. antitoxic sera, gonado-trophines, heparin, insulin and thyroid extract.
2. **Drugs** produced by genetic engineering (i.e. by DNA recombinant technology), e.g. human growth hormone and human insulin.
3. **Mineral,** e.g. zinc, aluminium hydroxide, liquid paraffin, lithium, magnesium trisilicate.
4. **Micro-organisms:** Important sources of antibacterial substances (e.g. penicillin and other antibiotics) are fungi and bacteria which are isolated from soil.
5. **Synthetic:** In clinical practice, majority of the drugs used are synthetic such as diazepam, paracetamol, clonidine, corticosteroids, etc.
6. **Plant:** For example atropine, emetine, quinine, morphine, digoxin and reserpine.

There are a number of pharmacologically active principles in plants such as:

i. **Oils:** They are of following types:
   a. *Fixed oils:* Chemically, the fixed oils are glycosides of palmitic, oleic and stearic acids. They are fats. Castor oil is pharmacologically active and is used as a laxative.
   b. *Volatile oils* are volatile, essential or flavouring oils. Chemically, they consist of hydrocarbon terpene or some polymer of it. They are not fats. They are useful as:
   - Antiseptic, e.g. used in mouth-washes and pastes.
   - Carminative, e.g. ginger and oil of eucalyptus.
   - Flavouring agents, e.g. oil of pep-permint.
   - Counter irritants, e.g. turpentine oil.
   - Analgesic, e.g. oil of clove in toothache.
   c. *Mineral oil,* e.g. liquid paraffin. It is a hydrocarbon. It is derived from petroleum and is used as a lubricant laxative. It is devoid of food value.

ii. **Alkaloids:** Alkaloids contain cyclic nitrogen. They are insoluble in water. They are basic substances. So they combine with acids to form well-defined water soluble salts, e.g. atropine, emetine and morphine.

iii. **Glycosides:** Chemically, these are ether like combinations of sugars with other organic structures. They are hydrolyzed to a sugar and non-sugar moiety (aglycon or genin) on heating with mineral acid, e.g. digoxin hydrolyses into digitoxose and digoxigenin. When a glycoside produces glucose on acid hydrolysis, it is called a glucoside, e.g. strophanthin.

iv. **Gums:** These are secretory products of plants, e.g. agar, gum acacia and gum tragacanth. Agar is employed as a bulk laxative while the other two are used in pharmacy as suspending and emulsifying agents.

v. **Resins:** They are formed in plants by oxidation or polymerization of volatile oils. They are insoluble in water but soluble in alcohol.

vi. **Oleoresins** are mixtures of volatile oil and resins, e.g. male fern extract.

vii. **Tannins:** These are non-nitrogenous constituents of plants. They have astringent action upon mucous mem-brane and thus exert a protective action. For example, tincture catechu releases tannic acid in the small intestine and so it is used in the treatment of diarrhea.

7. **Antibacterial substances:** These are derived from fungi and moulds, e.g. penicillin, kanamycin, tobramycin.

ROUTES OF DRUG ADMINISTRATION

The drugs may be either applied locally or administered systemically. It depends on nature of drug as well as patient. Factors, which govern the choice of route of administration of a drug, are:

- Physical and chemical nature of the drug.
- Rate and extent of absorption of the drug from different routes.
- Site of drug action.
- Desired onset of action.
- Condition of the patient.
- Effect of digestive juices and first pass metabolism.

Local Routes

These routes are used for localized lesion. The advantages are:

- Attainment of high concentration at the desired site.
- No or minimal systemic side effects.

The local routes are:

1. **Skin:** Drug may be applied on skin as ointment, dressings, cream, lotion, powder, paste, etc.
2. **Mucous membranes:** The dosage form depends on the site.
   a. *Anal canal:* As ointment, suppositories.
   b. *Bronchi and lungs:* As aerosols (nebulized solution or fine powder) inhalations.
   c. *Eyes, ear and nose:* As drops, ointment, irrigation, nasal spray.
   d. *Gastrointestinal tract:* As non-absorbable drugs given orally, e.g. kaolin, neomycin, aluminium hydroxide, etc.
   e. *Mouth and pharynx:* As paints, lozenges, mouthwashes, gargle.
   f. *Urethra:* As jelly, irrigation solution.
   g. *Vagina:* As cream, douches, pessaries, vaginal tablets, powders.
3. **Arterial supply:** This route can be used to infuse anticancer drugs through femoral or brachial artery for limb malignancies; for contrast in angiography.
4. **Deeper tissues:** Certain drugs can be administered by using syringe and needle to reach deeper tissue provided their systemic absorption is slow, e.g.
   a. Intra-arterial injection.
   b. Intrathecal injection.
   c. Retrobulbar injection.

Systemic Routes

Through systemic routes, drug is absorbed into blood. It is then distributed all over including the site of action through circulation.

1. Oral

Oral ingestion of a drug is the oldest and commonest mode of administration. Both solid and liquid dosage forms can be given orally.

Advantages

- Safer
- Convenient
- Non-invasive
- Often painless
- Does not need assistance
- Need not be sterile
- Cheaper

Limitations

- Onset of action is slow.
- May cause nausea and vomiting.
- Irritant and unpalatable drugs cannot be administered by this route.
- Cannot be used for uncooperative, unconscious, and vomiting patient.
- Certain drugs are destroyed by digestive juices (penicillin) or in liver (nitro-glycerine, testosterone, lidocaine, etc.).
- Certain drugs are not absorbed (streptomycin).
- Absorption of certain drugs is irregular and unpredictable.

Precautions

- In order to enhance the passage into stomach and permit rapid dissolution, the capsules and tablets should be washed down with a glass of water with the patient in upright posture (sitting or standing).
- To avoid damage to the esophageal mucosa, do not give drugs orally to a recumbent patient. The damage can be caused by drugs like tetracyclines, iron salts, and slow release potassium salts.

Sometimes pills and tablets are coated as under:

i. They are coated by sugars, gums, synthetic resins, polyhydric alcohols, waxes, colouring agents and flavouring agents to make them more palatable and acceptable.

ii. They are coated with gluten, cellulose acetate phthalate and anionic copolymers of methacrylic acid and its esters. These substances do not permit the acid juice of the stomach to disintegrate them but permit disintegration in the intestinal alkaline juice. So the purpose of enteric coating is:

   a. To get desired concentration of the drug in the small intestine.

   b. To retard the absorption of the drug.

However, there are certain disadvantages of enteric coating such as:

- Difficulty to maintain uniform body drug concentration.
- Required to administer large quantities of the drug to achieve a therapeutic concentration at the site of action.
- May cause more adverse actions.
- Necessity for frequent dosing and poor patient compliance.

Timsules/spansules: These are sustained release or time release preparations. They release the active drug over an extended period of time. To achieve this goal, the particles of the drug are covered with coatings which dissolve at different time intervals in order to provide uniform medication over a prolonged period. The basis for the so called controlled release, extended release, sustained release or prolonged action pharmaceutical preparation (oral dosage form) is dependent on its rate of dissolution in gastrointestinal tract fluids. *Potential advantages* of such preparations are:

- Reduction in the frequency of administration of the drug.
- Improved patients' compliance.
- Maintenance of therapeutic effect overnight.
- Decreased incidence and/or intensity of undesirable effects by elimination of the peaks in drug concentration.

However, such products have some drawbacks:

- During repeated drug administration, trough drug concentration resulting from controlled release dosage form may not be different from those observed with immediate-release preparations, although time interval between trough concentrations is greater for a well designed controlled release preparation.
- It is possible that dosage form may fail.
- "Dose-dumping" with resultant toxicity can occur, since the total dose of drug ingested at one time may be several times the amount present in the conventional preparation.

Controlled release preparations are most appropriate for drugs with short half-life (less than 4 hours).

2. Sublingual

The tablet or pellet containing the drug is placed under the tongue or crushed in the mouth in order to spread it over the buccal mucosa. Only lipid soluble and non-irritating drugs can be administered by this route.

Advantages

- Relatively rapid absorption.
- Quick onset of action.
- Drug can be spitted after the desired effect.

- Liver is bypassed; so drugs with high first pass metabolism can be absorbed directly into systemic circulation.

  Drugs given sublingually are nitroglycerine, clonidine, isoprenaline, nifedipine, methyl testosterone and buprenorphine.

3. Nasal

Many drugs may be absorbed readily through the mucous membrane of the nose. Examples are posterior pituitary powder, applied as a snuff; and spray of nebulized solutions.

4. Rectal

For systemic effect, drugs can be put into rectum. They are used as suppository or retention enema. Examples are aminophylline, diazepam, indomethacin, etc.

Advantages

- Certain irritant and unpleasant drugs can be given by this route.
- This route can be used in presence of recurrent vomiting.

Limitations

- Inconvenient and embarrassing.
- Absorption is slow, irregular and often unpredictable.
- Irritant drug may cause inflammation.

5. Inhalation

Gases and volatile liquids are given by inhalation, e.g. general anaesthetics, amyl nitrite.

Advantages

- Rapid absorption
- Controlled administration is possible
- Quick elimination

Limitations

Irritant vapours can cause:
- Inflammation of respiratory tract
- Increased secretion

6. Cutaneous

Drugs with high lipid solubility can be applied over the skin for slow and prolonged absorption after being incorporated in an ointment or impregnated in adhesive patches or strips. Examples are nitroglycerine, hyoscine, etc. Advantage is that liver is bypassed.

7. Parenteral

When a drug is administered by routes other than the gastrointestinal tract, it is called parenteral route.

Advantages

- Onset of action is faster and sure.
- Accuracy of dose is ensured.
- No gastric irritation and vomiting.
- Can be used in unconscious, uncooperative or vomiting patients.
- No interference by food or digestive juices.
- Irritant drugs to stomach can be given.
- Drugs which are not absorbed in the small intestine can be administered.
- Liver is by passed.
- Can be employed in case of diarrhoea and in patients unable to swallow.

Limitations

- Self-medication is difficult and often needs assistance.
- Less safe and more risky.
- Preparation has to be sterilized.
- Technique is invasive and painful.
- Local tissue injury is possible.
- Danger of infection, if proper care is not taken.
- Costlier.

Important parenteral routes are:

Subcutaneous (s.c.): Drug is deposited in the loose subcutaneous tissue. Self-injection is possible because deep penetration is not needed. The commonest drug used by this route is insulin. Repository (depot) preparation (oil solution or aqueous suspension) can be injected for prolonged action.

Limitations

- Absorption is slow because this tissue is richly supplied by nerves but is less vascular.
- Irritant drugs cannot be injected.
- This route should be avoided in patients of shock because the absorption is undependable.

Some special forms of this route are:

a. **Hypodermoclysis:** This procedure is used in paediatric practice to inject large quantity of saline subcutaneously. Drug absorption from the subcutaneous area can be enhanced by the addition of the enzyme hyaluronidase.

b. **Pellet implantation:** To provide sustained release of drug, solid pellet of the drug is introduced by a trochar and cannula, e.g. DOCA, testosterone.

c. **Dermojet:** A high velocity jet of drug solution is projected from a microfine orifice using a gun-like implement. Procedure is painless and suited for mass inoculation.

d. **Sialistic (non-biodegradable) and biodegradable implant:** Crystalline drug is packed in tubes made of suitable materials. It is implanted under the skin. Slow and uniform release of the drug occurs over months to provide constant blood levels. The non-biodegradable implants have to be removed later on but not the biodegradable ones. This has been tried for hormones and contraceptives.

Intramuscular (i.m.): The drug is injected in one of the large skeletal muscles such as deltoid, triceps, gluteus maximus, and rectus femoris. Volume of injection should not exceed 10 ml.

Advantages

- Mild irritants, suspensions and colloids can be injected.

- Absorption is faster so onset of action is rapid.
- Less painful.

Precautions

- Avoid injection near a nerve because an irritant solution can damage the nerve and cause severe pain and even paresis of the muscles supplied by it.
- Do not give i.m. injection into the buttock until the child starts to walk, because at this stage gluteus maximus is very tiny. So the lateral side of the thigh should be used in younger children.

Intravenous (i.v.): The drug is given in one of the superficial veins. It can be given intravenously: (a) as a bolous injection, e.g. frusemide, (b) over 5–10 minutes, e.g. aminophylline, (c) in an infusion which is 50–100 ml or more in volume.

Indications of infusion are:

- To slow the administration of the drug, e.g. morphine
- To maintain a constant plasma level of the drug, e.g. dopamine
- To administer large volumes either rapidly or over prolonged periods of time, e.g. fluids in dehydration or shock.

Advantages

- Onset of action is quick.
- Highly irritant drugs can be given.
- Smaller dose is required.
- Large volume can be infused.
- Response is accurately measurable, so titration of the dose with the response is possible.

Limitations

- Suspension cannot be injected.
- Thrombophlebitis of the injected vein may occur.
- Necrosis of adjacent tissue may develop if extravasation of irritant drug occurs.

- Hazardous route as vital organs are exposed to high concentration.

Precautions

- Ensure that needle is in the vein and then inject the drug.
- Inject minimum quantity of the drug to produce a particular effect.
- With certain drugs (iron, aminophylline, pentothal, calcium), injection is to be given slowly as sudden high blood concentration may be dangerous.
- Irritant solutions should be administered by piggybacking into a running intravenous drip or through a central line intravenous site which should be reselected at regular intervals, if irritating solutions are given through a peripheral vein.
- On extravasation of irritating fluid, it should be aspirated through the cannula before removing it.

Intradermal injection: The drug is injected into the skin raising a bleb (e.g. BCG vaccine, sensitivity test) or scarring (multiple puncture of the epidermis through a drop of drug (smallpox vaccination) is done. This route is employed for specific purpose only.

8. New Drug Delivery Systems

Various novel drug delivery systems have been developed.

1. **Drugs** are incorporated in a programmed dosage form. They administer the medicament at a predetermined rate over an extended period of time from a single application.

    Examples are:

    i. *Ocusert:* It is placed directly under the eyelid. It can deliver a steady amount of pilocarpine round the clock for seven days. It does not cause any discomfort. It obviates the need of repeated application of eyedrops.

    ii. *Progestasert:* It is an intrauterine contraceptive device. It causes controlled release of minute quantities of progesterone within the uterus for a year.

2. **Prodrug:** It is an inactive chemical derivative. After administration, it is converted into the pharmacologically active drug by biotransformation. The advantages of the use of prodrugs are:

    - It overcomes the barriers which limit the usefulness of a drug. Examples are propoxyphene, napsylate, chloramphenicol palmitate, L-dopa, talampicillin.
    - May be used to achieve longer duration of action, e.g. esters of phenothiazines and penicillin.
    - May be used to provide site specific delivery of drugs such as methenamine which is converted to formaldehyde and ammonia at the acidic urinary pH. It is used as a urinary antiseptic.

3. **For continuous or intermittent** (pulsed) administration of drugs, computerized, miniature syringe pumps have been developed. They are now being used for optimal drug effect of insulin and GnRH (gonadotropin releasing hormone).

4. **Monoclonal antibodies:** It is now possible to grow very large numbers of antibody producing cells from a single B cell. This is done by fusing a B cell to a myeloma cancer cell. The resulting hybridoma retains 2 main features from its 2 parent cells. It could grow indefinitely like the cancer cell yet also produce and secrete antibodies like the B cell. The antibodies produced by this technique are called monoclonal antibodies (MAbs) because they are derived from a single hybrid cell. Now monoclonal antibodies against cancer cell antigens have been developed for "targeted" delivery of anticancer drugs. These antibodies 'home in' on the cancer cells. Thus they deliver lethal concentration of the drug selectively to the cancer tissue.

5. **Packing in liposomes:** Liposomes are minute vesicles of certain phospholipids in aqueous suspension. Non-lipid soluble drugs may be filled in these vesicles. This is a mode of specific target orientated drug delivery system. Intravenous route is commonly used for the administration of liposomes. Liposomes have been utilized to administer:
   - Anticancer drugs, e.g. daunorubicin and doxorubicin
   - Antibiotic such as gentamicin
   - Antifungal drug like amphotericin-B

Points for Dental Students

1. Definitions introduce the various branches of pharmacology to the dental students.
2. Sources give an insight to the students regarding various types of drugs which will be used by them.
3. Theoretical knowledge of routes of administration of a drug is important for dental students in deciding an appropriate mode of administration of a particular drug.

TO REMEMBER

1. Pharmacology is the science of drugs.
2. Pharmacotherapeutics means use of a drug for prevention, mitigation or cure of the disease.
3. Chemotherapy deals with treatment of systemic infection/malignancy with specific drugs.
4. Pharmacy deals with collection, identification, purification, isolation, synthesis, standardization, compounding and dispensing of a drug.
5. Toxicology is the study of poisonous effects of drugs and other chemicals.

6. Drugs can be obtained from animals, minerals, micro-organisms, plants and by genetic engineering. However, in clinical practice majority of the drugs used, are synthetic.
7. There are number of pharmacologically active principles in plants such as fixed, volatile and mineral oils, alkaloids, glycosides, gums, resins, oleoresins and tannins.
8. Factors, which govern the choice of route of administration of a drug, are its physical and chemical nature, rate and extent of absorption, site of action, onset of action, condition of the patient, first pass metabolism and effect of digestive juices.
9. Local routes are used for localized lesion to attain high concentration at the desired site and no or minimal systemic side effects. Drugs are applied locally either on the skin and mucous membranes or through arterial supply and in deeper tissues directly.
10. Systemic routes will distribute the drug all over including the site of action through circulation. Various systemic routes are oral, sublingual, nasal, cutaneous, and parenteral (subcutaneous, intramuscular, intravenous, intradermal). Each one has its own advantages, disadvantages and limitations.
11. Various novel drug delivery systems have also been developed such as: (a) programmed dosage forms (ocusert, progestasert), (b) prodrug, (c) monoclonal antibodies, (d) packed in liposomes and (e) specially made for continuous or intermittent (pulsed) administration.

Chapter 2

Pharmacokinetics

The word pharmacokinetics is derived from Greek words *Pharmacon* (drug) and *kinein* (to move). Thus pharmacokinetics is the quantitative study of drug movement through and out of the body. To obtain the right effect with minimum risk of toxicity, the dose and mode of administration of the drug is determined by its pharmacokinetics. Its help is also taken to study latency of onset, time of peak action and frequency of administration of a drug.

All pharmacokinetic processes involve transport of the drug across biological membrane (bimolecular lipid layer). It is composed of phospholipids, cholesterol and small quantity of carbohydrates. It also contains pores and intercellular gaps (between certain interepithelial cells). Drugs are transported across the biological membranes by:

1. Passive diffusion.
2. Filtration.
3. Specialized transport.

> **Passive diffusion**
> a. It is a:
>   • Passive process
>   • Non-specific
>   • Non-energy dependent
> b. It depends upon:
>   • Concentration gradient
>   • Solubility of drug in the lipid layer
>   • pH

1. **Passive diffusion:** Diffusion is a passive process. The biological membrane plays no active role in the process. Thus the mechanism is non-specific and non-energy dependent. The drug diffuses across the membrane in the direction of its concentration gradient. It is dependent upon the solubility of the drug in the lipid layer. It is proportional to lipid: water partition coefficient of the drug. So a more lipid soluble drug can be absorbed by this process quickly. Further the diffusion of the drug is faster if the difference in the concentration of the drug on two sides of the membrane is greater. Influence of pH is equally important in passive diffusion of drugs. This is because most drugs are weak electrolytes, i.e. their ionization is pH dependent. As a general principle, basic drugs are more ionized and less diffusible in a relatively acidic medium while they are more lipid soluble and more diffusible in a relatively alkaline medium. Similarly acidic drugs are more ionized and less diffusible in a relatively alkaline medium while they are more lipid soluble and more diffusible in a relative acidic medium. Thus the non-ionized (non-polar) lipid soluble molecules can diffuse across the lipid membrane while the ionized (polar) water soluble molecules are unable to penetrate it. Weakly acidic drugs form salts with

cations, e.g. sodium sulfadiazine, sodium phenobarbitone, potassium penicillin V, etc. They are largely unionized at acid gastric pH. Hence they are absorbed from the stomach. Weekly basic drugs form salts with anions, e.g. atropine sulfate, ephedrine hydrochloride, chloroquin phosphate, etc. They are largely ionized in gastric pH. So they are poorly absorbed from stomach. In intestinal alkaline pH, they remain unionized and are mainly absorbed from that site.

Acidic drugs are ionized more in alkaline urine. They do not back diffuse in the kidney tubules and are excreted faster. On the other hand, basic drugs are excreted faster if urine is acidified. There are a few exceptions to the basic principles mentioned above as under:

i. Both ionized and non-ionized forms of some drugs are highly water soluble (e.g. penicillin). They are, therefore, excreted rapidly irrespective of the urine pH.

ii. Some drugs are permanently ionized at all values of body pH, e.g. heparin (acidic) or tubocurarine, suxamethonium, ipratopium (basic). These are non-diffusible polar drugs. They are neither absorbed from the gut nor diffuse into the tissues.

iii. On the other hand, some drugs are incapable of becoming ionized at any environmental pH (digoxin, and chloramphenicol). These are non-polar drugs that diffuse readily across the membrane.

2. **Filtration:** It is transportation of drugs with very low molecular weight (100–150), e.g. lithium and methanol, through aqueous pores in the biological membrane. Filtration of water soluble drugs can also take place through interepithelial gaps. Since capillary gaps are larger, they allow the filtration of drugs/chemicals with molecular weight up to 20,000–30,000 into extracellular spaces if not bound to plasma proteins. These gaps are still bigger in glomerular capillaries. So they allow filtration of drugs with molecular weight up to 69,000. No drug is filtered into the brain or placenta (blood brain/CSF and blood-placental barrier) because intercapillary gaps are missing at these sites.

3. **Specialized transport:** It may be:
   i. Carrier-mediated transport
   ii. Pinocytosis.

Carrier-mediated transport
Important features are:
- Active process.
- Occurs against concentration gradient.
- Specific.
- Energy dependent.
- Saturable.
- Competitive inhibition by analogues.

---

i. *Carrier-mediated transport:* In this case, the drug combines with a carrier (a specialized protein molecule) present in the membrane. The complex thus formed translocates from one face of the membrane to the other. Generally, such transport requires expenditure of energy. So it is called active transport. The transport is against concentration gradient. Metabolic poison inhibits this process. It is a specific, saturable process. It is competitively inhibited by analogues which utilize same carrier. Sometimes non-diffusible substances are translocated along their concentration gradient (e.g. vitamin B_{12}). It is called facilitated diffusion. It is not dependent on energy.

ii. *Pinocytosis:* In this case, the substance is transported across the cell in particulate form by formation of vesicles. Proteins and other big molecules are transported by this process. This is rarely applicable to drugs.

ABSORPTION AND BIOAVAILABILITY OF A DRUG

Absorption

Absorption means the movement of drug from its site of administration into the bloodstream. Clinical efficacy of drug depends on:

- The route of administration that determines the latent period between administration and onset of action.
- The fraction of the administered dose absorbed.
- Rate of absorption; its significance is given in the box.

> **Significance of information regarding the rate of absorption**
> - To decide the frequency of administration of a drug.
> - To determine the duration of effectiveness of a drug.
> - To forecast the onset of desired or undesired effects of a drug.

The drug has to cross biological membranes except when given i.v. So its absorption is governed by the above described principles. Other factors affecting absorption are:

1. **Physical properties:**
   - Concentrated solution of drug is absorbed faster than from diluted solution because passive transport depends on concentration gradient.
   - Drugs are absorbed in aqueous phase. So liquids are better absorbed than solids and crystalloids are better absorbed than colloids.
   - Drug is removed from the site of absorption by blood circulation. It is also responsible for the maintenance of

concentration gradient across the membrane. So increased blood flow hastens drug absorption.

2. **Dosage form:**
   - Smaller the particles of the drug in a tablet better is the absorption. So by reducing the particle size, the dosage of the active drug can be reduced without lowering efficacy, e.g. corticoids, chloramphenicol, griseofulvin, tolbutamide and spironolactone. On the other hand, in order to reduce absorption of anthelmintic (bephenium hydroxy-naphthoate), the particle size should be large.
   - To formulate powders or tablets, lactose, sucrose, starch and calcium phosphate or lactate is used as inert diluents. However, such substances may not be totally inert. They may influence the absorption as well as stability of the medicament. For example, calcium phosphate used as a diluent for calciferol may cause calcium toxicity, when given in large doses.
   - "Disintegration time" (rate of break up of the tablet or the capsule into the drug granules) and the dissolution rate (rate at which drug goes to solution) are important factors in determining the absorption of a drug.

3. Larger the area of absorbing surface faster is the absorption.

4. Each route of administration has its own peculiarities. It, therefore, affects drug absorption as under.

Oral

- Epithelial lining of the gastrointestinal tract is lipoidal. So it acts as effective barrier to orally administered drugs. The rate of absorption of non-ionized lipid soluble drugs (e.g. ethanol) from stomach as well as intestine is proportional to their lipid: water partition coefficient.

- Acidic drugs (e.g. salicylates, barbiturates, etc.) are absorbed from the stomach because they remain unionized in the gastric juice while basic drugs (e.g. morphine, quinine) are poorly absorbed as they remain ionized in the gastric juice. They are absorbed only on reaching the duodenum (alkaline pH). However, even absorption of acidic drugs from stomach is slower because of the following reasons:
  a. Thick mucosa.
  b. Mucous on mucosa.
  c. Small surface area.
- Presence of food retards/aids the absorption of drug by altering the gastric emptying time. It is observed that food retards the absorption of aspirin, ampicillin, captopril, digoxin, isoniazid, levodopa, penicillin G, rifampicin and tetracycline while it aids the absorption of carbamazepine, chloroquin, griseofulvin, lithium carbonate, nitrofurantoin, riboflavin, and spironolactone. However, rapid absorption occurs if most drugs are given on empty stomach.
- Certain drugs are ineffective orally because of the following reasons:
  a. Insulin and adrenocorticotrophic hormone (ACTH) are polypeptides. They undergo enzymatic degradation within the lumen of gastrointestinal tract.
  b. Poor absorption from the gastrointestinal tract, e.g. aminoglycoside antibiotics.
  c. Sex hormones and aldosterone are readily absorbed from the gut. However, they are inactivated in the gut wall as well as during the passage through liver before reaching to their site of action.
- Concurrently administered drugs may alter the absorption of a drug due to:
  a. *Luminal effect:* Insoluble complexes are formed, e.g. tetracycline with iron and antacids, phenytoin with sucralfate, cholesterol with liquid paraffin.

b. *Gut wall effects:* Number of drugs may alter motility of gut and thus alter the absorption of a drug, e.g. opioids, tricyclic antidepressants, metaclopramide, anticholinergics, etc. Further, absorption of a drug may be altered if mucosa of the gut wall is damaged by concurrent administration of a drug such as methotrexate, neomycin, and vinblastin.

Limitations of Oral Administrations

a. Onset of effect of the drug is delayed.
b. Peak effect occurs after a lapse of 30–60 minutes.
c. Peak plasma concentration is low because of slow rate of absorption and continuous elimination of the drug.
d. Drugs administered orally may give rise to oesophageal and gastric irritation or ulceration, nausea, vomiting and diarrhoea.

Subcutaneous and Intramuscular

- Many drugs are not absorbed on oral administration.
- However, they are absorbed on subcutaneous or intramuscular administration because they are deposited directly in the vicinity of capillaries on parenteral administration. Capillaries are highly porous. So they do not obstruct absorption of even large lipid insoluble molecules.
- Drug absorption is accelerated by application of heat and exercise by increasing blood flow.
- Vasoconstrictors, e.g. adrenaline retard absorption when injected along with the drug.
- Hyaluronidase facilitates drug absorption from subcutaneous site by promoting spread.
- Many depot preparations, e.g. benzathine penicillin, protamine zinc insulin, depot progestins can be given by these routes.
- Pellets and implants can be inserted subcutaneously for prolonged action.

Topical Sites (Skin, Cornea, Mucous Membranes)

On topical application, systemic absorption depends primarily on lipid solubility of the drugs. Mucous membranes of cornea, mouth, rectum and vagina absorb lipophylic drugs.

Lipid soluble unionized drugs are absorbed but lipid soluble ionized drugs are not absorbed. Abraded surfaces readily absorb drugs.

Few drugs such as corticosteroids, hyoscine, nitroglycerin, organophosphorous insecticides, etc. can be absorbed through intact skin. Absorption can be promoted by rubbing the drug incorporated in an oleaginous base or by use of occlusive dressing.

Bioavailability

Bioavailability of a drug means availability of biologically active drug. It is a determination of the amount or fraction of administered dose of the given dosage form that reaches the systemic circulation in the unchanged form. In other words, it is the rate at which and extent to which an active concentration of the drug is available at the site of action. On intravenous administration, all the drug is available for biological activity, i.e. bioavailability is 100%. However, it is lower after oral ingestion because it depends on the following factors:

- Rate of absorption.
- Gastrointestinal tract degradation.
- First pass metabolism by gut wall and hepatic enzymes.
- Enterohepatic circulation.
- Presence of food and other drugs.

Incomplete bioavailability after subcutaneous or intramuscular injection is less common but may occur due to local binding of the drug.

Oral pharmaceutical preparations from different manufacturers or different batches from the same manufacturer that satisfy the chemical and physical standards laid down in pharmacopoeia is called chemically equivalent. However, they may not yield similar blood levels, so they are biologically inequivalent. Due to this they may not provide equal therapeutic benefit, so they are therapeutically inequivalent also. Differences in bioavailability may be due to variations in disintegration and dissolution rates which may depend on manufacture process.

Clinical Significance of Bioavailability

Bioavailability variation is of practical significance under following circumstances:

- For drugs with low safety margin (digoxin).
- For precise control of doses of drugs (oral hypoglycemics, oral anticoagulants, etc.).
- For success or failure of antimicrobial regimen.

In general for a large number of drugs, bioavailability differences are negligible. So the risks of changing formulations have been often exaggerated.

DISTRIBUTION OF A DRUG

Once a drug has entered the bloodstream after absorption, it gets distributed to various fluid compartments such as (Fig. 2.1):

a. Plasma.
b. Interstitial fluid compartment (extracellular fluid space).
c. Transcellular fluid compartment, e.g. fluid in the gastrointestinal tract, bronchi, CSF.
d. Cellular fluid compartment (intracellular fluid compartment).

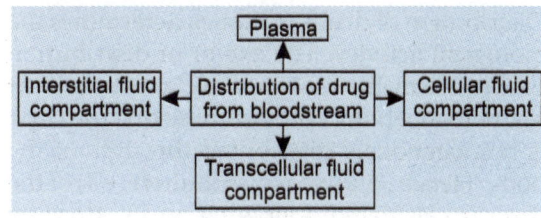

Fig. 2.1: Distribution of a drug

Every drug is distributed throughout the tissues of the body that initially has no drug. At this stage, concentration gradient is in the direction of plasma to tissues. The extent of distribution of drug depends on many factors such as:

- Lipid solubility.
- Ionization at physiological pH.
- Extent of binding to plasma and tissue proteins.
- Difference in regional blood flow.

Finally equilibrium is reached between unbound drug in plasma and tissue fluids and movement of drug is stopped. Some drugs pass into the cell, some remain on the cell membrane and some may be distributed extracellularly. Lipid insoluble drugs do not enter cells. Drugs extensively bound to plasma proteins are largely restricted to the vascular compartments.

When highly lipid soluble drugs are given intravenously or by inhalation, they initially get distributed to organs with rich blood supply such as brain, heart, kidney, etc. Later on less vascular but more bulky tissues (muscle, fat) take up the drug and plasma concentration falls. Due to this, drug is withdrawn from these organs with high blood flow. If the site of action of the drug is in one of the highly perfused organs, redistribution results in termination of drug action (e.g. thiopentone). However, on repeated or continuous administration of drug, the low perfusion high capacity sites get progressively saturated and the drug becomes longer acting.

Volume of Distribution

Distribution of drugs in tissues determines the biological activity. The extent of distribution of drug can be assessed by a convenient mathematical concept, assuming that the drug is homogenously distributed throughout the body. Hence volume of distribution (Vd) of the drug is calculated, following an i.v. dose by following formula:

$$Vd = \frac{Dose}{Cp} \text{ (in litres)}$$

Where Cp is the estimated plasma concentration per litre at the time of plasma-tissue equilibrium (zero-time) after i.v. injection. The Vd calculated by this method is not "real". It is hypothetical. It is, therefore, mentioned as "apparent volume of distribution".

Drugs with very low Vd are primarily confined in plasma, and those with high Vd are concentrated in tissues.

More precise multiple compartment models for drug distribution have been worked out, but the single compartment model, described above, is simple and fairly accurate.

Blood-brain and blood-CSF barrier: The endothelial cells of the capillaries of the brain and the cerebrospinal axis has tight inter-endothelial junctions and do not have intercellular pores or gaps. Also a sheet of glial cells lines these capillaries. So water soluble drugs cannot filter into CSF or brain. Drugs can either be transported into these areas by diffusion or by carrier mediated transport. Hence they allow the entry of lipoidal drugs while a large number of non-lipoid soluble drugs do not cross these barriers and have no central effect. However, this barrier is absent in hypothalamus, pineal gland, and the area postrema. So all circulating drugs come in contact with the vomiting centre and CTZ (chemoreceptor trigger zone) and may then initiate centrally mediating vomiting.

Placental barrier: A layer of trophoblastic cells in the chorionic villi separate the maternal and fetal bloodstreams. This lipid barrier allows the passage of lipid soluble drugs into fetal circulation by diffusion while water soluble drugs or essential nutrients cross the placental barrier by carrier mediated transport system. Placental transfer depends on:

- Properties of the drug.
- Evolving properties of the placenta.

- Altered maternal blood levels which are controlled by changing pharmacokinetics of pregnancy.

The knowledge of passage of drugs through placental barrier is important in a pregnant woman, because some drugs may have teratogenic properties and so are contra-indicated during pregnancy. Further, one has to be careful in administering drugs to the mother at the time of delivery because they may have adverse effect on the physiology of the newborn.

Plasma protein binding (Table 2.1): After absorption, the drug circulates in the blood either in the free form or bound to plasma proteins. Drugs may reversibly bind to non-specific non-functional sites on plasma proteins which serve no biological effect. Affinity of most drugs for plasma proteins depends on their physico-chemical properties as well as on the concentration of binding protein in the plasma. Thus, in pregnancy, the protein bound fraction of substances such as thyroxine increases due to a rise in the concentration of the specific binding protein in plasma. Conversely, free fraction of the drug is increased due to low plasma proteins in a patient of hypoproteinaemia. Acidic and neutral drugs bind to albumin fraction, e.g. salicylates, diazepam, phenytoin, warfarin. Basic drugs bind to orsomucoid (alfa-2-acid glycoprotein), lipoprotein, and beta-globulin. Examples of such drugs are lidocaine, propranolol and quinidine. Usual figures of percentage binding refer to the usual thera-peutic plasma concentration of a drug.

Clinical significance of plasma protein binding:

- Binding of drugs to plasma proteins assists absorption.
- Protein binding acts as temporary `store' of a drug. It, therefore, prevents large fluctuations in concentration of unbound drug in the body fluids.
- Protein binding reduces diffusion of the drug into the cell. So it delays its metabolic degradation and excretion.
- Highly plasma protein bound drugs are largely restricted to the vascular compartment. So it will have lower volume of distribution.
- Figures of plasma concentrations of the drug refer to bound as well as free drug. Bound fraction is not available for action. While prescribing any new drug such as an antibacterial agent claimed to have higher and longer plasma concentration than a previously available drug, one should ascertain the degree of protein binding. With extensively protein bound drugs, the therapeutic activity may be low.
- Various drugs get bound to the same binding sites on plasma proteins. This may lead to displacement interactions among drugs bound to the same site. Due to this sudden increase in the free concentration of one of them may occur to a dangerous toxic level.

Table 2.1: Plasma protein binding

Type of drug	Type of plasma protein	Examples
Acidic and neutral drugs	Albumin	Salicylates
		Diazepam
		Phenytoin
		Warfarin
Basic drugs	Orsomucoid (α_2-acid glycoprotein)	Lidocaine
	Lipoprotein	Propranolol
	β-globulin	Quinidine

Drug storage: After administration of a single dose of a drug, it may accumulate in specific organ or get bound to specific tissue constituents even when its plasma concentration is reduced to low or undetectable levels. For example, digoxin is accumulated in skeletal muscle, heart, liver and kidney. Many lipid soluble drugs are stored in the body fat depots such as thiopentone, DDT, ether, etc. Although the effect of a drug is mainly terminated by biotransformation and excretion, it may also result from redistribution of the drug from its site of action into other tissues or sites.

METABOLISM (BIOTRANSFORMATION)

Biotransformation means chemical change of a drug within a living organism. Drugs are foreign substances to the body. So body tries to get rid of them subjecting to various mechanisms.

After absorption, drugs could undergo three possible fates (Fig. 2.2):
- Excreted unchanged.
- Metabolized by enzymes.
- Spontaneously changed into other substances because of appropriate pH of body fluids.

Metabolism makes non-polar (lipid soluble) compounds to polar (lipid insoluble) substances so that they are not reabsorbed in the renal tubules and are excreted. The primary site for drug metabolism is liver. Other sites are kidney, intestine, lungs, and plasma. Biotransformation of drugs may lead to the following:
- Inactivation of drugs such as propranolol, morphine, etc.
- Formation of active metabolite from an active drug such as imipramine to desipramine; trimethadione to dimethadione. In this case, effect observed is due to the parent drug as well as active metabolite.

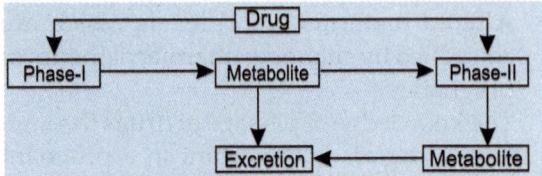

Fig. 2.2: Schematic representation of metabolism of a drug

- Formation of active metabolite from inactive drug. Such a drug is called prodrug. Its effect is then due to its active metabolite. Example is levodopa to dopamine.

Enzymes for Drug Biotransformation

Drug metabolizing enzymes are categorized into 2 groups:
- Microsomal enzymes
- Non-microsomal enzymes

Microsomal Enzymes

Microsomal enzymes are mainly present in the smooth surfaced endoplasmic reticulum of the liver. Main enzymes are mixed function oxidases and cytochrome P-450 (haem thiolate proteins). About 50 cytochrome P-450s are functionally active in human beings. These are categorized into families and sub-families. Term CYP (cytochrome P-450 mono-oxygenases) is used for their identification. About 8–10 isomers of CYP1, CYP2 and CYP3 families are associated in the majority of all drug metabolism reactions in human beings.

Microsomal enzymes are involved primarily with phase-I oxidation and reduction reactions. One exception to this is the involvement of microsomal enzymes system to carry out glucuronide acid conjugation, a phase-II synthetic reaction.

Non-microsomal Enzymes

These enzymes are present in plasma, cytoplasm, mitochondria of hepatic cells and other tissues. These enzymes are involved in all phase–II reactions (except glucuronide conjugation), certain oxidation, reduction and hydrolytic reactions.

Biotransformation reactions are of two types:

Phase–I non-synthetic reactions (Table 2.2): In this case, the metabolite may be active or inactive. It includes following reactions:

  i. Oxidation
 ii. Reduction
iii. Hydrolysis

These reactions introduce polar groups to drugs such as hydroxyl, amino, sulfhydryl and carboxy. Due to this, drugs are made water soluble and pharmacologically less active.

Oxidation: It is the most significant and important drug metabolizing reaction. Oxidation is carried out by microsomal "mixed function oxidase"(cytochrome P-450, NADPH, and haemoprotein enzymes) and non-microsomal oxidases (alcohol dehydrogenase, aldehyde dehydrogenase, diamine oxidase, monoamine oxidase and xanthine oxidase enzymes) in the liver. Oxidative reactions are hydroxylation, oxidation, deamination and dealkylation. Alcohol, barbiturates, diazepam, theophylline, morphine, paracetamol, steroids, etc. are metabolized by oxidative reactions.

Reduction: It is a reaction which is opposite to oxidation. It is very less common. Some of the drugs which are metabolized by this reaction are chloralhydrate, warfarin, halothane, chloramphenicol, naloxone and prednisone.

Hydrolysis: It occurs in plasma, liver, intestines and other tissues. It is carried out by esterases (e.g. plasma cholinesterase) or amidases. During this reaction, drug molecule is broken down into its two components. Examples are pethidine, cholinesters, procaine, procainamide, and lidocaine.

Conjugated metabolites may reach to intestine through the bile. They may be hydrolysed by the enzymes produced by intestinal organisms. During this reaction, free

Table 2.2: Phase-I non-synthetic reactions

Metabolic reaction	Examples of drugs metabolized
Oxidation	Alcohol
	Barbiturates
	Diazepam
	Theophylline
	Morphine
	Paracetamol
	Steroids
Reduction	Chloral hydrate
	Chloramphenicol
	Halothane
	Naloxone
	Prednisone
	Warfarin
Hydrolysis	Cholinesters
	Lidocaine
	Pethidine
	Procaine
	Procainamide
Cyclization	Proguanil
Decyclization	Barbiturates
	Phenytoin

drug is liberated which is reabsorbed (enterohepatic circulation).

Cyclization: In this reaction, a straight chain compound is converted to ring structure such as proguanil.

Decyclization: In this reaction, ring structure of the cyclic drug molecule opens up, e.g. phenytoin, barbiturates.

Phase–II synthetic (conjugation) reactions (Table 2.3): These reactions mostly give rise to inactive metabolites. There occurs conjugation of the drug or its phase-I metabolite with an endogenous substance. The later is derived from carbohydrate or amino acid. This reaction leads to the formation of a polar, highly ionized organic acid which is easily excreted in urine or bile. Various synthetic reactions are:

Glucuronide conjugation: Drugs with a hydroxyl or carboxylic acid group (e.g. aspirin, phenacetin, chloramphenicol, morphine,

Table 2.3: Phase-II synthetic (conjugation) reactions

Metabolic reaction	Examples of drugs metabolized
Glucuronide conjugation	Aspirin
	Chloramphenicol
	Phenacetin
	Metronidazole
	Morphine
	Thyroxine
Glycine conjugation	Salicylates
Glutathione conjugation	Quinone or
	Epoxide intermediates
	of certain drugs such
	as paracetamol
Acetylation	Hydralazine
	Isoniazid
	Para-amino-salicylic
	acid
Methylation	Adrenaline
	Histamine
	Nicotinic acid
Sulphate conjugation	Chloramphenicol
	Steroids
Ribonucleoside/nucleotide	Purine
	Pyrimidine

metronidazole) and endogenous substances like steroids, bilirubin and thyroxine are conjugated with glucuronic acid which is derived from glucose. It is the most important synthetic reaction.

Glycine conjugation: Compounds having carboxylic group such as salicylates are conjugated with glycine.

Glutathione conjugation: Certain drugs, e.g. paracetamol give rise to highly reactive quinone or epoxide intermediates during metabolism, which are inactivated by glutathione conjugation.

Acetylation: Drugs with amino or hydrazine residues (e.g. sulfonamides, hydralazine, PAS, isoniazid) are acetylated with the help of acetyl coenzyme-A. Rate of acetylation of these drugs is genetically controlled (slow and fast acetylators).

Methylation: The amines and phenols (e.g. adrenaline, histamine, and nicotinic acid) undergo methylation. The endogenous methyl

group for this reaction is derived from methionine and cysteine.

Sulfate conjugation: The phenolic compounds and steroids (e.g. chloramphenicol, adrenal and sex steroids) undergo sulfate conjugation by sulfokinases.

Ribonucleoside/ nucleotide synthesis: It plays an important role in the activation of purine and pyrimidine antimetabolites used in cancer therapy.

First-pass effect: On oral administration, a drug has to pass through the gut, gut wall and liver before reaching the systemic circulation. Some drugs may undergo substantial presystemic metabolism during their passage through these organs. This is called "first-pass effect". This is not seen when the same drug is given parenterally. First-pass effect consists of: (a) intestinal first pass effect and (b) hepatic first-pass effect.

a. *Intestinal first-pass effect:* Drugs may be metabolized by gastric acid, digestive enzymes or by enzymes in gut wall (e.g. catecholamine).

b. *Hepatic first-pass effect:* If a drug is rapidly metabolized in the liver, very little or no quantity of the orally administered drug reaches the systemic circulation. So to have desired therapeutic effect the drug has to be given either parenterally or orally in very large doses. Some drugs (e.g. propranolol, imipramine) give rise to active metabolites during hepatic metabolism. These drugs can be given orally. The bioavailability of drugs, which undergo extensive first-pass effect, may vary widely by number of factors. It may be increased and cause drug toxicity in case of hepatic disease, hepatic enzyme inhibition and saturation of metabolizing enzymes while it may be decreased in case of hepatic enzyme induction. Some of the drugs which undergo extensive first pass hepatic metabolism are sex hormones, morphine, labetalol, verapamil, terbutaline, lignocaine.

Inhibition of drug metabolism: Drug can inhibit metabolizing enzyme activity competitively if it utilizes the same enzyme or cofactors. Often enzyme inhibition produces undesirable drug-drug interactions. However, sometime specific enzyme inhibitors are used for therapeutic purpose, e.g. allopurinol, MAO inhibitors, disulfiram, CHE inhibitors, captopril, etc. Some other clinically important examples are:

- Cimetidine inhibits metabolism of propranolol, theophylline and lidocaine.
- Isoniazid, warfarin, chloramphenicol inhibit the metabolism of phenytoin.
- Ethanol inhibits methanol metabolism.
- Metronidazole and chlorpropamide interfere with alcohol metabolism.

Microsomal enzyme induction: On repeated administration, certain drugs stimulate the synthesis of microsomal metabolizing enzymes (generally mixed function oxidase enzymes and rarely conjugates). Drugs or chemicals which induce enzymes are called enzyme inducers. Some important enzyme inducers are ethanol, barbiturates, rifampicin, griseofulvin, tobacco, phenytoin, carbamazepine, etc. Drugs, whose metabolism is significantly affected by enzyme induction are phenytoin, warfarin, imipramine, tolbutamide, doxicycline, griseofulvin, oral contraceptives, chloramphenicol, phenylbutazone, and theophylline.

Clinical significance of enzyme induction:

- Development of tolerance (e.g. alcohol, barbiturates), if the drug induces its own metabolism.
- Reduction in some normal body constituents, e.g. adrenal steroids, bilirubin, sex hormones, vitamin D.
- Decreased pharmacological actions of a second drug due to enzyme induction by the first drug, e.g. failure of contraception with oral contraceptives.
- Increased drug toxicity, e.g. paracetamol, DDT, benzpyrene.

- Difficulty in dose adjustment of a drug prescribed on regular basis (e.g. oral anticoagulants, oral hypoglycaemics, antiepileptics, antihypertensives) along with intermittent use of an inducer drug.
- Since enzyme induction increases porphyrin synthesis, an acute intermittent porphyria attack may be precipitated.

Possible uses of enzyme induction:

i. Phenobarbitone is useful in congenital non-haemolytic jaundice because it causes rapid clearance of jaundice.

ii. Phenytoin may reduce the manifestations of Cushing's syndrome.

iii. Chronic poisoning.

iv. Liver disease.

There are a number of factors which affect the biotransformation of a drug such as:

a. At the extreme of life (old people and children) the rate of drug metabolism is slow. So the drug tends to produce greater and more prolonged effects.

b. In human beings, sex dependent variations in drug metabolism are less important. However, males may metabolize salicylates, benzodiazepines and oestrogens quicker than females.

c. Genetic factors and environment such as diet, weight, race, body temperature and specific genetic variation may influence the metabolism of drugs.

d. Many drugs may affect the biotransformation of other drugs either by enzyme induction (acceleration) or enzyme inhibition (delay).

e. Drug metabolic processes are inhibited in malnourished individuals as well as in patients with hepatic diseases (e.g. alcoholic hepatitis, biliary cirrhosis, viral hepatitis, and cancer liver). Oxidation reactions are affected the most because they are rate limiting. However, conjugation reactions are well preserved as they are less rapidly saturated.

f. Hepatic metabolic efficiency is impaired in congestive heart failure because it limits blood flow to the liver. It is enhanced in patients suffering from thyrotoxicosis. However, it is decreased in hypothyroidism and the half lives of practolol, digoxin and methimazole are increased.

EXCRETION

Drugs or their metabolites are eliminated through channels of excretion from the body. Important channels of excretion are:

1. **Kidney:** Most of the drugs are excreted through kidney. So this is the most important route of drug elimination. Following processes contribute to the excretion of a drug in the urine.

   i. *Passive glomerular filtration:* All non-protein bound drugs presented to the glomerulus are filtered. The rate of elimination of drug is dependent upon the glomerular filtration rate, molecular size of the drug and concentration of free drug in the plasma.

   ii. *Active tubular secretion:* This occurs at proximal tubules. This is the active transfer of organic acids and bases by organic acid transport and organic base transport respectively (non-selective saturable carrier systems). This transport is against electrochemical gradient. Further, this carrier system transports both free and protein bound drugs. Hence this is the most important mechanism of drug elimination by the kidney. There can be competitive inhibition if two drugs utilize the same carrier system for tubular secretion, e.g. simultaneous use of probenecid and penicillin prolongs the plasma t½ life of the later.

   iii. *Passive diffusion across the tubules:* This depends on lipid solubility and ionization of the drug at existing urinary pH. Since 99% of the glomerular filtrate is reabsorbed and only 1% is excreted in the urine, there is a concentration gradient of solutes between tubular fluid and plasma, which allows passive diffusion of weak acids and weak bases. Weak acids (e.g. barbiturates, aspirin) are reabsorbed in acidic urine but eliminated in alkaline urine. On the other hand, weak bases (e.g. amphetamine, pethidine) are reabsorbed in alkaline urine but excreted in acidic urine. Strong acids and strong bases are not reabsorbed because they remain ionized in the urine at all pH ranges. Similarly highly water soluble drugs (e.g. mannitol, quaternary ammonium compounds, penicillin, aminoglycosides) irrespective of urinary pH are not reabsorbed.

2. **Gastrointestinal tract:** Orally administered unabsorbed drugs and drugs excreted in the bile are eliminated in the faeces.

3. **Lungs:** Gases and volatile liquids (general anaesthetics, paraldehyde, alcohol) are eliminated by lungs irrespective of their solubility.

4. **Bile:** Unchanged drugs and their metabolized products may be excreted in bile. In gut, some of the metabolites specially glucuronides are deconjugated by intestinal bacteria and the released lipid-soluble drug is reabsorbed into circulation (enterohepatic circulation). Due to this, duration of action of the drug is prolonged. Examples of such drugs are rifampicin, benzodiazepines, stilbestrol and morphine. However, some amount of the drug or its metabolite is eliminated in the faeces.

5. **Breast milk:** Excretion of drugs in milk is important for the suckling infant who inadvertently receive the drugs. Most of the drugs are detectable in breast milk, but

usually their concentration is low. However, relatively significant concentrations of lipid soluble drugs enter into breast milk. So a few drugs, such as sulfonamides, tetracyclines, sedative hypnotics, etc. should be avoided or breast-feeding should be suspended.

6. **Skin and saliva:** Metalloids like arsenic and heavy metals like mercury are excreted in small quantity through skin. Certain drugs like iodides and metallic salts are excreted in the saliva.

Kinetics of Elimination

Time course of drug absorption, distribution and elimination can be determined in mathematical terms. Such a determination is important and its clinical significance is:

a. In understanding and planning drug regimes.

b. In deciding drug dose schedules.

c. In helping and supplementing to clinical monitoring and judgement.

In fact drug elimination is the sum total of metabolic inactivation and excretion. Clearance is the best measure of drug elimination. Drug clearance is the theoretical volume of plasma from which drug is completely removed in unit time. It is usually expressed as ml/min. For example, if clearance of verapamil is 1000 ml/min, it means that verapamil from 1000 ml of plasma is removed in one minute. Total body clearance is a total sum of all available routes of excretion of a drug, i.e.

Total body clearance (Cl) = Cl + Cl + Cl
renal liver other

A drug may be completely eliminated by glomerular filtration (e.g. aminoglycosides) or tubular secretion (e.g. penicillin). So rate of renal clearance of a drug cannot exceed glomerular filtration rate (120 ml/min) in case of former and renal plasma flow (700 ml/min) in case of later. However, a lipid soluble and diffusible drug is reabsorbed in the distal tubules in variable amount. This reabsorption process may decrease renal clearance to as low a level as 1 ml/min (rate of urine formation).

Kinetics of Clearance

1. **First order (exponential) kinetics:** In this case, the rate of elimination of a drug is directly proportional to its plasma concentration. It means that a constant fraction of the drug in the body disappears in unit time. These drugs have a constant plasma half-life (t½). Elimination of most drugs follows first order kinetics. In this case, the processes involved in removing most drugs are non-saturable over the clinically obtained plasma concentrations. Further, in this system log-plasma concentration-time curve is linear and near complete (97%) clearance is expected by the end of 5 t½ intervals after a single dose of a drug.

2. **Zero-order (linear) kinetics:** In this system, rate of elimination of a drug remains constant irrespective of its plasma concentration. It means constant amount of the drug is eliminated in unit time. This is also called dose-dependent elimination or saturation kinetics. In these cases, the reacting enzyme is limited and gets saturated (rate-limiting step). In this type of elimination of a drug, clearance decreases with increase in its plasma concentration. Further, the plasma t½ is not constant and there occurs increase in biological half-life with an increase in the dose of a drug. This will be associated with disproportionate increase in the plasma level of the drug. So to avoid adverse drug reactions the dose of the drugs which follow zero-order kinetics, should be increased carefully.

The elimination of certain drugs such as ethanol, oral propranolol, dicumarol is exponential with lower dosage level. However, their elimination becomes "zero-order", when dose exceeds a certain clinical level and elimination mechanism gets saturated.

3. **Plasma half-life (t½):** It is also called elimination half-life or biological half-life. It is defined as the time taken for the circulating plasma concentration of a drug to fall by 50%. When elimination of a drug is exponential, plasma half-life is independent of dose, route of administration and its plasma concentration. The duration of t½ is raised if drug is widely distributed in the body; highly protein bound; and follows enterohepatic circulation. Mostly t½ is indicative of duration of drug and helps in determining the dosage schedule. However, it is not always true as in case of:

a. Biotransformation of a drug into active metabolite.

b. Pathological conditions (renal or hepatic dysfunction).

c. Hit and run drugs (e.g. reserpine, MAO inhibitors).

d. Drugs which follow zero-order kinetics.

Steady State Level

When drug is given once, it follows the following phases:

a. **Absorptive phase:** There is a rise in plasma concentration.

b. **Distribution phase:** A rapid decline in plasma concentration.

c. **Elimination phase:** A steady decline in plasma concentration.

Most of the time, drug is given in a fixed dose at fixed intervals or given by infusion at a fixed rate. So on repeated administration, mean plasma concentration rises gradually. It depends on intake and elimination. Initially intake is higher than elimination. So there occurs continuous rise in mean plasma concentration during this period.

Subsequently intake of drug becomes equal to its elimination. At this stage, a steady state level of mean plasma concentration is reached. It is reached after 5 t½ in case of drugs which follow first order kinetics. It means the time to reach steady state level is a function of t½ (5 t½) irrespective of the dose or dose interval. However, the steady level reached is a function of the dose and dose intervals and not of t½. So it will be higher, if dose is increased or the dose interval is decreased.

Keeping the total daily dose constant, if the dose interval is increased, the mean steady state level will remain the same but there will be wide fluctuations in plasma concentration which may lead to toxicity at peak concentration and loss of biological activity in trough periods.

Drug Dosage

To produce a certain degree of response in a patient an appropriate amount of drug is required. This amount is called "dose". Dose of a drug varies in terms of chosen response and is called as prophylactic dose, therapeutic dose or a toxic dose. Further, a clinician has to keep following points in mind while deciding dosage regimen of a drug for a particular patient.

• Duration of treatment
• Frequency of administration of a drug
• Route of administration
• Amount of a single dose

In fact the decision of the physician will be based on the following pharmacokinetic considerations to individualize drug dosage.

i. **Standard dose:** It is one which is sufficient to produce desired therapeutic effect in most patients. This is possible with those drugs which have minor individual variation or wide safety margin, e.g.

amantadine, chloroquin, mebendazole, penicillin, oral contraceptives.

In certain clinical situations, a drug may have to be given in a single dose as and when required or at long intervals, e.g. analgesics, laxatives and hypnotics. There will be no accumulation of the drug and constant therapeutic plasma concentration is not essential. If patient does not respond, the dose of the drug is doubled.

ii. **Regulated dose:** Most of the drugs are administered in multiple doses. To avoid wide fluctuations in plasma, the clinician has to fix up the dose and frequency of its administration. It is better to give smaller doses at shorter intervals, rather than higher doses at longer intervals.

A finely regulated body function can be easily measured. When drug is to be employed to modify such a function, its dose can be regulated by repeated measurement of this body function. It is possible with the use of antihypertensives, anticoagulants, diuretics, general anaesthetics, hypoglycaemics, etc.

iii. **Titrated dose:** With few drugs, the dose required to achieve maximal therapeutic effect, cannot be given due to intolerable adverse effects. In such cases, dose of the drug is titrated to have therapeutic effect with an acceptable level of adverse effect. It can be practiced in two ways:
   a. In most non-critical situations, give low initial dose and titrate upwards.
   b. In critical situations, give high dose initially and titrate downwards.
   Examples are anticancer drugs, corticosteroids, and levodopa.

iv. **Target level dose:** In some cases, response is not easily measurable. Further, response occurs at a certain range of drug concentration in plasma. To achieve this plasma concentration initially, a loading dose is given.

v. **Loading dose:** It is a single dose or a few quickly repeated doses given in the beginning to attain target concentration rapidly. It is approximately equivalent to the anticipated total amount of the drug in the body at the time of desired therapeutic plasma concentration. This is seen with drugs which have the following characteristics:
   • Long $t\frac{1}{2}$
   • High volume of distribution
   • Slow rate of clearance
   • Cumulative in nature
   • Take several days for a steady state level to be reached.

Once the desired therapeutic plasma concentration of the drug has reached after giving loading dose, thereafter the effect is sustained by giving a maintenance dose. This dose is one that is to be repeated at specific intervals after the attainment of target steady state plasma concentration. Theoretically, it should be equivalent to daily excretion of the drug. Usually it is calculated by actual monitoring of plasma concentration, if facilities exist. If monitoring is not possible observe the effect of these drugs for a long period and make necessary adjustment in the maintenance doses. Examples are antidepressants, antiepileptics, digoxin, lithium and theophylline.

Therapeutic index or safety margin of a drug means the gap between its therapeutic effects and adverse effect. It is calculated in experimental animals as under:

Therapeutic index

$$= \frac{\text{Median lethal dose LD}_{50}}{\text{Median effective dose ED}_{50}}$$

Where LD_{50} is the dose which will be toxic to 50% of the animals of a treated group while ED_{50} will be a dose which is effective in 50% of the animals in a treated group. If it is one or more the drug is quite safe.

Fixed dose combination preparations:

These are the preparations which contain two or more drugs in a fixed dose ratio. It never means a concomitant drug therapy, where two or more drugs are used separately for treatment of disease. Rational or logical use of fixed dose combination of two or more drugs can be advantageous but illogical combination could be dangerous.

Pharmacokinetic rules for drug combinations are:
* If two drugs are to be combined in a single pharmaceutical formulation, they should have approximately equal plasma half-lives ($t\frac{1}{2}$).
* The ratio of the doses of two drugs, in such a formulation, will depend upon their apparent volume of distribution (aVd) and peak plasma concentration at steady state.

Examples of drug combinations:
* Sulphamethoxazole + trimethoprim (cotrimoxazole)
* Sulphadoxin + pyrimethamine for malaria
* Amoxycillin + clavulanic acid (augmentin)
* Carbidopa + levodopa for parkinsonism
* Ibuprofen + paracetamol as analgesic and anti-inflammatory agent
* Paracetamol + codeine as analgesic
* Beta blockers + diuretic as antihypertensive
  Drug combination may lead to summation of effects, additive effects or synergistic effects (for details see Chapter 3).

Advantages
* Convenient
* Better patient compliance
* Better effect among drugs combined
* Two drugs may counter the side effects of each other

Disadvantages
* All the drugs of combination may not be needed for treatment.
* Additional side effects and expense.
* Adjustment and individualization of doses is not possible.

* Time course of actions of its components may be different.
* Pharmacokinetics of its components may be differently affected under altered hepatic and renal function of the patient.
* The combination cannot be used if one of the components is contraindicated.
* Confusion of therapeutic aims and false sense of superiority of two drugs over one. This is particularly so in case of antimicrobial combinations. Corticosteroids should never be combined with any other drug.

In fact only handful of fixed dose combinations is rational and justified. However, present day situation is that far too many drug combinations are available and promoted. In fact this should be discouraged.

Monitoring of plasma concentration of drugs:

It is useful under the following conditions:
* To check patient compliance
* In case of poisoning
* In case of failure of response without any apparent reason, e.g. antimicrobials
* Drug with low safety margin
* Large individual variation in doses of a drug
* Use of potentially toxic drugs in presence of renal failure

It is not useful under the following situations:
* Drugs activated in the body, e.g. levodopa
* Drugs with irreversible action such as organophosphorus anticholinesterase
* With easily measurable response of drug e.g. antihypertensives, hypoglycaemics, diuretics, oral anticoagulants
* `Hit and run' drugs (whose effect lasts much longer than the drug itself), e.g. reserpine, MAO inhibitors.

Prolongation of drug action: The aims of prolongation of drug actions are:
* To avoid large fluctuations in plasma concentration
* To improve patient compliance
* To maintain drug effect overnight without disturbing sleep
* To reduce frequency of administration

Methods for prolonging drug action are:

1. By retarding drug absorption:
   i. *Oral:* By administering it full stomach or by giving it in sustained release tablets, spansules, capsules, etc.
   ii. *Parenteral:*
      a. Injecting drug in insoluble form or as oily solution subcutaneously and intramuscularly
      b. Pellet implantation
      c. Sialistic and biodegradable implants
      d. Transdermal drug delivery system: Drug is impregnated in adhesive patches, strips or as ointment and applied on the skin.
2. By increasing plasma protein binding
3. By decreasing rate of metabolism
4. By diminishing renal excretion.

Points for Dental Students

1. Knowledge of pharmacokinetics of each drug is important:
   - To obtain the right effect with minimum risk of toxicity.
   - To decide the appropriate dose and mode of administration of drug which will be based on the knowledge of latency of onset, time of peak action and duration of its action.
2. A dental student must learn the following pharmacokinetic points by heart because they will be useful in writing a rational prescription in dental practice.
   - When drugs, that are known inhibitors or inducers of metabolic enzymes, are added to therapy or taken together with other drugs, they will modify the rate of their own metabolism as well as of other drugs which use the same enzymes for their metabolism.
     For example, rifampicin (an enzyme inducer) accelerates the metabolic degradation of glucocorticoid and oral contraceptive pill. On the other hand, metabolism of tolbutamide is depressed by number of drugs such as salicylates, disulfiram, MAO inhibitor, chloramphenicol and probenecid. Due to this a dangerous hypoglycaemia may result if any of these drugs is given along with tolbutamide. This will need dose adjustment for desired therapeutic effect.
   - In case of drugs having a steep dose-response curve and/or narrow margin of safety, a small change in plasma concentration will lead to marked enhancement of drug effect or occurrence of toxicity, e.g. drugs like insulin, digoxin, anticoagulants, etc.
   - There are drugs that follow saturable metabolism (zero-order kinetics), e.g. alcohol, phenytoin, theophylline, etc. In such cases, a small interference in metabolism of the drug may lead to large alteration in plasma concentration that may lead to toxicity.
   - A reduction in plasma concentration of certain drugs, that are used chronically and which need precise plasma concentration for sustained effect, can result in therapeutic failure. For example, oral contraceptives, antiarrhythmics, antiepileptics, lithium, etc. are such drugs that require frequent plasma concentration monitoring.
   - Dose adjustment is needed in patients with significant impaired liver or hepatic disease.
   - Enhanced toxicity will be observed when two or more drugs, each having toxic effect on the same organ, are administered together, e.g. d-tubocurarine and aminoglycoside antibiotics may accentuate the block at neuromuscular junction.
   - Toxicity occurs when such two drugs, that are likely to interact, are given together for the treatment of same

disease, e.g. theophylline + salbutamol can cause cardiac dysrhythm when given together in the treatment of asthma.

- Modification of absorption of drug is of clinical significance. For example, epinepherine and norepinephrine are added to local anaesthetic to reduce their systemic absorption due to their vasoconstrictor effect. So this combination prolongs local anaesthetic action and decreases systemic toxicity. On the other hand, antibacterial action of tetracycline is decreased due to reduction in its absorption when administered along with iron and antacids.
- Protamine sulfate is an antidote to heparin while desferrioxamine is an antidote to iron overdose. They act by reducing distribution of heparin and iron.
- Dose adjustment and proper selection of drug are important in elderly. This is because they tend to have multiple pathology and so may receive several drugs concurrently.

TO REMEMBER

1. Pharmacokinetics is the quantitative study of drugs movement through and out of the body. All pharmacokinetic processes involve transport of the drug across biological membrane (bimolecular layer) by passive diffusion or filtration or specialized transport.
2. Passive diffusion is a non-specific, non-energy dependent passive process. In this process, the drug diffuses across the membrane in the direction of its concentration gradient.
3. Filtration is transportation of drugs with very low molecular weight through aqueous pores in the biological membrane, as well as of water soluble drugs through interepithelial gaps. No drugs are filtered into the brain or placenta because intercapillary gaps are missing at these sites.
4. Carrier-mediated transport (active transport) occurs against concentration gradient and requires expenditure of energy.
5. Drug absorption means the movement of drug from its site of administration into the bloodstream. It depends on route of administration, physical properties of drugs and dosage forms.
6. Bioavailability of a drug means availability of biologically active drug that reaches the systemic circulation in the unchanged form from the given dosage form.
7. Distribution of drug throughout the tissues of the body depends on lipid solubility, ionization at physiological pH, extent of binding to plasma and tissue proteins and difference in regional blood flow.
8. After absorption, the drug circulates in the blood either in the free form (biologically active) or bound to plasma proteins (biologically inactive). Binding of drugs to plasma proteins: (a) assists absorption, (b) acts as temporary store, (c) reduces diffusion of the drug into the cell and (d) may lead to displacement interactions among drugs bound to the same site.
9. Biotransformation (metabolism) means chemical change of a drug (non-polar lipid soluble compounds to polar lipid insoluble substances) within a living organism so that they are not reabsorbed in the renal tubules and are excreted.
10. Biotransformation reactions are of two types: Phase-I nonsynthetic reactions (oxidation, reduction, hydrolysis) and phase-II synthetic conjugation reactions.

11. Some drugs may undergo substantial presystemic metabolism during their passage through the gut, gutwall and liver before reaching the systemic circulation. This is called first pass effect.

12. On repeated administration, certain drugs stimulate the synthesis of microsomal metabolizing enzymes (generally mixed function oxidase enzymes and rarely conjugates). Drugs or chemicals which induce enzymes are called enzyme inducers and the process is known as microsomal enzyme induction.

13. Finally drugs or their metabolites are eliminated through channels of excretion (kidney, gut, lungs, bile, breast milk, skin and saliva) from the body.

14. Clearance is the best measure of drug elimination. Drug clearance is the theoretical volume of plasma from which drug is completely removed in unit time (ml/min.)

15. First order (exponential) kinetics means that the rate of elimination of a drug is directly proportional to its plasma concentration and these drugs have a constant plasma half-life (t½).

16. Zero-order (linear) kinetic means that the rate of elimination of a drug remains constant irrespective of its plasma concentration and the plasma half-life of the drug is not constant.

17. Plasma half-life (t½) is defined as the time taken for the circulating plasma concentration of a drug to fall by 50%.

18. Dose of a drug is the appropriate amount required to produce a certain degree of response in a patient.

19. To modify a finely regulated body function, the dose of a drug can be regulated by repeated measurement of this body function (regulated dose).

20. To achieve maximal therapeutic effect with few toxic drugs, its dose is titrated with an acceptable level of adverse effect (titrated dose).

21. Loading dose is a single dose or a few quickly repeated doses given in the beginning to attain target plasma concentration rapidly to achieve desired therapeutic effect in some cases where response is not easily measurable.

22. Therapeutic index (LD_{50}/ED_{50}) or safety margin of a drug means the gap between its therapeutic effect and adverse effect.

23. Fixed dose combinations are preparations which contain two or more drugs in a fixed dose ratio. In fact only handful of fixed dose combinations is rational and justified. Hence they should be discouraged.

Chapter 3

Pharmacodynamics

Pharmacodynamics is concerned with the actions, interactions and the mode of action of drugs. It deals with:

a. Quantitative study of the biological and therapeutic effects of drugs.
b. The mechanism of action of a drug.
c. Correlation of drug actions with the chemical structure.

An effect on a tissue is the end result of an interaction between drug molecules and some part of the tissue cells. So the terms 'action' and 'effect' are not synonymous. The action deals with the initial consequences of drug molecules-cell interaction and effect includes the remaining events. Interaction between drug molecules and some part of the tissue cell may be specific or non-specific. In former, the drugs act on pharmacological receptors situated on or within the cells while in case of later receptors are not involved. Specific features of two types of interactions are given in Table 3.1:

PRINCIPLES OF DRUG ACTION

Drugs do not create new functions to any system, cell or organ. They can only modify the inherent functions. They produce only a quantitative and not a qualitative change in the functions of the target organ. The basic types of drug action are:

1. **Stimulation:** Selective enhancement in the activity of specialized cells is called stimulation, e.g. caffeine stimulates central nervous system.

2. **Depression:** Selective diminution in the activity of specialized cells is called depression, e.g. barbiturates depress central nervous system.

3. **Irritation:** This indicates a non-selective and often noxious effect. It is particularly applied to less specialized cells such as epithelium, connective tissue, etc. Such drugs produce effects on the growth, nutrition, and morphology of living tissues. Mild irritation stimulates function, e.g. bitters increase salivary and gastric secretions. On the other hand, strong irritation leads to inflammation, corrosion, necrosis and morphological damage. Finally, this may result in diminution or loss of function.

Table 3.1: Comparison between drugs acting/not acting via receptors

Drugs acting via receptors	Drugs not acting via receptors
1. Act at low concentrations.	Act at higher concentrations.
2. React with specific receptors.	Do not react with specific receptors.
3. Show structure activity relationship.	Tend not to show structure-activity relationship.
4. Can be antagonized by specific antagonists.	Do not have any specific antagonists.
5. Examples: acetylcholine, histamine, adrenaline	Diuretics, halothane, detergents.

4. Use of natural metabolites, hormones or their congeners in deficiency states (e.g. levodopa in parkinsonism, insulin in diabetes mellitus) is called *replacement therapy*.
5. **As anti-infective agents:** Drugs are used for prevention, arrest and eradication of infection. They act specifically on the causative organisms and host cells are least affected, e.g. penicillin.
6. **Modification of immune status:** Sera, vaccines, and certain other drugs act by altering the immune status.

MECHANISM OF DRUG ACTION

Drugs produce their overt effects by a variety of fundamental actions:

1. **Outside the cell:**
   a. *Physical action:*
      i. **Colour** may exert a psychological effect.
      ii. **Smell:** Volatile oils like peppermint oil are used to mask the unpleasant smell of mixtures.
      iii. **Taste:** Compounds with bitter taste improve appetite by reflexly increasing flow of hydrochloride in the stomach.
      iv. **Physical mass:** Bulk purgatives
      v. **Adsorptive property:** Kaolin and activated charcoal
      vi. **Osmotic activity:** Magnesium sulfate, mannitol
      vii. **Soothing demulcent:** Syrup; calamine lotion
      viii. **Radioactivity:** ^{131}I and other radioactive isotopes
      ix. **Radio-opacity:** Contrast media
      x. **Reduction in surface tension:** Cationic surfactant
      xi. **Electric charge:** Heparin is strongly acidic compound. It probably exerts its anticoagulant effect by virtue of its negative charge.

   b. *Chemical properties:*
      i. Oxidizing agents are germicidal. They inactivate ingested alkalies.
      ii. Antacids neutralize gastric pH.
      iii. Chelating agents form a ring structure with the molecule of metalloid or the metal to give rise a non-toxic and highly water soluble compound. This helps in their excretion in urine.
2. **On intracellular constituents:**
   i. *Enzymes:* Monoamine oxidase, cholinesterase, or xanthine oxidase
   ii. Transport carrier molecules, e.g. probenecid on renal tubules
   iii. Cytosolic or nuclear receptors
   iv. DNA or RNA, e.g. with the use of different anticancer drugs
3. **Antimicrobial action:**
   i. Inhibition of cell wall synthesis, e.g. beta-lactam antibiotics.
   ii. Inhibition of cell membrane function, e.g. polymyxins.
   iii. Inhibition of protein synthesis, e.g. aminoglycosides.
   iv. Inhibition of nucleic acid synthesis and function, e.g. pyrimidine analogues, alkylating agents.
4. **On cell membrane:**
   i. Action on receptors of agonists and antagonists
   ii. Action on enzymes and pump, e.g. myocardial ATPase and neuronal noradrenaline uptake pumps; adenylyl cyclase enzyme, etc.
   iii. Action on ion channels, e.g. Ca^{++} channel
   iv. Physicochemical interaction with lipid, protein or water constituents of nerve cell membrane, e.g. with general and local anaesthetics, alcohol.

Targets of drug action
- Receptors
- Ion channels
- Structural proteins
- Carrier molecules
- Enzymes

Targets of Drug Action

Mostly drugs produce their effects by acting on specific macromolecular elements. Thus they alter their biochemical or biophysical activity. The following are important targets for drug action on mammalian cells.

Receptors: The functions of all the different cells in the body are regulated through their system of chemical communications. Receptors are the sensing elements of these chemical communications and the hormone or transmitter substances are chemical messengers. Receptor-mediated actions can indirectly activate or inhibit ion channels, enzymes and carrier molecules.

Drug receptor interactions are dealt later in this chapter.

Carrier molecules: These are carrier proteins which have "recognition sites". These sites act as targets for a drug. These carrier molecules transport ions and small organic molecules across cell membrane. Some carrier proteins are of proton pump, nor-adrenaline uptake and Na^+/K^+ pumps.

Ion channels: Mostly drugs modulate ion channels by binding with parts of the channel protein. However, some are ligand-gated receptor mediated ion channels while others are indirectly modulated through G-proteins or other intermediates. Na^+, K^+, Ca^{++}, and Cl^- are common ion channels.

Enzymes: Mostly drug molecules produce their effects by competitively inhibiting the enzymes.

A few drugs produce their effect acting on structural proteins, e.g. colchicine on tubulin.

Drug-Receptor Interactions

In the beginning of this century, Paul Ehrlic developed the concept of receptor. According to him the drug-receptor interaction is a lock (receptor) and key (drug) system. Most drug receptors (pharmacological receptors) are macromolecular proteins. They are specific in size, shape and structure. They occur at specific sites to which specific substances, i.e. drugs (sometimes called ligands) interact. Drug-receptor binding leads to a change in the macromolecule. This in turn triggers a sequence of events (transduction mechanisms or the signaling mechanisms) resulting in a biological response of the tissue or organ. Signaling mechanisms are different at different sites. So far four signaling mechanisms have been well understood.

1. **Ligand-gated channels:** GABA, n-ACh and the excitatory amino acids are natural ligands and synaptic transmitters. They produce their effects by regulating transmembrane flow of ions along with concentration gradient acting on specific receptor ion channel and opening the gate for relevant ion flow. ACh opens Na^+ channel and glutamate K^+ channel. There occurs depolarization of cell membrane due to the flow of ions.

2. **G-protein coupled receptors:** Most of the receptors (m-ACh, adrenergic, H_2, 5HT, opiate and many peptide hormones) in the body belong to this family. They are situated on the cell membrane. They are linked to the effector (enzyme/channel) carrier protein through one or more GTP activated proteins (G-proteins) for response effectuation. Among number of G-proteins, Gs and Gi are the two important ones. Gs and Gi produce opposite effects by causing stimulation and inhibition of adenylyl cyclase respectively. Stimulation of adenylyl cyclase enzyme leads to accumulation of cAMP while its inhibition is associated with decrease in concentration of cAMP. Gs protein is stimulated by β_1 adrenergic amine, H_2-agonists, 5-HT_1 agonists and polypeptide hormones while Gi protein is activated by β_2 adrenoceptor agonists,

M_2-ACh and δ-opioid receptor agonists. There are four major effector pathways through which G-protein coupled receptors function:

i. *Adenylyl cyclase cAMP pathway:* This system has a wide variety of receptor population and produces diverse effects. Activation of adenylyl cyclase leads to intracellular accumulation of second messenger cAMP, which functions almost exclusively through cAMP dependent protein kinase (PKa). Phosphodiesterases terminate the intracellular effects of cAMP by degrading it to 5-AMP. Methoxamines prolong the effects of cAMP by competitively inhibiting phospho-diesterases.

As observed there are different signaling mechanisms at a molecular level. These mechanisms modulate different cellular function or sometimes even the same cellular function. It means the effects may be complement or oppose each other. Examples are: There occurs release of glucose from liver by 2 different signaling mechanisms, i.e. stimulation of cAMP (beta-adrenoceptors) and phos-phoinositide (α_1—adrenoceptors) second messengers. Vasopressor drugs contract smooth muscles by IP3-mediated mobilization of Ca^{++} (alpha-1 adrenoceptors) whereas vasodilators act by elevation of cAMP (beta–adrenoceptors.

ii. *Phospholipase C-Ca^{++}/phosphoinositide system:* This system is more complex than the cAMP pathway due to two second messengers (inositotri-phosphate, IP3 and diacylglycerol, DAG) and multiplicity of protein kinases. This pathway is stimulated by 5HT$_2$, TRH, ACh(M$_1$), catecholamine (α_1), vasopressin and angiotensin.

iii. *cGMP pathway:* This pathway is limited to a few cell types. It is stimulated by ACh, histamine, peptide hormone, atrial natriuretic factor (ANF) and vascular endothelial nitric oxide. Activation of membrane bound guanylate cyclase leads to generation of cGMP. In turn it acts by stimulating a cGMP - dependent protein kinase.

iv. *Channel regulation:* The activated G-proteins can also open or close ionic channels specific for Ca^{++}, K^+, or Na^+, without involving any second messenger. In turn there occurs hyper-polarization/depolarization/changes in intracellular Ca^{++}. mACh receptors enhance K^+ permeability in cardiac muscle, and opiate analgesics open K^+ channels reducing neuronal excit-ability.

3. **Catalytic receptors (tyrosine kinase-linked receptors):** These receptors are enzymatic proteins themselves. The agonist binding site and the catalytic site lie respectively on the outer and inner face of the plasma membrane. Two sites are interconnected through a single trans-membrane stretch of peptide chain. These receptors mediate the actions of insulin, a variety of growth factors and peptide mediators which stimulate mitogenesis.

4. **Receptors regulating gene expression:** These receptors are intracellular (cytoplasmic or nuclear) soluble proteins. They respond to lipid soluble chemical messengers that penetrate the cell, e.g. steroid and thyroid hormones. The stimulation of these receptors results in stimulation of transcription of selected genes that in turn leads to the synthesis of particular proteins or enzymes. In turn, these proteins or enzymes produce the cellular effects. In this system, effect lasts for hours or days because of slow turnover of newly synthesized protein or enzyme.

Response of Drug-Receptor Interactions

Depending on the nature of drug molecule, the drug receptor interaction leads to a variety of responses. The ability of a drug to interact with a receptor is due to its affinity and the ability to produce a response (contraction of muscle or secretion from a gland) is called its 'intrinsic activity' or 'intrinsic efficacy'.

An agonist is a drug (neurotransmitter or hormone) which has affinity and intrinsic activity such as acetylcholine, noradrenaline, histamine, etc.

An antagonist is a drug which binds to the receptor but does not activate it. It means it has affinity but no intrinsic efficacy such as atropine. These drugs, however, compete with the endogenous ligand or exogenous agonists and prevent their receptor occupancy and response.

Some drugs have affinity but very low intrinsic efficacy. They are called partial agonists. They competitively block the effects of a full agonist. They produce a response by themselves which is much lower than that of a full agonist even at full receptor-occupancy.

Examples are pindolol (a beta blocker), saralasin, etc.

Inverse agonists are drugs which produce responses that are paradoxical in nature. For example, p-carbolines act on benzodiazepine receptors and produce anxiety, increased muscle tone and convulsions. On the other hand, the agonist benzodiazepines binding with same receptors produce sedation, anxiolysis, muscle relaxation and control of convulsions. Both the responses are mediated by modulating the effects of the neuro-transmitter GABA.

A mixed agonist-antagonist has also been described. It should not be confused with partial agonist. This type of drug acts simultaneously on a mixed group of receptors with an agonistic action on one set and with an antagonist action on another set. Examples are seen among the opioids.

There are binding forces in drug-receptor interactions such as covalent bonds (usually the strongest, producing almost irreversible effects), ionic bonds, hydrogen bonds and van der Waals forces (weakest attractive bonds producing a readily reversible effect).

It is also important to determine quantitative aspects of drug action. They help in deciding the mode of use of a drug. The most important aspects of quantitative nature is dose/concentration–effect/response relationship.

1. **Drug responses are of two types:**
    i. *Graded response:* This effect can be seen on a single subject, or discrete organ or tissue. In this case, the pharmacological response increases with an increase in the dose and it is measurable, e.g. contraction or relaxation of muscle, change in blood pressure, blood sugar, etc. The graded dose-response relation is partially a reflection of extent of occupancy of the receptors by the drug. However, the degree of pharmacological effect produced by increasing doses of a drug eventually reaches a steady level. This is termed as "ceiling effect" and the dose which produces this effect is called "ceiling dose". At this stage, there is no increase in therapeutic effect even if the dose of drug exceeds the ceiling dose. On the contrary, there may occur undesirable effects or different responses. Ceiling dose also helps in comparing the therapeutic efficacy of various pharmacologically active compounds.

    The graded dose response curve is usually sigmoid in shape. However, it is almost a straight line when drug response is plotted against the logarithm of the drug dose. The latter is useful for the comparison of the activity of various compounds, e.g. in bioassays.

ii. *Quantal response:* It is an 'all or none response'. It cannot be measured. Examples are analgesic, anticonvulsant or convulsant activity, death, etc. In this case also the log dose response curve is sigmoid in character. To make the relationship more linear, the responses are converted into probits (probability units) from statistical table and log-dose-probit response curve is plotted. This type of curve helps in determining LD_{50} or ED_{50} more accurately.

2. **Spare receptors:** Drug response is not directly proportional to the rate of receptor occupancy. A pure agonist may produce maximal response just by occupying even duly 1% of receptors. On the contrary, a partial agonist will not produce maximal response even after 100% receptor occupancy. So when the maximal response is produced by a pure agonist without occupying all the available receptors, the left over receptors are called spare receptors. Higher the spare receptor population, greater is the tissue sensitivity for the drug.

3. **Potency and efficacy:** A drug is said to be potent when it possesses high intrinsic activity at low unit weight doses. It depends on affinity of receptors and the efficiency of drug receptor coupling. The potency is determined by finding out ED_{50} or EC_{50}. Lower the ED_{50} or EC_{50}, higher is the potency. However, in drug selecting process efficacy of a drug plays more important role than potency. Efficacy refers to the maximum response or peak response produced by a drug. If a drug is more potent and has high efficacy than the older drug, it is certainly a better alternative. However, if it is more potent

but has low efficacy than the older drug, it is not a suitable alternative.

4. **Quantitative variation in drug response:** Due to normal "biological variations", responses to drugs vary from animal to animal, human to human. Sometimes a quantitative change in drug response may be observed in the same individual during the course of therapy. It is of great clinical importance. Depending on the change, a physician has to change either the dose or the drug itself. This may occur in the following circumstances:

a. *Down regulation:* On continuous exposure of tissues to an agonist, the number of receptors decreases (down regulation). This results in loss in efficacy. Down regulation of receptor occurs due to accelerated endocytosis of receptors (internalization) from the cell surface, which is faster than de novo synthesis of receptors. It is responsible for 'tolerance' or 'tachyphylaxis'.

b. *Up-regulation:* On continuous exposure of tissues to an antagonist, the formation of new receptors increases (up regulation) and is responsible for increased tissue sensitivity. This may be responsible for rebound hypertension/angina pectoris following withdrawal of beta-adrenoceptor blocker. Sometimes hormones may also cause up-regulation of receptors, e.g. increased cardiac sensitivity to catecholamines in thyrotoxicosis.

FACTORS MODIFYING THE EFFECT OF A DRUG

Degree and character of response of a drug varies from one individual to another individual. Hence to achieve desired therapeutic effect the optimum dose of a drug differs from person to person. This is why the

Factors modifying the effect of a drug
• Body weight and age
• Sex
• Genetic factors
• Diet and environment
• Metabolic disturbances
• Route of administration
• Emotional factors
• Cummulation
• Presence of disease
• Additive effect
• Synergism
• Antagonism
• Tolerance
• Drug dependence

doses of official preparations of drugs are always expressed in the form of range which gives therapeutic effect in the majority of subjects. However, these doses may not be applicable under all circumstances. So the important factors, which modify the effect of a drug, are:

1. **Body weight and age:** Determination of a proper dose of a drug is most important in therapeutics. The best way to calculate dosage is in terms of milligrams per kilogram body weight. However, doses calculated in this way may not be applicable to excessively obese patients or those suffering from oedema, dehydration, emaciation, cachetia and malnutrition. The dose in children may be calculated by the following formulae because they are more sensitive to drugs:

   i. Clark's formula (body weight):

   $$\frac{\text{Child's weight kg}}{70} \times \text{adult dose}$$

   $$= \text{child's dose}$$

   ii. Young's formula (age):

   $$\frac{\text{Age yrs}}{\text{Age yrs } 12} \times \text{adult dose}$$

   $$= \text{child's dose}$$

   iii. $$\frac{\text{Surface area m}^2}{1.8 *} \times \text{adult dose}$$

   $$= \text{child's dose}$$

   * (Average body surface area of 70 kg man is about 1.8 m²)

   The body surface area is calculated from the height and weight of the child. Infants are sensitive to many drugs because many drug metabolizing enzymes are either absent or deficient. So these drugs may show prolonged action in infants. Same is true in old individuals where metabolism of a drug may depend on the functional state of the liver, disease or previous exposure of the patient to the drug.

2. **Sex:** Sometimes excitement may be evoked in the females by central nervous system depressants like morphine or barbiturates. One has to be careful while prescribing a drug to a female patient during menstruation, pregnancy and lactation.

3. **Genetic factors:** To produce the same therapeutic effect, the dose of a drug may vary by 4 to 6-fold among different individuals. This is due to different rates of drug metabolism which is controlled by the amount of microsomal enzymes. The amount of microsomal enzymes are genetically determined. So there are now some specific genetic defects which are responsible for variation in drug responses, e.g.

   i. Glucose-6-phosphate dehydrogenase deficiency leads to haemolysis with primaquin and other oxidizing drugs.

   ii. Inability to hydroxylate phenytoin leads to toxicity at usual doses.

   iii. Atypical pseudocholinesterase causes succinylcholine apnoea.

   iv. Malignant hyperthermia occurs after halothane.

   v. Acetylator polymorphism causes isoniazid neuropathy, procainamide and hydralazine induced lupus.

vi. Acute intermittent porphyria is precipitated by barbiturates.

vii. Resistance to coumarine anticoagulants is due to an abnormal receptor for them.

viii. Mongolism-fatality is seen with therapeutic dose of atropine.

ix. Erythrocyte diaphorase methemo-globinemia is seen after administering certain drugs such as acetanilide, sulfonamide and nitrites.

4. **Diet and environment:** Although food interferes/decreases the rate and extent of drug absorption, most drugs are taken after meal to avoid the risk of gastric - irritation and associated nausea and vomiting. However, under special circumstances, drugs are given empty stomach, e.g.

   i. Antimotion sickness drugs for quick action

   ii. Anthelmintics to avoid mixing with food

   iii. Penicillin V to prevent inactivation in gut

   Dose of a hypnotic drug is more to produce sleep during day time than what is needed at bedtime in the night. DDT, polyhydrocarbons, and alcohol enhance biotransformation of drugs such as theophylline by inducing microsomal enzymes.

5. **Metabolic disturbances:** Alteration in physiological parameters of the body may modify the effect/dose of a drug, e.g.

   i. Metabolic acidosis reduces vasocons-triction effect of noradrenaline.

   ii. Salicylates decrease body temperature only in the presence of pyrexia (fever).

   iii. Maximum amount of iron is absorbed from gut in patients suffering from iron deficiency anemia.

6. **Route of administration:** Smaller doses are required for i.v. administration of a drug than oral doses. This is particularly so for drugs which are incompletely absorbed, e.g. morphine and digoxin. On i.v. administration, onset of action of a drug is quick but chances of drug toxicity is also more.

7. **Emotional factors:** The personality of a physician/patient may influence the drug effect, e.g.

   i. Placebos (inert dosage form) given by physician to patients of angina pectoris and bronchial asthma may produce beneficial therapeutic effect.

   ii. The dose of chlorpromazine will be ten times more than usual dose to produce quietening effect in some schizophrenic patients.

8. **Cummulation:** Some drugs are excreted slowly. So their continuous administration may lead to a sufficiently high concen-tration of the drug in the body to produce toxicity. Examples of such drugs are emetine, heavy metals, and digitalis. Most often cummulation is undesirable. Rarely may it be desirable such as use of pheno-barbitone in the treatment of epilepsy.

9. **Presence of disease:**

   i. Cirrhosis of liver prolongs the effect of barbiturates and chlorpromazine.

   ii. Impairment of kidney function may lead to toxicity of aminoglycoside antibiotics.

   iii. Myxoedema prolongs the action of morphine delaying its rate of oxidation.

10. **Summation effect:** On simultaneous administration, if two drugs produce same pharmacological effect by different mechanism of action and the total pharmacological effect is equal to the sum of their individual effect, it is called summation effect, e.g.

    • Paracetamol (inhibition of prosta-glandin synthesis) + codeine (opioid receptor agonist) as analgesic

- Ephedrine (adrenoceptor agonist) + theophylline (inhibition of phospho-diesterase enzyme) as bronchodilator

11. **Additive effect:** On simultaneous administration, if two drugs produce same pharmacological effect by same mechanism of action and the total pharmacological action of two drugs is equal to the sum of their individual effect, it is called additive effect, e.g.
    - Aspirin + paracetamol as analgesic/antipyretic (inhibition of prostaglandin synthesis)
    - Nitrous oxide + ether as general anaesthetic (inhibition of neuronal activity by a membrane effect).

12. **Synergism:** In this case, there occurs facilitation of pharmacological response by concomitant use of two drugs and their total effect will be more than the sum of their individual effect. Examples are:
    - Acetylcholine + physostigmine
    - Levodopa + carbidopa/benserazide
    - Sulfonamide + trimethoprim
    - Tyramine + MAO inhibitor
    - Adrenalin + cocaine/desipramine
    - Methyl alcohol + thiazide diuretic.

13. **Antagonism:** When two drugs, administered simultaneously, oppose the action of each other on the same physiological system, the phenomenon is called antagonism. It can be of following types:
    i. *Chemical antagonism:* It involves reduction or abolition of the biological activity of a drug by a chemical reaction with another agent, e.g. between acids and alkalies; BAL and arsenic.
    ii. *Functional antagonism:* In this case, two agonists oppose the action of each other acting independently of each other, e.g. acetylcholine and adrenaline on dogs blood pressure.
    iii. *Competitive or reversible antagonism (equilibrium type):* In this type of antagonism, the agonist and antagonist compete with each other for the same receptors. The extent of antagonism will depend by the relative number of receptors occupied by the two compounds. Other features are:
    a. Antagonist has chemical resemblance with agonist.
    b. Antagonism can be overcome by increasing the concentration of the agonist at receptor site. It means the maximal response to agonist is not impaired (surmountable).
    c. Antagonist shifts the dose response curve to right.
    d. E_{max} of agonist is obtained with high concentration of agonist.
    e. Duration of action is short. It depends on drug clearance.

    Examples:
    - Acetylcholine and atropine
    - Morphine and naloxan

    iv. *Non-competitive antagonism:* Here an antagonist inactivates the receptor (R) in such a way so that the effective complex with agonist cannot be formed irrespective of the concentration of the agonist. This can happen by various ways:
    a. The antagonist might combine with R at the same site in such a way that even higher concentration of the agonist cannot displace it.
    b. The antagonist might combine at a different site of R in such a way that agonist is unable to initiate characteristic biological response.
    c. The antagonist might itself induce a certain change in R so that the reactivity of the receptor site where agonist should interact is abolished.

    Other features of this antagonism are:
    a. Antagonist has no chemical resemblance with agonist.
    b. Maximum response is suppressed (insurmountable).

c. Although antagonist shifts the dose response curve to right, the slope of the curve is reduced.

d. The extent of antagonism depends on the characteristics of antagonist itself and agonist has no influence upon the degree of antagonism or its reversibility.

e. E_{max} of agonist is decreased even with high concentration of agonist.

f. Duration of action is long which depends upon new receptor synthesis. Examples are methysergide, phenoxybenzamine, and verapamil.

v. *Physiological antagonism:* In this interaction of two drugs, both are agonists. So they act at different receptor sites. They antagonize the action of each other because they produce opposite actions. Classical example of physiological antagonism is adrenalin and histamine. The former causes bronchodilatation while the latter causes bronchoconstriction. So adrenalin is a life saving drug in anaphylaxis.

Clinical significance of drug antagonism:

a. It helps to correct adverse effects of a drug, e.g. ephedrine antagonizes sedative effect of phenobarbitone.

b. It is useful to treat drug poisoning, e.g. naloxone is used to treat acute morphine poisoning.

c. It guides to avoid drug combinations with reduced drug efficacy such as penicillin and tetracycline combination.

14. **Drug tolerance:** It means requirement of a higher dose of a drug to produce a given therapeutic response. Drug tolerance may be:

a. *Natural:* In this case, the species/individual is inherently less sensitive to the drug, e.g. rabbits are tolerant to belladona; black races are tolerant to mydriatics.

b. *Acquired:* It occurs on repeated administration of a drug in an individual who was initially responsive. Body is capable of developing tolerance to most drugs. However, this phenomenon is very easily recognized in case of central nervous system depressants. Tolerance need not develop equally to all the actions of a drug, e.g.

   i. Tolerance develops to sedative action of chlorpromazine but not to its antipsychotic action.

   ii. Tolerance develops to sedative action of phenobarbitone but not to its anti-epileptic effect.

   iii. Tolerance develops to analgesic and euphoric effects of morphine but not to its constipating and miotic actions.

c. *Cross-tolerance:* It means development of tolerance among pharmacologically related compounds, e.g. alcoholics are tolerant to barbiturates and general anesthetics.

Mechanisms of development of tolerance:

i. *Pharmacokinetic/drug disposition tolerance:* In this case, there is decreased availability of drug at receptor site due to pharmacokinetic reasons, e.g.

   a. Due to enzyme induction as in case of repeated use of barbiturates, rifampicin, ethanol.

   b. Due to decreased rate of absorption.

   c. Due to rapid elimination of a drug such as phenylbutazone which is rapidly excreted in rodents, dogs and cats than in human beings. So these animals are relatively tolerant to phenylbutazone.

ii. *Pharmacodynamic/cellular tolerance:* In this type, cells of the target organs become less responsive. It may be of two types:

a. Physiological adaptation occurs due to activation of homeostatic (compensatory) mechanisms, e.g. with carbonic anhydrase inhibitor diuretics, vasodilator hypotensives.

b. Tissue tolerance is seen with many drugs, e.g. morphine, alcohol, barbiturates, psychotropic drugs. It may be due to down regulation of receptors.

Tachyphylaxis: It is a rapid development of tolerance. In this case, the effect diminishes rapidly when a drug is given continuously or repeatedly. It is a reversible phenomenon. The tissue regains its normal sensitivity following a drug free period of some minutes or hours. It may be due to:

a. Tight binding of agonist molecule leading to desensitization in ionic channel-coupled receptor, e.g. N-ACh receptors at the neuromuscular junction.

b. Down regulation of receptors.

c. Depletion of neuronal mediators as seen in case of indirectly acting sympathomimetics, e.g. tyramine, ephedrine, amphetamine.

15. **Drug dependence:** It is a condition in which an individual is dependent on a drug. It is seen with drugs which are capable of altering mood and feelings of an individual. These drugs are liable to be used repeatedly to derive euphoria, pleasure, and withdrawal from reality. Drug dependence is a biological phenomenon, which consists of: (a) psychic dependence and (b) physical dependence.

a. Psychic dependence is a condition in which drug produces a feeling of satisfaction and a psychic derive to take the drug periodically or continuously to have a feeling of pleasure or to avoid discomfort of life, e.g. heavy cigarette smoking.

b. Physical dependence is an altered physiological state which is produced by repeated administration of a drug. In this case, the body achieves an adaptive state. Hence intense physical disturbances (withdrawal syndrome) occur when drug is withdrawn, e.g. alcohol drinking.

When a drug is used for a "non-medical" purpose, it is supposed to be misused or abused. The drugs of abuse can be classified as under:

I. Drugs used or present in commonly used beverages:
   a. Caffeine in tea, coffee and cold drinks.
   b. Tobacco (nicotine) for smoking, chewing or intranasal administration.
   c. Ethyl alcohol.

II. Prescribed drugs, e.g. morphine, mepridine, barbiturates, tranquilizers, amphetamines.

III. Banned drugs such as heroin, cocaine, *ganja, charas*, LSD and other hallucinogens.

Principles of treatment of drug dependence:

1. Gradual or sudden withdrawal of the drug.
2. Substitution therapy.
3. Specific-drug therapy, e.g. antabuse in alcohol drug dependence.
4. Correction of nutritional deficiencies.
5. Psychotherapy and occupational therapy.
6. Community treatment and rehabilitation.

Points for Dental Students

It is essential for the dental students to have a basic knowledge of pharmacodynamics of each drug. This helps:

1. To select a suitable drug to be used in a particular situation with safety and maximum benefit to the patient.
2. To understand rational basis of use of a drug in a particular disease.
3. To know the various factors which modify the dose and effect of a drug so that necessary adjustments may be carried out for proper use of a drug.

4. To have knowledge of pharmacodynamic interactions in order to prescribe drugs rationally. For example, bronchial relaxation depends upon the formation of cyclic 3', 5'-AMP (cAMP). Catecholamines increase the formation of this 'second messenger' by stimulating adenylcyclase while aminophylline inhibits the breakdown of cAMP. So when two drugs are combined will be useful in the treatment of bronchial asthma. On the other hand, severe ototoxicity develops due to simultaneous use of amino-glycoside antibiotics and ethacrinic acid.

TO REMEMBER

1. Pharmacodynamics deals with the actions, interactions and the mode of action of drugs.
2. The terms 'action and effect' are not synonymous. The action deals with the initial consequences of drug molecules-cell interaction and effect includes the remaining events.
3. Drugs produce only a quantitative and not a qualitative change in the functions of the target organ, i.e. stimulation, depression, and irritation. They may modify immune status or used as anti-infective agents.
4. Drugs produce their overt effects by a variety of fundamental actions, viz.
   a. Acting outside the cell by their physical and chemical properties;
   b. Acting on intracellular constituents;
   c. Acting on cell membrane;
   d. By their antimicrobial action.
5. Drug receptor interaction is a lock (receptor) and key (drug) system. Pharmacological receptors are macro-molecular proteins on which drugs (ligand) interact and produce a biological response either by transduction or the signaling mechanisms.
6. Agonist is a drug which binds to the receptor (has affinity) and activate it (has intrinsic efficacy) while antagonist has affinity but no intrinsic efficacy. Inverse agonists are drugs which produce responses that are paradoxical in nature.
7. Mixed agonist-antagonist is a drug that acts simultaneously on a mixed group of receptors with agonistic action on one set and an antagonistic action on another set.
8. Drugs can produce a graded response (measurable and varies with dose) or quantal response (all or none response - not measurable).
9. A drug with high intrinsic activity at low unit weight doses is said to be potent while efficacy refers to the maximum or peak response produced by a drug.
10. Pharmacogenetics deals with genetically mediated variations in drug responses.
11. Additive/summation effect means the total pharmacological action of two drugs will be equal to the sum of their individual effect on simultaneous administration, while in case of synergism the total effect will be more than the sum of their individual effect.
12. Antagonism means two drugs oppose the action of each other on the same physiological system on simultaneous administration. It may be chemical, competitive, and non-competitive, functional or physiological.
13. Drug tolerance means requirement of a higher dose of a drug to produce a given therapeutic response. It may be natural or acquired.
14. Drug dependence is a condition in which an individual is dependent on a drug. It may be psychic dependence (psychic derive to take drug to have a feeling of pleasure) or physical dependence (altered physiological state due to repeated administration of a drug).

Chapter 4

Adverse Drug Reactions, Prescription Writing and Drug Interactions

ADVERSE DRUG REACTIONS

An adverse drug reaction is noxious and unintended response to a drug. It occurs at doses which are used in man for prophylaxis, diagnosis or therapy. Knowledge about drug adverse reactions and their mechanism is important in minimizing the undesirable effects of the drugs. Administration of a drug may lead to any of the following adverse drug reactions:

1. **Side effects:** They occur at therapeutic doses of a drug. They are the pharmacological actions, other than the one which is required for the treatment of a disease, e.g. dryness of mouth with atropine. A side effect may be troublesome in a particular condition but it may prove useful under other circumstances. So when atropine is used to treat peptic ulcer dryness of mouth is undesirable effect. However, this effect is useful when atropine is used as a preanaesthetic medication.

2. **Secondary effects:** These are the indirect consequences of primary drug action, e.g. resistant staphylococcal diarrhea following tetracycline therapy, potassium loss due to diuretic drugs, vitamin deficiency or super-infection during chemotherapy. They occur at therapeutic doses.

3. **Toxic effects:** They are observed on prolonged drug therapy or when drug is given in large doses (toxic doses). In fact

they are exaggerated pharmacological actions when drug is given in over doses. On the other hand, prolonged use of certain drugs, in therapeutic doses, may lead to delayed carcinogenicity, or teratogenicity or mutagenicity, or allergenicity or idiosyncrasy. It also includes reactions seen sometimes after sudden withdrawal of a drug such as:

- Rebound hypertension after clonidine withdrawal.
- Rebound adrenocortical insufficiency after withdrawal of corticosteroids.
- Myocardial infarction after withdrawal of propranolol in a patient of angina pectoris.

Large doses of drugs may cause poisoning. Poison may severely affect one or more vital functions and endanger life. There are specific antidotes only for a few drugs such as chelating agents, receptor-antagonists and specific antibodies. For others, the treatment includes general supportive and symptomatic measures only. General principles of treatment of poisoning are:

- Remove the patient to fresh air for inhaled poisons.
- Wash the eyes and skin for poisons entering from the surface.
- Induce emesis or perform gastric lavage for ingested poisons.
- Prevent absorption of ingested poison or suspension by activated charcoal

(20–40 gm in 200 ml of water) or universal antidote (2 parts of burned toast plus one part of strong tea plus one part of milk of magnesia).

- Artificial respiration for adequate ventilation and maintenance of patent airway.
- Maintain blood pressure by fluid infusion, pressor drugs and cardiac stimulants, etc. as the need may be.
- Eliminate poison by:
  a. Inducing diuresis with furosemide or mannitol.
  b. Altering urinary pH (alkalization for acidic drugs and acidification for basic drugs)
- Haemodialysis

4. **Intolerance:** Drug intolerance is inability of an individual to tolerate a drug. It may be further subdivided as:

i. *Quantitative intolerance:* Some individuals have a low threshold to pharmacological effects. Such individuals elicit exaggerated pharmacological effects in therapeutic or even smaller doses, e.g. vomiting with a single dose of salicylates or giddiness with one injection of streptomycin. So such individuals may be considered as hyper-reactors.

ii. *Qualitative intolerance:* In this case, symptoms and signs observed are totally different from those seen after administration of toxic dose of the drug. It may be of two types:

a. *Idiosyncrasy:* This is a qualitative type of intolerance. It is not due to immune mechanisms. In some cases, these abnormal reactions to drugs are due to genetically mediated variations in individuals (already explained earlier). However, in some other cases, the exact cause of these abnormal reactions to the drugs is not known, e.g. cholestatic jaundice following chlorpromazine or chloramphenicol induced aplastic anaemia.

b. *Allergic (hypersensitivity) reactions:* Allergic or hypersensitivity reactions may be produced by most of the drugs and sera used in therapeutics. They may be mild or very severe like anaphylaxis. They have immuno-logic basis. They develop in individuals who have been sensitized following the prior administration of the same drug. Drug allergy can be treated as under:

- Immediately stop administration of offending drug.
- H_1-antihistaminics are useful to treat urticaria, rhinitis, swelling of lips, etc. and some skin rashes.

Anaphylactic shock or angioedema of larynx is treated as under:

- Administer 0.5 mg of adrenaline subcutaneous/intramuscularly immediately (life saving drug).
- Subsequently administer H_1-anti-histaminics and i.v. glucocorticoids which act slowly.
- Use resuscitative measures.

Glucocorticoids are the only drugs which are useful in the treatment of cytolytic reactions (thrombocytopenia, agranulo-cytosis, aplastic anaemia, haemolysis, organ damage, and systemic lupus erythematosus), retarded arthus reactions (serum sickness, poly-arteritis nodosa, and Stevens-Johnson syndrome) and delayed hypersensitivity reactions.

5. **Photosensitivity:** It is a cutaneous reaction. It is due to sensitization of the skin to ultraviolet (UV) radiation. It is of 2 types:

i. *Phototoxic:* It is a photo-biological reaction. It occurs due to accumulation of drug or its metabolite in the skin which in turn absorbs light of shorter wavelength (290–320 nm UV-B) and undergoes a photochemical reaction. So there occurs sunburn like local tissue damage (eryhtema, oedema, blistering, hyperpigmentation and desquamation). Examples are tetracyclines (especially demeclocycline), tar products, amiodarone, fluoroquinolons, nalidixic acid, phenothiazines, sulphonamides, sulphones and thiazides.

ii. *Photoallergic:* It is a cell-mediated immune response. It is induced by drug or its metabolite on exposure to light of longer wavelengths (320–400 nm UV-A). The condition looks like papular or contact dermatitis. Examples are chloroquine, chlorpromazine, griseofulvin, sulphonyl urea and sulphonamides.

6. **Iatrogenic disease:** This means a disease which is induced by a drug. Iatrogenic disease may simulate a natural disease or syndrome. Some of the examples are:
   i. Hypertension and congestive cardiac failure precipitated by glucocorticoids.
   ii. Parkinsonian syndrome during therapy with reserpine or phenothiazines.
   iii. Gastric ulcer with NSAIDs.
   iv. Perforation of peptic ulcer may occur by glucocorticoids, aspirin, and indomethacin.
   v. SLE-like syndrome with hydralazine or procainamide.
   vi. Retrolental fibroplasia in premature infant with vigorous oxygen therapy.
   vii. Glaucoma with ocular corticoids.
   viii. Cushing's syndrome with vigorous glucocorticoids therapy.
   ix. Unspecific hepatitis by isoniazid or pyrazinamide or indomethacin.
   x. Oedema by cortisone and hydrocortisone.
   xi. Hypokalemia by diuretics like chlorothiazide and furosemide.
   xii. Haemopoietic toxicity:
      a. Leucopenia and agranulocytosis with chloramphenicol, chlorpromazine, procainamide, indomethacin, sulfonamides.
      b. Hemolytic reactions with primaquine, chloramphenicol, sulfones.

7. **Teratogenicity:** The word is derived from the Greek word *taros* which means "monster". Teratogenicity deals with production of various types of developmental anomalies in the newborn, which occur when some drugs are used in pregnant women. For example, thalidomide, a sedative when prescribed to pregnant women for giving relief from morning sickness, produced amelia (total absence of limbs) or phocomelia (absence of one or more limbs).

8. **Mutagenesis:** Drugs may cause abnormalities of genetic material (genes, chromosomes) of cells. Due to this a permanent change in the hereditary constitution (mutation) occurs. So potentially mutagenic drug such as metronidazole should be avoided in pregnant woman.

9. **Carcinogenesis:** Drug-induced malignant tumor is extremely complex and controversial topic. The numbers of drugs, which are known to be associated with increased cancer risk in man, are less, e.g. cytotoxic and immunosuppressant drugs; others are phenylbutazone, tetracycline, pyrimethamine, prolonged oestrogen therapy.

PRESCRIPTION WRITING

It is important that drugs are rationally prescribed. This is most needed in a country like ours where standards in medical practices are set. "Medicine" is not a perfect science. It is art of balancing probabilities. A general practitioner could, therefore, have serious problems when he defies the "standards".

There are many aspects in the treatment of a sick person. In practice, use of drugs is one of them. It is possible that drugs have only a minor role to play in treating certain patients while they are of the greatest importance in others. A clinician who prescribes drugs should know:

a. Nature and course of disease.

b. Basis for choosing a dosage form.

c. Pharmacological actions and toxicity of a drug.

d. Possible interactions, in case of multiple drug therapy.

e. Ways and means of assessing the efficiency and toxicity of the drug(s) used.

The most essential thing in drug prescribing is how a drug is used in clinical practice. It is less important what drug is used. For meticulous use of a drug, a physician must be familiar with both therapeutic and toxic effects of that preparation. It will only be possible if a clinician does not switch from one preparation to another preparation frequently. It is advisable to be slow in accepting a new drug. As time passes, it is observed that smaller doses of a newly introduced drug are equally effective, safer and more economical. At the time of its introduction, the doses suggested are those effective in majority of the cases. This is done purposely to ensure better effectiveness of a drug. Due to this, about one-fourth of the patients are needlessly over dosed. No doubt higher doses are highly effective but they are more prone to cause adverse reactions in few patients.

Another important factor in our country is the cost of medicine. Usually newer drugs are costly. Moreover, it is not always true that newer drugs are better than older, established, cheap preparations. It is, therefore, suggested that a particular drug should only be used when there is definite indication for doing so after outweighing the possible harm, immediate or remote. One should not prescribe them on the basis of advertisements and other modern sales promotion techniques.

There is no drug available which is devoid of adverse reactions. It is, therefore, necessary that doctors should not over prescribe drugs for minor ailments. Newer drugs should only be prescribed if the physician has studied its pharmacological actions and other precautions himself. They should not depend and be persuaded by the promotion material from the pharmaceutical industry. No doubt a clinician should have up-to-date knowledge about the latest drugs but for this he should read himself and do not depend on others who see their own interest for promoting the sale of new preparations.

Sometimes a combination of drugs is necessary and very useful. However, that does not mean that they should be used for every disease. Often they offer marginal advantage and expose the patient to additional toxicity. Sometimes they reduce the effectiveness of therapy. They should be used only when indicated. It is a better policy that physician should combine the drugs himself in doses required rather than using readymade mixtures with fixed doses.

While writing a prescription one should pay attention to the following points:

a. Select correct dosage form.

b. Indicate the dose to be administered clearly.

c. Specify frequency and manner of administration as well as duration of therapy.

This is not all. For purposeful future use of the drugs, a system of therapeutic audit should be followed. This will provide the physician fruitful information for the effective and rationale use of the drugs in future.

DRUG INTERACTIONS

When two or more drugs are used simultaneously there may occur interaction between them. Drug interaction may lead to:

a. Enhancement of intended effect of one or both drugs

b. Diminished effect of one or both drugs and
c. An unintended and potentially harmful reaction

Unfortunately harmful drug interactions are more numerous and the incidence of such reactions has increased due to:

a. Availability of potent drugs
b. Drug explosion and
c. Irrational polypharmacy

Drug interactions may occur outside or inside the body.

I. **Drug interaction outside the body:** These interactions (incompatibility) may occur during formulation and mixing of drugs. They may be due to:

1. *Physical interaction:* There occurs alteration in physical state of either drug, e.g. amphotericine is precipitated if mixed with normal saline instead of 5% dextrose solution.

2. *Chemical interaction:* In this case, interaction between the components of two drugs in solution leads to the formation of chemically altered product, e.g. dopamine and sodium bicarbonate; furosemide and ascorbic acid.

To avoid such in vitro interactions, a physician must follow general guidelines such as:

i. Do not add drugs to blood, plasma or amino acid solutions.

ii. Mix drugs with the infusion fluid immediately before use.

iii. In absence of special information, add the drug to simple solutions (normal saline, dextrose, dextrose-saline).

iv. Add single drug to simple solution (more safe).

v. Consult drug firm package inserts.

II. **Drug interactions in the body:** These interactions can be grouped as either pharmacokinetic or pharmacodynamic interactions.

Pharmacokinetic Interactions

A. **Altered absorption** from gastrointestinal tract due to interaction may lead to decrease/increase response of a therapeutic agent. Examples are:

i. Anticholinergic agents (e.g. atropine) decrease gut motility, so they increase the total absorption of drugs.

ii. Purgatives increase gastric emptying time and gut motility, so they decrease the total absorption of drugs.

iii. Antacids decrease the absorption of dicoumarol, warfarin, sulfonamides, and nalidixic acid, nitrofurantoin and tetracycline.

iv. Sorbital increases the absorption of paracetamol.

B. **Interaction during distribution:** Some drugs are highly bound to plasma proteins. In the bound form, the drug is pharmacologically inactive. Free molecules of a drug in plasma are transported to tissues and exert their effect. Certain group of drugs seems to share a limited number of protein binding sites. So they compete with each other for these sites and can displace each other in this process if administered simultaneously. This results in an increase in the free pharmacologically active form of one of the drugs and leads to toxicity. Usually drugs with higher binding affinity to plasma proteins displace agents with lower binding affinity. Some examples are:

i. Salicylates and sulfonamides displace tolbutamide and methotrexate from protein binding sites.

ii. Salicylates, clofibrate, phenytoin displace warfarin from protein binding site.

C. **Interaction during biotransformation:**
• Drugs are metabolized by liver microsomal enzymes. These enzymes can be

stimulated by number of commonly used drugs, insecticides and polycyclic hydrocarbons. Due to this, there occurs reduced therapeutic response to those drugs which are metabolized by microsomal enzymes. A few important examples are:

a. Phenobarbitone stimulates the metabolism of phenytoin and griseofulvin.

b. The metabolism of steroid hormones is increased by phenylbutazone, DDT and phenytoin.

c. Rifampicin accelerates the metabolic degradation of glucocorticoid and oral contraceptive pill.

- At present numerous cases of drug toxicity are due to inhibition of its metabolism in the body. A few examples are:

a. Metabolism of cyclophosphamide is inhibited by chloramphenicol.

b. Tolbutamide metabolism is depressed by salicylates, disulfiram, MAO inhibitor, chloramphenicol and probenecid. Due to this, a dangerous hypoglycaemia may result if any of these drugs is given along with tolbutamide.

c. Allopurinol inhibits the metabolism of 6-mercaptopurine and leads to bone marrow toxicity.

d. Oral contraceptives inhibit the metabolism of pethidine.

e. The p-hydroxylation of phenytoin is inhibited by p-aminosalicylic acid, disulfiram, dicoumarol, isoniazid and cycloserine.

D. **Interaction during excretion:** Any of the renal excretory processes may be involved in interactions occurring during excretion of drugs. However, most important drug interaction occurs due to either change in urinary pH or through competition for active tubular mechanisms. A few examples are:

a. Acidification of urine reduces the effectiveness of basic drugs (quinine, ganglionic blocking agents) as they will be largely ionized in acidic pH and readily excreted.

b. Alkalinization of urine with sodium bicarbonate, potassium citrate or acetazolamide enhances the excretion of acidic drugs (salicylates, barbiturates, anticoagulants).

c. Probenecid inhibits the tubular secretion of penicillin, indomethacin, thiazides and oral hypoglycaemics due to competition for the active secretory mechanisms.

d. Changes in electrolyte and fluid balance: Hypokalaemia produced by diuretics and corticosteroids increases digitalis toxicity. On the other hand, it antagonizes the antiarrhythmic activity of quinidine, lidocaine, procainamide, phenytoin and disopyramide.

Pharmacodynamic Interactions

1. Drugs acting on the same receptor site or at different active receptors may enhance or decrease the response, e.g. propranolol blocks the response of isoprenaline on vessel beta receptors; d-tubocurarine and aminoglycoside antibiotics may accentuate the block at neuromuscular junction; marked CNS depression by morphine and barbiturates; severe ototoxicity by aminoglycoside and frusemide.

2. Guanethidine and the related adrenergic neuron blocking drugs are actively transported into adrenergic neurons. This transport system is same that is responsible for the noradrenaline uptake into the neuron. Imipramine inhibits this system and interferes with the antihypertensive activity of guanethidine.

3. Bronchial relaxation depends upon the formation of cyclic 3', 5'-AMP (cAMP). Catecholamines increase the formation of this 'second messenger' by stimulating adenylcyclase while aminophylline inhibits the breakdown of cAMP. So when two drugs are combined, the combination will be useful in the treatment of bronchial asthma.

4. Bradycardia produced by beta-adreno-ceptor blockers due to unopposed action of the vagus nerve can be checked by concurrent administration of atropine.

Prevention of Adverse Drug Interactions

Unfortunately adverse drug interactions can not be predicted on the basis of animal studies. These drug interactions may cause life-threatening emergencies like hypertensive crisis, cardiac arrhythmias, hypoglycaemic coma, convulsions or, haemorrhage. So it is better to recognize and prevent such catastrophies. To achieve this goal, certain guidelines would be helpful:

1. Avoid irrational polypharmacy.
2. Enquire about alcohol consumption by the patient, because potentially severe reaction can occur when alcohol is consumed concomitantly with analgesics, hypnotics, tranquilizers, antihistaminics, anticonvulsants, antidiabetics, or oral anticoagulants.
3. For proper and safe use, adjust the dosages of combined drugs which are highly protein bound.
4. Appropriately adjust the dosage of any drug that is lipid-soluble at physiological pH because usually it is capable of causing enzyme induction.

Points for Dental Students

1. Every dental student must have knowledge about adverse reactions of a drug and their mechanism. This will help him in minimizing the undesirable effects of the drug.

2. This chapter is also important for dental students because in routine practice they may be administering two drugs together or one after the other or a new drug is added to therapy in a patient already taking a drug. In such cases, the response to one drug may be modified (increased or decreased) and it may be beneficial or harmful.

3. Beneficial drug-drug interactions are desirable. They form the basis of rational polypharmacy. Usually drugs are combined to increase the efficacy of therapy, reduce toxicity of individual and delay the occurrence of drug resistance.

4. Undesirable or harmful interactions may result in therapeutic failure or enhanced toxicity of interacting drugs.

5. So it is important to know about drug interactions and their mechanism of development.

Unfortunately, harmful drug interactions are more numerous. Their incidence has increased due to:
- Availability of potent drugs
- Drug explosion
- Irrational polypharmacy

6. Some times these drug interactions may cause life-threatening emergencies. So it is better to recognize and prevent such catastrophies. To achieve this goal, every dentist must keep certain guidelines in his mind such as:
- Avoid irrational polypharmacy.
- Adjust the dosages of combined drugs which are highly protein bound.
- To avoid enzyme induction, appropriately adjust the dosage of lipid soluble drug at physiological pH.

7. It is important that drugs are rationally prescribed. For this standards in medical

practices are set. 'Medicine' is not a perfect science. It is art of balancing probabilities. A general dentist could, therefore, have serious problems when he defies the standards. It is, therefore, important that a dental student must learn these standards as described in this chapter for rational drug prescribing.

TO REMEMBER

1. Adverse drug reaction is noxious and unintended response to a drug.
2. Side effects are the pharmacological actions other than the one which is required for therapeutic purpose.
3. Secondary effects are the indirect consequences of primary drug action.
4. Toxic effects are seen on prolonged drug therapy or when drug is given in large doses (toxic doses).
5. Drug intolerance is inability of an individual to tolerate a drug. It may be quantitative intolerance (due to low threshold to pharmacological effects - exaggerated pharmacological response in therapeutic or even smaller doses), or qualitative intolerance (different responses from those observed after administration of toxic dose).
6. Idiosyncrasy (qualitative intolerance) may be due to either genetically mediated variation in individuals or unknown reasons. It is devoid of immunological basis.
7. Allergic reactions (qualitative intolerance) have immunologic basis and may be produced by most of the drugs and sera.
8. Iatrogenic disease is induced by a drug and may simulate a natural disease or syndrome.
9. Teratogenicity deals with production of various types of developmental anomalies in the newborn by some drugs used during pregnancy.
10. Mutagenesis deals with abnormalities of genetic material of cells by drugs; so mutagenic drug should be avoided during pregnancy.
11. Carcinogenesis means drug-induced malignant tumor.
12. It is important that drugs are rationally prescribed. While writing a prescription a physician should pay attention to: (a) selection of correct dosage form, (b) clear indication of the dose to be administered and (c) specify frequency and manner of administration as well as duration of therapy.
13. Drug interactions may occur when two or more drugs are used simultaneously. These interactions (incompatibility) may occur during formulation and mixing due to alteration in physical state of either drug or formation of chemically altered product.
14. Drug interactions in the body can be grouped as either pharmacokinetic or pharmacodynamic interactions.

Section 2

Gastrointestinal Drugs

Chapter 5

Drugs used in Constipation and Diarrhoea

MILD AND STRONG PURGATIVES

Constipation is a condition in which the bowel is evacuated at a longer interval or with difficulty. Causes of constipation are:
1. Change of environment
2. Emotional tension
3. Disregard of the call to pass motion
4. Disease or abnormality of gastrointestinal tract
5. Adverse effects of drugs
6. Drying of stools (faecal impaction)
7. Obstruction of intestine and
8. Severe illness with too small food intake

Classification

Mild Purgatives (Laxatives)

1. **Bulk producing drugs:**
   i. *Isapgol:* 4 to 5 gm once or twice a day.
   ii. *Agar-agar:* 1 to 6 gm in divided doses.
   iii. *Bran:* 12–24 gm daily in divided doses
   iv. *Methyl cellulose:* 1 gm, 1–4 times daily
   v. *Sodium carboxy methyl cellulose:* 1.5 gm, 1–4 times daily
2. **Stool softeners:** Dioctyl sodium sulfosuccinate: 50–500 mg daily
3. **Lubricant laxative:** Liquid paraffin: 15 ml per day
4. **Mild saline purgatives:**
   i. *Magnesium hydroxide (as 8% W/W suspension–milk of magnesia):* 30 ml
   ii. *Sodium potassium tartrate (Rochelle salt):* 8–15 gm

Strong Purgatives (Cathartics)

1. **Osmotic purgatives:**
   i. *Magnesium sulfate (magsulf):* 5–15 gm daily
   ii. *Lactulose:* 30–50 ml (3.5 gm per 5 ml) 3 times a day
   iii. *Glycerine:*
      a. As rectal suppositories: 3 gm
      b. As glycerine-edible oil enema: 30–50 ml of each
   iv. *Polyethylene glycol:* 250 ml every 15–20 minutes up to 4 litres over a period of 4 hours.
2. **Irritant purgatives:**
   i. *Phenolphthalein:* 60–120 mg daily.
   ii. *Senna glycosides:* 0.6 gm (1–2 tabs daily).
   iii. *Bisacodyl:* 5–15 mg daily.
   iv. *Cascara sagarada:* 1–2 tab at bedtime.
   v. *Castor oil:* 15–25 ml daily.

General Mechanisms of Actions

Purgatives generally may act in one of the following ways:
1. By either inhibiting segmenting non-propulsive contractions or stimulating propulsive contractions
2. By retention of intraluminal fluid due to hydrophilic or osmotic mechanisms
3. By decreasing net absorption of fluid due to effects on small and large bowel fluid and electrolyte transport

MILD PURGATIVES (LAXATIVES)

Uses of Laxatives

They are used:
- To treat constipation.
- To avoid undue straining at defaecation in cases having hernia, haemorrhoids or cardiovascular disease.
- Before or after surgery of anorectal disease.
- In bedridden patients.

1. Bulk Producing Drugs

These drugs absorb water and increase bulk in the intestine. So they make the stool soft and help in the evacuation. The onset of their action is slow, about 12–24 hours. They are the safest purgatives. In our country, isapgol is most commonly used. Adverse effects are rare. Occasionally, flatulence may occur. This can be relieved by increasing the fluid intake. On chronic use, isapgol decreases plasma cholesterol by interfering with the absorption of bile acids. So to obtain maximum benefit and to avoid the possibility of intestinal obstruction (rarely reported), plenty of fluids should be taken along with these drugs.

Bulk forming laxatives decrease the absortion of other drugs such as salicylates, warfarin, and tetracycline by binding with them. So while prescribing these drugs the dentists should ask the patient to take them 2 hours after the administration of bulk purgatives.

2. Stool Softeners

Dioctyl sodium sulfosuccinate: It is an effective stool softener. It is a detergent. It is an anionic surfactant. By reducing the surface tension of fluids in the bowl, it softens the stool and permits easier defaecation. It also acts as a wetting agent for the bowl because it facilitates the penetration of water into faeces by emulsifying the colonic contents. It increases the absorption of mineral oils, so it should not be taken simultaneously with mineral oils.

3. Lubricant Laxative

Liquid paraffin: It is an inert mineral oil. It lubricates the intestines. It makes the passage of stools smooth and comfortable by forming a film or coating around the stools. It softens the stool by retarding the absorption of water from the stool. It is often recommended in cases in which straining to evacuate may be harmful, e.g. piles, heart attack, pregnant women, after surgery on the rectum or abdomen.

Indiscriminate and prolonged use of liquid paraffin is not desirable because it dissolves the fat-soluble vitamins, e.g. A, D and K and impairs their absorption. So it may cause deficiency of fat soluble vitamins. It prevents complete evacuation of bowels because its presence in rectum inhibits the stimulatory reflexes to the intestine. On aspiration (in dysphagia patients or rarely in normal elderly and weak person on oral ingestion), liquid paraffin has also been reported to cause lipoid pneumonia. Its use is not preferred after surgery for piles because it delays healing. Lastly, leakage of oil per rectum is annoying and embarrassing and may also be a cause of pruritus ani. It should not be taken along with dioctyl sodium sulfosuccinate as the latter promotes its absorption from the intestine.

4. Mild Saline Purgatives

Magnesium hydroxide: It is a mild laxative so it can be used even by pregnant women and children. On oral ingestion, it builds up an osmotic pressure in the intestinal lumen and draws water into it from the mucosal blood vessels to form the bulk. Thus it makes the stools soft and stimulates peristalsis. Besides purgative action, it counteracts acidity in the stomach. Its action starts after 2 to 6 hours. It may produce flatulence in some people. Plenty of fluid must be taken along with this purgative. Milk of magnesia should be avoided in patients with chronic kidney disease because of difficulty of its excretion.

Sodium potassium tartrate: It is the basic ingredient of commonly used ENO's fruit salt and Seidlitz powder. The latter consists of two packets; the blue packet contains 2.5 gm of sodium bicarbonate and 7.5 gm of sodium potassium tartrate, the white packet contains 2.2 gm of tartaric acid. The contents of white packet are dissolved in a glass of water and then the contents of blue packet are added to the solution. The interaction between sodium bicarbonate and tartaric acid yields carbon dioxide and so the drink effervesces. It is pleasant to take and is drunk while it is effervescing. The gas present in the solution distends the stomach and reflexly stimulates movements of the intestines. It also absorbs water from the intestines which assists in forming the bulk and softening of the stools. Its action starts after 3–6 hours. It should not be taken by those who are on a sodium restricted diet, e.g. patients of heart failure, hypertension, etc.

STRONG PURGATIVES (CATHARTICS)

Strong purgatives are used for causing complete evacuation of the bowel. They should only be used under medical supervision. These purgatives should not be used for treatment of constipation because fully evacuated bowels become inactive (atonic) and after constipation usually follows for which a milder purgative is again needed. However, their indications are:

- As post-purge to flush out worms after the use of an anthelmintic drug.
- To induce labour if the delivery does not occur at the expected time.
- For complete colonic cleansing prior to gastrointestinal procedures.
- To prepare the bowel before surgery or abdominal X-ray.
- For postoperative or post-myocardial infarction and bedridden patients.

There are two types of strong purgatives:
- Osmotic purgatives
- Irritant purgatives

Osmotic Purgatives

On oral administration certain salts are not much absorbed from gastrointestinal tract. They are retained there and exert an osmotic effect. So they hold considerable amounts of water and increase the intestinal bulk. In turn, they cause increase in the intestinal motor activity and evacuation by mechanical stimulus.

i. **Magnesium sulfate (magsulf):** It causes total evacuation of bowel in 1 to 3 hours. So it is usually taken in the morning. It may cause dehydration because of excessive loss of fluids. It may cause serious depression of central nervous system, even if a minute amount of magnesium is absorbed into the bloodstream from the intestines.

ii. **Lactulose:** This is a synthetic non-absorbable disaccharide. It is metabolized into lactic acid and other organic acids by bacteria in the distal ileum and colon. So lactulose and its metabolites produce evacuation of the bowel by osmotic effect. Further, lactic acid can bind ammonia. Due to this it is used in the treatment of hepatic coma to produce 2–3 soft stools per day.
   Lactilol: It is a synthetic disaccharide. It is more palatable than lactulose and has similar actions.

Important features of osmotic purgatives
- Act in the small and large intestines.
- Produce watery evacuation within 3–6 hours.
- Given early in the morning before breakfast.
- Do not cause irritation.
- To avoid dehydration plenty of water is to be taken.

iii. **Glycerine:** It softens and lubricates the dried up faeces by its osmotic action. It also stimulates rectal contractions. It is employed in the form of suppositories as well as a glycerine-edible oil enema.

iv. **Polyethylene glycol:** It is a non-absorbable electrolyte sugar that retains water due to its high osmotic nature. It is used orally in form of a balanced isotonic solution prepared by adding sodium chloride, sodium sulfate, sodium bicarbonate and potassium chloride so that no electrolyte shift occurs across the intestinal wall. So it does not cause dehydration. It is used to clean the bowel before surgery, colonoscopy and radiological procedures.

Irritant Purgatives

Phenolphthalein, senna, glycosides, bisacodyl, cascara sagarada and castor oil are irritant

---

Therapeutic uses of purgatives
- In constipation due to diminished intestinal tone.
- In drug induced constipation.
- In food or drug poisoning.
- In patients with severe neuromuscular disease.
- In patients with hepatic encephalopathy.
- To reduce the absorption of ammonia and toxins from colon.
- In patients with painful anal conditions (fissure, thrombosed piles) and in cardiac disease (acute myocardial infarction), in order to avoid straining during defaecation.
- In patients with an i-leostomy or colostomy to modify the effluent.
- In children with encopresis and congenital/acquired mega colon.
- To eliminate the parasites following anthelmintic therapy.
- To clean the bowel before surgery, colonoscopy and radiological procedures.

---

purgatives. They act by causing irritation of the intestines. They usually produce purgation in 3 to 6 hours. Phenolphthalein has a long duration of action as it is absorbed and re-excreted in the intestines (effective for 2 to 3 days).

They may cause gripping or cramping pains in the abdomen. Sometimes there may be erosion of inflamed mucosa leading to passage of mucous in stools. They may cause excessive loss of fluids and electrolytes. Phenolphthalein may induce allergic reactions in 0.01% cases in the form of rashes and pigmentation of the skin. Important precautions in the use of irritant purgatives are that they should not be used:

- For treatment of chronic constipation
- In pregnant women
- In cases with previous history of abdominal pain
- In feeding mothers because these are secreted in milk
- If allergic reactions occur by phenolphthalein

DRUGS USED IN DIARRHOEA (NON-SPECIFIC ANTIDIARRHOEAL AGENTS)

Frequent passage of liquid or semisolid stools is called diarrhoea. It may be accompanied by abdominal pain. It can be caused by enteric infection, food toxins, malnutrition, inflammation and drugs like reserpine, synthetic prostaglandins, metoclopramide, domperidon, cholinergic drugs, quinidine and purgatives. Dysentery is characterized by abdominal pain and passage of blood and mucous due to infection or inflammation. For infective diarrhoeas, specific chemotherapy is required.

Diarrhoea may be non-specific. It may be caused by fear, anxiety or apprehension, indigestion and in people on the move. This type of diarrhoea can be treated by non-specific measures. These measures provide symptomatic relief and do not treat the underlying cause. They reduce the frequency of stools and change the consistency, from liquid to semisolid.

1. **Oral rehydration therapy:** This therapy is effective in majority of patients with watery diarrhoea which lead to symptoms due to loss of fluid and electrolytes. As per WHO/UNICEF recommendations, this therapy consists of:

   Rx

Sodium chloride	3.5 gm
Potassium chloride	1.5 gm
Sodium citrate	2.9 gm
Glucose	20 gm
Water ad	1 ltrs.

   If oral rehydration therapy is not adequate or the patient is severely dehydrated, administer intravenous fluid and electrolytes.

2. **Antimotility agents:** These drugs reduce peristalsis. So they help reabsorption of water by delaying intestinal transit time. They also increase tone of the rectal sphincter. Tincture of opium and codeine was used earlier but its use has been discontinued because of tolerance and chances of physical dependence. At present, opioid agonists are used. They act on μ (mu) and δ (delta) recep-tors. By stimulating μ-receptors they decrease peristaltic movements while by stimulating δ receptors they have antisecretory effect. Following drugs are used.

   Diphenoxylate is a congener of pethidine. It acts on opioid mu and δ receptors. It is combined with atropine (diphenoxylate 1 mg + atropine 0.025 mg) to discourage abuse. This combination (lomotil) is given in doses of 1 tablet every 3–4 hours. It may cause nausea, vomiting, abdominal discomfort, dryness of mouth and drowsiness. Since these symptoms appear

in children even at near therapeutic doses, its use has been banned in children below the age of six years. Diphenoxin is an active metabolite of diphenoxylate and is available for treatment of diarrhoea.

Loperamide is also pethidine congener. It is sparingly absorbed. It also acts through stimulation of mu and δ receptors. It does not cause physical dependence and respiratory depression in therapeutic doses. However, it may cause nausea, vomiting and abdominal discomfort. Recommended dose is 4–8 mg per day. Antimotility agents are contraindicated in infants and children because of danger of induction of paralytic ileus.

Racecadotril acts by increasing local concentration of enkephalins in intestinal mucosa due to inhibition of enkephalinase enzyme. Then enkephalins stimulate μ and δ opioid receptors to produce antidior-rhoeal effects. It is given in doses of 100–300 mg three times a day. Important side effects are nausea, constipation and headache. Avoid its use in lactating mothers because it is secreted through breast milk.

3. **Adsorbents:** Kaolin, pectin and chalk are adsorbents. They absorb toxins. They have marginal antidiarrhoeal effect. Hence nowadays they are rarely used. Bismuth subsalicylate is an adsorbent as well as exerts local anti-inflammatory effect due to salicylate. It is recommended for traveler's diarrhoea in doses of 520 mg four times a day.

4. **Antispasmodic drugs:** Atropine and oxyphenonium (antrenyl): These drugs decrease cramps, abdominal pain and diarrhoea associated with spasms of the intestines. They may be used alone or in combination with other antidiarrhoeal and antidysentery drugs. Atropine is used in doses of 0.125 and 0.5 mg twice a day while

oxyphenonium in doses of 5 mg twice a day. Occasional use is devoid of adverse effects. However, its continuous use or its larger dose may cause dryness of mouth, urinary retention and blurring of vision.

5. **Other antidiarrhoeal agents:** Clonidine is α_2-adrenergic agonist. Its antidiarrhoeal effect is due to:
   - Facilitation of absorption of fluids from gastrointestinal tract
   - Inhibition of secretion of fluids
   - Increase in intestinal transit time

It is used to treat diabetic diarrhoea as well as in diarrhoea caused by opiate withdrawal in doses of 0.1 mg twice daily.

Berberin is a quaternary plant alkaloid. Its antidiarrhoeal effect is due to its antimicrobial (*E. coli* and *Vibrio cholera*) as well as antisecretory and antimotility activity.

Octreotide is a synthetic octapeptide. It has similar actions as that of somatostatin. It is more potent and has longer half-life (1.5–2 hrs) than somatostatin (3 min). It reduces gastrointestinal tract motility, intestinal fluid and electrolyte secretion, pancreatic secretion and gallbladder contractions. It is mainly used to treat diarrhoeas associated with carcinoid tumours and vasoactive intestinal peptide (VIP) secretion tumours as well as to treat acromegaly and to prevent variceal bleeding. It is administered in doses of 100 µg s.c. twice or three times a day. Common side effects are nausea, abdominal discomfort and pain at site of injection. On long-term therapy gallbladder stone formation and hypothyroidism may occur.

Points for Dental Students

1. Since bulk forming laxatives bind with other drugs such as salicylates, warfarin and tetracycline, they should not be taken within 2 hours of taking these drugs. This point must be kept in mind by dentist while prescribing these drugs.

2. Stool softeners (e.g. liquid paraffin) inhibit absorption of fat soluble vitamins on prolonged use. This point should be remembered by dentists who often use these vitamins in dentistry.

TO REMEMBER

1. Constipation is a condition in which the bowels are evacuated at a longer interval or with difficulty. It may require treatment with purgatives (laxatives).

2. Purgatives are contraindicated in patients suffering from organic (secondary) constipation or in individuals of undiagnosed abdominal pain, colic or vomiting.

3. In spastic constipation (irritable colon), stimulant purgatives are contraindicated. This is treated by administering dietary fiber (first choice) or any of the bulk forming agents.

4. In resistant cases of atonic constipation (irritable bowel), a bulk forming purgative should be prescribed. However, if patient is not satisfied bisacodyl or senna may be given once or twice a week for a short period only.

5. Purgatives may be required for bedridden patients (enema, liquid paraffin, bisacodyl or senna), to avoid straining at stools (bulk forming agent or docusates), to prepare bowl for surgery, colonoscopy, abdominal X-ray (saline purgative, bisacodyl or senna), after certain anthelmintics (saline purgative or senna) and in patients of food/drug poisoning (saline purgatives).

6. Chronic use of purgatives must be discouraged because of the danger of:
   (a) flaring of intestinal pathology;
   (b) rupture of inflamed appendix;
   (c) fluid and electrolyte imbalance;
   (d) spastic colitis; (e) protein loosing

enteropathy; (f) steatorrhoea and (g) malabsorption syndrome.

7. Frequent passage of liquid or semi-solid stools is called diarrhoea. It may be infective or non-specific. The former needs specific chemotherapy while latter can be treated by non-specific measures which provide symptomatic relief.

8. Oral rehydration therapy (glucose + electrolyte solutions) is effective in majority of patients with watery diarrhoeas. If it fails or the patient is severely dehydrated administer i.v. fluid and electrolytes.

9. Antimotility agents (diphenoxylate and loperamide) reduce peristalsis and increase tone of the rectal sphincter. They help reabsorption of the water by delaying intestinal transit time. They are contraindicated in infants and children because of danger of induction of paralytic ileus.

10. Antispasmodic drugs (atropine and oxyphenonium) are used to decrease cramps, abdominal pain and diarrhoea associated with spasms of the intestines.

11. Nowadays adsorbents (kaolin, pectin and chalk) are rarely used because of their marginal antidiarrhoeal effect.

Chapter 6

Emetics, Antiemetics and other Gastrointestinal Drugs

Nausea is a desire to vomit. It may or may not culminate in vomiting. Emesis or vomiting is a protective mechanism. It serves to eliminate harmful substances from the stomach and duodenum. Emesis is a coordinated act of medullary vomiting centre (VC) and the chemoreceptor trigger zone (CTZ), situated in the area postrema in the floor of the fourth ventricle. The major afferent inputs to VC are routed through CTZ which has dopaminergic (D_2), histaminergic (H_1), muscarinic (M_1), opioid (μ) and serotonergic ($5HT_3$) receptors. The vestibular apparatus (rich in muscarinic M_1 and histaminic H_1 receptors) generates impulses during motion sickness which reach VC mainly through cerebellum and also through CTZ (though D_2 receptor antagonists do not control motion sickness). Irritation of gastrointestinal mucosa by irritants, chemotherapeutic agents, radiation therapy, endogenous toxins and poisons leads to activation of $5\text{-}HT_3$ receptors of vagal and splanchnic afferents of gut by releasing mucosal serotonin from enterochromaffin like cells. This then sends vagal afferent inputs to nucleus tractus solitarius (NTS) for onward transmission to VC either directly or through CTZ. Vomiting centre contains mainly muscarinic M_1, histamine H_1 and serotonin $5\text{-}HT_3$ receptors.

Nausea and vomiting may occur even to a healthy person due to indigestion, unpleasant smell, unpalatable food, drugs and chemicals, motion sickness and pregnancy. Various diseases such as food poisoning, acute abdominal emergencies (appendicitis, obstruction of intestine), diseases of the gallbladder, liver, peritoneum, acute infective illnesses (hepatitis, cholera, meningitis, and malaria), heart diseases (myocardial infarction), etc. may cause nausea and vomiting. These various unpleasant sensory stimuli can cause nausea and vomiting by stimulation of VC via higher centres.

Emetics

These are the drugs which cause vomiting. Nowadays, they are not indicated in the treatment of poisoning. Apomorphine is a DA receptor agonist. It stimulates CTZ and is used as an experimental emetic agent. A large number of drugs (morphine, cytotoxic agents, digitalis glycosides, bromocriptine, NSAIDs, theophylline, etc.) are known to stimulate CTZ and induce nausea and vomiting as side effects.

Antiemetics

They are employed for symptomatic relief of nausea and vomiting. The important antiemetics are:

1. **Phenothiazines (prochlorperazine, triflupromazine, promethazine, chlorpromazine):** These drugs act by blocking D_2 receptors in CTZ. These agents are very

effective in preventing vomiting due to almost any cause including radiotherapy and cytotoxic agents. They produce extrapyramidal symptoms, drowsiness, and hepatotoxicity as adverse effects.

2. **Metoclopramide and domperidone:** These drugs block D_2 receptors in CTZ. They also act peripherally (prokinetic action) by raising the tone of cardiac sphincter, relaxing pyloric sphincter and increasing peristalsis of proximal ileum. They are useful to treat vomiting due to wide range of causes. They are of specific benefit in vomiting during anaesthesia and after surgery. Metoclopramide induces extrapyramidal symptoms on prolonged use, drowsiness, infantile convulsions in large doses and hyperprolactinaemia. Domperidone has lesser extrapyramidal side effects and hyperprolactinaemia. Hence it is preferred over metoclopramide.

3. **Cisapride:** Although it is structurally related to metoclopramide, it is devoid of DA receptor blocking action. It increases gastrointestinal cholinergic activity and may produce abdominal cramps and diarrhoea. It has prokinetic effect like domperidone.

4. **Antihistaminics:** Dimenhydrinate, promethazine, cyclizine, meclizine, cinnarizine are H_1 receptor antagonists. They may act as antiemetic agents by virtue of significant anticholinergic activity. They are used in motion sickness and labyrinthine disorders. Drowsiness, dry mouth, blurred vision may occur as side effects.

5. **5HT$_3$ receptor antagonists (ondansetron, granisetron, zacopride):** They act by blocking the 5-HT heteroreceptors modulating DA synthesis and release. They are used to control emesis due to radiotherapy and cytotoxic agents. They also have antianxiety effect. Flushing,

headache, and constipation may occur as side effects. Most commonly used drug is granisetron (10 µg/kg i.v. 30 min prior to chemotherapy or 2 mg orally 1 hour before chemotherapy). This is the one which is also used by dentist during chemotherapy- or radiation-induced nausea and vomiting in patients suffering from different oral cancers. These are also preferred by them to control postoperative nausea and vomiting.

6. **Other drugs:** Dexamethasone (inhibits PGE_2 induced nausea and vomiting by decreasing PGE_2 synthesis by inhibiting phospholipase A_2) + metoclopramide (D_2 receptor blocking effects) + lorazepam (for enhancing the inhibitory effect of GABA on CTZ) are used with granisetron to treat refectory emesis due to cytotoxic agents by doctors including dentists.

Treatment of vomiting associated with pregnancy: Usually no therapy is required during morning sickness. However, in severe cases promethazine is used. In hyperemesis, gravidarum pyridoxine supplement along with phenothiazines may be required.

Carminatives

Certain drugs promote the expulsion of gases from the gastrointestinal tract. They are called carminatives. Common carminatives are :

i. Sodium bicarbonate (Dose: 0.6–1.5 g); It reacts with gastric hydrochloride and carbon dioxide is produced. Carbon dioxide distends the stomach, relaxes lower oesophageal sphincter and causes eructation.

ii. Others (oil of peppermint: 0.06–0.1 ml; Tr. cardamom Co: 1–2 ml; oil of dil: 0.06–0.2 ml; Tr. ginger: 0.6–1 ml) are condiments and spices. They contain volatile oil which relaxes the lower oesophageal sphincter and increases gastrointestinal motility due to their mild irritant action and flavour.

They give a feeling of warmth and comfort in the epigastrium. Carminatives are used to treat flatulent dyspepsia and to prevent regurgitation of milk in infants.

Bitters

Bitters are used before meals in dyspepsia. Due to their bitter taste, they reflexly promote gastric secretion and improve appetite. Commonly used bitters are Tr. gentian (2–3 ml); picrorrhiza (1–4 ml liquid extract of its powdered root); chirata (2–4 ml of infusion in 25% alcohol); ethyl alcohol (20–30 ml of 7–12%); Tr. aurantii (2–4 ml). However, their efficacy is unreliable.

Digestants

A number of proteolytic, amylolytic and lipolytic enzymes are believed to promote digestion of food. However, they are only effective when their production in gastro-intestinal tract is deficient. Their routine use in tonics and appetite improving mixtures is irrational. Commonly used digestants are hydrochloric acid, pepsin, papain, pancreatin, diastase and taka-diastase.

Points for Dental Students

A dental student must learn thoroughly about the drugs which are used in gastro-enterology. This is important due to following reasons:

1. Many drugs used by dentists produce gastrointestinal disturbances such as anorexia, nausea, vomiting, diarrhoea, constipation, gastric erosions, etc. They require suitable management.
2. Cytotoxic drugs and radiotherapy are used to treat oral squamous cell carcinoma by dentists. Common adverse effects of these procedures are anorexia, nausea and vomiting which are to be prevented and treated by suitable drugs as discussed above.

TO REMEMBER

1. Nausea is a desire to vomit. Emesis or vomiting is a protective mechanism which serves to eliminate harmful substances from the stomach and duodenum.
2. Emetics (e.g. apomorphine) are drugs which cause vomiting. Nowadays they are not indicated in the treatment of poisoning. Antiemetics are employed for symptomatic relief of nausea and vomiting.
3. Phenothiazines, metoclopramide and domperidone act as antiemetics by blocking D_2-receptors in chemoreceptor trigger zone, while cisapride and antihistaminics (H_1 receptor antagonists) produce this effect by increasing gastrointestinal cholinergic activity.
4. Granisetron is a 5-HT_3 receptor antagonist which acts as antiemetic by blocking the 5-HT heteroreceptors modulating dopamine synthesis and release.

Chapter 7

Drugs used in Peptic Ulcer

Peptic ulcer is a major health problem. It is a wound inside the stomach or duodenum. It occurs due to localized destruction of the inner wall (mucosa) of the stomach (gastric ulcer) or the upper part of the small intestine (duodenal ulcer). It is usually associated with the hyperacidity. The causes of peptic ulcer are complex. Major factors in the genesis of peptic ulcer are: (a) increased acid and pepsin secretion, (b) decreased gastroduodenal epithelial and mucosal resistance, (c) *Helicobactor pylori* infection. Excessive smoking and excessive use of alcohol, tea, coffee and certain drugs like corticosteroids, phenylbutazone, indomethacin, reserpine, etc. may also be responsible for peptic ulcer. Important symptom is sharp, penetrating and burning type of pain in the upper part of the abdomen which may be aggravated by food.

Some drugs, which are used to treat peptic ulcer, act by reducing the gastric acid. It is, therefore, worthwhile to know the important physiological features of gastric acid secretion. Gastric acid is secreted by the parietal cells in gastric mucosa due to stimulation of proton pump (H^+K^+ ATPase pump). The basolateral membrane of these cells contain receptors for the three main stimulants of acid secretion, namely gastrin (from antral G-cells), histamine (from enterochromaffin-like cells) and acetylcholine (from vagal efferents). Histamine binds to H_2 receptors and increases intracellular cAMP by activating adenylyl cyclase enzyme; acetylcholine and gastrin cause increase in cytosolic Ca^{++}. In turn both cAMP and cytosolic Ca^{++} activate protein kinases which stimulate acid secretion from H^+K^+ ATPase pump.

Gastric acid secretion is stimulated in three phases:

- **Cephalic phase:** Sight, smell or taste of the food stimulates acid secretion via vagus.
- **Gastric phase:** Amino acids and peptides in the food stimulate G-cells of antrum to release gastrin which binds to the parietal cell receptors. Due to this, there occurs increase in cytosolic Ca^{++} which stimulates protein kinases to promote acid secretion through an H^+K^+ ATPase pump (proton pump) into the lumen of the stomach.
- **Intestinal phase:** Gastric acid secretion starts due to luminal distention and nutrient assimilation of food in the intestine.

Gastric acid production is inhibited by somatostatin hormone which is released by D-cells of gastric mucosa in response to H^+. It acts either by decreasing histamine release from enterochromaffin-like cells (ECL) or by decreasing gastrin release from G-cells. Secretin and cholecystokinin are other hormonal factors which provide negative feedback to gastrin release in response to raised gastric H^+ concentration.

ANTIPEPTIC ULCER DRUGS

1. **Antacids:** These are classified into two groups:
   i. *Non-absorbable antacids:* (a) Aluminium salts such as aluminium hydroxide, aluminium phosphate, dihydroxy aluminium aminoacetate and aluminium carbonate. (Dose: 200–600 mg every hour during acute attacks). (b) Magnesium salts such as magnesium trisilicate, magnesium hydroxide (milk of magnesia), magnesium oxide and magnesium carbonate (Dose: 250–500 mg every hour during the acute attacks). (c) Calcium carbonate.
   ii. Absorbable antacid such as sodium bicarbonate.

   Mode of action: They neutralize gastric hydrochloric acid and prevent activation of pepsin. Aluminium also binds pepsin. The trisilicate salt of magnesium and aluminium hydroxide form protective coating over ulcer surface by forming hydrated silicon gel.

   Use: Antacids mainly provide symptomatic relief by reducing acid irritation of ulcers and to a lesser extent promote healing.

   Adverse reactions: Although sodium bicarbonate causes rapid relief from pain, it is not used clinically because it causes systemic alkalosis, gastric distension, rebound acidity and milk alkali syndrome. Aluminium salts induce constipation, phosphate depletion on prolonged use and aluminium encephalopathy on prolonged use in presence of renal failure. Magnesium salts produce diarrhoea and hypermagnesaemia in the presence of renal failure. Calcium salts cause constipation, milk alkali syndrome, rebound acidity and perforation of ulcer due to production of carbon dioxide. Clinically, aluminium and magnesium salts are used in combination to counteract the side effects of each other.

   Drug interactions:
   a. Sodium containing antacid reduces the antihypertensive effect of drugs.
   b. Aluminium decreases the absorption of digoxin, tetracycline, isoniazid, iron salts and prednisolone.
   c. Magnesium retards the absorption of tetracycline, digoxin and dicoumarol.
   d. Calcium carbonate containing antacid decreases the absorption of scopolamine, glycopyrrolate, and propantheline, which are used to control excessive salivation in dentistry.

2. **Anticholinergic agents:**
   i. Non-selective M_1 and M_2 receptor blockers like probanthine, oxyphenonium and dicyclomine.
   ii. Selective M_1 receptor blockers like pirenzepine and telenzepine. They have minimum effect on heart, intestine, and urinary bladder. So the adverse effects such as dryness of mouth, blurred vision and headache are less common.

   Mode of action: They act by reducing gastric acid secretion. They also inhibit gastric motility which may be helpful in ulcer healing.

   Use: Since they have weak antisecretory effect, they are used only as adjunct to other antiulcer drugs. Commonly used drug is pirenzepine. It is given in doses of 50 mg orally twice or thrice daily for 4–6 weeks.

   Drug interactions: Non-selective anticholinergic drugs increase the absorption of digoxin, prednisolone, and phenytoin by delaying intestinal transit time.

3. **Histamine H_2 antagonists (cimetidine, ranitidine, famotidine, nizatidine, roxatidine):** These drugs block histamine H_2 receptors. They block histamine-mediated acid secretion from gastric parietal cells

and also reduce gastrin and cholinergic acid secretion. They reduce both quantity and concentration of acid but have no effect on mucous secretion and gastric motility.

Uses: These are used in:

- Gastric and duodenal ulcers. They help in ulcer healing and prevent recurrence of ulcers.
- Gastric erosions with or without bleeding.
- Reflux oesophagitis.
- Stress ulcers (burns).
- Zollinger-Ellison syndrome.
- Chronic gastritis.
- Chronic urticaria as they increase the effect of H_1 antagonists.
- Protection of aspiration pneumonia. This is achieved by giving them preoperatively to decrease the risk of aspiration of gastric acid content.

Dosage:

Ranitidine: 150 mg twice daily or 300 mg at bedtime for 4–6 weeks.

Famotidine: 20 mg twice daily or 40 mg at bedtime for 4–6 weeks.

Roxatidine: 75 mg twice daily or 150 mg at bedtime.

Nizatidine: 150 mg twice daily or 300 mg at bedtime for 4–6 weeks.

Loxatidine: Recently developed powerful non-competitive H_2 antagonist.

Side effects: Cimetidine is no more used, due to gynecomastia and impotency which are produced in males by cimetidine because of its weak antiandrogenic activity. Cimetidine may produce mental confusion, hallucinations, drowsiness and convulsions also because it crosses blood–brain barrier.

Newer H_2 blockers do not have antiandrogenic activity and have minimal access across the blood–brain barrier. They occasionally induce diarrhoea, headache, and vertigo, mild disorientation and skin rashes.

Drug interactions: Cimetidine potentiates the toxicity of propranolol, diazepam, theophylline, imipramine, lignocaine, phenytoin, warfarin and phenobarbitone by inhibiting hepatic microsomal oxidase enzyme. However, in therapeutic doses newer H_2 antagonists have minimal hepatic enzyme inhibiting activity. They retard absorption of ketoconazole due to reduction in gastric acidity.

4. **Proton pump inhibitors:** They inhibit the so called proton pump by inhibiting the enzyme H^+K^+ ATPase of the gastric parietal cells. The important members of this group are omeprazole, esomeprazole, lansoprazole, pantoprazole and rabeprazole. All are prodrugs. Their active entity is a sulfonamide cation that is produced within gastric parietal cells. All are given orally except pantoprazole which can also be given i.v.

Uses:

- These are used to treat gastric and duodenal ulcers, not responding to H_2 antagonists because there long-term use is likely to be hazardous.
- These are drug of choice for Zollinger-Ellison syndrome.
- Reflux oesophagitis.
- NSAIDs induced ulcerations and bleeding.
- For prevention of acid aspiration during general anaesthesia. For this purpose, these are given in doses of 40 mg oral an evening before surgery and further a 40 mg oral 6 hrs before surgery.

Doses: Therapeutic doses of these drugs are in range of 20 to 40 mg once daily for 4–6 weeks. However, for the treatment of Zollinger-Ellison syndrome, higher doses (in range of 60 to 120 mg daily) may be required to be given for longer period.

Side effects: During short-term therapy, it causes nausea, diarrhoea, pain in abdomen, dizziness, headache. They are generally mild and do not require reduction in doses.

During long-term therapy there occurs gastrin stimulated hyperplasia of gastric epithelium and bacterial overgrowth due to sustained decrease in gastric acidity which converts ingested nitrates into carcinogenic nitrosamines.

5. **Drugs providing protection to mucosa:**
   i. *Sucralfate:* It is an aluminium containing salt of sucrose octasulfate.

      Mode of action:
      - It becomes highly viscous gel in acid pH of the stomach. The gel binds to proteins in the ulcer crater and forms a protective coating. Due to this, it checks the diffusion of H^+ ions and pepsin.
      - It protects parietal cells by increasing endogenous prostaglandin synthesis.
      - It attenuates peptic activity by binding with pepsin.
      - It also binds with bile salts and provides an ideal physical barrier. Thus it protects ulcer site from offensive intraluminal acid.

      Uses:
      - Chronic gastric and duodenal ulcer
      - Chronic gastritis.

      Since sucralfate is effective only in acid medium, it should not be given along with antacids, omeprazole or H_2 antagonists. It effectively prevents ulcer recurrence.

      Dose: 1 gm 6 hourly or 2 gm 12 hourly.

      Side effects: It may cause constipation, nausea, dyspepsia, headache, itching and swelling of skin due to allergy. Rarely aluminium toxicity may occur in renal failure.

   ii. *Carbenoxalone:* It is extracted from roots of the plant liquorice. It increases mucus and promotes healing by increasing endogenous prostaglandin levels. However, this drug has little or no place in the treatment of peptic ulcer because it retains water and salt causing high blood pressure. Spironolactone (an aldosterone antagonist) reduces the ulcer healing effect of carbenoxolone.

   iii. *Prostaglandins:* Prostaglandins (PGE_2 and PGI_2) maintain gastroduodenal mucosal integrity. Hence their reduction (endogenous PG levels) leads to mucosal damage and ulceration. Natural PGs have transient effects. Hence synthetic analogues are used. They are:
      - Misoprostol (methyl ester of 15 methyl PGE_1),
      - Enprostil (dehydro-PGE_2, derivative),
      - Rioprostil (methyl PGE_1, derivative),
      - Arboprostil (15-methyl PGE_2), and
      - Trimoprostil (trimethyl-11 deoxy derivative of PGE_2)

      Out of these, misoprostal is available for clinical use. It is given in doses of 200 µg four times a day.

      Mode of action:
      - They strengthen the so-called mucus bicarbonate barrier by increasing secretion of mucus and bicarbonate.
      - They prevent acid assault on mucosa by increasing phospholipid content of surface epithelium.
      - They accelerate ulcer healing by increasing mucosal repair and restitution.
      - They have protective effect on parietal cells of the stomach by increasing mucosal blood flow.

Uses:

- Chronic gastritis
- Duodenal ulcer
- NSAIDs induced ulceration and bleeding

Side effects: Diarrhoea, abdominal pain, nausea, dysmenorrhea are fairly common. PGs are contraindicated in pregnancy because they stimulate uterine muscles and can cause abortion or premature labour.

6. **Anti-*Helicobacter pylori* drugs:** *H. pylori* is a gram-negative bacillus. It has uniquely adopted to survival in the hostile environment of stomach. It attaches to the surface epithelium beneath the mucus. It has high urease activity. So it produces ammonia which maintains a neutral micro-environment around the bacteria and promotes back diffusion of H^+ ions.

It is now well know that *Helicobacter pylori* infection is one of the most important etiological factors for peptic ulcer. So it is appropriate to treat *H. pylori* in patients with peptic ulcer or low-grade mucosa associated lymph oil tissue (MALT) lymphoma. Single drug regimens are not advocated due to the potential for the development of antibiotic resistance. This is particularly true to macrolides and nitroimidazoles, which are the key antimicrobials in the multi-drug regimes for *H. pylori*. At present, dual treatment combining a proton pump inhibitor(PPI) with either clarithromycin or amoxicillin are also not used because of unacceptable low eradication rates. Possible regimens for *H.Pylori* infection are given in Table 7.1.

Comments

Although bismuth based triple therapy consisting of colloidal bismuth subcitrate,

Table 7.1: Regimen for eradication of *H. pylori*

Regimens	Dosage	Duration (In weeks)	H. pylori eradication (In %)
Omeprazole Clarithromycin	20 mg b.i.d. 500 mg b.i.d.	2	60–80
Colloidal bismuth subcitrate Tetracycline Metronidazole	120 mg q.i.d. 500 mg q.i.d. 400 mg q.i.d.	2	30–95
Omeprazole Amoxicillin Metronidazole	40 mg o.d. 500 mg t.i.d. 400 mg t.i.d.	1–2	75–90
Omeprazole Clarithromycin Metronidazole	40 mg o.d. or 20 mg b.i.d. 250 mg b.i.d. 400 mg b.i.d/t.i.d.	1–2	85–95
Omeprazole Amoxicillin Clarithromycin	40 mg o.d. or 20 mg b.i.d. 1 gm b.i.d. 250–500 mg b.i.d.	1–2	85–95
Omeprazole Colloidal bismuth subcitrate Tetracycline Metronidazole	20 mg o.d or b.i.d. 120 mg q.i.d. 500 mg q.i.d. 400–500 mg q.i.d. or t.i.d.	1	86–98
Ranitidine bismuth citrate Clarithromycin Metronidazole	400 mg b.i.d. 500 mg b.i.d 500 mg b.i.d /t.i.d.	1–2	>90

tetracycline and metronidazole for 2 weeks is cheap, well investigated having high cure rate, it is not used in developing countries because 80–90% of *H. pylori* strains are resistant to metronidazole. So triple therapies with a combination of a proton pump inhibitor and 2 antibiotics have largely replaced the use of the classical bismuth based triple therapy in almost all countries. A new group of triple regimen has been developed which replaces proton pump inhibitor with ranitidine bismuth citrate. This regimen causes less acid suppression and also provides additional antimicrobial action of bismuth. In an attempt to achieve 100 % eradication of *H. pylori*, a quadruple therapy combination has been developed. The major advantages of this regimen over the classical triple therapy are:

a. High and consistent eradication rate

b. A 1 week treatment offering a cure rate similar to the classical triple therapy.

c. A significant reduction in complications seen with the 2 weeks bismuth based triple therapy.

d. This regimen is also recommended as the rescue line therapy when the first line therapy fails.

Points for Dental Students

1. Patients suffering from gastroesophagial reflux disease may complain of dysgeusia (foul taste), dental sensitivity (due to the erosion of enamel by gastric acid), and/or pulpitis. These patients should be treated in a semisupine position and premedicated with H_2 receptor antagonists. To minimize dysgeusia, the mouth may be rinsed with mild bicarbonate mouth rinse (½ teaspoon of sodium bicarbonate in 8 ounces of water).

2. Dentist may have to treat patients with history of peptic ulcer disease. In such cases, dentist should pay attention to the following points:

- Avoid lengthy dental procedures or spread out over shorter appointments to minimize stress.

- Avoid administering drugs that exacerbate ulceration and cause gastro-intestinal distress such as NSAIDs. In such cases, acetaminophen products are recommended.

- Dry mouth occurs when patient is taking anticholinergic drugs. This may be problematic for denture wearers. To retain these prostheses, the patient should be advised to take help of denture adhesives and artificial saliva. Further, in such cases to prevent dental caries, artificial saliva and/or chewing sugarless gum to stimulate saliva flow may help.

- Aluminium, magnesium and calcium containing antacids bind with certain antibiotics/drugs, e.g. erythromycin, tetracycline, iron, itraconazole, digoxin, ketoconazole, ciprofloxacin, etc. and decrease absorption of these drugs significantly. So such antibiotics should be taken 2 hours before or 2 hours after administration of antacids.

- Glucocorticoids are commonly used in dental practice. They may precipitate peptic ulcer. So these are contraindicated. It is also better to avoid topical use of glucocorticoids as in stomatitis because it may be absorbed through oral mucosa.

- Antacids increase renal clearance of salicylates. A patient may be using them and they interfere with the effect of salicylates. So a dentist must enquire about it while taking history of the patient.

- Cimetidine, an H_2 receptor blocker, decreases the metabolism of number of drugs used in dental practice such as benzodiazepines, beta adrenoceptor blocking agents, lidocaine, phenytoin.

TO REMEMBER

1. Peptic ulcer is a wound inside the stomach or duodenum.

2. Now antacids have a limited and secondary role in peptic ulcer. They mainly provide symptomatic relief by reducing acid irritation of ulcers and to a lesser extent promote healing. A combination of two or more antacids is frequently used to have prompt as well as sustained effect; to counter the side effects of each other; and to have least effect on gastric emptying.

3. Anticholinergic drugs act by reducing gastric acid secretion and inhibiting gastric motility. Being weak antisecretory agents, they are used only as adjunct to other antiulcer drugs.

4. H_2 receptor antagonists are currently the most popular drugs for peptic ulcer. They act by suppressing gastric acid secretion through blockade of H_2 receptors.

5. Proton pump inhibitors (omeprazole): Omeprazole is used to treat gastric and duodenal ulcers, not responding to H_2 antagonists because its long-term use is likely to be hazardous.

6. Sucralfate, carbenoxolone sodium and deglycyrrhizinized liquorice are used to promote healing of peptic ulcer.

7. It is now well known that *Helicobacter pylori* infection is one of the most important etiological factors for peptic ulcer. So it is appropriate to treat *H. pylori* in patients with peptic ulcer. Single and dual drug regimens are not advocated due to the potential for the development of antibiotic resistance. So possible regimes for *H. pylori* infection are given in Table 7.1.

8. H_2 receptor antagonists and omeprazole are also used to treat reflex oesophagitis, Zollinger-Ellison syndrome and stress ulcers.

Section 3

Drugs Acting on Central Nervous System

Chapter 8

General Anaesthetics

General anaesthetics are drugs which produce a state of reversible unconsciousness, analgesia, variable degree of skeletal muscle relaxation and abolition of reflexes. The aim is to make the patient unaware of and unresponsive to pain during surgical procedures. At present, anaesthesia is a highly specialized science itself. In modern practice balance anaesthesia is achieved by using combination of drugs.

Classification (Based on the Route of Administration)

1. **Inhalation anaesthesia**
   a. *Gases:* Nitrous oxide, cyclopropane
   b. *Volatile liquids:* Diethyl ether, halothane, methoxyflurane, enflurane, isoflurane, desflurane, sevoflurane, trichloro-ethylene, chloroform (obsolete).
2. **Intravenous anaesthetics**
   i. *Inducing agents:* Thiopentone sodium, methohexitone, sodium propofol, etomidate.
   ii. *Slower acting agents:*
      a. Benzodiazepines: diazepam, loraze-pam, midazolam.
      b. Dissociative anaesthesia: ketamine
      c. Neurolept analgesia: fentanyl + droperidol

THEORIES OF GENERAL ANAESTHESIA

General anaesthesia is induced by a wide variety of chemical agents. So it is known to be due to inhibition of central nervous system neuronal activity by a more generalized membrane action; transmitter and receptor functions may be affected secondarily. Actually precise mechanism of neuronal inhibition is unknown. Several theories have been postulated. No doubt these theories are interesting but conjectural.

1. **Lipid theory (Overten and Meyer theory):** According to this theory, anaesthetic potency varies with lipid solubility of the drug and minimal alveolar concentration is shown to be inversely proportional to potency of the anaesthetic agent. It is now proposed that anaesthetic agent impedes the opening up of the fast Na^+ channels of neuronal cell membrane, required for generation of the action potential.
2. **Hydrate theory:** This theory states that inhalation anaesthetics impede the opening up of Na^+ channels by freezing water molecules to form anaesthetic hydrate crystals (clathrates) close to the surface of the neuronal membrane.
3. **Protein theory:** This theory suggests that anaesthetics alter membrane function by binding to hydrophobic sites on protein molecules of the neuronal membrane.

STAGES OF ANAESTHESIA

An inhalation anaesthetic induces well-defined stages in a patient who has not received any premeditation. Signs of different stages of anaesthesia vary with the type of general anaesthetic agent. These stages are seen as the blood concentration of the anaesthetic agent gradually increases. In modern practice, these clear-cut stages are not seen due to the use of faster acting general anaesthetics, premeditation and many other drugs together. So the classical signs of these stages of anaesthesia (produced by ether) have lost diagnostic importance but they still serve to define the effects of light and deep anaesthesia.

Stage-I or stage of analgesia: This is the period from the beginning of anaesthetic administration to the loss of consciousness. There occurs drowsiness, analgesia and amnesia. Motor activity and reflexes remain normal.

Stage-II or stage of delirium or excitement: Its salient features are: consciousness–lost; respiration–normal but irregular; muscle tone–increased; pupils–dilated, roving eyeballs; conjunctival reflex abolished; augmented release of endogenous catecholamines (tachycardia, hypertension and ventricular arrhythmias).

Stage-III or stage of surgical anaesthesia: This extends from onset of regular breathing to cessation of spontaneous breathing. This is divided into four planes. Distinguished features of each plane are:

Plane 1: Roving eyeballs; eyes become fixed at the end of this plane.

Plane 2: Loss of corneal and laryngeal reflexes.

Plane 3: Loss of light reflex and pupil starts dilating; respiration abdominal and marked muscle relaxation.

Plane 4: Dilated pupil; shallow abdominal respiration; intercostal paralysis.

Stage-IV or stage of medullary paralysis: Completely dilated pupil; totally flabby muscles; death occurs due to respiratory arrest and circulatory failure.

PROPERTIES OF AN IDEAL GENERAL ANAESTHETIC

1. Should produce rapid and smooth induction.
2. Should have good analgesic and muscular relaxant effects.
3. Should be non-irritant to mucous membrane.
4. Should be non-toxic to heart, liver, kidney and brain.
5. Should be non-inflammable.
6. Should have prompt recovery of the patient once the administration of anaesthesia is stopped.
7. Should be cheap and easy to preserve.

However, none of the anaesthetic agent fulfils all the above criteria.

PREANAESTHETIC MEDICATION

To make general anaesthesia more pleasant and safe, certain drugs are administered before exposing the patient to anaesthetic agent. The aims of preanaesthetic medication are:

- To reduce anxiety.
- To overcome the secretory effects of general anaesthetics.
- To facilitate smooth and rapid induction.
- To induce amnesia for pre- and post-operative events.
- To supplement analgesic action of anaesthetic.
- To potentiate them so that less anaesthetic is needed.
- To have antiemetic effect extending to the postoperative period.
- To decrease acidity and volume of gastric juice so that it is less damaging if aspirated.
- To relieve postoperative pain.

Generally, anticholinergic drugs (for anti-secretory effect and to prevent reflex bradycardia and hypotension), narcotic analgesics and antianxiety drugs (to induce sedation and analgesia), prokinetic agents (to have antiemetic effect and to inhibit reflux aspiration) and antacids or H$_2$ receptor antagonists are used as preanesthetic agents.

A typical preanaesthetic regime consists of:

i. Atropine sulfate (0.4–0.6 mg) or hyoscine hydrobromide (0.4 –0.6 mg) i.m. one hour prior to surgery.

ii. Morphine sulfate (8–12 mg) or pethidine (50–100 mg) i.m. one hour before surgery.

iii. Diazepam (5–10 mg oral) or lorazepam (2–4 mg) i.m. one hour prior to surgery.

iv. H$_2$ receptor blockers (ranitidine 150 mg or famotidine 20 mg given orally night before and in the morning).

v. Metoclopramide (10–20 mg i.m.) or ondansetron (4–8 mg i.v.).

Basal anesthesia is a type of preanaesthetic medication. At present, it is induced by administering diazepam (i.v.) and ketamine (i.v.) which produce marked sedation and reduce the dose of inhalation anaesthetic. Neuroleptoanalgesia (described later) is also a type of basal anaesthesia.

Generally, loss of consciousness is induced with the help of thiopentone or another intravenous anaesthetic and there after anaesthesia is maintained by inhalation anaesthetic agent. To ensure adequate muscle relaxation, a neuromuscular blocking agent is used.

INHALATION ANAESTHETICS

Ether (diethyl ether): It is a volatile liquid. It has characteristic odour. The minimum alveolar concentration of ether for anaesthesia is 1.9%.

Advantages:

• It is a safest inhalation anaesthetic.

• It produces good analgesia and muscular relaxation.

• It has no hepatotoxicity, renal toxicity and does not affect blood pressure, pulse and cardiac rhythm during light to moderate anaesthesia.

• It is cheap and quite stable under proper storage conditions.

Disadvantages:

• It is explosive with oxygen or air.

• Its vapours are irritating to mucous membranes of the respiratory tract.

• Induction is slow and stormy.

• Recovery is also slow.

Although ether is a safe anaesthetic, it is not commonly used.

Halothane: It is a volatile, non-inflammable, very potent and relatively non-toxic fluorinated hydrocarbon. It is the most widely used inhalation anaesthetic.

Advantages:

• Induction is smooth, rapid and pleasant.

• It is non-irritant to mucous membranes of the respiratory tract and no bronchoconstriction.

• Recovery is also smooth.

Disadvantages:

• It sensitizes the heart to sympathetic amines (adrenaline) and causes fall in blood pressure.

• It is hepatotoxic being a halogenated compound.

• It causes poor analgesia and poor muscle relaxation.

• It is expensive.

• Rarely it causes malignant hyperthermia (genetic anomaly).

• It is not suitable for neurosurgery as it raises intracranial tension.

Its main uses are: (a) To maintain anaesthesia during major surgery and (b) To supplement to anaesthetic action of nitrous oxide oxygen mixture.

Nitrous oxide: It is a colourless and relatively odourless gas. As it causes laughing during induction of anaesthesia it is called "laughing gas". It is incapable of producing surgical anaesthesia. So it is used as a supplement to other agents for induction and maintenance of anaesthesia.

Nitrous oxide is used to produce conscious sedation in paediatric patients to induce relaxation and to modify the noxious stimuli of dental treatment.

Advantages:
- Rapid onset.
- Profound analgesia.
- Lack of irritation to mucous membrane of respiratory tract.
- Non-inflammable.

Disadvantages:
- Low potency.
- Hypoxia.
- Poor muscle relaxation.

Enflurane

Advantages:
- It is non-irritating and non-inflammable liquid.
- It does not sensitize the heart to adrenaline.
- It has good skeletal muscle relaxant effect.
- Recovery is pleasant.

Disadvantages:
- Induction of anaesthesia is not smooth.
- It has marked respiratory depressant effect.
- Brief clonic seizures occur at deeper levels if respiration is not assisted.

Isoflurane, desflurane and sevoflurane are other fluorinated congeners of enflurane. Their common features are:
- They have very rapid induction and recovery of anaesthesia. They do not sensitize the heart to adrenergic arrhythmias.
- They do not provoke seizures.
- They cause respiratory depression.

Their differentiating features are:
- **Isoflurane:** It is preferred for neurosurgery.
- **Desflurane:** It is irritant to air passage; may cause brief sympathetic stimulation and tachycardia; very useful anaesthetic for out patient surgery as well as routine surgery.

- **Sevoflurane:** It has properties intermediate between isoflurane and desflurane; very useful for out patient surgery as well as routine surgery.

Cyclopropane, chloroform, trichloro-ethylene and methoxyflurane are no longer used as a general anaesthetic because of hepatotoxicity, hypotension, cardiac irregularities, respiratory depression and low margin of safety.

INTRAVENOUS ANAESTHETICS (INDUCING AGENTS)

To obviate the unpleasant experience of anaesthetist and the patient during stages I and II, anaesthesia is induced by intravenous anaesthetics which produce unconsciousness smoothly within 15–20 seconds, i.e. as soon as the drug reaches the brain from its site of administration. They may also be used alone to produce a light level of narcosis for short surgical procedures.

Thiopental sodium: It is one of the most widely used intravenous anaesthetics. As it is unstable, the drug must be dissolved immediately before use. Thiopental is used as 2.5% solution. On i.v. injection (100--200 mg), it causes unconsciousness within 10 to 30 seconds which lasts for 5–10 minutes. Blood concentration of thiopental is rapidly declined due to its redistribution to liver, kidney and muscles, and later to body fat. It is slowly eliminated by hepatic metabolism. It may cause laryngospasm, respiratory depression and cardiovascular depression. It should be used cautiously in patients of asthma, urticaria, angioedema and is contraindicated in acute intermittent porphyria. Extravasation at the injection site may lead to tissue necrosis and arterial spasm (gangrene).

Benzodiazepines (BZDs): These are frequently used for inducing, maintaining and supplementing anaesthesia. On i.v. adminis-tration, they produce sedation (for 6 hours), amnesia (for 2–3 hours) and unconsciousness (for 1 hr.) within 5–10 minutes. These are now commonly used for endoscopies, cardiac catheterization, angiographies, sedation, during local/regional anaesthesia, fracture setting, electroconvulsive therapy. They are a frequent component of balanced anaesthesia. The advantage is that the anaesthetic action of BZDs can be rapidly reversed by flumazenil (0.5–2 mg i.v.). For this purpose, commonly used BZDs are:

- Diazepam—0.2–0.5 mg/kg: By slow undiluted injection in running i.v. drip in order to reduce the burning sensation in the vein and incidence of thrombophlebitis.
- Lorazepam—0.04 mg/kg i.v.: It is 3 times more potent and less irritating than diazepam.
- Midazolam—0.2 mg/kg i.v.: It is water soluble, non-irritating faster and short acting and 3 times more potent than diazepam.

Ketamine: It is a non-barbiturate compound and is chemically related to phencyclidine, a psychotomimetic drug. It is a useful inducing agent in children and asthmatics. It is also used to produce dissociative anaesthesia. Unlike other intravenous anaesthetics, ketamine produces analgesia and is valuable for replacing opioids. On i.v. injection, onset of its effect is slow (2–5 minutes). It acts by selectively blocking excitatory amino acid receptor (NMDA-receptor). It can also be administered by intramuscular route. It does not affect cardiovascular and respiratory systems and does not cause muscle relaxation. It produces hallucination, vomiting, salivation and skin rash. It is contraindicated in epilepsy and hypertension. Its i.v. dose is 2 mg/kg while i.m. dose is 10 mg/kg.

Methohexitone: It is an ultrashort acting barbiturate similar to thiopental.

Etomidate is similar to thiopental but is more quickly metabolized. There is less risk of cardiovascular depression.

Propofol: It is oily liquid (1% emulsion). On bolus i.v. administration (2 mg/kg), anaesthesia is produced within 15–45 sec and lasts for 15 minutes. However, intermittent injection (9 mg/kg/hr) or continuous infusion has been used for total i.v. anaesthesia when supplemented by fentanyl. Since residual impairment is less marked and incidence of postoperative nausea and vomiting are low, it is particularly suitable for out patient surgery. Side effects are excitatory effects, involuntary movement, induction apnoea and fall in blood pressure. Dose dependent respiratory depression occurs on maintenance anaesthesia.

Adverse Reactions of General Anaesthetics

A. **Immediate adverse effects (during anaesthesia):**
   1. Fall in blood pressure
   2. Cardiac arrhythmias, asystole
   3. Respiratory depression and hypercarbia
   4. Asphyxia and laryngospasm
   5. Salivation and respiratory secretions
   6. Aspiration of gastric contents leading to acid pneumonitis
   7. Delirium and convulsions; often seen with i.v. anaesthetics
   8. Fire and explosion

B. **After anaesthesia (delayed adverse effects):**
   1. Nausea and vomiting
   2. Pneumonia, atelectasis
   3. Persisting sedation, impaired psychomotor function
   4. Organ toxicities: liver and kidney damage
   5. Nerve palsies due to faulty positioning
   6. Emergence delirium.

SOME SPECIAL TYPES OF ANAESTHESIA

1. **Neuroleptanalgesia:** It is produced by a combination of a neuroleptic droperidol

(2.5 mg) and a potent narcotic analgesic, fentanyl (0.05 mg) in 1 ml, administered in i.v. drip (0.1 ml/kg). It is an induced state of analgesia, where the patient is cooperative. This combination along with nitrous oxide is called neurolept-anaesthesia and is used for general anaesthesia.

Droperidol causes antianxiety effect, indifference and reduced motor activity whereas fentanyl provides sedation and analgesia. Alfentanil and sulfentanil are still short acting congeners. They can be used in place of fentanyl.

2. **Dissociative anaesthesia:** It is produced by ketamine (5 mg/kg i.m. or 2 mg/kg i.v.). It is characterized by a state of light hypnosis, amnesia and analgesia for about 30 minutes, without actual loss of consciousness.

3. **Balance anaesthesia:** For surgical intervention, there will be full loss of consciousness, analgesia and adequate muscle relaxation. To achieve this (balanced anaesthesia), a combination of pharmacological agents are used as under:
   a. Thiopental sodium.
   b. Narcotic analgesic like morphine or pethidine or fentanyl.
   c. Nitrous oxide.
   d. Skeletal muscle relaxants like d-tubocurarine, gallamine, pancuronium, etc.

Points for Dental Students

1. General anaesthetics may be used in dental practice for various surgical procedures. Before using them, special attention is needed for patients suffering from diabetes or on antihypertensive and corticoid therapy.

2. Anaesthetic effect is also increased by simultaneous use of certain drugs such as opioids, alcohol, neuroleptics, etc.

3. It means certain following points must be kept in mind before administering general anaesthesia.
   - Insulin need of a diabetic is increased during general anaesthesia; so give plain insulin even if the patient is on oral hypoglycaemics.
   - Halothane, cyclopropane and trichloro-ethylene sensitize heart to adrenaline. They may precipitate arrhythmias.
   - If general anaesthetics are given to patients on antihypertensives, blood pressure may fall. Necessary measures should be taken to avoid it.
   - If a patient on corticosteroid is to be anaesthetized, give 100 mg hydro-cortisone intraoperatively to prevent precipitation of adrenal insufficiency due to anaesthetic stress.

4. Since anaesthetic effect is potentiated by neuroleptics, opioids and monoamine oxidase inhibitors, this requires dose adjustment.

5. General anaesthesia should be avoided in patients with sickle cell trait or sickle cell anaemia; when used it is imperative to avoid episodes of hypoxia because cerebral or myocardial thrombosis can result.

6. Short general anaesthesia in the dental chair may be administered. It is recommended that inhalation general anaes-thesia in the dental chair should not be maintained for longer than 10 minutes and maximum up to 15 to 20 minutes.

7. In children, for oral surgical procedures on an out patient basis are conducted with inhalation anaesthesia, generally utilizing halothane, nitrous oxide and oxygen. A full facemask is used for induction and if the procedure is short, maintenance is accompanied with the same agents using a nosepiece. If procedure is lengthy an i.v. infusion may be started and patient is maintained on i.v. barbiturates in addition to inhalation agents with nasopharyngeal tube.

8. In adult, induction is generally accomplished with an i.v. barbiturate (generally methohexital 1%). The maintenance of general anaesthesia is done by methohexital supplemented with inhalation agents.

9. After the extraction, all excess blood and saliva are removed from the mouth by either suction or swabbing. The operator must be sure that no oozing of blood occurs postoperatively from the socket. If found any bleeding from the socket, sutures are placed.

10. The patient must have recovered from the effects of anaesthesia and have stopped bleeding before he is discharged.

TO REMEMBER

1. General anaesthetics are drugs which produce a state of reversible unconsciousness, analgesia, variable degree of skeletal muscle relaxation and abolition of reflexes.

2. Preanaesthetic medication: To make general anaesthesia more pleasant and safe, certain drugs are administered before exposing the patient to anaesthetic agent. A typical preanaethetic regime consists of: (i) atropine sulfate (0.4–0.6 mg) i.m., (ii) morphine sulfate (8–12 mg) or pethidine (50–100 mg) i.m., (iii) diazepam (5–10 mg) or lorazepam (2–4 mg) i.m. and (iv) H_2 receptor blockers. These drugs are given one hour prior to surgery.

3. Halothane is commonly used inhalation anaesthetic. It is a volatile, non-inflammable, very potent and relatively non-toxic fluorinated hydrocarbon.

4. Nitrous oxide is a colourless and relatively odourless gas which is used as a supplement to other agents for induction and maintenance of anaesthesia.

5. Isoflurane is more potent, more volatile and less soluble in blood and its induction and recovery are rapid. Since it is less toxic and has higher margin of safety then halothane and enflurane, it is preferred in neurosurgery.

6. Desflurane and sevoflurane are recently introduced fluorinated congeners of enflurane. They are very useful for out patient surgery.

7. Intravenous anaesthetics are inducing agents as well as used to produce a light level of narcosis for short surgical procedures.

8. Neuroleptanalgesia is produced by a combination of a neuroleptic, droperidol (2.5 mg) and a potent narcotic analgesic, fentanyl (0.05 mg) in 1 ml; administered in i.v. drip (0.1 ml/kg).

9. Dissociative anaesthesia is characterized by a state of light hypnosis, amnesia and analgesia for about 30 minutes, without actual loss of consciousness. It is produced by ketamine (5 mg/kg i.m. or 2 mg/kg i.v.)

10. For surgical intervention, at present, a balanced anaesthesia is produced. It is induced by administering: (a) thiopental sodium, (b) narcotic analgesic like morphine, or pethidine, or fentanyl, (c) nitrous oxide and (d) skeletal muscle relaxant.

Chapter 9

Antiepileptics

Epilepsy is a Greek word for seizures. It is a common chronic neurological problem. It affects about 0.5% of the population. In most of the patients, the aetiology is unknown. It is characterized with brief episode of seizures which appear with or without loss of consciousness. An epileptic seizure is precipitated by high frequency electrical discharge of certain neurons in the brain. The abnormal electrical activity during a seizure can be recorded by an electro-encephalograph (EEG). The exact pathophysiology of epileptic seizure is not known. However, it is believed to be either due to lack of GABA (an inhibitory neurotransmitter) or increase in glutamate (an excitatory neurotransmitter) in brain. The epileptic seizures are classified on the basis of locus, nature and spread of the abnormal discharge.

1. Grandmal type (tonic, clonic seizures).
2. Petitmal type (clonic-clonic; also known as absence seizures).
3. Psychomotor or temporal lobe epilepsy (partial seizures and repetitive bizarre behaviour).
4. Infantile myoclonus type.
5. Status epilepticus (rapid repetitive grandmal seizures).

Classification

1. **Hydantoin derivatives:** Diphenyl hydantoin (phenytoin), ethotoin, mephenytoin.

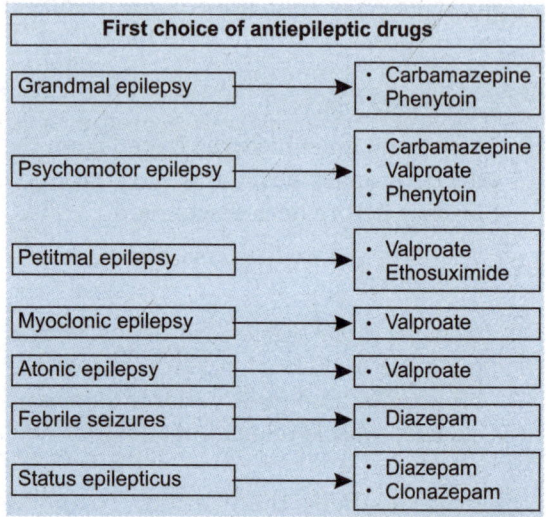

First choice of antiepileptic drugs	
Grandmal epilepsy	• Carbamazepine • Phenytoin
Psychomotor epilepsy	• Carbamazepine • Valproate • Phenytoin
Petitmal epilepsy	• Valproate • Ethosuximide
Myoclonic epilepsy	• Valproate
Atonic epilepsy	• Valproate
Febrile seizures	• Diazepam
Status epilepticus	• Diazepam • Clonazepam

2. **Barbiturates:** Phenobarbitone, mephobarbitone.
3. **Deoxybarbiturate:** Primidone.
4. **Iminostilbenes:** Carbamazepine.
5. **Benzodiazepines:** Diazepam, clonazepam, clobazepam.
6. **Succinimides:** Ethosuximide, methosuximide.
7. **GABA transaminase inhibitors:** Sodium valproate, vigabatrin.
8. **GABA reuptake inhibitors:** Tiagabine.
9. **GABA agonists:** Gabapentin.
10. **Others:** Lamotrizine, felbamate, topiramate, zonisamide, acetazolamide (carbonic anhydrase inhibitor), oxazolidinediones (trimethadione) and phenacemide are no longer used due to toxicity.

80

Phenytoin (diphenyl hydantoin): It is effective in all types of epilepsy except petitmal. It does not produce sedation. It has stabilizing effect on excitable cell membranes. It reduces Na$^+$ conductance and reduces Ca^{++} influx. So it will attenuate action potential generation in excitable cells and increase seizure threshold. Phenytoin reduces the spread of the seizure process from an active focus into adjacent normal brain tissue through an increase in the activity of the inhibitory neurotransmitters like GABA and possibly glycine. It is well absorbed from gut. 80–90% is bound to plasma proteins. It is metabolized in the liver by oxidation and conjugation. Rate of inactivation follows saturation kinetics.

Gum hyperplasia is the most common side effect in children. The other side effects include gastric distress, ataxia, nystagmus, vertigo, muscle incoordination, dizziness, skin rashes and drug allergy.

It is given in a dose of 150–300 mg per day. It has narrow range of safety. So plasma levels should be checked up periodically. In children, its dose is 5–8 mg/kg daily.

Phenobarbitone: It is effective in all types of epilepsy except petitmal epilepsy. Like phenytoin, it reduces spread of the seizure process and seizure discharge. It is well absorbed from gut and about 50% is bound to plasma proteins. 75% of the drug is metabolized in liver by oxidation and conjugation while rest of it is excreted unchanged in urine. The dose is 90–375 mg daily in divided doses by oral route. It may be given as a single dose at bedtime. In children below 12 years of age, up to 90 mg is the daily dose. Important side effects are sedation, ataxia, nystagmus, folic acid deficiency anaemia.

Primidone: It is also effective in all types of epilepsy except petitmal epilepsy. It acts by reducing seizure discharge and spread of

seizure process. It is well absorbed from gut and is metabolized into phenobarbitone and phenyl-ethyl malonamide by liver. Activity is mainly due to these active metabolites. About one-third primidone is excreted unchanged by kidney. Its side effects are similar to phenobarbitone. However, rarely it may cause anaemia, leukopenia, and lymph node enlargement.

Dose: 250–500 mg twice a day; children 10–20 mg/kg/day.

Carbamazepine (tegretol; mezetol): It is structurally similar to phenothiazines or tricyclic antidepressant drug. However, it causes less sedation than phenothiazine and has questionable mood elevating property. It acts by reducing spread of seizure discharge. It is effective in all types of epilepsy. It is drug of choice for psychomotor epilepsy. It is also useful in trigeminal neuralgia and manic depressive psychosis. It is well absorbed from gut and is metabolized in liver. Its initial half-life is reduced over first few weeks from 30 to 15 hours due to enzyme induction. Side effects include visual and gastrointestinal disturbances, dizziness, allergic reactions and blood dyscrasias.

Dose: 200–400 mg three times a day.

Benzodiazepines: They act as anticonvulsant agents by enhancing GABA activity and inhibiting seizure discharge.

Clonazepam: Its oral absorption is slow and erratic. It is completely metabolized in liver and conjugated metabolites are excreted in urine. It is primarily used in petitmal epilepsy. It is also useful as an adjunct in myoclonic and akinetic epilepsy and may afford some benefit in infantile spasm. Important adverse effects are sedation and tolerance. Due to later side effect, its value in epilepsy is limited.

Dose: Adults 0.5–4 mg three times daily; children 0.2 mg/kg/day.

Diazepam: It is a potent anticonvulsant drug. But it is not used for long-term therapy of epilepsy because of prominent sedative effect and rapid development of tolerance to the anti-epileptic effect. However, it is drug of choice for emergency control of convulsions, e.g. status epilepticus, tetanus, eclampsia, covulsant drug poisoning, etc. For this purpose, it is given by slow i.v. injection in doses of 0.2–0.5 mg/kg. Dose may be repeated as required (maximum 100 mg/day). It may cause thrombophlebitis of injected vein, marked fall in blood pressure and respiration. For febrile convulsions in children, it is preferably administered by rectal instillation.

Clobazepam: Its actions and advantages are similar to diazepam. It is used as an adjunct in treatment of epilepsy. It is useful:

- In short courses in patients in whom seizure occurs in clusters
- To prevent exacerbations around menstruation in catamanial epilepsy
- To ensure seizure control during examination and marriage

Ethosuximide: It is a succinimide. Its mechanism of action is not clear. Clinically, it is effective only in petitmal epilepsy. It is rather slowly and completely absorbed from gut. It is largely metabolized in liver by hydroxylation and glucuronide conjugation. It is excreted in urine as conjugates. It may cause anorexia, hallucinations, anxiety, hypersensitivity reactions like Stevens-Johnson syndrome, lupus erythematosus, pancytopenia, aplastic anaemia.

Dose: 20–30 mg/kg/day.

Valproic acid (sodium valproate): It is a propylacetic acid derivative. It increases GABA activity by inhibiting GABA transaminase. It is a broad-spectrum anticonvulsant and is used in all types of epilepsy. It is well absorbed from gut. It is 90% bound with plasma proteins. It is metabolized in liver and excreted in urine as glucuronide conjugates. Its adverse effects are hair loss, rarely hepatitis and acute pancreatitis. Coagulation defects due to reduced prothrombin fibrinogen and platelet levels may be seen.

Dose: Adults–initial: 200 mg three times daily; maximum 800 mg/day in three divided doses; children; 15–30 mg/kg/day.

Vigabatrin: It is an analog of GABA. It inhibits the enzyme GABA transaminase and thus enhances GABA activity. It is well absorbed from gut and is excreted unchanged in urine. It is effective in all types of epilepsy. It has also been used in seizures not controlled by conventional antiepileptic agents. Important side effects are ataxia, drowsiness, dizziness, and behavioural changes.

Tiagabine: This is a nipecotic acid analogue. Tiagabine decreases neuronal and astrocytic reuptake of inhibitory transmitter GABA. Thus it leads to an increase in synaptic GABA which is responsible for its antiepileptic action. It is mainly used as an "add-on" drug for the treatment of partial seizures in doses of 4–12 mg 3 times a day. Common side effects are headache, dizziness and somnolence.

Gabapentin: It acts by increasing the release of GABA by unknown mechanism. It is used in combination with other drugs in partial seizures resistant to other drug therapy in the dose of 900–1800 mg per day in 3 divided doses. Common adverse effects are: Somnolence, dizziness, ataxia and fatigue.

Lamotrizine: It is phenyltriazine derivative. Its anti-seizure effect is due to its ability to suppress sustained rapid firing of neurons and to produce a voltage and use dependent inactivation of sodium channels. It also reduces voltage-activated low threshold Ca^{++} current.

On oral administration, the drug is completely absorbed. It is metabolized primarily by glucuronidation to the 2-N-glucuronide, which is excreted in the urine.

Uses: It is used:

- As an add-on therapy
- As monotherapy for partial seizures
- In absence and monoclonic seizures in children

Its side effects are dizziness, headache, diplopia, nausea, somnolence and skin rash.

Dose: 100–300 mg per day: Valproate causes 2 fold increases in the drug's half-life. In patients receiving valproate, the initial dosage of lamotrizine must be reduced to 25 mg every other day.

Felbamate: It is recommended only as a third line drug for refractory cases of partial seizure because it causes aplastic anaemia and severe hepatitis at unexpectedly high rates. Probably it acts by blocking NMDA receptor via the glycine binding site. It is readily absorbed on oral administration. It is metabolized by hydroxylation and conjugation; a significant percentage of drug is excreted unchanged in the urine. Usual dosages are 1–4 gm/day. It is also effective against the seizures that occur in Lennox-Gastaut syndrome.

Topiramate: It is a substituted monosaccharide. Its antiseizure effect is due to:

• Blocking of voltage-dependent sodium channels
• Potentiation of inhibitory effect of GABA and
• Depression of the excitatory action of kainite on AMP_A receptors.

On oral administration, it is rapidly absorbed. It is minimally plasma protein bound and is moderately metabolized. The drug is primarily excreted unchanged in the urine.

Topiramate is effective against partial and general tonic-clonic seizures. It is also effective against Lennox-Gastaut syndrome, West's syndrome and even absence seizures.

Dose: 200–600 mg/day. Dose related side effects occur most frequently in the first 4 weeks and include somnolence, fatigue, dizziness, cognitive slowing, paraesthesia, nervousness and confusion.

Zonisamide: It is a sulfonamide derivative. It acts primarily by prolonging inactive state of voltage-dependent Na^+ channels with a concomitant prolongation of refractiveness. It also reduces low threshold Ca^{++} current. The drug is effective against partial and general tonic-clonic seizures and may also be useful against infantile spasms and certain myoclonias. It has good bioavailability, linear kinetics, low protein binding, renal excretion and a half-life of 1–3 days. Doses range from 100 to 600 mg/day in adults and from 4–12 mg/day in children. Adverse effects are drowsiness and cognitive impairment.

Levetiracetam: Levetiracetam is a piracetam analog. Its mechanism of action against seizures is unknown. It is used for the treatment of partial seizures in doses of 500 mg orally twice a day. It has excellent bioavailability, linear kinetics, low protein binding, renal excretion and a half-life of 6–8 hours. Adverse effects include somnolence, asthenia and dizziness.

Treatment of status epilepticus: Status epilepticus is an emergency condition. Its treatment consists of i.v. diazepam infusion (2 mg/min; maximum dose given in adults is 20 mg) plus phenytoin i.v. infusion (50 mg /min; maximum dose in adults is 100 mg). Diazepam has rapid onset and short duration of action while phenytoin has slow onset but sustained duration of action. If seizures are not controlled, increase the i.v. dose of phenytoin to 100 mg/min (maximum dose 1000 mg). As these drugs induce hypotension and respiratory depression, keep adequate measures ready for cardiorespiratory support. ECG monitoring is desirable.

Alternative drugs are clonazepam and lorazepam. During pregnancy, chlormethiazole is preferred in seizures because of virtual absence of teratogenicity.

Points for Dental Students

During history taking, ask the patient whether he is suffering from epilepsy. If so find out whether he is taking an antiepileptic drug. This is important due to following reasons:

1. Most of the antiepileptic drugs may induce displacement of other drugs from plasma protein binding site (e.g. phenytoin displaces aspirin) and increases their activity.
2. Most of the antiepileptic drugs (e.g. phenytoin, phenobarbitone, carbamazepine, etc.) induce hepatic microsomal enzymes. So they increase the metabolism of other drugs (e.g. doxycycline, gresiofulvin, chloramphenicol, warfarin, etc.) and often their own metabolism. Due to this, they decrease activity of these drugs and require dose adjustment.
3. Phenobarbitone, phenytoin, sodium valproate and to a lesser extent carbamazepine may lead to folate deficiency which is responsible for spina bifida and folic acid deficiency anaemia. As such folate supplements are essential.
4. When valproate is used, evaluate for clotting ability during gingival instrumentation because inhibition of platelet aggregation may occur and may be responsible for increased bleeding.
5. If a patient of epilepsy is not taking any antiepileptic drug, dental surgical intervention may precipitate an attack of seizure due to stress. So this aspect must be taken care of before dental surgery.
6. If a patient of epilepsy is taking regular treatment, the dentist should give an appointment when his or her plasma concentration of epileptic drug is therapeutically optimal. Further, if such a patient is forewarn about the seizure attack by sensing the aura and he or she tells the dentist for the same, all precautions should be taken to protect the patient from injury.
7. Over dose of local anaesthetic may precipitate seizures which may be prolonged in a patient of epilepsy and need anticonvulsant treatment with slow i.v. diazepam or midazolam administration. If such facility is not available, midazolam can be given by buccal route which provide seizure control within 10 minutes.

TO REMEMBER

1. Epilepsy is a common chronic neurological problem which is characterized by brief episodes of seizures that appear with or without loss of consciousness.
2. Phenytoin (diphenyl hydantoin) is effective in all types of epilepsy except petitmal. It acts by reducing the seizure process through an increase in the activity of the inhibitory neurotransmitters like GABA and possibly glycine. Commonest side effects are gum hyperplasia and cerebellar disturbances.
3. Phenobarbitone and primidone are also effective in all types of epilepsy except petitmal. They also act by reducing spread of the seizure process and seizure discharge. Commonest side effects are sedation, ataxia, nystagmus and folic acid deficiency anaemia.
4. Carbamazepine is effective in all types of epilepsy, trigeminal neuralgia and manic depressive psychosis.
5. Benzodiazepines act as anticonvulsant agents enhancing GABA activity and inhibiting seizure. (a) Clonazepam is primarily used in petitmal epilepsy and an adjunct in myoclonic and akinetic epilepsy. (b) Diazepam is the drug of choice for emergency control of status epilepsy.
6. Valproic acid is a broad-spectrum antiepileptic agent and is effective in all types of epilepsy. It acts by inhibiting

GABA transaminase enzyme and thereby increasing GABA activity.

7. Most of the antiepileptic drugs may displace other drugs from plasma protein binding site or induce hepatic microsomal enzymes.

8. Tiagabine decreases neuronal and astrocytic reuptake of inhibitory transmitter GABA leading to an increase in synaptic GABA which is responsible for its antiepileptic action.

9. Gabapentin acts as antiepileptic by increasing the release of GABA by unknown mechanism.

10. Lamotrizine has anti-seizure effect by:
    * Suppressing sustained rapid firing of neurons
    * Producing a voltage and use dependent inactivation of sodium channels
    * Reducing voltage-activated low threshold Ca^{++} current.

11. Felbamate acts as antiepileptic drug by blocking NMDA receptor via the glycine binding site.

12. Topiramate acts as an antiseizure drug by:
    * Blocking of voltage-dependent sodium channels
    * Potentiation of inhibitory effect of GABA
    * Depression of the excitatory action of kainite on AMP_A receptors.

13. Zonisamide acts as an antiepileptic drug by:
    * Prolonging inactive state of voltage-dependent Na^+ channels with a concomitant prolongation of refractiveness
    * It also reduces low threshold Ca^{++} current.

14. Folate supplements are essential with the use of phenobarabitone, phenytoin sodium valproate and carbamazepine.

Chapter 10

Sedative-Hypnotics

Sedative is a drug that induces calmness without inducing sleep. However, the drug may produce drowsiness.

Hypnotic is a drug that induces and/or maintains sleep which resemble with natural sleep from which the individual is arousable by external stimuli. In small doses, hypnotics are sedatives.

Sleep is a physiological cyclical depression of consciousness. It is essential to maintain normal body function. It is broadly divided into two types:

a. Rapid eye movement (REM) sleep (paradoxical or fast wave EEG sleep).

b. Non-rapid eye movement (NREM) sleep (slow wave EEG sleep).

Insomnia means inadequate sleep. There may be difficulty in falling sleep or difficulty in maintaining sleep. Insomnia may occur due to physiological causes (exhaustion or tension, etc.) or neuropsychiatric disease (anxiety and depression).

Classification

1. **Benzodiazepines:** Classification is given in Chapter 14 (Antianxiety Drugs).
2. **Barbiturates:**
   a. *Those used to maintain sleep in insomnia:* Amylobarbitone and butobarbitone.
   b. *Those used to induce sleep in insomnia:* Secobarbitone and pentobarbitone.

3. **Other drugs:**
   a. Old sedatives and hypnotics:
      - *Chloral derivative:* Chloral hydrate
      - *Aldehydes:* Paraldehyde
      - *Thiazide derivative:* Chlormethiazole
      - *Piperidinediones:* Glutethemide
      - *Alcohol:* Ethchlorvynol
      - *Phenothiazine:* Promethazine
      - *Antihistaminics:* Promethazine, diphenhydramine.
   b. New sedative and hypnotics:
      - Zopiclone
      - Zolpidem

Benzodiazepines

Selected benzodiazepines are drug of choice as sedatives and hypnotics. They have replaced barbiturates which were earlier widely used for this purpose due to the following reasons.

- They produce sleep that resembles normal sleep with little hangover.
- They cause less suppression of REM sleep. So there is less chance of rebound increase in REM sleep (nightmare) on withdrawal.
- They produce mild tolerance and physical dependence.
- Withdrawal symptoms are minor.
- They may induce amnesia but drug automatism is not reported.
- Therapeutic index is high. So overdose is rarely lethal.

- Enzyme induction is minimal with these drugs.
- Same drugs can be used for induction and maintenance of sleep.
- They can be used as sedative and anxiolytics during day time in subhypnotic doses.
- They do not affect respiration or cardiovascular function in hypnotic doses.
- In case of poisoning, a specific benzodiazepine antagonist, flumazenil is available.

Details of benzodiazepines have been given under antianxiety agents. Commonly used benzodiazepines as hypnotics are:

I. For chronic insomnia, short-term insomnia with anxiety; frequent nocturnal awakening; night before operation (long acting benzodiazepines):
   Diazepam 5–10 mg oral
   Flurazepam 15–30 mg oral
   Flunitrazepam 1–2 mg oral
   Nitrazepam 5–10 mg oral

II. For individuals who react unfavourably to unfamiliar surroundings or unusual timings of sleep; sleep onset difficulties (short acting benzodiazepines):
   Temazepam 10–20 mg oral
   Triazolam 0.125–0.25 mg oral
   Midazolam 7.5 mg oral

Barbiturates

Barbiturates are non-selective central nervous system depressants. They induce effects ranging from sedation and hypnosis to general anaesthesia. Probably they act by increasing the inhibitory activity of GABA. Thus they increase GABA mediated increase in chloride conductance. They are believed to act on picrotoxin receptor site because the action is blocked by picrotoxin.

Classification (Based on Duration of Action)

i. **Long acting (12–16 hours):** Phenobarbitone and mephobarbitone; used as antiepileptics and anticonvulsants; used as hypnotics.

ii. **Intermediate acting (4–6 hours):** Amylobarbitone and butobarbitone.

iii. **Short acting (2–3 hours):** Secobarbitone and pentobarbitone; used as hypnotics.

iv. **Ultrashort acting (15–30 minutes):** Thiopentone; used as intravenous general anaesthetic.

Pharmacological Actions

Central nervous system depression: Depending on the dose they produce mild sedation to profound central depression. Death occurs due to depression of the vital medullary centres including vasomotor and respiratory centres. "Drug automatism" and unintended poisoning by barbiturates is due to the amnesia. Further, they decrease the effect of narcotic analgesics.

Cardiovascular system: Hypnotic doses may decrease cardiac output and induce vasodilatation and peripheral pooling of blood, leading to lowering of blood pressure. Higher doses cause depression of vasomotor centre, marked hypotension and depression of compensatory vascular sympathetic reflexes.

Pharmacokinetics: Barbiturates are well absorbed from the gastrointestinal tract. They are widely distributed in the body. Plasma protein binding varies with the compound. They cross the placenta and are secreted in milk. Short acting barbiturates are primarily metabolized in liver by oxidation, dealkylation and conjugation. Long acting barbiturates are significantly excreted unchanged in urine. Alkalinization of urine increases ionization and excretion.

Therapeutic Uses

i. Barbiturates are rarely used as sedatives or hypnotics due to following reasons:
   - Hangover is common.
   - They cause marked suppression of REM sleep. So nightmare occurs on withdrawal.

- They cause marked tolerance to their hypnotic effect and physical dependence is marked. Life-threatening withdrawal symptoms are precipitated.
- Therapeutic index is low; so overdose may be lethal.
- They cause drug automatism that is characterized by repeated drug intake due to loss of short-term memory (amnesia); may lead to overdosage and death.
- They cause marked enzyme induction which is responsible for serious drug interactions.
- Not preferred as sedative because they cause drowsiness.

ii. Phenobarbitone is used as an anti-convulsant and antiepileptic drug.

iii. Thiopentone is used as an i.v. anaesthetic agent.

iv. Phenobarbitone is used in the treatment of hyperbilirubinaemia and resultant kernicterus in neonates due to its ability to cause enzyme induction.

Adverse Reactions

Acute overdosage, suicidal or accidental, may cause marked respiratory and vasomotor depression, coma and renal failure. No specific antidote is available.

  Treatment: (i) Gastric lavage and use of activated charcoal to prevent absorption of remnant drug from gut. (ii) Forced alkaline diuresis is produced by frusemide i.v. infusion (3–4 mg/min) up to a dose of 250 mg in 25 ml of sodium bicarbonate (1.4%) or sodium lactate (M/6 or 1.85%). (iii) Supportive measures for maintenance of respiration and reversal of hypotension. (iv) Doxapram may be used initially before instituting respiratory support.

Contraindications

- Liver and kidney disease
- Acute intermittent porphyria
- Chronic pulmonary insufficiency.

Drug Interactions

i. Barbiturates reduce the effectiveness of warfarin, steroids (including contraceptives) tolbutamide, griseofulvin, chloramphenicol by inducing their metabolism.

ii. The absorption of griseofulvin from gut is decreased by phenobarbitone.

iii. It has additive effect with other central nervous system depressants such as alcohol, antihistaminics, opioids, etc.

iv. Phenobarbitone has complex interaction with phenytoin and imipramine, i.e. it competitively inhibits as well as increases their metabolism by enzyme induction.

v. Plasma concentration of phenobarbitone is increased by sodium valproate.

Other Drugs

a. **Old sedatives and hypnotics:** All these drugs produce respiratory and cardiovascular depression, tolerance and physical dependence.

  i. *Chloral hydrate:* It does not cause enzyme induction and has mild addictive potential. It is a useful hypnotic drug but can induce nausea, jaundice and proteinuria.

  ii. *Chlormethiazole:* It has moderate addictive potential and does not cause enzyme induction. It is useful hypnotic in elderly patients. It is also used as anticonvulsant drug.

  iii. *Glutethimide and ethchlorvynol:* They are not recommended as hypnotic drugs because of marked addiction potential and their ability to cause enzyme induction.

  iv. *Promethazine:* It has mild addiction potential and causes enzyme induction. It is useful as hypnotic in children. Vertigo and delirium are important side effects.

  v. *Methaqualone:* It is not recommended as hypnotic because of marked addiction liability and hepatotoxic potential.

vi. *Paraldehyde:* It does not cause enzyme induction and has mild addiction liability. It is useful hypnotic and anticonvulsant in children. It can be given per rectum. Important side effects are bad smell and taste, hepatic, respiratory (pulmonary oedema) and renal toxicity. Injection abscess may occur.

b. **New sedative and hypnotics:**

i. *Zopiclone:* It is a cyclopyrrolone hypnotic. Its actions on sleep are similar to those of benzodiazepines. However, it does not alter REM sleep. It tends to prolong stages 3 and 4 of sleep. It acts by potentiating GABA by binding to a different site than benzodiazepines. It does not:

- Disturb sleep architecture
- Produce hangover
- Have withdrawal phenomenon.

It is used:

- For short-term treatment of insomnia
- To wean off insomniacs taking regular benzodiazepines.
- Its side effects are metallic aftertaste, impaired judgment and alertness, psychological disturbances, dry mouth and rarely dependence.

Dose: 7.5 mg at bedtime for not more than 2–4 weeks.

ii. *Zolpidem:* It is imidazopyridine hypnotic. It reduces sleep latency and increases sleep duration. It does not act on benzodiazepine receptors. Its advantages are:

- Relative lack of effects on sleep stages.
- Minimal residual day time sedation.
- No rebound on withdrawal.
- Low abuse potential.

Dose: 10–20 mg at bedtime.

Points for Dental Students

1. At present benzodiazepines are used as sedative and hypnotics in place of barbiturates.
2. However, phenobarbitone is indicated in epilepsy. When it is being used a dentist must take precautions for rational use of following drugs:
   - Doxycycline, corticosteroids, itraconazole and ketoconazole: Dose adjustment is required because phenobarbitone increases their metabolism due to enzyme induction.
   - Antihistaminics, opioids and alcohol: Dose adjustment is needed because phenobarbitone has additive effect with these central nervous system depressant drugs.
3. Diazepam, midazolam and triazolam may be used to produce conscious sedation in children for paediatric dental treatment. Out of these, midazolam (0.2 to 0.3 mg/kg) has been administered commonly through intranasal route to produce conscious sedation in children with minimum respiratory depression and delay in recovery.

TO REMEMBER

1. A sedative drug induces calmness without inducing sleep.
2. A hypnotic drug induces and/or maintains sleep which resembles with natural sleep.
3. For sedation and hypnosis, benzodiazepines are preferred over barbiturates because they: (a) induce sleep with little hangover; (b) do not cause nightmare, automatism, enzyme induction; (c) produce mild tolerance and physical dependence with minor withdrawal symptoms; have high therapeutic index.

4. Phenobarbitone is still used as an anticonvulsant and antiepileptic drug. It is also used in the treatment of hyperbilirubinaemia and resultant kernicterus in neonates due to its ability to cause enzyme induction.

5. Thiopentone sodium is used as an i.v. anaesthetic.

6. Chloral hydrate, chlormethiazol and paraldehyde do not cause enzyme induction. Chlormethiazol is useful hypnotic agent in elderly patients while paraldehyde is useful hypnotic and anticonvulsant in children.

7. Gultethimide, ethchlorvynol and promethazine cause enzyme induction. First two are not used as hypnotic due to marked addiction potential while promethazine is employed as hypnotic in children.

8. Zopiclone is a new sedative and hypnotic. It acts by potentiating GABA by binding to a different site than benzodiazepines.

9. Zolpidem is another new sedative and hypnotic. It does not act on benzodiazepine receptors.

Chapter 11

Opioid (Narcotic) Analgesics

Pain (algesia) is an unpleasant, ill-defined subjective symptom. It is usually evoked by an external or internal noxious stimulus. The pain inducing endogenous substances are called algogenic agents. They are released during ischaemia, inflammation, tissue injury, and by thermal or mechanical stimuli. These algogenic agents are acetylcholine, histamine, kallidin, bradykinin and leukotrienes. Bradykinin acts partly by releasing prostaglandins (PGs) which do not produce pain themselves but sensitize pain terminals to the action of other algogenic chemicals. Although pain causes discomfort, it is a warning signal and mainly protective in nature. Unbearable excessive pain may be associated with apprehension, nausea, palpitation, sweating, sinking sensation, techypnoea, and rise or fall in blood pressure. As a symptom, pain demands instant relief by drugs. A drug that selectively relieves pain without significantly altering consciousness is called analgesic. An analgesic may achieve this goal by acting in the central nervous system or on peripheral pain mechanisms.

Analgesics are classified into opioid (narcotic) and non-opioid (non-narcotic) groups.

OPIOID ANALGESICS

These are potent analgesics. Since they cause variable degree of sedation, they are also called narcotic analgesics. All of them act by stimulation of central opiate receptors {mu(μ); kappa (κ) and delta (δ)} which are widely distributed in central nervous system and other tissues. Subtypes of mu (μ_1 and μ_2) and kappa (κ_1 and κ_3) receptors have been identified. Morphine and its congeners have high affinity for mu receptors. The μ_1 has higher affinity for morphine. It mediates supraspinal analgesia and is selectively blocked by naloxone. The μ_2 has lower affinity for morphine. It mediates spinal analgesia, respiratory depression and constipation actions. The kappa agonists primarily cause spinal analgesia through κ_1 receptors while κ_3 receptors mediate lower ceiling supraspinal analgesia. The delta receptors are responsible to mediate spinal analgesia mainly. These receptors are also responsible for dependence reinforcing actions, proconvulsant action and gastrointestinal motility.

Endogenous opioid peptides (beta-endorphin, enkephalins, and beta-dynorphin) have been identified. They are derived from distinct precursor polypeptides (pro-opiomelanocortin, proenkephalin, and prodynorphin respectively). In the central nervous system, they are believed to act as endogenous analgesics, as neurotransmitters and as behaviour modulators. In fact they form part of the complex-pain inhibiting mechanisms in the brain and spinal cord.

91

All opioid receptors are G-protein coupled receptors. These are situated mostly on prejunctional neurons. They generally cause inhibitory modulation. So they decrease release of the junctional transmitter such as noradrenaline, dopamine, 5-hydroxy-tryptamine, GABA, glutamate, etc.

Activation of opioid receptor decreases intracellular cAMP. This in turn opens up K^{++} channels (mainly through μ and δ receptors)or suppresses voltage gated N type Ca^{++} channels (mainly κ receptors). So there occurs neuronal hyperpolarization and reduction in intracellular Ca^{++} followed by decrease neurotransmitter release by central nervous system and myenteric neurons.

The sigma (σ) receptor is no longer considered as opioid receptor. However, certain opioids (pentazocine, butorphanol, etc.) bind to this receptor and produce dysphoria, psychotomimetic action, tachycardia and mydriasis.

DRUGS ACTING ON OPIOID RECEPTORS

These drugs are classified as under on the basis of their receptor activity.

I. **Agonists:** They have main affinity for mu-receptors and some affinity for kappa and delta receptors.
1. *Natural opium alkaloids:* Morphine and codeine.
2. *Semisynthetic opiates:* Heroin (diacetyl morphine), ethylmorphin, phlocodeine. (Not used in India: Hydromorphone, oxmorphone, hydrocodone, oxycodone).
3. *Synthetic opioids:* Pethidine (meperidine), fentanyl, methadone, dextropropoxyphene and ethoheptazine. (Not used in India: Alphaprodine, anileridine, dextromoramide, dipipanone, alfentanil, sulfentanil).

II. **Mixed agonist antagonists:** These have agonistic activity at kappa receptors and antagonistic effect on mu-receptors. They also have affinity for sigma-receptors.
1. *Not used as analgesics:* Nalorphine, levallorphan
2. *Used as analgesics:* Pentazocine, nalbuphine
3. *Partial/weak agonists:* Buprenorphine, butorphanol

III. **Antagonists:** These drugs mainly block mu-receptors. In higher doses, they also block kappa and delta receptors. They are naloxone and naltrexone.

Agonists

Opium alkaloids: Opium is obtained by incising the unripe seed capsule of the poppy plant, Papaver somniferum. On the basis of chemical structure, the pharmacologically active alkaloids can be divided into two groups:
1. Phenantherine alkaloids:
   a. Morphine
   b. Codeine
   c. Thebaine.
2. Benzyl isoquinoline alkaloids (devoid of analgesic activity; act as smooth muscle relaxants):
   a. Papaverine
   b. Noscapine
   c. Narcine

1. Morphine

It is the most important alkaloid of opium and will be discussed as prototype of this group.

Pharmacokinetics: On oral administration, the absorption of morphine from gut is slow and incomplete. Further, it is extensively metabolized during first pass through liver. Hence systemic availability is poor. It is, therefore, administered parenterally (i.m. or s.c.). On intramuscular administration, half-life is 2.5 hours. About 30% is bound to plasma proteins. Only a small fraction enters brain rather slowly. It freely crosses placenta. It is metabolized by N-dealkylation and oxidation, followed by glucuronide or sulfate conjugation. Approximately 90% (small amounts of free morphine and large amounts of conjugated morphine) is excreted in urine within 24 hours. A small amount of the drug is excreted in sweat. Seven to 10% of conjugated morphine appears in bile and is excreted in faeces.

Mechanism of action: Major pharmacological actions of morphine are due to its agonistic action on opioid receptors. Other pharmacological actions may be due to its influence on major neurotransmitter systems such as:

a. It releases histamine but inhibits the release of substance P.

b. It increases cholinergic and 5-HT activity.

c. It inhibits dopaminergic, noradrenergic and GABAergic activity.

Pharmacological Actions

Central nervous system: Morphine has site specific depressant and stimulant actions in the central nervous system.

Depressant effects:

i. **Analgesia:** Morphine relieves acute and chronic pain due to its effect on endogenous opioid receptors in supraspinal pain processing sites and on midbrain (periaqueductal grey) and brainstem (nucleus raphe megnus) areas. Due to its action at these sites, there occurs alteration in processing and interpretation of pain impulses. Further they send inhibitory impulses through descending pathways to the spinal cord. In addition morphine also acts directly on the dorsal horn, where it inhibits the release of substance P.

Morphine raises pain threshold and so it reduces the perception of pain. The patient frequently regards pain with detachment because it modifies the emotional reaction to pain. Euphoria and hypnosis produced by morphine may also help in raising the pain threshold.

ii. **Euphoria:** Morphine produces a marked sense of well-being, which is termed euphoria. It relieves anxiety and apprehension. Rarely morphine may produce restlessness, fear or anxiety which is termed as dysphoria. It is particularly seen in pain free individuals.

iii. **Sedation** is produced by morphine in analgesic doses and is useful when pain is accompanied by insomnia.

iv. **Respiration:** Morphine depresses respiratory centre in a dose dependent manner through its effect on mu-receptors. It decreases both rate and tidal volume. The cause of death in morphine poisoning is respiratory failure. Neurogenic, hypercapneic and later hypoxic drives to respiratory centres are suppressed in succession.

v. It depresses cough centre, temperature regulating centre (hypothermia occurs in cold surroundings) and vasomotor centre (at higher doses).

Stimulant effects: Morphine stimulates the following centres/sites and leads to:

i. Vagal centre → bradycardia.

ii. Chemoreceptor trigger zone (CTZ) → nausea and vomiting. However, larger doses of morphine depress the vomiting centre directly; so emetics should not be used in acute morphine poisoning.

iii. Edinger-Westphal nucleus of III cranial nerve → miosis; however, no miosis occurs on topical application.

iv. Certain cortical areas and hippocampus cells → muscular rigidity and convulsions may occur in morphine poisoning.

Gastrointestinal tract: Morphine causes constipation which is due to:

• Spasm of duodenum and colon

• Decreased propulsive movements

• Spasm of pyloric, ileocaecal and anal sphincters.

- Inattention to defaecation reflex by its central action
- Decrease in all gastrointestinal secretions. Since tolerance does not develop to this action, an addict remains chronically constipated.

Other Smooth Muscles

i. **Bronchi:** Morphine causes bronchoconstriction by releasing histamine.
ii. **Biliary tract:** Morphine produces:
   - Spasm of sphincter of Oddi
   - Increase in intrabiliary pressure
   - Biliary colic

   Atropine counteracts this action of morphine partially, while naloxone (opioid antagonist), nitrates and theophylline counteract it more completely.
iii. **Uterus:** It may slightly prolong labour.
iv. **Urinary bladder:** Morphine causes urinary urgency and difficulty in micturition by increasing the tone of both detrusor muscle and sphincter. It also increases the contractions of ureters.

Cardiovascular system: Morphine causes:
i. Vasodilatation due to:
   - Depression of vasomotor centre
   - Decreased tone of blood vessels by direct effect
   - Histamine release
ii. Reduction in cardiac work due to decrease in peripheral resistance.
iii. Postural hypotension and fainting due to impairment of vascular reflexes. However, therapeutic doses cause little change in blood pressure of recumbent normovolemic patient.
iv. Shift of blood from pulmonary to systemic circuit due to greater vasodilatation in the latter.
v. Increase in intracranial tension due to CO_2 retention. This then leads to cerebral vasodilatation.
vi. Heart rate may increase reflexly due to fall in BP or decrease due to stimulation of vagal centre.

Morphine produces slight fall in body temperature due to:
- Decreased metabolic rate
- Reduced respiratory rate
- Decreased muscular activity
- Peripheral vasodilatation

Miscellaneous

i. Morphine causes increased release of ADH and increased plasma prolactin levels.
ii. Morphine decreases release of ACTH, growth hormone and gonadotrophins.
iii. Morphine has immunosuppressant effect probably due to central action.

Therapeutic Uses

i. **As analgesic:** Morphine is indicated in severe pain of any type (burn, trauma, postoperative pain, and myocardial infarction). It is also used to relieve renal and intestinal colic with atropine). In routine, morphine is not used in chronic pain because it causes tolerance and physical dependence. However, it is employed to relieve pain associated with terminal cancer patients.
ii. **Morphine may be used for preanaesthetic medication:**
   - To allay anxiety and apprehension of the operation
   - To produce pre- and postoperative analgesia
   - To smoothen the induction
   - To reduce the dose of anaesthetic required
   - To supplement poor analgesic (thiopentone, halothane) or weak (NO_2) anaesthetics
   - To reduce postoperative restlessness

iii. **Acute left ventricular failure (cardiac asthma):** Morphine (i.v.) affords dramatic relief by:

- Inducing marked venodilatation and fall in preload
- Arteriolar dilatation and fall in afterload
- Relieving pulmonary congestion and oedema by shifting blood from pulmonary to systemic circuits
- Allaying air hunger by causing depression of respiratory centre
- Calming the patient, it cuts down sympathetic stimulation and reduces cardiac work

iv. **Obsolete uses:** It may be used as anxiolytic, antidiarrhoeal and antitussive agent.

Dose: 10–15 mg i.m. or s.c. (rarely orally); or 2–10 mg i.v.; 2–3 mg epidural/intrathecal; children 0.1–0.2 mg/kg.

Contraindications: They are enumerated in Table 11.1.

Adverse effects: They may occur due to pharmacological actions of morphine. Important side effects are sedation, nausea, vomiting, mental clouding, lethargy, sweating, constipation, dysphoria, respiratory depression, blurring of vision, urinary retention, pruritus, piloerection, bradycardia, hypotension, bronchospasm.

Apnoea may occur in newborn when morphine is given to mother during labour because morphine attains higher concentration in fetal brain than in that of mother due to undeveloped blood–brain barrier.

Acute morphine poisoning may be accidental, suicidal or seen in drug addicts. Lethal dose is about 250 mg. Signs and symptoms are stupor or coma, cyanosis, pinpoint pupil, flaccidity, shallow and occasional breathing, convulsions, hypotension and shock. Pulmonary oedema occurs at terminal stages. Death is due to respiratory and circulatory failure. Treatment is given in the box.

Tolerance and Dependence

On repeated use, high degree of tolerance can be developed to morphine and related opioids. It is partly pharmacokinetic (enhanced rate of metabolism) but mainly pharmacodynamic (cellular tolerance). An addict can tolerate very high dose of morphine (500–600 mg). Cross-tolerance exists among opioids and to other CNS depressants as well.

Morphine produces predominantly physical dependence. It is characterized by

Table 11.1: Contraindications of morphine

Contraindications	Reasons for contraindication
1. Head injury	a. Respiratory depression
	b. Miosis and vomiting, interfering in prognosis
	c. Rise in intracranial tension
2. Acute abdomen (undiagnosed)	Can mask symptoms of the major pathology
3. Chronic lung disease	Respiratory insufficiency may aggravate symptoms
4. Bronchial asthma	a. Bronchospasm
	b. Respiratory depression
5. Enlarged prostate	Precipitation of urinary retention
6. Ulcerative colitis	Production of colonic dilatation
7. Biliary colic and after cholecystectomy	Increases tone of biliary tract
8. In obstetrics	Respiratory depression of neonate
9. Hypothyroidism	Slow metabolism of morphine and increased toxicity
10. Hepatic failure	Reduced metabolism and increased toxicity. Small doses can produce hepatic coma
11. Cautious use in elderly and in hypovolemic shock.	

Treatment of Ac poisoning

i. Gastric lavage with potassium perman-ganate to remove unabsorbed drug. It is indicated even when morphine has been injected.

ii. Respiratory support (positive pressure respiration). It also decreases pulmonary oedema formation.

iii. Maintenance of blood pressure by i.v. fluids and use of vasoconstrictors.

iv. Specific antidote is naloxone. It is given in doses of 0.4–0.8 mg. i.v., repeated every 2–3 minutes till respiration picks up or till 10 mg has been administered. It is preferred because it is devoid of any agonistic action and does not perse depress respiration. Since it has short duration of action, injection should be repeated every 1–4 hours later on, according to response.

Treatment of dependence

i. Gradual withdrawal of morphine and substitution of methadone (long acting, orally effective opioid)

ii. In order to reduce the severity of with-drawal symptoms, the help of following drugs is taken:
a. Diazepam or chlorpromazine
b. Clonidine

iii. The doses of methadone and clonidine are gradually reduced and tailed off.

iv. Naltrexone (100–200 mg on alternate days) or buprenorphine (0.4 mg three times a day sublingually) has been used to prevent relapse of addiction.

severe withdrawal syndrome which can also be precipitated by naloxone. Withdrawal of morphine in an addict will cause lacrymation, yawning, anxiety, fear, sweating, insomnia, restlessness, severe diarrhoea, mydriasis, palpitation and tremors. Delirium and convulsions are seen only occasionally. The withdrawal symptoms are probably due to rebound increase in noradrenergic and dopaminergic activity. Treatment is given in the box.

Interactions

- The actions of morphine and other opioids on respiration are potentiated by phenothia-zines, tricyclic antidepressants, MAO inhibitors, amphetamine and neostigmine either by retarding its metabolism or by a pharmacodynamic interaction at the level of central neurotransmitters.
- Hypotension is aggravated by antihyper-tensives.
- Cimetidine inhibits metabolism of morphine.

- Morphine retards absorption of many orally administered drugs by delaying gastric emptying.

2. Codeine

It occurs naturally in opium. It is methyl-morphine. In the body, part of it is demethy-lated to morphine and is responsible for its analgesic action. It is less potent analgesic than morphine. However, it is more selective cough suppressant (only one-third as potent as morphine). It is given orally and its effect lasts for 4–6 hours after a single oral dose. Its abuse liability is low. Constipation is a prominent side effect. Codeine or its substitutes are widely used for suppressing dry, irritating cough.

3. Ethylmorphine and Pholocodeine

These drugs have codeine like actions. They are claimed to be less constipating than codeine. They have been used mainly as antitussive agents.

4. Heroin

It is diacetylmorphine (diamorphine), which is more lipid soluble. It is 3 times more potent analgesic than morphine. It has better access across the blood–brain barrier and is biotransformed into morphine in the brain. Heroin is not used clinically being the most potent addicting drug.

5. Apomorphine

It is prepared by acid-catalyzed arrangement of morphine. It acts as potent emetic due to activation of dopaminergic receptors on the chemoreceptor trigger zone situated in the area postrema. This in turn stimulates an emetic centre located in the area of the nucleus fasciculi sediterrii. Neuroleptics like chlorpromazine block this effect. However, this effect is not blocked by antihistaminics. It produces a variety of behavioural, neuropharmacological and endocrinal effects in large doses due to its effect on both pre- and post synaptic dopamine receptors located in the neostriatum. In man, vomiting occurs promptly (with in 5 minutes)in a dose of 6 mg injected i.m/s.c. It is mainly used as experimental tool in study of psychopharmacological drugs.

6. Pethidine (Meperidine)

It is about one-tenth as potent as analgesic than morphine. However, in equianalgesic doses, it produces the same degree of respiratory depression and vomiting. Important differences from morphine are:

- Less sedative, antitussive and constipative effect.
- Shorter duration of action but onset of action is quick.
- Has atropine like actions such as spasmolytic, mydriatic and other visual effects.
- Causes less histamine release.
- Has local anaesthetic action; corneal anaesthesia is seen after systemic doses.
- Overdose of pethidine produces many excitatory effects due to accumulation of norpethidine (metabolite).

It is used as an analgesic and in preanaesthetic medication.

7. Fentanyl and Sufentanil

They are pethidine congeners. They are more potent than morphine, both in analgesic and respiratory depression. They have shorter duration of action (30–60 min). So they are used in combination with the neuroleptic droperidol to induce neuroleptanalgesia.

Oral Transmucosal Fentanyl Citrate (OTFC) is available as a lozenge on a plastic stick (fentanyl oralet) and terms lollipop. It is used to produce conscious sedation in paediatric patients to induce relaxation and to modify the noxious stimuli of dental treatment. The principle of formulation is to permit the child to suck on the lozenge and slowly releases the active drug, fentanyl, which is absorbed across the mucous membranes of the oral cavity. The advantages of OTFC are patient's acceptance, rapid onset and a much higher bioavailability compared with oral administration. Dose: 5–15 µg/kg; doses higher than 15 µg/kg are contraindicated due to an excessive frequency of hypoventilation. The lozenge should be removed once the desired level of preoperative sedation is achieved. Respiratory depression, hypotension, itching of the eyes and nose, nausea and vomiting have been reported.

8. Methadone

It is a synthetic opioid. It is chemically dissimilar but pharmacologically very similar to morphine. It is effective orally and has a longer duration of action than morphine. It has abuse liability. Withdrawal syndrome is of gradual onset (appears after 1–2 days), prolonged and less severe. So it has been used primarily as substitution therapy of opioid dependence; 1 mg of oral methadone can be substituted for 4 mg of morphine, 2 mg of heroin, and 20 mg of pethidine.

9. Dextropropoxyphene

It is chemically related to methadone. It has less analgesic, antitussive, respiratory depressant and addictive properties than methadone. Overdose can lead to respiratory arrest, hypotension, and cardiac arrhythmia within one hour. It is usually combined with paracetamol for use as an analgesic.

10. Ethoheptazine

It is chemically related to pethidine. It is a low efficacy orally active analgesic which is often combined with aspirin like drugs.

AGONIST-ANTAGONISTS

1. **Nalorphine (N-allyl normorphine):** It has structural resemblance to morphine. At lower doses, it competitively antagonizes most of the actions of morphine. However, at higher doses, it induces analgesia and other morphine like actions and pentazocine-like dysphoria (not suitable as analgesic). Nalorphine acts as an antagonist at mu-receptors. It has partial agonist activity at kappa and delta receptors. On chronic use, tolerance to its agonistic actions and physical dependence develops. Since large doses are required to antagonise the effect of overdoses of morphine or heroin and such doses themselves cause respiratory depression, it is no more used for this purpose

2. **Levallorphan:** Another similar agonist-antagonist; longer acting and more potent than nalorphine, not marketed in India.

3. **Pentazocine:** It acts at kappa receptors (responsible for agonistic actions) and mu-receptors (responsible for antagonistic actions). It has weak antagonistic and more marked agonistic effects. Its profile of action is similar to morphine; important differences are:
   • Less potent and shorter acting analgesic
   • Causes tachycardia and rise in blood pressure due to sympathetic stimulation
   • Less sedation and respiratory depression
   • Less constipating and induces less spasm of biliary sphincter

• Induces dysphoria rather than euphoria
• Induces mydriasis rather than miosis due to sympathetic stimulation
• Less addiction liability and less severe withdrawal symptoms

Pentazocine is effective orally. It is oxidized and undergoes glucuronide conjugation in liver. It is excreted in urine. Plasma t½ is 3–4 hours; duration of action of a single dose is 4–6 hours. Important adverse effects are vomiting, dysphoria, hallucinations, palpitations, hypertension, respiratory depression, dizziness. It can precipitate morphine withdrawal symptoms.

Pentazocine is indicated for post operative and chronic/recurrent, moderately severe pain. It is useful in obstetrics since it has less access across placenta.

Dose: Oral 25–100 mg, 4 hourly; i.m. 30–60 mg, 4 hourly.

4. **Nalbuphine:** It is pentazocine like agonist-antagonist. It has stronger mu-antagonistic action. It induces less sympathomimetic, dysphoric and psychotomimetic effects. It is not available in India.

5. **Buprenorphine:** It is a synthetic thebaine congener. It is a partial agonist at mu-receptors and can precipitate morphine withdrawal. It has slower onset and longer duration of action. It is a potent analgesic. It induces significant respiratory depression. It is less euphoric than morphine and less dysphoric than pentazocine. The effects of buprenorphine are partially reversed by naloxone (at high dose) because of its more tight binding to mu-receptors. Sublingual route is preferred because bioavailability on oral administration is unpredictable. Abuse liability is rated lower than morphine. It is used as an analgesic and for treatment of morphine addiction. Its doses are:

0.3–0.6 mg i.m., s.c. or slow i.v.,also sublingual 0.2–0.4 mg 6–8 hourly.

6. **Butorphanol:** It is a kappa analgesic. It is more potent analgesic than pentazocine. It is similar in action and side effects as that of pentazocine. However, it has less dysphoric and psychotomimetic effects. It has been employed in a dose of 1–4 mg i.m. or i.v. for postoperative and other short lasting (e.g. renal colic)painfull conditions. Meptazinol and dozocine are newer agonist-antagonist opioids.

PURE OPIOID ANTAGONISTS

1. **Naloxone (N-alylnor-oxymorphone):** It is a competitive antagonist on all types of opioid receptors; has highest affinity for the mu-receptor subtype. It has no subjective or autonomic effects of its own. It can antagonize the actions of morphine-like and pentazacine-like analgesics and precipitate withdrawal symptoms in dependent individuals. It is inactive orally because of high first pass metabolism in liver. It is a drug of choice for narcotic poisoning (0.4–0.8 mg i.v. very 2–3 min, maximum 10 mg) and to reverse opioid effects in neonates (10 mg/kg in the chord) and after surgical anaesthesia. It is also used to diagnose opioid dependence.

2. **Naltrexone:** It is chemically related to naloxone and has actions similar to naloxone. It is more potent than naloxone and is effective orally. It has longer duration of action. It is not useful in the treatment of acute opioid drug overdosage. It is employed for "opioid blockade" therapy of post-addicts (50–100 mg/day) so that if the patient takes his usual shot of the opioid, no subjective effects are produced and he loses the craving.

Points for Dental Students

1. Narcotic analgesics are used in dental practice:
   a. To relieve pain of terminal cancer in oral cavity
   b. As preanaesthetic medication before administration of general anaesthesia

2. These are drugs of abuse. So they should be used carefully for the period during which they are indicated.

3. There are important contraindications, e.g. head injury, bronchial asthma, enlarged prostate, etc. and important drug interactions such as inhibition of morphine metabolism by cimetidine, aggravation of hypotension by antihypertensive drugs, etc.

4. So dental students must learn thoroughly all the aspects of narcotic analgesics for their safe and judicious use.

TO REMEMBER

1. Pain: Although it is an unpleasant, ill-defined subjective symptom, it is a warning signal and mainly protective in nature. It demands instant relief by drugs.

2. Analgesic is a drug that selectively relieves pain without significantly altering consciousness either by acting in the central nervous system or on peripheral pain mechanisms.

3. Opioid agonists have main affinity for mu-receptors and some affinity for kappa and delta receptors.

4. Opioid mixed agonist antagonist have agonistic activity at kappa receptors and antagonistic effect on mu-receptors. They also have affinity for sigma-receptors.

5. Opioid antagonists mainly block mu-receptors. In higher doses, they also block kappa and delta receptors.

6. a. Emetics should not be used in acute morphine poisoning because morphine depresses the vomiting centre directly. However, gastric lavage with potassium permanganate is carried out to remove unabsorbed drug even when morphine has been injected because it is excreted through bile also.
   b. Morphine does not cause miosis on topical application because it occurs due to stimulation of Edinger-Westphal nucleus of third cranial nerve on systemic administration.
   c. Naloxone, nitrates and theophylline counteracts the effect of morphine on biliary tract completely while atropine counteracts partially.
7. Important indications of opioids are given in Table 11.2.

Table 11.2: Important indications of opioids

Drug	Uses
i. Morphine	a. Left ventricular failure (cardiac asthma) b. Severe visceral pain
ii. Codeine or its substitutes	To suppress dry, irritating cough
iii. Pethidine	a. Severe visceral pain b. Preanaesthetic medication
iv. Fentanyl and sufentanil	To induce neuroleptanalgesia (For this combine one of them with droperidol)
v. Methadone	Used as substitution therapy of opioid dependence
vi. Pentazocine	Postoperative and chronic/recurrent moderately severe pain Useful in obstetrics since it has less access across placenta
vii. Buprenorphine	a. As an analgesic b. To treat morphine addiction
viii. Naloxone	Narcotic poisoning (acute)
ix. Naltrexone	For "opioid blockade" therapy of post-addicts

Chapter 12

Non-opioid (Non-narcotic) Analgesics and Non-steroids

ANTI-INFLAMMATORY DRUGS

The characteristic features of this group of drugs are:

1. These drugs are weak analgesics than narcotic analgesics.
2. Unlike narcotic (opioid) analgesics, they do not induce central depressant and sedative activity, so they are called non-narcotic (non-opioid) analgesics.
3. Most of them have additional anti-inflammatory and antipyretic effects.
4. They do not produce physical dependence and have no abuse liability.
5. They act primarily on peripheral pain mechanisms; they also raise pain threshold in central nervous system.
6. The major pharmacological actions of these drugs are believed to be due to their ability to inhibit the synthesis of prostaglandins (PGs) by inhibiting cyclogenase (COX) enzyme in arachidonic acid cascade (PGs, PGI_2, and TXA_2, etc.). Mainly there are two types of cyclo-oxygenase enzymes, namely COX–1 and COX–2. COX–1 is constitutionally expres-sed that means it is always present in most of the cells. Traditional non-steroidal anti-inflammatory drugs (NSAIDs) inhibit both COX–1 and COX–2. It appears that their analgesic, antipyretic and platelet aggregation effects are due to their ability to inhibit COX–1 while the anti-inflam-matory effect is mainly related to their inhibition of COX–2. The COX–2 is not constitutively expressed. It is induced in inflammatory cells by an inflammatory stimulus such as endotoxins, cytokines, and tumour promoters. It is not predominant at the sites of gastrointestinal tract and platelets.

7. They exhibit anti-inflammatory activity but are not steroids like anti-inflammatory glucocorticoids; so they are popularly known as non-steroidal anti-inflammatory drugs.
8. These drugs are chemically different; however, most of them are organic acids.

Classification

I. **Non-selective COX inhibitors:**
   a. Drugs with marked antipyretic but weak anti-inflammatory activity: Paracetamol.
   b. Drugs with marked analgesic and anti-inflammatory activity:
   - *Salicylic acid derivatives:* Aspirin, benorylate, choline magnesium tricyclate, diflunisal, salicylamide, salsalate.
   - *Arylacetic acid derivatives:* Diclofenac, tolmetin, fenclofence.
   - *Indole derivatives:* Indomethacin, sulindac.
   - *Pyrazolone derivatives:* Phenylbuta-zone, oxyphen-butazone, azapropa-zone.

101

- *Oxicam derivatives:* Piroxicam, tenoxicam.
- *Pyrrolo-pyrole derivative:* Ketoralac.

c. Drugs with analgesic and mild to moderate anti-inflammatory activity:
- *Fenamic acid derivatives:* Mefenamic acid, enfenamic acid
- *Propionic acid derivatives:* Ibuprofen, fenprofen, flurbiprofen, indopr ofen, ketoprofen, naproxen.

II. **Selective COX–2 inhibitors:**
- Nimesulide
- Etodolac
- Meloxicam
- Nabumeton
- Rofecoxib
- Celecoxib
- Valdecoxib
- Etoricoxib

III. **Others:** Nefopam

Aspirin (Acetylsalicylic Acid)

Aspirin was initially obtained from willowbark. Now it is synthesized. In the body, it is rapidly converted into salicylic acid. So most of the actions of aspirin are due to salicylic acid.

Pharmacological Actions

1. **Analgesia:** Aspirin is less potent analgesic than pethidine. It is effective in relieving non-visceral pain, such as inflammatory, tissue injury related, connective tissue and integumental pain. Its analgesic effect is due to its ability:
   a. To inhibit peripheral prostaglandin synthesis
   b. To raise the threshold to pain perception at central subcortical level.

2. **Antipyretic action:** Aspirin does not cause hypothermia in individuals with normal body temperature. It rapidly reduces body temperature of patients having pyrexia by inhibiting prostaglandin synthesis in hypothalamus. Aspirin lowers raised body temperature by promoting heat loss (peripheral vasodilatation and sweating). It does not decrease heat production.

3. **Anti-inflammatory action:** This occurs at high doses. Aspirin is a potent anti-inflammatory agent. It acts by causing inhibition of PG synthesis. However, there may be other mechanisms such as: (a) stabilization of lysosomal membrane in leukocytes and (b) antagonism of certain actions of bradykinin.

4. **Respiration:** In therapeutic doses, aspirin stimulates the respiratory centre due to increased CO_2 production by its metabolic effects. Larger doses (anti-inflammatory doses) stimulate respiration by peripheral (increased CO_2 production) and central (increased sensitivity of respiratory centre to CO_2) actions and increase the rate and depth of respiration. Respiratory alkalosis may develop which is compensated by renal loss of bicarbonates along with sodium, potassium and water. So overdosage of aspirin can lead to hypokalaemia, dehydration and respiratory depression; death is due to respiratory failure.

5. **Metabolic effects:**
   a. Due to uncoupling of oxidative phosphorylation in skeletal muscles, aspirin causes increased O_2 consumption and CO_2 production.
   b. In severe poisoning, metabolic acidosis will occur due to:
      i. Accumulation of lactic and pyruvic acids, caused by interference with enzymes of Kreb's cycle; and
      ii. Accumulation of acetoacetic acid, caused by increase in lipid metabolism.
   c. Aspirin decreases blood sugar (especially in diabetics) due to increased utilization of glucose and causes

depletion of liver glycogen. However, there occurs hyperglycaemia at toxic doses of aspirin due to central sympathetic stimulation and release of adrenaline and corticoids.

d. Chronic use of large doses of aspirin causes:

   i. Negative N_2 balance by increased conversion of proteins to carbohydrates;

   ii. Reduction in plasma free fatty acids and cholesterol.

6. **Gastrointestinal tract:** Aspirin inhibits mucoprotective PG of gastrointestinal tract. So it can cause gastric and intestinal erosions and hemorrhage. It also stimulates chemoreceptor trigger zone; so vomiting, caused by aspirin, has also a central component at higher doses.

7. **Cardiovascular system:** In therapeutic doses, aspirin has no direct effect on cardiovascular system. At larger doses, cardiac output is increased to meet with increased peripheral oxygen demand. It also causes direct vasodilatation. Toxic doses cause fall in blood pressure by depressing vasomotor centre and it may precipitate congestive heart failure in patients with low cardiac reserve due to increased cardiac work and sodium + water retention.

8. **Effect on coagulation:** At therapeutic doses, aspirin does not significantly modify coagulation because it inhibits the generation of both eicosanoids (thromboxane A_2 induces platelet aggregation; and PGI_2 inhibits platelet aggregation). However, low doses of aspirin specifically inhibit thromboxane A_2 (TXA_2) synthesis and do not affect levels of PGI_2. So it may reduce intravascular clotting and prevent thrombogenesis. Hypoprothrombinaemia occurs at large doses of aspirin. It can be reversed by vitamin K.

9. **Uric acid excretion:** The effects of aspirin are dose dependent.

   i. Therapeutic doses of aspirin (less than 2 g/day) may cause hyperuricaemia by inhibiting tubular secretion of uric acid.

   ii. Larger doses (8–10 g/day) inhibit uric acid reabsorption in renal tubules and produce a uricosuric effect.

Pharmacokinetics: On oral administration, aspirin is absorbed from stomach and small intestine. Its absorption can be enhanced by microfining drug particles and inclusion of an alkali. Alkalinization of urine would also lead to increased elimination of aspirin.

Aspirin is rapidly deacetylated in the gut wall, liver, plasma and other tissues to release salicylic acid which is the major circulating and active form. Half-life of aspirin is only 15 minutes but half-life of salicylic acid is 3 hours. Both aspirin and salicylic acid are metabolized in liver (glycine and glucuronide conjugation) and are excreted in urine.

Therapeutic Uses

1. As an analgesic in mild to moderate pain of non-visceral aetiology. It is, therefore, used for headache, backache, myalgia, joint pain, toothache, neuralgias and dysmenorrhoea (primary dysmenorrhoea may be due to increased uterine PG activity).

2. As an antipyretic for symptomatic relief of fever of any origin.

3. As an anti-inflammatory agent in rheumatic fever, rheumatoid arthritis, osteoarthritis, Dressler's syndrome.

4. Cardioprotective: In low doses, aspirin has been employed for primary or secondary prevention of myocardial infarction.

5. Aspirin has also been used in the treatment of cerebral ischaemia and for prevention of cerebral stroke.

6. Miscellaneous uses:
   - In radiation induced diarrhoea: Prostaglandins are probably involved.
   - Patent ductus arteriosus: Aspirin may bring about closure and avoid surgery.
   - Pregnancy associated hypertension and pre-eclampsia: They are believed to be due to imbalance between TXA_2 and PGI_2. Aspirin 100 mg/day may benefit by selectively suppressing TXA_2 production.

Doses (Oral)

Analgesia/Antipyretic: 300–900 mg 4–6 hourly
Rheumatic fever: 900–1200 mg 4–6 hourly
Rheumatoid arthritis: 600–900 mg 4–6 hourly
Cardioprotective: 50–75 mg per day.

Adverse Effects

1. **Side effects:** Commonest adverse effects are nausea, vomiting, epigastric distress, heartburn, abdominal pain and increased occult blood loss in stools. Aspirin causes gastric mucosal damage and peptic ulceration by:
   - Back diffusion of H^+ ions in the gastric mucosa
   - Decreased secretion of mucus and bicarbonates
   - Decreased synthesis of cytoprotective prostaglandins
   - Occurrence of local mucosal ischaemia
2. **Salicylism** (a syndrome) occurs at high doses or with chronic use of aspirin. It is characterized by tinitus, hearing defects, blurring of vision, dizziness, mental confusion and headache. It is reversible.
3. **Hypersensitivity and idiosyncrasy (infrequent):** Aspirin may cause rashes, fixed drug eruptions, severe rhinitis, bronchospasm, urticaria, angioneurotic oedema and anaphylactic shock.

4. Rarely aspirin can cause irreversible renal damage (analgesic nephropathy) due to inhibition of local vasodilator PGs, resulting in focal ischaemia. The condition is characterized by chronic interestitial nephritis, papillary necrosis and acute renal failure.
5. Reye's syndrome (liver damage and encephalopathy) may be precipitated in infants and children by aspirin who are recovering from febrile viral infection. Hence paracetamol is preferred in pyrexia of uncertain origin in children under the age of 12 years.
6. During pregnancy, aspirin may prolong gestation and delay labour due to inhibition of PG synthesis in uterus.
7. Aspirin may aggravate acute gout due to retention of uric acid in therapeutic doses.
8. Acute salicylate poisoning: It is more common in children. Manifestations are vomiting, dehydration, restlessness, hyperpyrexia, electrolyte imbalance, delirium, hallucinations, acidotic breathing, convulsions and coma. Death occurs due to respiratory failure and cardiovascular collapse.

Treatment

- Gastric lavage
- External cooling
- Intravenous infusion of sodium bicarbonate (1.26%) with dextrose (5%). Potassium chloride may be added to infusion (20 mM/h)
- Vitamin K 10 mg i.v.
- Peritoneal dialysis or haemodialysis

Contraindications

- Gout
- Ulcerative colitis
- Peptic ulcer
- Renal failure
- Hypersensitive patients.

Drug interactions: Important drug interactions are given in the Table 12.1.

Other Clinically used Salicylates

1. **Salicylic acid:** It is a keratolytic agent. It is used to remove corn. It is used locally in epidermophytosis in combination with benzoic acid (Whitfield ointment).
2. **Methylsalicylate:** It acts as a counterirritant. It is used topically in the form of liniments and ointments in muscle and joint pain. Systemic absorption can lead to toxicity.
3. **Salicylamide:** It is not recommended now because its anti-inflammatory effects are rather unreliable.
4. **Benorylate:** It is an ester of aspirin and paracetamol; well absorbed from GIT; broken within the body into its constituents; causes less gastric irritation and bleeding. So it is a better tolerated alternative to aspirin (Dose: 4 g/day).
5. **Diflunisal:** It is fluorine containing, long acting salicylate. It is not marketed in India.

Other NSAIDs

A large number of non-steroidal anti-inflammatory drugs are now available.

Qualitatively they possess similar pharmacological actions, clinical uses and adverse effects as that of aspirin. So salient features of these clinically important drugs will be described in brief.

1. **Paracetamol (acetaminophen):** It is a good analgesic and antipyretic drug but has negligible anti-inflammatory action. A new third form of COX–3 mRNA is expressed most abundantly in cerebral cortex and heart of humans. It is involved in pain perception and fever but not in inflammation. Paracetamol is reported to be selective COX–3 inhibitor. Another reason for lack of anti-inflammatory effect of paracetamol is its poor ability to inhibit COX–1 in the presence of peroxides, generated at inflammatory sites by leukocytes. Plasma half-life of paracetamol is 2–4 hours. It is a safe drug with mild gastric toxicity. However, in paracetamol overdosage or on prolonged use, N-acetyl-p-benzoquinone (minor, toxic metabolite) tends to accumulate and can induce hepatic and acute tubular necrosis. There is delay in the appearance of clinical signs of acute toxicity such as jaundice, liver tenderness, (1–2 days) and hepatic failure

Table 12.1: Drug interactions of aspirin

Name of the drug	Mechanism of interaction	Outcome/effect
1. Oral anticoagulant	i. Displacement of plasma protein binding ii. Inhibition of platelet aggregation by aspirin	Increased risk of haemorrhage
2. Sulphonylurea	Displacement from plasma protein binding	Potentiation of hypoglycaemic effect
3. Phenytoin	Displacement from plasma protein binding increased toxicity	Potentiation of its effects
4. Methotrexate	Displacement from plasma protein binding	Increased toxicity
5. Furosemide and thiazide	Blunts diuretic action	Attenuation of diuresis
6. Spironolactone	Competition between canrenone (active metabolite of spironolactone) and aspirin for active transport in proximal tubules	Attenuation of diuresis
7. Probenecid	Inhibition of tubular secretion of uric acid (at low doses of aspirin)	Antagonism of its uricosuric effect
8. Sulfinpyrazone	Inhibition of tubular secretion of uric acid	Antagonism of its uricosuric effect

(3–7 days). So it is vital to provide effective and energetic anticipatory treatment as given in the box.

a. **Acetylcystein:** It is administered i.v. in a phased manner:
   - 150 mg/kg in 200 ml 5% dextrose - administered over 15 min.
   - 50 mg/kg in 500 ml 5% dextrose - administered over 4 hours
   - 100 mg/kg in 100 ml 5% dextrose - administered over 16 hrs.

b. **Methionine:** It may be administered orally in doses of 10 gm in divided doses in patients who are unlikely to have severe hepatic damage. Limiting factor is vomiting.

Hepatic microsomal enzyme inducers (phenobarbitone, phenytoin, rifampicin and griseofulvin) may enhance paracetamol toxicity.

2. **Diclofenac:** It is a potent analgesic, antipyretic and anti-inflammatory drug; similar in efficacy to ibuprofen. Adverse effects are common. It is also available as gel for topical use. It may also inhibit lipoxygenase. Its plasma half-life is 2–3 hours.

3. **Tolmetin:** It is a potent analgesic, antipyretic and anti-inflammatory drug. Side effects are frequent. Plasma half-life is 3–5 hours.

4. **Indomethacin:** Clinically very effective potent anti-inflammatory and antipyretic drug. As an analgesic, it mainly relieves inflammatory or tissue injury related pain. It has high incidence of adverse effects. It may aggravate pre-existing renal disease and induce mental confusion and hallucinations. Its plasma half-life is 2–3 hours. It reduces efficacy of diuretics and antihypertensive action of propranolol by causing inhibition of renal prostaglandins.

5. **Sulindac:** It is a prodrug. In the body, it is converted into active metabolite (a sulphide) by gut flora and hepatic enzymes. It is less potent and less toxic than indomethacin. It is safe in presence of renal disease because it does not inhibit renal PGs. It is a long acting drug.

6. **Phenylbutazone:** It is a potent anti-inflammatory agent but poor analgesic and antipyretic drug. It is uricosuric by virtue of a metabolite which inhibits renal tubular reabsorption of uric acid. Its clinical use is limited because of bone marrow depression and other severe adverse effects. Plasma half-life is 50–100 hours.

7. **Oxyphenbutazone:** It is a biotransformation product of phenylbutazone and has similar actions as that of parent drug but not a uricosuric agent. Its clinical use is limited because it causes bone marrow depression. Plasma half-life is 10–14 hours.

8. **Piroxicam:** It is a long acting potent anti-inflammatory, analgesic and antipyretic drug. It has enterohepatic circulation. It can be used safely in renal disease. Adverse effects are common. Plasma half-life is 45 hours.

9. **Tenoxicam:** It is a congener of piroxicam with similar properties and uses.

10. **Ketorolac:** It is a potent analgesic and modest anti-inflammatory agent. In postoperative pain, its efficacy is equal to morphine but it does not interact with opioid receptors and free from morphine like adverse effects. It is used for short-term management of moderate pain. Continuous use for more than 5 days is not at present recommended.

11. **Ibuprofen:** It is better tolerated than aspirin as analgesic, antipyretic and anti-inflammatory drug. It is a drug of choice in the treatment of rheumatoid arthritis because of lesser adverse effects. Plasma half-life is 2–3 hours.

12. **Naproxen:** It is better tolerated than aspirin as analgesic, antipyretic and anti-inflammatory agent. It is long acting and

its half-life is 12–14 hours. It is second choice after ibuprofen in the treatment of rheumatoid arthritis.

13. **Fenprofen:** Prodrug; activated in liver, hence less gastric toxicity; plasma half-life is 8–12 hours.

14. **Flubiprofen:** No special advantage over ibuprofen.

15. **Ketoprofen:** It inhibits both cyclooxygenase and lipooxygenase.

16. **Mephenamic acid:** It has not gained popularity because of lower efficacy as analgesic, antipyretic and anti-inflammatory agent.

17. **Enphenamic acid:** It has modest analgesic, antipyretic and weak anti-inflammatory action. It is claimed not to cause sodium and water retention like other non-steroidal anti-inflammatory drugs.

18. **Selective COX–2 inhibitor non-steroidal anti-inflammatory drugs:**

General features are:

- These drugs selectively block COX–2 activity more than COX–1 activity.
- They interfere less with the protective action of COX–1 in the stomach, blood vessels, and kidneys.
- On oral administration, they are completely absorbed.
- They are as effective as the established analgesic-anti-inflammatory non-steroidal anti-inflammatory drugs.
- They cause fewer gastric ulcers.
- They do not inhibit platelet aggregation.
- On long-term use, coxibs can reduce whole body PGI_2 production without affecting TXA_2 content of platelets. Due to this, they disturb the cardioprotective $PGI_2 : TXA_2$ ratio. Hence increased TXA_2 concentration may exert prothrombotic influence. So they are responsible for higher incidence of cardiovascular side effects during their long-term use.

- Common side effects are nausea, vomiting, dyspepsia, diarrhea, abdominal pain and oedema of the lower extremities. Since celecoxib and valdecoxib are sulfonamide derivatives, they may cause rashes and hypersensitivity reactions.
- Like non-steroidal anti-inflammatory COX inhibitors, they may cause renal toxicity because COX–2 is constitutively present in kidney.
- They may interfere with wound (ulcer) healing, bone-remodeling, ovulation and prenatal renal development.
- They should not be used in children, lactating mothers and women of child bearing age.

The characteristic features of each drug are as under:

  i. *Nimesulide:* It is a weak PG synthesis inhibitor with 5 to 10-fold more COX–2 selective inhibition than COX–1 inhibition. So other important actions are involved for its anti-inflammatory action such as:

- Reduction of superoxide generation.
- Free radical scavenging action.
- Inhibition of platelet activation factor synthesis.
- Inhibition of metalloproteinase activity in cartilage.

The advantages are:

- Causes no bronchospasm.
- Shows no cross-resistance to aspirin.

Following are preferential COX–2 inhibitors with 10 to 20-fold more COX–2 inhibition than COX–1 inhibition:

 ii. Etodolac is more potent than aspirin but has less gastrointestinal toxicity.

iii. Meloxicam is longer acting. It is less toxic than piroxicam and other non-steroidal anti-inflammatory drugs.

iv. Nabumetone is a prodrug which is convertated to active acetic acid derivative (6-methoxy-2-naphthyl acetate acid). It is long acting. It is more potent antipyretic than aspirin with less marked side effects.

v. Coxibs (celecoxib, roficoxib, valdecoxib, and etoricoxib) are selective COX–2 inhibitors (>50-fold COX–2 selective). These drugs selectively inhibit COX–2 isoenzyme that is induced at the site of inflammation. They do not affect the action of COX–1 present in gastrointestinal tract and platelets. Coxibs have analgesic, antipyretic and anti-inflammatory actions similar to that of non-steroidal anti-inflammatory drugs. These are mainly used to treat osteoarthritis, rheumatoid arthritis, gouty arthritis, acute musculo-skeletal pain, dysmenorrhoea and familial colonic polyposis.

Oral doses (mg):
- Nimesulide: 200–300 daily in divided doses
- Etodolac: 200–400 three times or four times a day
- Nabumeton: 500–1000 once daily
- Meloxican: 7.5–15 once daily
- Celecoxib: 200–400 once daily or twice a day
- Rofecoxib: 12.5–50 once daily
- Valdicoxib: 10–20 once daily
- Etoricoxib: 60 once daily

19. Nefopam: It is a non-opioid analgesic. It does not inhibit prostaglandin synthesis. It has been found useful to relieve traumatic and musculoskeletal pain. Important side effects are blurred vision, urinary retention, tachycardia, nervousness. It should not be used in epileptic patients. Its oral dose is 30–60 mg three times a day.

OTHER RHEUMATOID ARTHRITIS MODIFYING DRUGS AND DRUGS FOR GOUT

Rheumatoid Arthritis Modifying Drugs

Rheumatoid arthritis is a chronic, progressive autoimmune disease. Although its pathogenesis remains unclear, it is now proposed that activated macrophages release interleukin-1 (IL-1) which is an important factor in the initiation and perpetuation of rheumatoid arthritis. Initially non-steroidal anti-inflammatory drugs (NSAIDs) are used in the treatment of this disease. When NSAIDs do not provide relief to the patient even after 6 months of use, the arthritis modifying drugs are employed. Following are important drugs used for this purpose.

Gold: It has anti-inflammatory and immunosuppressive actions. It causes inhibition of IL-1 release and reduces circulating rheumatoid factors. Sodium aurothiomalate is given by deep intramuscular injection. Initially a test dose of 10 mg is given to detect hypersensitivity. If patient is not hypersensitive, give 50 mg weekly till response is observed. Usually 8 doses are required before beneficial effect is seen. If there is no clinical response within 4 months, it is best to discontinue gold therapy. Important adverse effects are mouth ulcers, skin rashes, and proteinuria and blood dyscrasias

Penicillamine: It is a chelating agent. In rheumatoid arthritis, it is proposed to act by inhibiting release of IL-1 and preventing the maturation of newly synthesized collagen. It is effective (125–250 mg daily) in plain dromic rheumatism and juvenile chronic arthritis. It is generally used when the patient has problems with excessive doses of corticoids. Adverse effects are anorexia, nausea, vomiting, impaired taste and buccal ulcers. Less commonly, it causes renal damage, myositis, lupus erythematosus, skin rashes and blood dyscrasias.

Chloroquine: It is indicated in active rheumatoid arthritis. It is given in a dose of 150–300 mg orally daily preferably after meals for one year with gradual withdrawal thereafter. Although the mechanism of action is not clear, it may be useful due to:

a. Anti-inflammatory action
b. Immunosuppressive action
c. Inhibition of phospholipase A
d. Reduction of synthesis and release of IL-1
e. Stabilization of lysosomes and
f. Inhibition of breakdown of collagen.

Sulphasalazine (sulphapyridine + salicylate): It is of value in remission of active rheumatoid arthritis in doses of 500–1000 mg, 6 hourly, orally.

Methotrexate, cyclophosphamide, and azathioprine: These drugs are reserved for patients with rapidly progressive disease not responding to other drugs. They are not used routinely because of their toxicity.

Glucocorticoids: Systemic steroid therapy in rheumatoid arthritis is usually restricted to patients not responding to NSAIDs or the 'rheumatoid arthritis modifying drugs' or unable to tolerate adverse effects of the latter group. There is evidence that they may be able to slow down rapid progress of the disease. So they have been used with success in acute exacerbation of symptoms. When 1–2 major joints are involved and pain, swelling, and immobility are very marked, intra-articular corticosteroid therapy is advocated. Injection into particular joint should not exceed 2–3 per year.

Anti-TNF-α-Drugs

Cytokines play a central part in the human immune response and therefore rheumatoid arthritis. Out of wide range of cytokines TNF-α (tissue necrosing factor-alfa) appears to be at the heart of the inflammatory process in the joints of rheumatoid arthritis patients.

TNF-α is produced by macrophages and activated T cells. It stimulates the release of other inflammatory cytokines, including inter-leukins-IL-a,-6, and -8, and proteases such as collagenase and neutral metalloprotienases. These TNF-α cytokines require activation of specific membrane bound TNF-receptors for their effect. So anti-TNF-α drugs have been developed to treat rheumatoid arthritis.

1. **Infliximab:** It is a chimeric (25% mouse and 75% human) monoclonal antibody. It binds with high affinity and specificity to human TNF-α. The drug is given as i.v. infusion in doses of 3 or 10 mg/kg at 0, 2 and 6 weeks and thereafter at interval of 4 or 8 weeks. The median duration of response after a single infusion is 6 to 8 weeks. It has been given in severe cases of rheumatoid arthritis along with metho-trexate. This combination significantly slows down radiographic damage compared with methotrexate alone.

   Common adverse effects are upper respiratory tract infection, headache, nausea, sinusitis, rash and cough. Infliximab leads to the formation of human antichimeric antibodies (HACA). However, concurrent therapy with methotrexate greatly decreases the prevalence of HACA. Rarely it causes mild reversible drug induced lupus like illness.

2. **Etanercept:** It is a recombination fusion protein. It binds with two TNF-α molecules. It is usually administered as 25 mg s.c. twice weekly. It is used to treat:
   • Serious rheumatoid arthritis
   • Psoriatic arthritis
   • Juvenile chronic arthritis
   It is equally effective as that of metho-trexate. Radiographic progression is slowed more by the methotrexate - evanescent combination. Adverse effects at injection site are mild erythema, local pain, swelling and itching.

3. **Leflunomide:** It is a new immunosuppressive prodrug. It undergoes rapid conversion to its active metabolite (A77–1726) predominately in the intestinal mucosa and plasma. Its metabolite acts by inhibiting dihydroorotate dehydrogenase (DHODH) enzyme. Finally, it inhibits autoimmune T cells proliferation and production of autoantibodies by B cells. It also increases the mRNA level of IL-10 receptor, decreases IL-8 receptor type A mRNA concentrations and blocks TNF dependent nuclear factor-kappa B activation.

Leflunomide is given orally. It is rapidly and completely absorbed from the intestinal tract. It has been found effective in patients with early rheumatoid arthritis. Patients who do not respond to methotrexate alone benefit from combination therapy with leflunomide and methotrexate. Common side effects are diarrhea and elevation of liver enzymes.

Drugs for Gout

Gout is a hereditary metabolic disease. It occurs due to over-production of uric acid. There occurs intermittent attacks of acute arthritis due to deposition of urate crystals in synovial tissue of joints. Acute attacks of gout are most often treated with anti-inflammatory analgesics like indomethacin, naproxen, piroxicam, diclofenac, sulindac and azopropazone. Out of this, indomethacin (75–200 mg orally in divided doses) is highly effective. Aspirin is avoided because of uric cid retention. If required, prednisolone (40 mg orally in divided doses) can be used.

Colchicine: It is an alkaloid from colchicum autumnale. It is essentially indicated in acute gout. It is not an analgesic. It is concentrated in neutrophils and reduces inflammation. Initial dose of 1 mg followed by 0.5 mg every 2–3 hours relieves pain. A maximum of 10 mg can be used. Most common side effects include nausea, vomiting, abdominal pain and diarrhoea. With safer alternatives (NSAIDs) available, there is little place now for colchicine in acute gout.

Probenecid (250–500 mg orally twice daily): It is used in chronic gout. It has a uricosuric action by inhibiting uric acid reabsorption in the renal tubules. Salicylates interfere with the uricosuric effect of probenecid and sulphinpyrazone. Therefore, aspirin should not be employed concurrently.

Nausea, vomiting and hypersensitivity reactions may appear as side effects.

Sulphinpyrazone: It is similar in action and side effects as that of probenecid. It is also used in chronic gout in doses of 100–200 mg daily.

Allopurinol: It is a purine compound. It has chemical resemblance to hypoxanthine. It acts by inhibiting the enzyme xanthine oxidase and thus decreases the synthesis of uric acid from hypoxanthine and xanthine. It is used in chronic gout and in prevention of acute exacerbations. It is given initially in a dose of 100 mg and gradually increased to 300 mg daily. Rashes, fever, gastrointestinal disorders and drowsiness may occur as side effects.

Points for Dental Students

1. Since non-steroidal anti-inflammatory drugs are used by the dentist in routine to relieve pain, the dental students must learn in detail the pharmacodynamics and pharmacokinetics of these drugs for judicious use. For example, NSAIDs (ibuprofen, naproxen, diclofenac, nabumetone, celecoxib and rofecoxib) are commonly prescribed for control of myofacial pain of masticatory muscles, articular disc disorders, arthritis of the temporomandibular joint, intraoral pain disorders (related to dental pulp, periodontium, mucogingival tissues and tongue); salicylate gel is applied for temporary relief of aphthous ulcer; topical

diclofenac is used to relieve pain of mild cases of recurrent aphthous stomatitis.

2. Most of the time these drugs may be prescribed to patients who are receiving other drugs for the treatment of some other chronic diseases. Due to this, important drug interactions may occur, e.g. increased risk of haemorrhage if oral anti-coagulants are being used; potentiation of hypoglycaemic effect of sulfonylureas, etc. So important drug interactions should be learnt as given in the Table 12.1.

3. If dental surgery is anticipated, avoid use of analgesic and anti-inflammatory doses of NSAIDs such as aspirin, ibuprofen, etc. before operative procedure due to risk of bleeding.

4. Indomethacin reduces efficacy of diuretics and antihypertensive action of propranolol causing inhibition of prostaglandins.

5. For oral pain in cancer patients, narcotic analgesics, when required, should be provided on a regular scheduled or time-contingent basis. However, in general, non-narcotic analgesics should be provided to all patients even if potent opioids are required because this may allow a lower dose of narcotic medication.

6. Primaquine is contraindicated in patients receiving NSAIDs to avoid haemolysis.

TO REMEMBER

1. Non-opioid (non-narcotic) drugs are weak analgesics of different chemical structure and have additional anti-inflammatory and antipyretic activity. Since they do not have central depressant and sedative activity, and they do not cause physical dependence, they have no abuse liability.

2. Paracetamol is the drug of choice in pyrexia (fever).

3. Ibuprofen is the first drug of choice in rheumatoid arthritis and naproxen is the second drug of choice in this disease.

4. Although enphenamic acid is modest analgesic, antipyretic and weak anti-inflammatory agent, it is claimed not to cause sodium and water retention like other non-steroidal anti-inflammatory drugs.

5. Selective COX–2 inhibitors are nabumeton, nimesulide, meloxicam, celecoxib and rofecoxib. Amongst these drugs, celecoxib and rofecoxib are highly selective and long acting COX–2 inhibitors. These drugs are believed to be stomach friendly. Since these are costly drugs, they should be used in patients who do not tolerate other non-steroidal anti-inflammatory drugs for some reasons.

6. Aspirin: In addition to its use as analgesic, antipyretic and anti-inflammatory agent, it is also indicated: (a) for primary or secondary prevention of myocardial infarction (in low doses), (b) in the treatment of cerebral ischaemia and for prevention of stroke, (c) in radiation induced diarrhoea and (d) in patent ductus arteriosus. Reye's syndrome (liver damage and encephalopathy) may be precipitated in infants and children by aspirin who are recovering from febrile viral infection.

7. Paracetamol can induce hepatic and acute renal tubular necrosis on prolonged use or in overdose due to accumulation of N-acetyl-p-benzo-quinon (minor toxic metabolite). It requires urgent treatment with acetylcysteine and methionine.

8. Interleukin-1 (IL-1), released by activated macrophages, is an important factor in the initiation and perpetuation of rheumatoid arthritis.

9. Gold, penicillamine, chloroquine, sulphasalazine, and methotrexate, are rheumatoid arthritis modifying drugs. They are used in this clinical condition when NSAIDs do not provide relief.

10. Glucocorticoids are only used in rheumatoid arthritis when the patients do not respond to NSAIDs or the disease modifying drugs, or unable to tolerate adverse effects of the latter group.

11. Gout is a hereditary metabolic disease which occurs due to over production of uric acid.

12. With safer alternatives (NSAIDs) available, there is little place for colchicine in acute gout.

13. Probenecid, sulphinpyrazone and allopurinol are indicated for the treatment of chronic gout.

14. Probenecid and sulphinpyrazone are uricosuric drugs while allopurinol inhibits the synthesis of uric acid.

Chapter 13

Psychopharmacological Agents

The drugs, which are employed to treat mental or behavioural diseases (psychiatric illnesses), are called psychotropic drugs, psycho-therapeutic agents or psychoactive agents. They can be divided into the following groups:

1. **Antipsychotics (neuroleptics; major tranquilizers):** They are used to treat patients of psychosis or schizophrenia.
2. **Antianxiety drugs (anxiolytics; minor tranquilizer):** These drugs treat anxiety states. They are also used as sedative or hypnotics.
3. **Antidepressant drugs:** They are used in the treatment of depression.
4. **Hallucinogens:** These substances cause hallucinations. They are not used therapeutically.

ANTIPSYCHOTICS

In schizophrenia (psychosis), the mental function is sufficiently impaired. So the patient is unable to meet the demands of day to day life. There occurs distortion in thought and perception, hallucination and delusion. Following circumstantial evidences suggest that dopamine (DA) overactivity is responsible for most manifestations of schizophrenia:

- The typical antipsychotic drugs like haloperidol and pimozide act by blocking post-synaptic DA receptors (D_2) strongly in mesolimbic frontal system.
- Drugs that increase the central DA activity, e.g. levodopa (DA precursor) or ampheta-mine (DA releaser) or apomorphine (DA receptor agonist) either aggravate schizophrenia or precipitate the symptoms of schizophrenia in normal individual.

Apart from this, abnormal 5-HT metabolism, endogenous opioides, prostaglandins, and noradrenaline have also been implicated in psychosis because typical antipsychotic drugs do not provide absolute cure of schizophrenia. Further, atypical neuroleptics like clozapine and olanzepine have little effect on D_1 or D_2 receptors but bind more avidly to 5-HT$_2$, D_4, α_1 and H_1 receptors. 5-HT has a modulatory role on DA pathways. Another neurotransmitter implicated in pathophysiology of schizophrenia is glutamate because glutamate NMDA receptor antagonists such as phencyclidine and ketamine produce psychotic symptoms on administration to normal subjects, e.g. hallucinations and thought disorders.

Antipsychotics are classified on their chemical groupings as:

I. Typical or classical neuroleptics which block both D_1 and D_2 receptors:
1. *Phenothiazines:* Chlorpromazine, triflupromazine, thioridazine, trifluoperazine.
2. *Butyrophenones:* Haloperidol, droperidol, trifluperidol, penfluridol.
3. *Thioxanthines:* Flupenthixol, chlorprothizene, thiothixene.

113

4. *Miscellaneous*:
   - Diphenylpiperidines: Pimozide
   - Benzamides : Sulpride
   - Dihydroindoles: Molindone
II. Atypical neuroleptics which have selectivity towards dopamine D_2 receptors.
   1. *Dinenzodiazepines:* Clozapine, olanzapine, loxapine
   2. *Miscellaneous:* Risperidone, quetiapine, ziaprasidone, aripiprazole
III. Rauwolfia alkaloids (act by depleting DA, NA and 5-HT): reserpine.

Pharmacokinetics

On oral administration, most of the neuroleptics including chlorpromazine are erratically and incompletely absorbed. These drugs are highly lipophilic. They are extensively protein bound. They cross the blood–brain and placental barriers freely. They are metabolized in liver by oxidation followed by glucuronide conjugation. The half-life of most of the neuroleptics ranges between 20–40 hours. Metabolites are usually inactive and are eliminated by kidney.

Mechanism of Action

The antipsychotic action of typical neuroleptics is due to their ability to competitively block postsynaptic D_2 receptors in mesolimbic system. These drugs also have a variety of other therapeutically useful and unwanted effects as a result of blockade of DA receptors as under:

- Competitive blockade of D_1 and D_2 receptors in nigrostriatal pathway leads to unwanted extrapyramidal effects.
- Blockade of D_2 receptors in the turbero-infundibular pathway (connects arcuate nuclei and periventricular neurons to hypothalamus and posterior pituitary) leads to endocrine effects.
- Blockade of D_2 receptor in CTZ leads to antiemetic effect.

- Many of their autonomic side effects are due to α–adrenergic blocking and anticholinergic properties.

The antipsychotic effects of atypical neuroleptics are due to a combination of 5-HT$_2$, D_4 and D_2 receptor blockade. Lower affinity for D_1 and D_2 receptors appears to be responsible for the absence of extrapyramidal side effects. They also antagonize α_1, M_1 and H_1 receptors.

Aripiprazole is a new atypical neuroleptic drug. It is a partial agonist at D_2 and 5-HT$_1$A while antagonist at 5-HT$_2$A receptors (vaguely referred to as DA: 5-HT stabilizer in CNS). Extrapyramidal symptoms are very low but it may cause neurolept-malignant syndrome (NMS).

Atypical neuroleptics differ from typical neuroleptics as under:

- Unique receptor affinity profile
- Effectiveness against the negative as well as positive symptoms of schizophrenia
- Effectiveness in patients refractory to typical neuroleptics
- Lesser liability for inducing extrapyramidal side effects

Pharmacological Actions of Neuroleptics

Qualitatively, the pharmacological actions of the various neuroleptics are similar with only minor differences.

Chlorpromazine (CPZ) is the first effective phenothiazine neuroleptic. It is a three ring structure where two benzene rings are linked by sulphur and nitrogen atoms. It can be taken as the prototype and its pharmacological actions will be discussed.

1. Although it causes sedation, tolerance develops to this effect much faster than tolerance to its antipsychotic effect. So it is not a serious drawback in the long-term therapy. Even in very high doses, it does not cause real hypnosis or anaesthesia.

2. In psychotic patients, it causes emotional quietening, psychomotor slowing and affective indifference (neuroleptic syndrome).

3. In normal individuals, it brings about quietening and psychomotor slowing.

4. Acting on the chemoreceptor trigger zone, it has antiemetic effect.

5. It causes hypothermia by acting on hypothalamus.

6. In women, it inhibits ovulation and release of prolactin release inhibiting hormone. So it promotes lactation due to its later effect. In fact all phenothiazines promote lactation and weight gain.

7. Chlorpromazine lowers seizure threshold. So it may exacerbate epileptic fits. Atypical neuroleptics have minimal effect on seizure threshold.

8. Chlorpromazine induces muscle relaxation and attenuate schizophrenic catatonia.

9. Neuroleptics potentiate narcotic and non-narcotic analgesia. Haloperidol has significant analgesic action.

10. It has weak anti-histaminic and antiserotonin action.

11. Phenothiazines have anticholinergic activity.

12. Phenothiazines block alpha-adrenergic receptors and cause hypotension and failure of ejaculation.

13. Chlorpromazine exhibits a quinidine like effect on cardiac potential. So it can cause bradyarrhythmias.

14. Chlorpromazine inhibits the secretion of ACTH, growth hormone, gonadotropins, ADH and insulin (neuroendocrine blocking effect).

Side Effects

Neuroleptics have a very high therapeutic index. So acute toxicity is not a problem. However, drugs of this group are used for long period, i.e. for months or some times for years. So these can produce adverse effects which are attributed to the extension of pharmacological effects and receptor activity.

Important side effects are:

1. Parkinson like syndrome causing akinesia, rigidity and tremors.

2. Tardive dyskinesia develops in 10 to 20% of patients on classical neuroleptics after interval of a few months to several years of therapy. It is due to nigrostriated DA-receptor up regulation and supersensitivity following prolonged use of DA receptor blocking neuroleptics. *Such patients may approach to dentist. So dentist must be able to recognize it and explain the patient that it is not a dental problem.*

3. Anticholinergic effects: Dryness of mouth, blurring of the vision, diminished sweating, decreased gastric secretion. *Dryness of mouth may lead to dental caries and candidiasis.*

4. Adrenergic blocking effect: Postural hypotension and inhibition of ejaculation in males.

5. Pseudo pregnancy in women due to inhibition of prolactin-releasing inhibitory hormone as a result of its blocking effect on dopamine receptors in the anterior pituitary.

6. Weight gain in both men and women.

7. Rare side effects: Skin rashes, jaundice, blood dyscrasias, photosensitivity and coloration.

Drug Interactions

1. Chlorpromazine and other neuroleptics potentiate the actions of central nervous system depressants like alcohol, barbiturates, opioids, antihistaminics and analgesics.

2. Chlorpromazine antagonizes the action of guanethidine, methyldopa and clonidine.

3. Antacids decrease absorption of neuro-leptics from gut and anticholinergics increase intestinal metabolism.

4. Barbiturates and phenytoin increase metabolism of neuroleptics by causing induction of hepatic microsomal enzymes.

Therapeutic Uses

1. Schizophrenia and allied psychiatric disorders.

2. Acute mania in bipolar depression along with lithium.

3. Preanaesthetic medication: Mainly prome-thazine is used due to its sedative, antihistaminic, anticholinergic and antie-metic effects.

4. Droperidol in combination with fentanyl, a narcotic analgesic, is employed to induce neuroleptanalgesia.

5. Aggressive behaviour: Haloperidol is effective in violent aggressives and in self-mutilated syndrome.

6. Chlorpromazine and selected phenothia-zines are used to treat intractable hiccough.

7. Almost all neuroleptics, except thiori-dazine, molindone and atypical agents, are used to control a wide range of drug and disease induced vomiting at doses much lower than those required for psychosis due to D_2 receptor blockade in CTZ as well as gastrointestinal tract.

8. Phenothiazines, like promethazine, can be used for relief of pruritus due to their antihistaminic effects (Table 13.1).

Important Features of other Neuroleptics

Butyrophenones

- **Haloperidol:** It is most widely used butyrophenon. Its pharmacological pro-perties are similar to phenothiazines. It has less anticholinergic and alpha-receptor blocking actions in comparison to chlorpro-mazine. It has very potent dopamine antagonistic effect and is a potent

Table 13.1: Commonly used phenothiazines

Compound	Daily dose (mg)	Therapeutic uses
Group I		
Chlorpromazine	500–1000	Antipsychotic, antiemetic
Promazine		Antipsychotic, antiemetic
Triflupromazine	10–30	Antipsychotic, antiemetic
Group II		
Thioridazine	100–500	Antipsychotic, hiccough
Group III		
Fluphenazine	2.5–10	Antipsychotic
Trifluoperazine	5–10	Antipsychotic
Perphenazine	12–24	Antipsychotic, antiemetic
Prochlorperazine	10–30	Antipsychotic, antiemetic
Thiethylperazine maleate	10–30	Antiemetic
Group IV		
Diethazine		Parkinsonism
Ethopropazine		Parkinsonism
Group V		
Promethazine	25–50	Antihistaminic

antipsychotic drug. Its oral dose is 2–6 mg daily and intramuscular dose is 3–5 mg.

- **Trifluperidol:** It is similar to but slightly more potent than haloperidol. Oral dose is 0.5–8 mg daily.
- **Droperidol:** It is a short acting potent neuroleptic which is mostly used in combination with fantanil to induce leptanalgesia.
- **Penfluridol:** It is a long acting neuroleptic which is useful for chronic schizophrenia, affective withdrawal and social maladjustment.
- **Chlorprothixene:** It is a thioxanthine analogue of CPZ. It has similar properties to CPZ.
- **Flupenthixole:** It causes less sedation than CPZ. It is useful in schizophrenia and other psychoses particularly in withdrawn and apathetic patients. However, it should not be given to patients having psychomotor agitation or mania. It is also used in depression at lower doses for a short period.
- **Clopenthixol:** It is a thiozanthine derivative. Like chlorpromazine it also has anxiolytic and antidepressant effect. It is devoid of antiemetic effect. It causes mild sedation and hypotension. It produces moderate extrapyramidal effects.
- **Clozapine:** It is a dinenzodiazepine. It produces moderate sedation, mild postural hypotension and has no antiemetic effect. Extrapyramidal effects are minimal. It may produce tremors, convulsions, salivation and hypertension. The major limiting factor is higher incidence of agranulocytosis.
- **Olanzapine:** It has similar properties as that of clozapine but is devoid of agranulocytosis. Main disadvantage is that it causes weight gain.
- **Ziprasidone:** It is like olanzapine but causes less weight gain. Depot injection is available. It causes QT prolongation.
- **Pimozide:** It is a diphenylpiperidine. It is an antiemetic drug. It produces mild sedation. Extrapyramidal effects are also

minimal. It can produce hypothermia and hyperprolactinaemia.

- **Loxapine:** It is a dibenzoxazepine which is similar in action as that of CPZ. Its onset of action is quick and duration of action is up to 12 hours. It has no advantage over other antipsychotics.
- **Sulpiride:** It is a benzamide. It has mild extrapyramidal effects and produces mild sedation, hypothermia and hyperprolactinaemia. It is an antiemetic drug also.
- **Risperidone:** Its antipsychotic activity is due to D_2 + 5-HT_2 receptor blockade. It also blocks α_1, α_2 and H_1 receptors. It has few extrapyramidal side effects.
- **Quetiapine:** It has similar properties as that of risperidone but less potent. So it is given twice a day. Important adverse effects are postural hypotension and dry mouth.
- **Reserpine:** It is a principal alkaloid of Rauwolfia serpentine. Its central nervous system effects are similar to chlorpromazine so it produces tranquilization, sedation and extrapyramidal effects. Now it is hardly used in psychiatry because of its serious toxicity.
- **Aripiprazole:** It is a recent atypical neuroleptic with a noval mechanism of action. It does not block central dopaminergic receptors. It is a partial agonist at D_2 and 5-HT_2A receptors while antagonist at 5-HT_2A receptor. It is vaguely considered as DA: 5-HTstabiliser in CNS. Extrapyramidal symptoms are low but it may cause genetically mediated neurolept-malignant syndrome (NMS) in some individuals.

Points for Dental Students

1. Concurrent use of following drugs should be avoided by dentist in a patient receiving classical antipsychotic drugs:
   - Erythromycin + pimozide—to avoid prolongation of QT interval and cardiac arrhythmias

- Tramadol (an opioid analgesic) + phenothiazines/butyrophenones—to avoid lowering of seizure threshold
- Hydroxazine (an antihistamine) + thioridazine—to avoid prolongation of QT interval and cardiac arrhythmias

2. Clozapine (atypical antipsychotic drug) induces paradoxical hypersalivation particular in night. So inorder to provide dry field in such patients during dental procedures scopolamine (300 mg) should be chewed and swallowed.

3. A patient on classical neuroleptics may develop bruxism which leads to dental attrition due to grinding of teeth. This can be reduced by a dentist using a suitable antianxiety drug.

TO REMEMBER

1. Schizophrenia (psychosis) may be due to limbic dopaminergic hyperactivity together with increased density and supersensitivity of mesolimbic dopamine D_2 receptors. Apart from this, abnormal 5-HT metabolism, endogenous opioids, prostaglandins, and noradrenaline have also been implicated in psychosis.

2. Dopamine D_2 receptor block is responsible for antipsychotic, antiemetic and neuroendocrine effects of neuroleptics while blockade of D_1 receptors of the extrapyramidal system is responsible for motor disturbances. 5-HT block may contribute to antipsychotic action. Noradrenaline block is responsible for hypotension and muscarinic M_1 receptor block affords protection against extrapyramidal effects.

3. Important indications of antipsychotics are:

Drugs	Uses
a. Phenothiazines	Schizophrenia, acute mania in bipolar depression, preanaesthetic medication, intractable hiccough, senile psychosis.
b. Haloperidol	Violent aggressives and self-mutilated syndrome.
c. Droperidol	Neuroleptanalgesia.

4. Important side effects are:
   a. Parkinsonism-like syndrome
   b. Tardive dyskinesia
   c. Weight gain
   d. Pseudopregnancy
   e. Anticholinergic and adrenergic blocking effects.

5. Important drug interactions are:
   a. Antacids decrease the absorption of neuroleptics
   b. Anticholinergics increase intestinal metabolism of neuroleptics
   c. Barbiturates and phenytoin increase metabolism of neuroleptics
   d. Chlorpromazine potentiates the effects of alcohol, barbiturates and other central nervous system depressants while antagonize the actions of guanethidine, methyldopa and clonidine.

6. Antipsychotic effects of clozapine and risperidone are due to D_2 and $5\text{-}HT_2$ receptor blocked.

Chapter 14

Antianxiety Drugs (Anxiolytics)

Anxiety may be due to minor maladjustments in day to day life. Such individuals complain of 'tension' with vague symptoms without any obvious signs of illness. In fact they do not really need drug therapy. In pathological anxiety, behavioural and mental functions are often severely impaired. So anxiety becomes excessive, inappropriate and it interferes with the well-being of individual. These patients may complain of digestive disorders, headache, backache lowering of sexual function, and may have continuous high blood pressure. Earlier barbiturates were used as sedative. However, they are no more used for this purpose because they cause marked sedation, respiratory depression, and drug dependence. At present, benzo-diazepines are employed for this purpose. Further, anxiety can lead to augmented autonomic activity which may also be treated simultaneously.

Classification

A. Benzodiazepines (Table 14.1)

B. Non-benzodiazepine anxiolytics

1. **5-HT$_1$A partial agonist:** Buspirone, ipsap-irone, gepirone

2. **5-HT$_3$ *antagonist:*** Ondansetron

3. **Adrenergic beta-blocker:** Propranolol (used to control somatic symptoms)

4. **Tri- and tetracyclic antidepressants** are used in generalized disorders, phobia and panic attacks.

5. **Other sedatives:** Meprobamate, hydroxy-zine, chlomazanon.

BENZODIAZEPINE ANXIOLYTICS

All the benzodiazepines have certain common pharmacological actions. They all show:

1. Calming effect (antianxiety)
2. Muscle relaxant property

Table 14.1: Benzodiazepines

	Long (>20 hr)	Intermediate (6–20 hr)	Short (< 6 hr)
1. Anxiolytics	Diazepam Chlordiazepoxide Flurazepam Nitrazepam	Lorazepam Temazepam Alprazolam	Oxazepam Triazolam
2. Sedative hypnotics	Flurazepam Nitrazepam	Temazepam	Triazolam
3. Antiepileptic	Clonazepam Clobazepam	—	—
4. Antidepressant	—	—	Alprazolam

119

3. Anticonvulsant action
4. Hypnotic-sedative effect

Mechanism of action: These drugs act on benzodiazepine (BDZ) receptors in brain. These receptors are in proximity of $GABA_A$ receptors and Cl^- channel. Benzodiazepines modulate the activity of GABA, an inhibitory neurotransmitter, and increase Cl^- conductance. BDZ receptors are blocked by flumezenil (BDZ antagonist) and is employed as antidote to benzodiazepine overdosing. Further skeletal muscle relaxant and sedative effects are useful in inducing a sense of relaxation in patients of anxiety.

Pharmacokinetics: On oral administration, most of the benzodiazepines are rapidly and completely absorbed from gut. Usually peak plasma concentrations are reached within 30–60 min. However, absorption following intramuscular administration is unpredictable except for lorazepam. Secondary plasma peaks may occur due to enterohepatic circulation. Benzodiazepines are highly plasma protein bound. Many benzodiazepines are biotransformed to clinically active metabolites such as desmethyldiazepam, desalkyl flumazepam, oxazepam, etc. Renal excretion of metabolites occurs usually after hepatic glucuronidation.

Side effects: They are safe drugs. Minor side effects are sedation, lethargy, ataxia, weight gain, and skin rashes. Toxicity due to over dosage is rare. The action of benzodiazepines may be potentiated by central nervous system depressants and sedatives. Physical or psychological dependence is rarely seen with benzodiazepines. However, the dependence can develop to short acting drugs and diazepam when taken for long duration in low doses. In such case, withdrawal symptoms occur on sudden stoppage of the drug.

Therapeutic Uses

1. Anxiety: The best results are seen in acute and recurrent anxiety reactions, and in

Drug	Oral dose (mg)
Diazepam	5–10
Oxazepam	10
Chlordiazepoxide	10–30
Alprazolam	0.25–0.5
Nitrazepam	5–10
Lorazepam	1–4
Clonazepam	1.5–10
Flurazepam	15–30
Ketozolam	15–30
Medazepam	10–50
Temazepam	15–30
Trizolam	0.25–1

generalized anxiety disorders. Since newer benzodiazepines do not offer any added advantage, diazepam is the drug of choice. Alprazolam and clonazepam may be used to treat panic and phobic disorders.

2. Effective disorders: Alprazolam is effective in mild depression associated with anxiety and insomnia. Clonazepam may be used to treat manic depression.

3. Due to anxiolytic, sedative, amnesic, and muscle relaxant actions diazepam or lorazepam is used in preanaesthetic medication.

4. Benzodiazepines have replaced barbiturates as hypnotics.

5. Diazepam and chlordiazepoxide are given i.v. in tetanus, strychnine poisoning, atropine poisoning, delirium tremens and infantile convulsions to control convulsions.

6. Diazepam and chlordiazepoxide have been used to reduce alcohol, barbiturate, cocaine and opiate withdrawal symptoms.

7. Clonazepam and clobazepam have a wide spectrum of antiepileptic effect. So they are used in major and minor form of epilepsy. Diazepam is used i.v. in status epilepticus (initial dose 5–10 mg; repeat at 10–15 min up to maximum of 30–35 mg).

8. Benzodiazepines are also employed in irritable bowel syndrome, peptic ulcer, and hypertension to allay anxiety.

9. Diazepam (0.25 mg/kg, i.v.) and medazolam (0.15 mg/kg, i.v.) have been used to induce anaesthesia.

10. Antianxiety agents are useful, especially during acute exacerbations of myofacial pain of the masticatory muscle in dental practice. For oral therapy, timazepam is used due to its longer duration of action (10–18 hrs).

11. Midazolam (i.v. or i.m.) is used by dent ist to induce anterograde amnesia; to depress gag reflex; and to manage seizures due to over dose of local anaesthetic.

Benzodiazepine antagonist is **flumazenil**. It is given parenterally to treat benzodiazepine overdosage, to counteract benzodiazepine sedation and to reduce drowsiness and coma associated with hepatic encephalopathy and alcohol intoxication.

Precautions

i. The use of antiallergic drugs, alcohol, and phenothiazine shall be avoided while taking these drugs as the sedative effect is potentiated.

ii. These should not ordinarily be given to patients of kidney or liver disease.

iii. When used with opioid analgesics reduce dose of opioid by one-third.

iv. Use lower doses in elderly patients because they are more prone to orthostatic hypotension.

Other Antianxiety Drugs

1. **Buspiron :** It is a new non-benzodiazepine anxiolytic agent. It is a partial agonist at 5-HT$_1$A receptors and reduces 5-HT release since these receptors are autoreceptors. It does not have sedative, hypnotic, muscle relaxant and anticonvulsant properties. It causes less impairment of memory and has a very low dependence potential. However, its onset of action is slow. It takes 4–6 weeks to show its

optimal clinical benefit. Important side effects are headache, dizziness, insomnia, dysphoria and gastrointestinal upsets. It is useful in general anxiety neurosis and is given in a dose of 15–30 mg daily.

2. **Ondansetron:** It is 5-HT$_3$ receptors antagonist which are heteroreceptors.These receptors modulate dopaminergic and cholinergic activity. Its profile of action and advantages are similar as that of buspiron. Its onset of clinical response is quick. It does not have central nervous system stimulant effect. It is particularly useful to control anxiety associated with withdrawal of addicting drugs such as morphine, barbiturates, cocaine and benzodiazepines being able to reduce central dopaminergic activity.

3. Propranolol is a non-specific beta-adrenoceptor antagonist. It reduces the peripheral autonomic manifestations of anxiety. It may also have central activity. Dose: 40–160 mg 6 hourly.

4. Meprobamate, hydroxyzine and chlormezanon are old anxiolytic drugs. They are no more used because of severe sedation and high addiction liability.

Points for Dental Students

1. A dental student must learn pharmacokinetic and pharmacodynamic properties of benzodiazepines thoroughly because these are commonly used drugs in dentistry as:
   a. Sedative and hypnotic
   b. Anxiolytic agent (diazepam, alprazolam, clonazepam)
   c. Preanaesthetic medication (diazepam, lorazepam)
   d. Induction of general anaesthesia (diazepam and midazolam)

2. Avoid use of antiallergic drugs along with benzodiazepines because they potentiate the sedative effect.

3. Ordinarily avoid use of benzodiazepines in presence of kidney and liver disease because these organs are involved in biotransformation and excretion. However, if these drugs are to be used in presence of liver disease oxazepam and lorazepam may be used because these are metabolized by phase II conjugation reactions which are least affected by hepatic disease.

4. Use lower doses of benzodiazepines in elderly because they are more prone to orthostatic hypotension.

TO REMEMBER

1. Anxiety may be due to minor maladjustments in day to day life. Such individuals complain of tension with vague symptoms and do not really need drug therapy.

2. In pathological anxiety, behaviour and mental functions are often severely impaired. So it becomes excessive, inappropriate, and interferes with the well being of individual. It is treated with antianxiety drugs.

3. Barbiturates are no more used to treat anxiety because they cause marked sedation, respiratory depression and drug dependence.

4. Common pharmacological actions of benzodiazepines are: (a) calming effect (antianxiety), (b) muscle relaxant, (c) anticonvulsant and (d) hypnotic sedative effects.

5. Benzodiazepines act on benzodiazepine (BDZ) receptors in brain and modulate activity of GABA, an inhibitory neurotransmitter and increase Cl⁻ conductance.

6. Flumezenil is BDZ antagonist which is employed as antidote to benzodiazepine overdosing.

7. Important therapeutic uses of benzodiazepines are: (a) anxiety (diazepam), (b) panic and phobic disorders (alprazolam or clonazepam), (c) mild depression with anxiety and insomnia (alprazolam), (d) manic depression (clonazepam), (e) preanaesthetic medication (diazepam or lorazepam), (f) anticonvulsant (diazepam or chlordiazepoxide), (g) antiepileptic (clonazepam or clobazepam), (h) status epilepticus (diazepam) and (i) sedative and hypnotic (BDZ).

8. Buspiron is a new non-benzodiazepine anxiolytic agent which is a partial agonist at $5\text{-HT}_1\text{A}$ receptors and reduces 5-HT release being autoreceptors.

9. Ondansetron is a 5-HT_3 receptor antagonist which modulates dopaminergic and cholinergic activity. It is useful to control anxiety associated with withdrawal of addicting drugs.

Chapter 15

Antidepressants, Psychostimulants and Hallucinogenic Agents

Mental depression is a serious condition because it can disrupt the normal social life and may derive the individual to commit suicide. Broadly it can be divided into two main groups:

1. **Unipolar (major) depression:** In this disorder, the mood swings in one direction only, i.e. either depression with a feeling of worthlessness or depression with groundless irritability. It may be of two types:

   a. Reactive, neurotic or psychological depression: It is characterized by feeling of guilt, tension, anxiety, emotional withdrawal. It is self-limiting. It can be treated by antianxiety drugs like alprazolam.

   b. Endogenous (melancholic) depression: In this type in addition to above mentioned symptoms there are motor retardation and there is a greater tendency to commit suicide. It occurs due to genetic cause or due to deranged neurotransmission of norepinephrine or 5-HT or both/and possibly DA in certain areas of brain.

2. **Bipolar depression or manic depression psychosis:** It is a cyclic bipolar affective disorder. In this case, mood swings between "extreme excitement" (manic phase) and "profound depression" (depressive phase). It is characterized by mania (mood elevation, hyperactivity, uncontrolled thought, pressured speech and a little need for sleep followed by severe depression). Suicidal tendencies are also observed.

The antidepressant drugs are classified into the following groups:

Drug	Dose (mg/24 hr.)
I. Old antidepressants	
1. Monoamines reuptake inhibitors:	
i. Tricyclic antidepressants	
• Imipramine	75–200
• Desipramine	75–200
• Trimipramine	75–200
• Amitriptyline	75–200
• Nortriptyline	75–200
• Amoxapine	120–480
• Doxepin	50–100
• Dothiepin	50–100
ii. Heterocyclic antidepressants:	
• Trazodone	100–300
• Mainserine	30–40
2. Selective serotonin (5-HT) reuptake inhibitors:	
• Fluoxetine	20
• Fluvoxamine	100–300
• Paroxetine	20–40
• Citalopram	10–40
3. Monoamine oxidase inhibitors:	
i. Non-selective MAO inhibitors:	
• Non-hydrazine: Tranylcypromine 20	
• Hydrazine: Phenelzine 10–30	
ii. Selective MAO inhibitors:	
• MAO-A inhibitor : Logline and moclobamide	
• MAO-B inhibitor : Selegiline (deprenyl)	

4. Antimanic (mind stabilizing) drugs:
   - Lithium carbonate   250–2000
   - Carbamazepine   400–600
   - Sodium valproate   600–800

II. **New antidepressants**
   - Venlafaxin   75–225
   - Nefazodone   200–600
   - Mirtazapine   15–60
   - Roboxetine

Mode of Action of Antidepressants

A. Antidepressant effect of these drugs depends on their effect on biogenic amine neurotransmitters:

1. Imipramine, clomipramine, amitriptyline and doxepin are tricyclic antidepressants. They block the amines norepinephrine (NE) or serotonin reuptake pumps and permit a longer sojourn of neurotransmitter at the receptor site. They also bind to α–adrenergic, histaminergic (H_1) and cholinergic receptors (responsible for many of the side effects). Desipramine and nortriptyline are also tricyclic antidepressants. They act predominantly inhibiting norepinephrine reuptake.

2. Amoxapine and maprotiline are tetracyclic antidepressants. They also act by inhibiting NE reuptake leading to increased concentration of NE in the synaptic cleft in the central nervous system.

3. Some of the second generation antidepressants such as trazodone, nefazodone, and mirtazapine mainly act by antagonizing subtypes of serotonin receptors (5-HT_2A or 5-HT_2C). Mirtazapine also causes antagonism of $α_2$–adrenergic receptors; bupropion alters the output of norepinephrine. Thus newest antidepressants of this group act through serotonergic and nor-adrenergic effects.

4. Monoamine oxidase inhibitors act by blocking a major degradative pathway for the amine neurotransmitters. So they permit more amines to accumulate in presynaptic stores and more to be released.

5. Recently selective serotonin reuptake inhibitors (SSRIs) such as sertraline, fluoxetine, fluvoxamine, paroxetine and citalopram have been developed. These antidepressant drugs have minimal autonomic toxicity. They act selectively by blocking serotonin reuptake and increasing the levels of serotonin in the synaptic cleft.

B. Receptor and post-receptor effects:

1. There occurs decrease in norepinephrine stimulated cAMP. Beta-adrenoceptor binding is also decreased by selective norepinephrine uptake inhibitors, those with mixed action on norepinephrine, serotonin, monoamine oxidase inhibitors and even electroconvulsive therapy. Such changes do not consistently occur after selective serotonin uptake inhibitors, $α_2$ receptor antagonists and mixed serotonin antagonists.

2. It is suggested that enhanced stimulation or responsiveness of post-synaptic 5-HT_1A receptors are particularly important in the action of antidepressants.

3. It is possible that antidepressant effect of these drugs may be due to long-term intracellular changes which involve phosphorylation of various regulating elements including those within the nucleus.

4. It is suggested that enhanced serotonin throughput is necessary for the antidepressant action of serotonin but not for norepinephrine uptake inhibitors while enhanced norepinephrine throughput is needed of norepinephrine uptake inhibitors.

Tricyclic and Heterocyclic Antidepressants

Imipramine is a dibenzazepine derivative and is commonly used tricyclic antidepressant drug. So it is discussed as a prototype. The advantages and limitations of other drugs will also be dealt.

Pharmacological Actions

1. **Central nervous system:** In therapeutic doses, it induces sedation. In depressed individual, changes in mood and behaviour are noticed after a lag period of 2–3 weeks.
2. **Autonomic nervous system:** The drug has central as well as peripheral anticholinergic effects such as dryness of mouth, constipation, blurred vision and palpitation.
3. **Cardiovascular system:** Orthostatic hypotension (due to peripheral adrenergic blockade) and sinus tachycardia (due to blockage of noradrenaline uptake and anticholinergic effect) are common effects. It causes cardiac depression followed by ventricular arrhythmias at toxic dose levels.

Desipramine appears to be better tolerated because of lesser sedative, anticholinergic and adrenergic blocking actions. Amitriptyline has marked sedative and anticholinergic effects which are less in biotransformed metabolite nortriptyline. Doxepin has prominent sedative effect and can be used as an antianxiety agent as well. Protriptyline has anticholinergic effect but has the least sedative effect.

Amoxapine is a metabolite of the antipsychotic drug loxapine. So it retains some of the antipsychotic action and dopamine receptor antagonism. It is, therefore, suitable drug for depression in psychotic patients. However, it may cause akathisia, parkinsonism, amenorrhoea, galactorrhoea syndrome and perhaps tardive dyskinesia due to dopamine antagonism.

Trazodone has antidepressant and hypnotic effects. So sometimes it is combined with monoamine oxidase inhibitors, which disturb sleep.

Pharmacokinetics

On oral administration tricyclic antidepressants are well absorbed. They are bound to plasma proteins. They are metabolized in liver. Imipramine and amitriptyline are metabolized to active metabolites like desipramine and nortriptyline, respectively. They are slowly excreted in urine. They take 2–3 weeks to achieve the full therapeutic effect, which represent the time interval to down-regulate these receptors. The half-life of these agents is long, ranging from a few hours to several days. To attain steady-state plasma levels, the repeated administration of drug is essential.

Therapeutic Uses

1. These are the drugs of choice for patients of melancholic (endogenous major) depression. The clinical response occurs after 14–21 days. Abrupt drug withdrawal is not advisable. Drug should be gradually withdrawn over a 3–4 weeks period.
2. They are also used in nocturnal enuresis (bed wetting) in children.
3. **Other uses:**
   i. Chronic pain such as neuralgias, fibromyalgia and migraine; so amitryptyline and dothiepin have proven effect in managing chronic orofacial pain including temporomandibular joint dysfunction in dental practice due to its analgesic (at low dose), sedative and hypnotic effects. These drugs should be used at night to avoid day time sedation.
   ii. Severe anxiety states, with panic reactions and obsessive compulsive disorder

  iii. Chronic alcoholism
  iv. Irritable bowel syndrome
   v. Hyperkinesia in children
  vi. Bulimia
 vii. Cataplexy with narcolepsy.

Side Effects

- **Anticholinergic:** Dry mouth, blurred vision, nausea, vomiting, constipation and urinary retention. Dry mouth (xerostomia) may lead to dental caries and candidiasis. This risk is more with tricyclic antidepressants while atypical antidepressants and selective serotonin reuptake inhibitors are comparatively safe.
- **Central nervous system:** Parkinson's like symptoms (tremors and rigidity) and convulsions at high doses; drowsiness, sedation and dizziness.
- **Cardiovascular:** Postural hypotension, arrhythmias.
- **Rare:** Reversible obstructive jaundice and leukopenia.

Drug Interactions

1. These drugs cause dangerous depression of the central nervous system if combined with barbiturates, benzodiazepines and alcohol.
2. These drugs block the antihypertensive effects of guanethidine, methyldopa and clonidine by inhibiting the amine pump.
3. Concurrent administration of tricyclic antidepressants and MAO inhibitors can result in severe toxicity including high fever, depression of respiration, and marked excitement.
4. Metabolism of tricyclic antidepressants is increased by enzyme inducers.
5. Plasma protein bound tricyclic antidepressant can be displaced by aspirin, chlorpromazine, hyoscine, phenytoin and phenylbutazone.
6. They potentiate the effects of exogenously administered noradrenaline.

Selective serotonin reuptake inhibitors lack many of the toxicities of the tricyclic and hetrocyclic antidepressants. So patient compliance is better despite adverse effects such as nausea, decreased libido and even decreased sexual function. They should not be given along with MAOI because combination may lead to serotonin syndrome due to marked increase of serotonin in synapses.

Monoamine Oxidase Inhibitors

Monoamine oxidase inhibitors are as effective as tricyclic antidepressants in treating endogenous depression. However, they are to be used only after the therapy with tricyclic has failed because of their toxicity and potentially lethal interactions with other drugs and with tyramine containing foods. Other important pharmacological actions are central nervous system stimulation, lowering of blood pressure and antianginal effects.

Side Effects

- **Common:** Orthostatic hypotension, weakness, dizziness, fatigue, vertigo, headache, dry mouth and difficulty in urination.
- **Rare:** Hepatotoxicity, tremors, agitation, insomnia and hallucination.

Drug interactions

MAO inhibitors cause:
1. Potentiation of effects of sympathomimetics, central nervous system depressants, L-dopa and L-tryptophan
2. Fatal hyperpyrexia with narcotic analgesics (pethidine)
3. Hypertensive crisis and hallucination with tricyclic antidepressants
4. Reduction in the antihypertensive effect of alphamethyldopa, guanethidine and reserpine
5. Hypertensive crisis with food preparations containing sympathomimetic amines (tyramine in cheese, beer, wine, yeast, chocolate, etc.)

Newer Selective MAO Inhibitors

1. **MAO-A inhibitors** are being re-evaluated for use as antidepressant. Moclobemide is a reversible, short acting MAO-A inhibitor. It appears to be relatively free to a very high risk of hypertensive reactions to tyramine ingested in food.
2. **MAO-B inhibitors** (e.g. deprenyl) are used as an adjunct drug in Parkinsonism and are also believed having antiaging action due to its free radical scavenging action.

New Antidepressants

1. **Nefazodone:** It is closely related to trazodone but less sedating; produces fewer adverse sexual effects than SSRIs; should not be used along with cisapride, terfenadine or estimazole because all inhibit CYP3A4 enzyme in the liver.
2. **Venlafaxine:** It is a potent inhibitor of serotonin reuptake and a weak inhibitor of norepinephrine transport.
3. **Mirtazepine:** It is a derivative of mianserin. It has antidepressant and antihistaminic effects. Its use is associated with weight gain.

Name	Mechanism of action of newer antidepressants
Venlafaxine	Potent 5-HT and NA reuptake inhibitor
Nefazodone	5-HT$_2$ receptor antagonist. Increases 5-HT neurotransmission at 5-HT$_1$A receptor. Limited 5-HT and NA reuptake inhibition
Mirtazapine	Antagonism of both 5-HT$_2$ and 5-HT$_3$ receptors. Potent antagonism of central α-2-adrenergic receptors. High affinity for H$_1$ receptors
Reboxetine	Selective inhibitor of NA reuptake

Antimanic Agents

Lithium: It is a monovalent cation. It has the tendency to substitute for one or more electrolytes, like sodium, potassium, calcium and magnesium. It does not modify the neurological and behavioural processes in normal individuals. However, it definitely has mood stabilizing effect in different types of psychiatric illness. Although the exact mechanism of its antimanic action is not known, it is postulated that lithium increases 5-HT release and postsynaptic activity and concomitantly increases neuronal uptake of noradrenaline. Further, recently it is suggested that lithium interferes with a second messenger system, the phosphatidylinositol cycle (intraneuronal signaling system) to normalization of neurotransmitter function. This in turn may be the basis of mood stabilization by lithium.

Lithium ions are completely absorbed from gastrointestinal tract. It is distributed non-uniformly throughout extracellular and intracellular fluids. It is not bound to plasma proteins. The half-life is about 20 hours and equilibrium is reached by one week of continuous administration. It is entirely eliminated by the kidneys. Lithium salts have narrow therapeutic ratio. Therefore, it is essential to regulate plasma concentration of lithium in patients within 0.9 to 1.4 mEq/litre. Over dosage may be fatal.

Adverse reactions: Side effects include gastrointestinal disturbances, tremors, polyurea, muscle weakness and central nervous system disturbances. Lithium toxicity is made worse by salt depletion and by simultaneous use of thiazide diuretics. Lithium is contraindicated during pregnancy and in lactating mothers.

Xerostomia is manifested by lithium in patients of manic depressive psychosis due to lithium induced polyuria. This may lead to dental caries in about 70% cases. Lithium toxicity is precipitated by NSAIDs and metronidazole due to decreased renal excretion of lithium. So these drugs should not be used along with lithium.

Therapeutic Uses

1. Used for the treatment of mania and prevention of manic depressive illness.
2. Used to treat schizophrenia and schizo-affective disorders in combination with neuroleptics.
3. Used to convert a patient of endogenous depression, not responding to conventional antidepressant treatment, into a responder.
4. Used to prevent episodic outbursts of anger and violence in mentally disturbed patients.

Other Antimanic Drugs

1. **Antipsychotic agents (chlorpromazine, haloperidol and pimozide)** are used in severely manic patients for initial urgent treatment. Since high doses of neuroleptics are employed, anticholinergic anti-Parkinson drugs (benzhexol or orphenadrine) are coadministered to prevent the occurrence of iatrogenic Parkinsonism.
2. **Carbamazepine:** It has been found to be effective in prophylaxis of bipolar depression. It may be used alone or in combination with lithium. It may be effective by reducing the influx of sodium into neurons, increasing serotonergic and dopaminergic postsynaptic activity and blocking adenosine receptors.

   Dose: Initial—200 mg twice daily; increasing to a daily dose of 600–1200 mg by daily increment of 200 mg.
3. **Sodium valproate:** It is not a strong antimanic as carbamazepine. It can be useful in prevention and treatment of acute mania patients who are not responding to lithium or carbamazepine. It is particularly useful in patients with rapid cycling pattern. Lithium and valproate combination may succeed in cases resistant to monotherapy with either drug.

PSYCHOSTIMULANTS

This group includes amphetamine, congeners of amphetamine and cocaine. They have no clinical utility. They are only drugs of abuse.

Psychostimulants cause: (1) elevation of mood (euphoria); (2) a sense of increased self-esteem; (3) physical and mental well-being; (4) decreased appetite, and (5) sleep.

Chronic use of these drugs may lead to reversible psychosis. These drugs also unmask psychotic symptoms in latent schizophrenia. These drugs produce their effects by augmenting central noradrenergic and dopaminergic activity. Amphetamine acts as a dopamine receptor agonist. It also induces neuronal release of dopamine and nor-adrenaline. Cocaine inhibits the neuronal reuptake of dopamine and noradrenaline. So these drugs cause marked increase in the sympathetic activity.

These drugs produce tolerance, and physical dependence. However, abstinence symptoms are not severe.

HALLUCINOGENIC (PSYCHODYSLEPTIC) AGENTS

As these drugs are capable of producing psychosis-like symptoms, they are also called psychotomimetic drugs. They are also known as hallucinogenic agents because of their ability to cause hallucinations. These drugs produce alteration in mood, depersonalization, and a variety of effects on memory and learned behaviour.

Following hallucinogenic agents are commonly abused:

1. Cannabis sativa (marijuana, hashish, ganja, bhang, charas)
2. Lysergic acid diethylamide (LSD)
3. Phencyclidine
4. Mescaline
5. Psilocybin and psilocin
6. Ololinque
7. Tryptamine derivatives.

Cannabis (Marijuana)

Cannabis is obtained from the hemp plants, cannabis sativa and cannabis indica. The resinous exudate of the tops of the female plant contains the active ingredient, i.e. tetrahydrocannabinol. The resin is known as hashish or charas. Bhang is prepared from the dried leaves and the flowering shoots. Ganja is the resinous mass which is obtained from the small leaves and brackets of inflorescence.

Cannabis induces euphoria, calmness and drowsiness. The individual becomes more sensitive to external stimuli and colour looks more vivid and brighter. The drug causes depersonalization and difficulty in concentration and thinking. Other acute pharmacological effects are bronchodilatation, tachycardia, hypotension, conjunctival vascular congestion, and decrease in intraocular pressure, antiemetic, analgesic and anticonvulsant effects. Cannabis produces psychological dependence with mild abstinence symptoms (nausea, insomnia, sweating, and tremors).

Potential therapeutic uses: Cannabis, tetrahydrocanabinol (THC) or its synthetic derivative, nabilone have potential use in cancer patients on cytotoxic drug therapy due to their antiemetic, analgesic and euphoria actions. Other possible uses are in glaucoma, bronchial asthma and as an anticonvulsant.

Lysergic Acid Diethylamide (LSD) and other Hallucinogens

These psychodyspleptic agents induce a qualitatively similar behavioral profile of actions. They have a disintegrating effect on both inborn and learned behaviour. These drugs cause marked changes in mood with emotional outbursts. Individuals my laugh or cry on slightest provocation. Motivation is impaired. Many subjects experience a fear of disintegration of self. All these drugs may have some sympathomimetic actions such as mydriasis, piloerection, tachycardia, tremor and hyperglycemia.

Phencyclidine is related to ketamine. Initially it was introduced to produce dissociative anaesthesia. But now it is a popular drug of abuse because of low cost and easy synthesis.

Tolerance to all hallucinogens occurs quickly. Cross-tolerance is seen between LSD, mescaline and psilocybin but is not present between LSD and phencyclidine. These drugs produce psychological dependence because the withdrawal symptoms (nausea, diarrhea, sleep disturbances, and tremors) are minor.

Neotropic Agents

They are a new class of psychotherapeutic agents. They facilitate the acquisition of learning and enhance memory retention. Cognition is defined as the process of acquiring, storing and utilizing intellectual knowledge. These drugs can overcome or retard cognitive decline which occurs in old age and in some diseased conditions. The disruption of the process of memory consolidation by hypoxia, trauma, seizures, hypoglycaemia and other aversive factors can also be preserved by these drugs. Some neotropic drugs are piracetam, aniracetam, oxiracetam, hydergine, vincamine, meclo-fenoxate, pentoxiflylline, pyritinol, cyclandate, nicergoline.

Mechanism of Action

Pentoxifylline, pyritinol, cyclandate and nicergoline may act as cerebral protectors by improving cerebral circulation and microcirculation. Other drugs may induce neurotransmitter environment conducive to learning, acquisition and memory retention by causing an increase in central cholinergic, noradrenergic and dopaminergic activity with concomitant reduction in serotonin function.

Piracetam is a cyclized derivative of GABA. It was the first nootropic agent to be introduced. It is believed to augment energy utilization and resistance to adverse cellular changes induced by anoxia. It also alters the central neurotransmitter as mentioned above. It is shown to improve mental performance in children and aging individuals with memory deficit. It is devoid of autonomic, motor or behavioural effects.

Dose: 2–3 gm daily in divided doses.

Therapeutic Uses

1. Cognitive deficits seen in Alzheimer's disease and during aging.
2. Learning and attention deficit in children.
3. Coexisting memory deficits in neurological and psychiatric illness.
4. Amnesia following cerebral trauma, drug abuse including alcoholism, seizures, etc.

Points for Dental Students

The drugs of this group have important side effects and drug interactions. So if a drug is selected by dentist to be used, he must take care of following important drug interactions and side effects for its safe use:

1. The use of selective serotonin receptor inhibitors should be avoided with: (a) NSAIDs (e.g. aspirin) to avoid the surgery related bleeding because they also impair platelet aggregation; (b) tramadol (an opioid analgesic) to avoid "serotonin syndrome" (hyperthermia, muscle rigidity, tremors, mental confusion and cardiovascular collapse).
2. The antidepressants should not be used with macrolide antibiotics (e.g. erythromycin) to avoid QT prolongation and precipitation of cardiac arrhythmias.
3. Fluoxetine prolongs the sedative effect of alprazolam, midazolam, and triazolam.

TO REMEMBER

1. Mental depression can disrupt the normal social life and may derive the individual to commit suicide.
2. One group of antidepressants is monoamine reuptake inhibitors, e.g. tricyclic and heterocyclic antidepressants, selective serotonin reuptake inhibitors. The other group acts by preventing the oxidative deamination of catecholamines and serotonin. Thus both groups of drugs increase the functional availability of these monoamines in the brain. However, newest antidepressants (trazodone, nefazodone, mirtazapine) act by antagonizing subtypes of serotonin receptors (5-HT_2A or 5-HT_2C), and α_2–adrenergic receptors or altering the output of norepinephrine. So they act through serotonergic and noradrenergic effects.
3. Tricyclic antidepressants are the drugs of choice for patients of melancholic (endogenous major) depression. MAO inhibitors are only used when tricyclic antidepressants fail because they are very toxic and have potentially lethal interactions with other drugs and with tyramine containing foods.
4. Lithium is a monovalent cation. Its antimanic effect may be due to its ability to increase 5-HT release and post-

synaptic activity as well as it concomitantly increases neuronal uptake of nor-adrenaline. Further, recently it is suggested that lithium interferes with a second messenger system (phosphatidylinositol cycle interneuronal signaling system) to normalization of neurotransmitter function.

5. Amphetamine and its congeners and cocaine are psychostimulants. They have no clinical utility and are only drugs of abuse. They act by augmenting central noradrenergic and dopaminergic activity.

6. Hallucinogenic (psychodysleptic) agents are also called psychotomimetic drugs because they produce psychosis like alteration in mood, depersonalization and a variety of effects on memory and learned behaviour. Out of all, LSD is the most dangerous agent because it may cause permanent psychosis in a few individuals and damage to sex chromosomes.

7. Neotropic agents facilitate the acquisition of learning and enhance memory retention. They have been used in Alzheimer's disease, learning and attention deficit in children, coexisting memory deficits in neurological and psychiatric illness and amnesia following cerebral trauma, drug abuse, and seizures.

Chapter 16

Alcohols

ETHYL ALCOHOL (ETHANOL)

Ethanol is hydroxy derivative of aliphatic hydrocarbons. Pharmacology of ethanol is important because of extensive consumption of alcoholic beverages, alcohol abuse and its interaction with other therapeutic agents. Alcohol is produced by fermentation of sugars. Fermentation stops when alcohol content reaches 15% because the process is inhibited by alcohol itself. There is large variety of alcoholic beverages (Table 16.1).

Table 16.1: Beverages, alcoholic
contents and their sources

Beverage	Approx. % of alcohol	Source
Beer	4–8	Cereals
Brandy	43–57	Wine
Cider	8–12	Apple juice
Champagne	12–13	Grape juice
Claret	9–12	Apple juice
Gin	51–59	Cereals
Port	16–22	Wine
Rum	51–59	Molasses
Sherry	16–22	Wine
Whisky	51–59	Cereals
Rectified spirit	95	Cereals

Pharmacological Actions

Local actions: Ethanol is a mild rubifacient, counter irritant and astringent when rubbed on skin. It acts as an antiseptic by precipitating bacterial proteins. On subcutaneous injection, it causes pain, inflammation and necrosis followed by fibrosis.

Systemic actions: Alcohol is primarily neuronal depressant. Degree of depression depends on the quantity of ethanol consumed. The cortex and reticular activating system are more sensitive to alcohol; other areas get depressed as concentration rises. The behavioural stimulation (euphoria) is seen after alcohol consumption. It is apparently due to depression of the inhibitory pathways of the brain, which control behaviour. Though alcohol can induce anaesthesia but margin of safety is narrow.

Cardiovascular system is not affected significantly with moderate amount of alcohol. Larger doses cause fall in blood pressure due to direct myocardial as well as vasomotor centre depression. Chronic alcoholics show cardiomyopathy and cardiac arrhythmias. Ethanol inhibits the secretion of antidiuretic hormone from the posterior pituitary and causes diuresis. However, diuretic action disappears on chronic use of ethanol. It interferes with the renal excretion of uric acid. So it may precipitate gout by elevating the uric acid level. Often amenorrhea and infertility occur in alcoholic women and lowering of the motility of sperm cells in men. Ethanol has aphrodisiac (sex stimulation) property due to loss of inhibitions. However, performance of the sexual act is often impaired.

Moderate amount of ethanol dilates peripheral skin blood vessels causing the feel of warmth and stimulates salivary and gastric secretion. It causes irritation of gastric mucosa, chronic gastritis and peptic ulcer in heavy drinkers. Chronic alcoholism leads to mental and physical disability, malnutrition, vitamin deficiency and constipation. Hepatic cirrhosis and fatty infiltration may also occur. Within limit, alcohol has certain food value, i.e. one gram of alcohol supplies 7 calories. However, it cannot be used as a food because it is quickly metabolized and does not serve as a reserve food.

Ethanol adversely affects the performance of skilled tasks and in vehicle driving the judgement is impaired, the reaction time increases and is the major cause of road accidents. Typing or workmanship is also affected.

Pharmacokinetics: On oral ingestion, about 25% of ethanol is absorbed from stomach and the remaining amount is absorbed from small intestine. The rate of ethanol absorption is determined by the presence of food in the stomach. Ethanol absorption is decreased by food with high lipid content. Ethanol is primarily metabolized in the liver by the enzymes alcohol dehydrogenase and aldehyde dehydrogenase into CO_2 and water at a rate of 10 ml/hour in adults. Since alcohol metabolism follows zero-order kinetics, its rate of metabolism is not affected by the amount ingested. Disulfiram inhibits the enzyme aldehyde dehydrogenase. Thus it increases the plasma concentration of acetaldehyde which gives rise to unpleasant aldehyde syndrome. About 90–98% of ethanol is metabolized and excreted in urine.

Clinical uses: The uses of ethanol can be divided into external and internal.

1. **External:** 5% alcohol is used as a preservative for many drugs, 25% as a solvent, 50% for application on the surface to prevent bedsores and 70% is popularly used as a disinfectant.

2. **Internal:**
   - It is used as an appetizer in the form of beverages containing less than 10% ethanol.
   - Injection of alcohol round the nerve causes permanent loss of transmission and is used to treat intractable neuralgias (trigeminal and others) and severe cancer pain.
   - It is also used in methanol poisoning.

Ethanol is contraindicated in:
- Hepatic and renal diseases
- Peptic ulcer
- Epilepsy
- Pregnant women

Drug Interactions

- Ethanol causes marked central nervous system depression with tranquilizers, hypnotics, opioids and antihistaminics (synergistic action).
- It induces disulfiram like reaction with sulfonylureas, metronidazole and certain cephalosporins.
- It enhances the hypoglycemic effect of insulin and oral antidiabetics.
- Acute alcohol ingestion inhibits while chronic intake induces tolbutamide and phenytoin metabolism.

Acute alcohol intoxication: An individual is said to be under the influence of alcohol if his blood concentration is 50–100 mg%. If the blood alcohol concentration is more than 100 mg% the chances of accidents due to drunken driving are high. The characteristic features of acute alcohol intoxication are:
- Cold clammy skin
- Fall in body temperature
- Depressed respiration
- Normal or dilated pupil
- Finally there may occur coma and death

The treatment consists of
- Gastric lavage
- Maintenance of patency of airways
- Prevention of aspiration of vomitus
- Positive pressure respiration
- 50 ml of 50% glucose i.v. for hypoglycemia
- 100 mg of thiamine i.v. (bolus)
- 2–4 gm of magnesium sulphate by i.v. infusion over 1–2 hours
- If the individual is agitated and violent give sedative.

Chronic alcoholism: Chronic ethanol abuse is one of the greatest drug problem. It produces pharmacodynamic type of tolerance. There also exists cross-tolerance between general anaesthetics, sedative and hypnotics. Sudden stoppage of ethanol will lead to withdrawal symptoms such as restlessness, muscle cramps, purposive behaviour and convulsions. Such cases are managed with:

- Maintenance of nutrition and electrolytes
- Administration of glucose i.v. to combat hypoglycemia
- Administration of 100 mg of thiamine i.v.
- Prevention of autonomic hyperactivity with either clonidine (0.1–4 mg q.i.d. orally) or atenolol (50–100 mg daily orally)
- Diazepam or chlordiazepoxide for sedation
- IV diazepam to control convulsions

Treatment of alcohol dependence is done under medical supervision.

It is divided into: (a) detoxification and (b) rehabilitation.

Drugs used for detoxification are
- Disulfiram, citrated calcium cyanamide (CCC)
- Naltrexone, nalmephene
- Tiapride
- Acamposate
- Lithium carbamazepine and selective 5HT reuptake inhibitors

Disulfiram (antabuse) and carbimide (citrated calcium cyanamide) are used as aversion drugs. These drugs interfere with the oxidation of acetaldehyde which is formed during the metabolism of alcohol by alcohol dehydrogenase enzyme. They achieve this by inhibiting aldehyde dehydrogenase enzyme and preventing the conversion of acetaldehyde into CO_2 and water. They also cause depletion of catecholamines by inhibiting dopamine beta oxidase and thus interfering with synthesis of noradrenaline. Before administering these drugs, ensure that alcohol has not been consumed for at least 12 hours.

Disulfiram treatment is initiated with 800 mg as a single dose on the first day. This dose is gradually reduced over 5 days to a maintenance dose of 100–200 mg daily. Treatment may be continued for up to 1 year. After a week's treatment, a small amount of alcohol is given to the patient to produce toxic reactions such as flushing, perspiration, palpitation, marked nausea, vomiting, fall of blood pressure and even collapse. This is done to realize the patient that while on this drug he cannot tolerate even a small amount of alcohol.

Side effects of disulfiram are drowsiness, nausea, headache, cramps, fatigue and a metallic taste. Carbimide has similar properties as that of disulfiram. However, it has shorter duration of action and less side effects but causes leukocytosis and hypothyroidism.

These drugs are contraindicated in:
- Uncontrolled diabetes mellitus
- Hepatic and circulating diseases
- Alcoholics with obvious personality changes

Naltrexone and nalmephene are μ-opioid antagonists which block alcohol induced release of dopamine in the nucleus accumbers. These are used to reduce alcohol consumption and craving for alcohol along with psychosocial treatment.

Other drugs which are available to reduce craving and excitement that occur during alcohol withdrawal are:

- **Tiapride:** It has neuroleptic and anxiolytic properties due to its ability to antagonize D_2 receptors.
- **Acamprosate:** It acts as GABA receptor agonist and N-methyl D-aspartate (NMDA) receptor inhibitor. Common side effects are headache and diarrhea. It is given in doses of 2–3 gm per day in divided doses.
- **Lithium, carbamazepine and fluoxetine** are mood stabilizers. They are used as supportive drugs for alcohol conversion therapy.

Rehabilitation therapy consists of psychotherapy and institutional therapy. In the former, an individual must be convinced that he is a sick person like others and if willing, he can be treated. In case of latter, the patient can see for himself the ex-alcoholics who have become abstainers and are leading a happy life.

METHYL ALCOHOL (METHANOL)

Methanol has similar properties as that of ethanol. It is often employed as industrial solvent and denaturant. It has no clinical use. Although methanol is readily absorbed, it is slowly metabolized (oxidized) to formaldehyde and formic acid, which are responsible for methanol poisoning. Methanol has led to accidental poisoning. Signs of acute intoxication occurs generally after 8–36 hours such as headache, dizziness, nausea, vomiting, severe abdominal and back pain and visual impairment. There may occur partial or total blindness due to damage of optic nerve. Pupils do not react to light. There also occurs acidosis and respiratory depression.

Treatment of methanol poisoning is:
- Hospitalize the patient
- Proper nursing care
- Gastric lavage

- Administer activated charcoal
- Administer ethyl alcohol: 0.6 gm per kg i.v. loading dose; followed by 10 gm/hour by infusion
- Treatment of acidosis with i.v. sodium bicarbonate infusion (3 gm/hour) until urine pH reaches 7.5
- Treatment of hypokalemia (if present)
- Maintain nutrition
- Accelerate metabolic degradation of formate by administering folinic acid 1 mg/kg (maximum 50 mg) i.v. + folic acid 1 mg/kg i.v. 4 hourly for 6 doses
- Administer 4-methyl pyrazole (alcohol dehydrogenase inhibitor) 100 mg diluted in 250 ml of isotonic saline and infused slowly over 45 minutes
- Perform hemodialysis in severe cases

Isopropyl alcohol: It is a constituent of various industrial or home-cleaning products, antifreeze preparations and skin lotions. On oral administration, it is absorbed within 30 minutes. Abdominal pain, gastritis, vomiting and hypotension may occur as toxic manifestations. Treatment consists of giving an emetic and gastric lavage.

Points for Dental Students

1. Alcohol is often used in dental practice:
   - As solubilizing agent and preservative in mouthwashes
   - As obtundent (70%)
   - As antiseptic (70%)
   - To treat intractable neuralgias (trigeminal and other neuralgias)
   - To treat severe cancer pain
2. Dental students must have the knowledge of drug interactions with alcohol for safe prescribing of drugs to alcoholics.
3. So a dentist always enquires about alcohol consumption by the patient. This is because potentially severe reactions can occur when alcohol is consumed concomitantly with other drugs. For example,

alcohol enhances effect of insulin and oral antidiabetics (need dose adjustment); it induces disulfiram like reaction with sulfonylureas, metronidazole, and certain cephalosporins such as cefamandole, cefoperazone, cefotetan, and moxalactam (contraindicated or stop use of alcohol for more than 12 hours before their administration); marked central nervous system depression with antihistaminics and hypnotics (synergistic action).

TO REMEMBER

1. Ethanol is hydroxy derivative of aliphatic hydrocarbons. It is produced by fermentation of sugars. Fermentation stops when alcohol content reaches 15% because of inhibitory effects of alcohol itself.
2. Although 1 gm of alcohol supplies seven calories, it cannot be used as a food because it is quickly metabolized and does not serve as a reserve food.
3. Important uses of ethanol are: (a) as a preservative (5%); (b) as a solvent (25%); (c) to prevent bedsores (50%); (d) as a disinfectant (70%), (e) to treat intractable neuralgias and severe cancer pain; and (f) in methanol poisoning.
4. Ethanol is a drug of abuse. It produces pharmacodynamic type of tolerance and drug dependence. The acute withdrawal symptoms are controlled by the use of benzodiazepines or barbiturates. In periodic drinkers, disulfiram may be helpful.
5. Methyl alcohol is often employed as industrial solvent and denaturant. Often methanol is led to accidental poisoning. It is treated by correcting acidosis by sodium bicarbonate and administration of ethyl alcohol.
6. Isopropyl alcohol is a constituent of cleaning products, antifreeze preparations and skin lotions. Treatment of its acute toxicity consists of giving an emetic and performing gastric lavage.

Chapter 17

Pharmacologic Management of Parkinsonism

Parkinsonism is characterized by rigidity, bradykinesia, tremors and postural instability. It is usually idiopathic but can also occur by a wide variety of reasons. It may have genetic background. Idiopathic disorder may be due to exposure to some unrecognized or neurotoxin or to the occurrence of oxidation reactions with the generation of free radicals. The normally high concentration of dopamine in the basal ganglia of the brain is reduced in parkinsonism. Due to this, there occurs imbalance between the cholinergic and dopaminergic influences on the basal ganglia. Further dopaminergic neurons in the substantia nigra that normally inhibit the output of GABAergic cells in the corpus striatum are lost.

Classification

I. Drugs acting through the dopaminergic system
  i. Dopamine precursor: Levodopa (L-dopa)
  ii. Dopamine metabolism inhibitors:
     a. MAO-B inhibitors: Selegiline
     b. COMT inhibitors: Talcapone, entacapone
  iii. Dopaminergic agonists: Bromocriptine, lisuride, pergolide, piribedil
  iv. Drugs that facilitates dopaminergic transmission: Amantadine
  v. Peripheral decarboxylase inhibitors: carbidopa, benserazide

II. Drugs acting through cholinergic system
  i. Central anticholinergic: Trihexyphenidyl (benzhexol), procyclidine, biperiden
  ii. Antihistaminics: Orphenadrine, promethazine

Levodopa

It is [(-) -3-(3, 4-dihydroxylphenyl) L-alanine]. Dopamine does not cross the blood–brain barrier while levodopa penetrates the brain. Levodopa is the immediate metabolic precursor of dopamine which is decarboxylated to dopamine in the brain. Dopaminergic antiparkinsonian drugs produce beneficial effects in patients of parkinsonism by stimulation of dopamine D_2 receptors but dopamine D_1 receptor stimulation may also be required for maximum benefit.

Levodopa is rapidly absorbed from the small intestine. Peak plasma concentration occurs between 1 and 2 hours after an oral dose and the plasma half-life is usually between 1 and 3 hours. About two-thirds of the dose appears in the urine as metabolites (homovanillic acid and dihydroxyphenyl acetic acid). Unfortunately, only about 1–3% of the administered levodopa actually enters the brain unaltered, the remainder being metabolized extracerebrally, predominantly by decarboxylation to dopamine. Hence levodopa is always administered along with the dopa decarboxylase inhibitor which may reduce the daily requirements of levodopa by approximately 75%.

Levodopa can ameliorate all of the clinical features of parkinsonism but it is particularly effective in relieving bradykinesia and any disabilities resulting from it. It is given in combination with carbidopa. Dose: carbidopa 25 mg + levodopa 100 mg three times daily. Later on the dose of levodopa may have to be gradually increased to 250 mg.

Adverse effects: Anorexia, nausea, vomiting, dyskinesia (chorea, ballismus, athetosis, dystonia, myoclonus, tics and tremors), behavioural effects (depression, anxiety, agitation, insomnia, somnolence, confusion, delusions, hallucinations, night-mares, euphoria and other changes in mood or personality), mydriasis, blood dyscrasias, hot flushes, aggravation or precipitation of gout, abnormalities of smell and taste, brownish discolouration of saliva, urine or vaginal secretion, priapism, elevation of blood urea nitrogen and of serum transaminases, alkaline phosphatase and bilirubin.

Certain fluctuations in response to levodopa occur with increasing frequency as treatment continues. These fluctuations may be related to the timing of levodopa intake (weaning of reactions or end-of-dose akinesia) or unrelated to the timing of doses (on-off phenomenon). The exact mechanism of on-off phenomenon is not known. It is characterized by off periods of marked akinesia that alternate over the course of a few hours with on periods of improved motility. The situation can be handled by: (a) taking medication at more frequent interval; (b) reducing dietary intake of protein; (c) using controlled release formulations.

Levodopa should not be given along with pyridoxine (enhances extracellular metabolism of levodopa) and monoamine oxidase A inhibitors (precipitate hypertensive crisis).

Levodopa is contraindicated in psychotic patients (exacerbate the mental disturbance), in patients with angle-closure glaucoma and history of melanoma. It should be given carefully in patients with active peptic ulcer.

Dopamine Agonists

The enzymes responsible for synthesizing dopamine are depleted in the brains of parkinsonism patients. So dopamine agonists have a beneficial effect and an important role as first line therapy for Parkinson's disease. They lower incidence of the response fluctuations and dyskinesia occurring with long-term levodopa therapy.

i. **Bromocriptine** is an ergot derivative. It is widely used in patients with parkinsonism in doses between 7.5 and 30 mg. Peak plasma levels are reached within 1–2 hours after an oral dose. It is excreted in the bile and faeces. It is a D_2 agonist.

ii. **Pergolide** is another ergot derivative. It directly stimulates both D_1 and D_2 receptors. The average dose is 3 mg daily. The doses of both drugs should be small in the beginning of the treatment and gradually increased to full dose in order to avoid adverse effects. When these drugs are used the dose of levodopa is gradually reduced to about half of the previously required dose.

Important adverse effects are anorexia, nausea, vomiting, dyspepsia, postural hypotension, dyskinesia, confusion, delusions, hallucinations, headache, nasal congestion and erythromelagia. They are contraindicated in patients with history of psychotic illness and recent myocardial infarction. They are best avoided in patients with peripheral vascular disease or peptic ulceration.

iii. **Non-ergot dopamine agonists:** Prami-pexole and ropinirole are newer non-ergot dopamine agonists. Due to non-ergoline structure, adverse effects such as erythro-melagia, vasospasm and pleural or retro-peritoneal fibrosis are unlikely to occur.

Pramipexole acts on D_3 receptors preferentially. It may ameliorate effective symptoms of parkinsonism by its ability to scavenge hydrogen peroxide and enhance neurotropic activity in mesencephalic dopaminergic cultures. On oral administration, it is rapidly absorbed and peak plasma concentration occurs approximately in 2 hours. It is excreted largely in the urine. It may be used as monotherapy for mild parkinsonism as well as an adjunct to levodopa therapy to reduce and to smooth response fluctuations. It is given in doses of 0.5–1.5 mg three times daily. Treatment is started with 0.125 mg three times daily and the dose is gradually increased depending on response and tolerance.

Ropinirole is a relatively pure D_2 receptor agonist. It may be used as monotherapy in mild parkinsonism as well as an adjunct to levodopa therapy. It is given initially on doses of 0.25 mg three times daily. The dose is gradually increased up to 2–8 mg three times daily depending upon the response. The drug is neutralized in the liver.

The adverse effects of both the drugs are postural hypotension, fatigue, somnolence or insomnia, peripheral edema, nausea, constipation, dyskinesia and confusion.

Monoamine Oxidase Inhibitors

i. **Seligiline (deprenyl)** is a selective inhibitor of monoamine oxidase B. So it retards the breakdown of dopamine and enhances and prolongs the antiparkinsonian effect of levodopa. It is, therefore, indicated as adjunctive therapy for patients with a declining or fluctuating response to levodopa. Dose: 5 mg with breakfast and 5 mg with lunch. It should not be given to patients receiving meperidine, tricyclic agents or serotonin uptake inhibitors because of the risk of acute toxic interactions. Its neuroprotective effect may be due to its metabolite desmethylseligiline. It is believed to slow down disease progression.

ii. **Rasagiline:** It is another monoamine oxidase B inhibitor. It is more potent than seligiline in preventing MPTP-induced parkinsonism.

Catechol-O-Methyltransferase Inhibitors

Tolcapone and entacopone are selective COMT inhibitors. They prolong the duration of levodopa by diminishing its peripheral metabolism. Clearance of levodopa is decreased and relative bioavailability of levodopa is thus increased. They are useful in patients of parkinsonism receiving levodopa who have developed response fluctuations. They will, thus, lead to smooth response, more prolonged "on time" and the option of reducing total daily dose of levodopa. Out of the two, entacopone is preferred because it does not cause hepatotoxicity.

Entacopone is rapidly absorbed, bound to plasma proteins and metabolized prior to excretion. It has peripheral effect only. It is given in doses of 200 mg along with each dose of levodopa, i.e. 4–6 times daily. Adverse effects are dyskinesia, nausea, vomiting, confusion, diarrhea, abdominal pain, orthostatic hypotension, sleep disturbance and an orange discolouration of urine.

Amantadine

Amantadine is an antiviral drug. Its antiparkinsonian effect may be due to its ability to potentiate dopaminergic function by influencing the synthesis, release or uptake of dopamine. Peak plasma concentration occurs within 1–4 hours after an oral dose and its plasma half-life is between 2 and 4 hours. Most of the drug is excreted unchanged in urine.

Amantadine reduces bradykinesia, rigidity and tremor of parkinsonism. Disadvantages of the drug are that its desired effect disappears within a few weeks of treatment.

Common adverse effects are restlessness, depression, irritability, insomnia, agitation, excitement, hallucinations and confusion. It may also cause headache, congestive heart failure, postural hypotension, urinary retention and gastrointestinal disturbances. Overdose may produce an acute toxic psychosis and convulsions. Livedo reticularis sometimes occurs. It is due to local release of catecholamines resulting in vasoconstriction.

Acetylcholine Blocking Drugs

Centrally acting antimuscarinic preparations are used in the treatment of parkinsonism. They may improve tremor and rigidity but have little effect on bradykinesia. Some of the commonly used drugs are:

i. Benztropine mesylate: 1–6 mg/day
ii. Procyclidine: 7.5–30 mg/day
iii. Biperidine: 2–12 mg/day
iv. Trihexyphenydyl: 6–20 mg/day
v. Orphenadrine: 150–400 mg/day.

Treatment is started with a low dose of one of the above drugs. The dose is then gradually increased until benefits occur or adverse effects appear. Important adverse effects are drowsiness, mental slowness, inattention, restlessness, confusion, agitation, delusions, hallucinations and mood changes. Other adverse effects are dryness of the mouth, blurring of vision, mydriasis, urinary retention, nausea and vomiting, constipation, tachycardia, tachypnea, increased intraocular pressure, palpitations and cardiac arrhythmias. Dyskinesia may occur rarely. These drugs should be withdrawn gradually. These drugs are contraindicated in patients with prostatic hyperplasia, pyloric stenosis, paralytic ileus and angle-closure glaucoma.

Drug-induced Parkinsonism

Following drugs induce parkinsonism:
i. **Reserpine and tetrabenazine:** Due to depletion of biogenic monoamines from their storage sites.
ii. **Haloperidol and phenothiazines:** Due to their ability to block dopamine receptors. These drugs produce parkinsonism syndrome usually within three months of starting therapy with them. The syndrome clears over a few weeks or months after withdrawal. It may be treated with antimuscarinic drugs, if necessary. However, levodopa is of no help if neuroleptics are continued.
iii. **MPTP:** It is 1-mthyl-4-phenyl-1, 2, 3, 6-tetrahydropyridine. It is nephridine analogue. It is a protoxin. In the body, it is converted by MAO B to N-methyl-4-phenylpyridinium (MPP^+). MPP^+ is selectively taken up by cells in substantia nigra through an active mechanism normally responsible for dopamine reuptake. MPP^+ inhibits mitochondrial complex, thereby inhibiting oxidative phosphorylation. This probably leads to cell death and thus to striatal dopamine depletion and parkinsonism.

Recognition of the effects of MPTP suggests:
- Spontaneously occurring Parkinson's disease may result from exposure to an environmental toxin that is similarly selective to its target—no such toxin has been identified.
- A successful means of producing an experimental model of Parkinson's disease in animal, especially non-human primates.

Points for Dental Students

1. Most of antiparkinson drugs cause xerostomia which is aggravated by antimuscarinic drugs used to treat

parkinsonism. It may increase the incidence of dental caries, pain in swallowing and difficulty in speech.

2. Xerostomia is also increased with concurrent use of antihistaminics, tricyclic antidepressants and dicyclomine. This point is to be kept in mind by dentists while prescribing these drugs to patients of Parkinsonism during dental procedures.

3. Oral tremors provide difficulty during prosthetic restoration.

4. Patients with parkinsonism always suffer with orthostatic hypotension. So to avoid instant fall and injury, they should be asked to change the position in dental chair slowly.

5. Use of adrenaline containing local anaesthetic in Parkinson's patients on levodopa may precipitate cardiac arrhythmias due to peripheral conversion of levodopa to dopamine which stimulates the β_1 receptors of the heart.

TO REMEMBER

1. Parkinsonism (paralysis agitance) is characterized by rigidity, bradykinesia, tremor and postural instability. It is due to imbalance between cholinergic and dopaminergic influences on the basal ganglia and loss of dopaminergic neurons in the substantia nigra.

2. Levodopa, immediate metabolic precursor of dopamine, is the drug of choice in the treatment of parkinsonism.

It is always given with carbidopa (dopa decarboxylase inhibitor) which may reduce the daily requirement of levodopa by reducing its peripheral metabolism.

3. Dopamine agonists are used as first line therapy for parkinsonism. They are ergot derivatives (bromocriptine and pergolide) as well as non-ergot dopamine agonists (pramipexole and ropinirol).

4. Selegiline (deprenyl) and rasogiline are selective inhibitor of monoamine oxidase B. They prolong the antiparkinsonian effect of levodopa by reducing the breakdown of dopamine.

5. Tolcapone and entacopone are selective catechol-O-methyltransferase inhibitors. They also prolong the duration of levodopa by diminishing its peripheral metabolism.

6. Amantadine has antiparkinsonian effect due to its ability to potentiate dopaminergic function by influencing synthesis, release or output of dopamine.

7. Centrally acting antimuscarinic preparations (benzotropine, mesylate, procyclidine, biperidine, trihexyphenydyl and orphenadrine) are used to improve tremor and rigidity in parkinsonism.

8. Parkinsonism may be precipitated by certain drugs such as reserpine, tetrabenazine, haloperidol, phenothiazine and MPTP.

Section 4

Drugs Acting on Autonomic Nervous System

Chapter 18

General Considerations

Autonomic nervous system (ANS) is divided into sympathetic (adrenergic) and parasympathetic (cholinergic) divisions. It maintains homeostasis by integrating with sensory, somatomotor, endocrinal, metabolic, immunological and emotional activities. The limbic system and hypothalamus coordinate autonomic reactions with emotions. Anteromedial and posterolateral nuclei of hypothalamus are associated with cholinergic and adrenergic activities respectively. Vital centres in the medulla, e.g. vagal, vasomotor, vomiting, respiratory and cough centres play an important role in the coordination. The ANS has a property to regulate organ function automatically, largely independent of consciousness and has voluntary control (Autos—self, nomos—regulating). The characteristic features of autonomic nerves are:

1. They innervate smooth muscles, heart, blood vessels, and exocrine glands.
2. Their preganglionic neurone is myelinated while postganglionic fibres are non-myelinated.
3. The effector cells do not undergo atrophy on nerve damage and can maintain independent activity.
4. The chemical transmitter is acetylcholine or noradrenaline depending on the site of release.
5. The two divisions of ANS remain in a state of dynamic equilibrium to maintain homeostasis.

Parasympathetic system participates in conserving the body energy while sympathetic system participates in utilizing the body energy.

Autonomic nervous system consists of afferent and efferent fibres with central connections for their integration. Autonomic afferent fibres conduct impulses from the peripheral organs to the central nervous system. They are non-myelinated and run in the same nerve bundles as the efferent fibres. Autonomic efferent fibres conduct impulses from the central nervous system to the periphery. They are of two types, i.e. cholinergic and adrenergic. They differ from each other and important differences are given below:

Cholinergic Fibres

- They originate from central nervous system (craniosacral outflow: Cranial—3, 7, 9, 10, 11 and sacral—2, 3, 4).
- Their preganglionic fibres are long and myelinated.
- The ganglia are located very close to the tissue, innervated.
- Their postganglionic fibres are short and non-myelinated.
- On stimulation, resultant reaction is localized and they produce changes that tend to conserve energy.

The neurotransmitter at preganglionic and postganglionic neurones is acetylcholine.

Adrenergic Fibres

- They also originate from central nervous system (thoracolumbar outflow: T_1 to T_{12}, L_1 to L_3).
- Their postganglionic fibres are long and non-myelinated (except adrenal medulla).
- Their ganglia are located away from organ as under:
  a. A pair of paravertebral ganglion chains.
  b. Prevertebral ganglia
  c. Adrenal medulla
  d. Terminal ganglia to urinary bladder and rectum.

On stimulation, they produce diffused or generalized reaction and they prepare the body for active exertion (fight or flight). The neurotransmitter at preganglionic fibres is acetylcholine, while mainly noradrenaline at postganglionic neuron except those which innervate sweat glands and some blood vessels in skeletal muscles where acetylcholine is neurotransmitter.

Cholinergic Receptors

The actions of acetylcholine on visceral effectors resemble the actions of naturally occurring plant alkaloid muscarine. Therefore, these receptors are called muscarinic receptors, which are blocked by atropine. The cholinergic receptors at autonomic ganglia (sympathetic and parasympathetic) and neuromuscular junction are known as nicotinic receptors because the responses on these receptors resemble with the effects of naturally occurring alkaloid nicotine. Hexamethonium blocks the ganglionic nicotinic receptors and d-tubocurarine blocks these receptors in the skeletal muscle. Recently the cholinergic receptors have been classified into subtypes as under:

1. **M_1 (neural):**
   - Distributed in autonomic ganglia, myentric plexus of stomach, presynaptic and postganglionic parasympathetic nerve to SA node and cerebral cortex.
   - They are excitatory in nature.
   - They stimulate membrane phospholipase C-Ca^{++} Phosphoinositide system.
   - They induce gastric acid secretion and increase gastrointestinal motility.
   - Oxotremorine, acetylcholine and carbachol are agonists and pirenzepine, telenzepine, atropine and dicyclomine are antagonists.

2. **M_2 (cardiac):**
   - Distributed in myocardium and smooth muscles.
   - They produce inhibitory effect by inhibiting adenylate cyclase and activating K^+ channels.
   - They produce negative chronotropic and inotropic effects.
   - Acetylcholine and carbachol are agonists while atropine, gallamine and methoetramine are antagonists.

3. **M_3 (glandular):**
   - Distributed in smooth muscles and exocrine glands.
   - They are excitatory in nature and the mechanism of action is same as that of M_1 receptors.
   - They cause contraction of smooth muscles and secretion of exocrine glands.
   - Acetylcholine and carbachol are agonists while atropine, difenidol and hexahydrosila are antagonists.

4. **ACh-NM (N_1):**
   - Distributed in neuromuscular junction.
   - They cause contraction of skeletal muscle by opening up of cationic channels (Na^+, K^+), resulting in depolarization on stimulation.
   - Acetylcholine, nicotine and phenyl trimethylammonium are agonists while d-tubocurarine and alpha-bungarotoxin are antagonists.

5. **ACh-NN (N_2):**
   - Distributed in autonomic ganglia, suprarenal medulla, and CNS.
   - On stimulation at various sites, they produce transmission of impulse in

ANG, release of catecholamine and excitation or inhibition of CNS by opening up of cationic channels (Na^+, K^+, Ca^{++}) resulting in depolarization.

- Nicotine, ACh, dimethyl-phenyl piperazinium are agonists while hexamethonium and trimetaphan are antagonists.

Adrenergic Receptors

Norepinephrine is the neurotransmitter at the sympathetic postganglionic nerve terminals that innervate visceral effectors. Based on the nature and physiological response obtained, adrenoceptors are classified as alpha (α_1 and α_2) and beta (β_1 and β_2) receptors. Generally, alpha receptors are excitatory (vasoconstric-

tion) and beta receptors are inhibitory (vasodilatation) in nature with the exception of heart (β_1- stimulatory) and visceral smooth muscles (alpha and beta receptors are inhibitory).

Transmission in ANS: Two chemical transmitters have been established as neurotransmitters in the ANS. These are acetylcholine and norepinephrine. Both the transmitters are synthesized primarily in the nerve terminals and stored in the synaptic or varicosity vesicles until released by a nerve impulse. The effects of stimulating autonomic nerves on different organs are summarized in Table 18.1.

Drugs: Drugs acting on adrenergic receptor subtypes are listed in Table 18.2.

Table 18.1: Effects of stimulating autonomic nervous system on different organs

Tissue or organ	Adrenergic		Cholinergic
	Response	Receptor	Response
1	2	3	4
1. Blood vessels			
i. Arterioles			
a. Skin, splanchnic, cerebral, coronary	Constriction	α_1	Generalized vasodilatation and fall in blood pressure
b. Skeletal	Dilatation	β_2	
	Constriction	α	
ii. Veins			
a. Coronary	Constriction	α	
	Dilatation	β_2	
b. Pulmonary	Constriction	α	
	Dilatation	β_2	
c. Abdominal viscera	Constriction	α	
	Dilatation	β_2	
d. Renal	Constriction	α	
	Dilatation	β_2	
2. Heart			
i. SA node	Tachycardia	β_1, β_2	Bradycardia
ii. AV node	Tachycardia	β_1, β_2	Bradycardia
iii. Atria	Increased contraction	β_1, β_2	Decreased contraction
iv. Ventricles	Increased contraction	β_1, β_2	Slight decrease in contraction
v. Contractility	Increased	β_1, β_2	Decreased
vi. Automaticity	Increased	β_1, β_2	—
vii. Overall effect	Tachycardia and increase in cardiac output		Bradycardia and decrease in cardiac output.

3. Bronchial				
i. Muscles	Relaxation	β_2	Contraction	
ii. Glands	Decreased secretion	α_1,	Increased	
	Increased secretion	β_2	secretion	
4. Skin				
i. Pilomotor muscles	Contraction	α_1	—	
ii. Sweat gland	Increased secretion	α_1	—	
5. Eye				
i. Radial muscles, iris	Contraction	α_1	—	
ii. Circular muscle	—		Contraction	
iii. Ciliary muscle	Relaxation for far vision	β_2	Contraction	
iv. Pupil	Dilatation	α_1	Contraction	
v. Lachrymal glands	Secretion	α	Increased secretion	
6. Gastrointestinal tract				
i. Muscle	Relaxation	$\alpha_1, \alpha_2, \beta_1, \beta_2$	Contraction	
ii. Sphincter	Constriction	α_1	Relaxation	
iii. Glands	Decreased secretion	α_2	Increased secretion	
iv. Peristalsis	Decreased	$\alpha_1, \alpha_2, \beta_1, \beta_2$	Increased	
7. Urinary system				
i. Kidney (renin secretion)	Decreased; increased	α_1, β_1	—	
ii. Ureter (motility and tone)	Increased	α_1	—	
iii. Bladder				
a. Trigone	Contraction	α_1	—	
b. Detrusor	Relaxation	β_1	Contraction	
iv. Sphincter	Constriction	α_1	Relaxation	
8. Reproductive system				
i. Male sex organ	Ejaculation	α_1	Erection	
ii. Female sex organ	Relaxation	α_1, β_2	Contraction	
a. Uterus, pregnant	Contraction			
b. Uterus, non-pregnant	Relaxation	β_2		
9. Metabolism				
i. Liver	Glycogenolysis	β_2, α_1	—	
	Neoglucogenesis		—	
ii. Adipose cell	Lipolysis:	$\beta_1, \beta_2, \beta_3$	—	
	Inhibition of lipolysis	α_2		
10. Spleen capsule	Contraction; relaxation	α_1, β_2	—	
11. Lymphocyte	Stimulation		—	
12. Mast cell	Stabilization of membrane	β_2	—	
13. Pancreas				
i. Acini	Decreased secretion	α	Secretion	
ii. Islets	Decreased secretion:	α_2, β_2	—	
(β cells)	Increased secretion			
14. Salivary glands	K^+ and water secretion	α_1	K^+ and water secretion	
	Amylase secretion	β	—	
15. Pineal gland	Melatonin synthesis	β	—	
16. Posterior pituitary	ADH secretion	β_1	—	
17. Skeletal muscle	Increased contractility	β_2	—	
	Glycogenolysis: K^+ uptake			
18. Adrenal medulla	—	—	Secretion of epinephrine and norepinephrine	

Table 18.2:Drugs acting on adrenergic receptor subtypes

Receptor with location	Agonists	Antagonists	Mechanism of action
α_1 • Postsynaptic	Methoxamine Phenylephrine	Prazocin	Alteration of cellular Ca^{++} fluxes
α_2 • Presynaptic • Postsynaptic • Nonsynaptic (platelets)	Clonidine	Yohimbine	Inhibition of adenylatecyclase
β_1 • Postsynaptic	Dobutamine	Atenolol Metoprolol Propranolol Pindolol	Stimulation of adenylatecyclase
β_2 • Presynaptic • Postsynaptic • Nonsynaptic (Lymphocytes and poly- morphonuclear cells)	Isoetharine Orciprenaline Salbutamol Terbutaline	Propranolol Pindolol	Stimulation of adenylatecyclase

TO REMEMBER

1. Autonomic nervous system (ANS) maintains homeostasis by integrating with sensory, somatomotor, endocrinal, metabolic, immunological and emotional activities. It is divided into sympathetic (adrenergic) and parasympathetic (cholinergic) divisions.

2. ANS consists of afferent (conducts impulses from periphery to CNS) and efferent (conducts impulses from CNS to periphery) fibres. Efferent fibres may be cholinergic or adrenergic.

3. Cholinergic fibres have long and myelinated preganglionic fibres while short and non-myelinated postganglionic fibres. The neurotransmitter at pregang-lionic and postganglionic neuron is acetylcholine. The ganglia are located very close to the tissue, innervated.

4. Adrenergic fibres have long and non-myelinated postganglionic fibres (except adrenal medulla) and their ganglia are located away from organ. The neuro-transmitter at preganglionic fibres is acetylcholine, while mainly noradrena-line at postganglionic neuron except those which innervate sweat glands and some blood vessels in skeletal muscles where it is acetylcholine.

5. Cholinergic receptors are divided into muscarinic (M_1, M_2 and M_3 subtypes) and nicotinic (ACh-NM (N_1) and ACh-NN (N_2) subtypes) receptors.

6. Muscarinic receptors (M_1, M_2 and M_3) are blocked by atropine.

7. ACh-NM (N_1) nicotinic receptors are blocked by d-tubocurarine, while ACh-NN (N_2) nicotinic receptors are blocked by hexamethonium and trimetaphan.

8. Adrenergic receptors are classified as alpha (α_1 and α_2) and beta (β_1 and β_2) receptors. Generally, alpha receptors are excitatory and beta receptors are inhibitory with the exception of beta-1 receptors of heart (stimulatory)and alpha and beta receptors of visceral smooth muscles (inhibitory).

9. Norepinephrine is the neurotransmitter at the sympathetic postganglionic nerve terminals.

10. Both the neurotransmitters (ACh and NE) are synthesized primarily in the nerve terminals and stored in the synaptic or varicosity vesicles until released by a nerve impulse.

Chapter 19

Cholinergic Agonists (Parasympathomimetics)

Acetylcholine is a physiological neurotransmitter which acts on both muscarinic and nicotinic receptors. It is not useful as a drug being non-specific and having short duration of action. So such compounds have been developed which are more selective and have longer duration of action than acetylcholine. Drugs, which combine with acetylcholine receptors and mimic the effects of parasympathetic stimulation, are called parasympathomimetics or cholinergic agonists or cholinomimetic drugs. On the basis of their mode of action, they can be classified as under:

I. **Directly acting**
   1. *Cholinesters:*
      - Acetylcholine
      - Methacholine
      - Carbachol
      - Bethanechol.
   2. *Cholinomimetic alkaloids:*
      - Pilocarpine
      - Muscarine
      - Arecoline.
   3. *Miscellaneous:*
      - Oxotremorine
      - Metoclopramide.

II. **Indirectly acting (anticholinesterase agents)**
   1. *Reversible anticholinesterases (carbamates)*
      - Tertiary amine: Physostigmine (eserine)
      - Quaternary ammonium compounds:
        i. Neostigmine (prostigmine)

ii. Pyridostigmine(mestinone)
iii. Ambenonium(mytelase)
iv. Edrophonium(tensilon)
v. Demecarium (humorosol)
   2. *Irreversible anticholinesterases (organophosphorus compounds):*
      - DFP (dyflos)
      - Echothiophate

Besides these agents, ganglionic stimulants also have parasympathomimetic action.

Directly Acting Drugs

Acetylcholine: It is an ester of choline and acetic acid. It is synthesized with the help of an enzyme cholineacetylase. It is stored in vesicles within the nerve and is released on nerve stimulation by exocytosis. It is rapidly hydrolyzed in the body by acetylcholinesterase and pseudocholinesterase enzymes. Acetylcholinesterase is present in all the sites of action of acetylcholine and has high specificity for acetylcholine. Pseudocholinesterase is found in plasma and liver and it is non-specific because it can break number of drugs with ester linkage.

The actions of acetylcholine are divided into two groups depending on its action on muscarinic or nicotinic receptors.

1. **Muscarinic actions** of acetylcholine are:
   - Stimulation of exocrine glands such as sweat, salivary, mucous, and lacrimal glands

- Stimulation of smooth muscle in bronchi, gastrointestinal tract, bile duct, urinary bladder and ureters
- Stimulation of circular muscle of the iris and the muscles of accommodation so that the pupil is constricted and the lens is fixed for near vision
- Relaxation of the smooth muscles of the blood vessels
- Slowing of the heart (bradycardia)
2. **Nicotinic actions** of acetylcholine are:
   - Stimulation of sympathetic and para-sympathetic ganglia
   - Stimulation of adrenal medulla to discharge epinephrine and norepine-phrine
   - Contraction of skeletal muscle.

Acetylcholine is not effective by oral route. The nicotinic effects are not seen in ordinary doses. On intravenous administration, it causes transient fall in blood pressure, bradycardia, flushing, sweating, salivation, lacrimation and increased mucous secretions. It is only employed in experimental pharma-cology as a tool to study parasympatho-mimetic effects.

Methacholine is a synthetic drug. It has similar muscarinic effects as that of acetylcholine. However, it has no nicotinic action. It has longer duration of action than

acetylcholine as three times more resistant to cholinesterases. It is poorly absorbed from gastrointestinal tract and is usually administered by subcutaneous route. It is rarely used now.

Carbachol is also synthetic drug. It has more potent muscarinic actions than acetylcholine on the gastrointestinal tract, urinary bladder and the iris. However, it has less pronounced effects on heart than acetylcholine. It is not hydrolyzed by cholinesterase enzymes. It has potent nicotinic actions also. It is employed to lower intraocular pressure in glaucoma (0.75–3% solution). It is less commonly used for the treatment of urinary retention.

Bethanechol is a synthetic drug. Its muscarinic effects are similar as that of carbachol. However, it is devoid of nicotinic activity. It has more selective action on gastrointestinal tract and the urinary bladder, but has slight effect on cardiovascular system. It is not hydrolyzed by cholinesterases. It is used orally in a dose of 2.5 to 5 mg to treat postoperative or neurogenic urinary retention.

Pilocarpine is an alkaloid. It is obtained from the leaves of *Pilocarpus jaborandi*. Like acetylcholine, it has muscarinic effects. However, it has prominent effect on the sweat glands and salivary glands. It also enhances gastric secretion but has less marked effects on cardiovascular system. Pilocarpine hydrochloride or nitrate (0.5 to 4% solution) is used for the treatment of glaucoma every 4–6 hours. It has also employed to produce miosis for counteracting the mydriatic and cycloplegic actions of atropine.

Important uses of directly acting cholinergic drugs

- *Methacholine:* May be used for the diagnosis of bronchial hyperactivity and asthmatic conditions.
- *Carbachol:* To lower intraocular pressure in glaucoma.
- *Bethanechol:* Urinary retention; post-operative abdominal distension; gastric atony and retention or gastroparesis.
- *Pilocarpine:* Glaucoma; xerostomia, following head and neck radiation or associated with Sjogren's syndrome in women; to counteract the mydriatic and cycloplegic actions of atropine

---

Contraindications in the use of choline esters

- *Bronchial asthma:* Precipitation of bronchospasm
- *Hyperthyroidism:* Precipitation of cardiac arrhythmias
- *Myocardial infarction:* Precipitation of hypotension and conduction block
- *Peptic ulcer:* Increase gastric acid secretion

Muscarine is an alkaloid that is obtained from the mushroom *Amanita muscaria*. It has 100 times more marked muscarinic effects than acetylcholine and has a prolonged effect because not destroyed by cholinesterases. Muscarinic poisoning is effectively treated by atropine.

Oxotremorine: It is an extremely potent synthetic compound. It stimulates central muscarinic receptors more than peripheral muscarinic receptors and produces tremors and extrapyramidal symptoms. It is used as an experimental tool.

Metoclopramide: It is a synthetic drug, that has cholinomimetic and anti-dopaminergic (D_2 receptor blocking) actions. It blocks D_2 receptors on chemoreceptor trigger zone and has antiemetic effect. Metoclopramide increases gastro-oesophageal sphincter pressure and prevents gastro-oesophageal reflux. It enhances gastric emptying and intestinal peristalsis. Atropine blocks its action on gastrointestinal tract being cholinomimetic in nature. However, this effect is not blocked by chlorpromazine like anti-dopaminergic drugs. It is well absorbed orally, and metabolized in liver; it crosses blood–brain barrier. Its uses are:

i. As an antiemetic

ii. Reflux oesophagitis

iii. Prior to radiological investigations of gastrointestinal tract

Dose: 10 mg 3 three times a day.

Indirectly Acting Drugs

Reversible Anticholinesterases (Carbamates)

Physostigmine (eserine): It is an alkaloid, obtained from the dried ripe seeds of *Physostigma venenosum*. It crosses the blood brain barrier and is well absorbed from gastrointestinal tract and conjunctiva. It is

Uses of reversible anticholinesterases	
Disease	*Drug of choice*
1. Glaucoma	Physostigmine
2. Myasthenia gravis	Pyridostigmine
	Ambenonium
	Neostigmine
3. Postoperative paralytic ileus and urinary retention	Neostigmine
4. Snake venom poisoning	Edrophonium
5. Atropine poisoning	Physostigmine

mainly used as a miotic and to treat glaucoma either alone (physostigmine sulphate—0.25–0.5%) or in combination with pilocarpine hydrochloride (2–4%). Physostigmine is used in the treatment of atropine, tricyclic antidepressant (imipramine), and antipsychotic (chlorpromazine) poisoning in doses of 0.5–2 mg i.v. bolus, repeated at 5–10 minute interval till the clinical signs of poisoning disappear. Physostigmine is used because it can antagonize both central and peripheral effects of these drugs.

Neostigmine (prostigmine): It is a synthetic quaternary ammonium compound with a quick onset of action. Although it has similar anticholinesterase activity to physostigmine but differs from it in that it is poorly absorbed orally, does not cross the blood-brain barrier and has direct skeletal muscle stimulant action. So it is particularly effective as an anticurare agent (0.5–2 mg i.m. or s.c.) and in the treatment of myasthenia gravis (15–30 mg orally 3 to 4 times daily).

Pyridostigmine: It closely resembles neostigmine. Its onset of action is slow but duration of action is longer. It is used in myasthenia gravis in doses of 60–240 mg per day orally or 1–5 mg intramuscularly or subcutaneously.

Edrophonium: It has a very short duration of action. So it is mainly used as a diagnostic agent to differentiate between cholinergic crisis and myasthenia crisis (10 mg i.v.).

Ambenonium: It is more potent and has a more sustained effect than neostigmine. It may be used for myasthenia gravis in a dose of 10–25 mg orally.

Demecarium: It is more potent and has a very prolonged effect. It is used in glaucoma in a dose of (0.25% solution) 2 drops twice weekly. Miosis occurs within 20 minutes and persists for a week.

Irreversible Anticholinesterases

Organophosphorus compounds cause irreversible inhibition of cholinesterase enzyme. Most of the insecticides and war gasses (nerve gasses) like tabun, sarin and soman belong to this category and are more of toxicological importance. DFP (di-isopropyl fluorophosphate) is used clinically as topical application (0.1% solution in arechis oil) for glaucoma (one drop instilled once or twice daily).

Ecothiophate has longer duration of action and is used in concentration of 0.06 to 0.25% solutions.

Treatment of organophosphorus poisoning: Since organophosphorus compounds are widely used as house hold and agricultural insecticides, acute and chronic poisoning with them are quite common. The acute intoxication is manifested by muscarinic and nicotinic signs and symptoms. The cause of death is central as well as peripheral respiratory paralysis followed by cardiovascular collapse. To save life, patient should be immediately given artificial respiration and treatment of shock should be started. The autonomic effects such as excessive salivation, bronchial secretion and bronchoconstriction are controlled by atropine (2–4 mg i.m. or i.v.). Administer pralidoxime (2PAM) i.v. in a dose of 1 to 2 gm to regenerate cholinesterase enzyme. The dose may be repeated if necessary. Administer suitable antibiotic to prevent secondary infection. Patient should be kept under vigilance for 72 hours to prevent relapse.

Myasthenia gravis: It is a chronic disease. It is characterized by abnormal skeletal muscle weakness and fatigue. It is now generally believed that myasthenia gravis is an autoimmune disease (antibody mediated). It occurs due to blockade of the acetylcholine receptors on the motor end plate of skeletal muscle. It is diagnosed by intravenous injection of the short acting anticholinesterase agent edrophonium that produces a brief increase in the muscle strength of the extremities. After proper diagnosis, treatment is started with oral administration of neostigmine, pyridostigmine or ambinonium.

Glaucoma: It is a major cause of blindness in persons over 40 years of age. There are two main types, i.e. open angle (wide angle) and narrow angle glaucoma. Open angle glaucoma is more common. In these patients, the aqueous humor fails to drain and continues to accumulate leading to increase intraocular pressure that in turn causes compression of the retina and optic nerve. Due to this, there occurs visual loss and blindness. Drugs are used to contract the ciliary muscles and constrict the pupil in order to enhance the drainage of aqueous humor (cholinergic and adrenergic drugs).

Some drugs also reduce the formation of aqueous humor.

Points for Dental Students

1. Many drugs produce side effects related to cholinergic system. These may be due to stimulation of muscarinic or nicotinic receptors. Hence the knowledge of basic principles of this system will be useful to understand them and minimize them.

2. Pilocarpine (5–10 mg TDS) or cervimeline (30 mg TDS) is used to treat xerostomia to avoid development of dental caries and oral candidiasis.

TO REMEMBER

1. Acetylcholine is not useful as a drug being non-specific and having short duration of action because it is rapidly hydrolyzed in the body by acetylcholinesterase and pseudocholinesterase enzymes.

2. Methacholine is a synthetic cholinergic drug, which is rarely used now.

3. Carbechol is also a synthetic cholinergic drug, which is less commonly used for the treatment of urinary retention.

4. Bethanochol is a synthetic drug which is used orally in a dose of 2.5 to 5 mg to treat postoperative or neurogenic urinary retention.

5. Pilocarpine is an alkaloid which is used in glaucoma and as miotic to counteract the mydriatic and cycloplegic actions of atropine.

6. Muscarine is an alkaloid. Its poisoning is effectively treated by atropine.

7. Oxotremorine is an extremely potent, synthetic compound which is used as an experimental tool.

8. Metoclopramide (synthetic drug) has cholinomimetic and antidopaminergic actions. It is used as an antiemetic, in reflux oesophagitis and prior to radiological investigations of gastrointestinal tract.

9. Physostigmine (eserine) is an alkaloid which is mainly used as a miotic in glaucoma and to treat atropine poisoning.

10. Neostigmine (prostigmine) is a synthetic quaternary ammonium compound which is particularly effective as an anticurare agent and in the treatment of myasthenia gravis.

11. Pyridostigmine is used in myasthenia gravis.

12. Edrophonium has short duration of action. So it is used to differentiate between cholinergic and myasthenia crisis.

13. Ambenonium may be used for myasthenia gravis.

14. Demecarium is used in glaucoma.

15. Acute or chronic organophosphorus poisoning is quite common because these compounds are widely used as house hold and agricultural insecticides. Treatment consists of: (a) artificial respiration, (b) treatment of shock and (c) administration of atropine and pralidoxime.

16. Myasthenia gravis is a chronic disease which is treated by neostigmine or pyridostigmine or ambinonium.

Chapter 20

Anticholinergic Drugs

Anticholinergic drugs selectively reduce or abolish the muscarinic receptor mediated effects of acetylcholine and parasympathetic stimulation. So these drugs are also called antimuscarinic or parasympatholytic agents. These drugs inhibit the actions of endogenous acetylcholine and muscarinic agonists at muscarinic receptor sites in peripheral tissues and in the central nervous system. The actions of acetylcholine at the nicotinic sites (neuromuscular junction, autonomic ganglia and adrenal medulla) are, however, not blocked by anticholinergic drugs. The nicotinic actions of acetylcholine are blocked by neuromuscular blocking (d-tubocurarine) and ganglionic blocking (mecamylamine) agents.

Belladona Alkaloids

Clinically two natural alkaloids, atropine (from *Atropa belladona*, *Datura stramonium* and *Atropa accuminata*) and hyoscine (from *Hyoscyamus niger* and *Scopala carniolica*) are used. The pharmacological effects of atropine are described below as a prototype of cholinergic antagonists.

1. **Exocrine glands:** Atropine inhibits salivary, lacrimal and bronchial glands. So it causes dryness of mucous membranes. It also reduces total acidity and volume of basal (fasting) gastric secretion, pepsin and mucous secretions. Sweating is diminished by atropine leading to an increase in body temperature.

2. **Gastrointestinal system:** Atropine effectively reduces the tone and motility of the gut. It, therefore, causes prolongation of gastric emptying time, closure of the sphincters and decrease in tone, amplitude and frequency of peristaltic movements. Atropine has little effect on biliary tract.

3. **Respiratory tract:** The smooth muscles of bronchioles are relaxed. However, it is not useful in bronchial asthma because of the involvement of other spasmogens.

4. **Urinary tract:** Atropine reduces tone of the ureter and relaxes detrusor muscle of the urinary bladder with increased tone of trigonal sphincter.

5. **Eye:**
   - Atropine causes passive dilatation of the pupil by blocking the muscarinic receptors of circular muscle of the iris.
   - It causes cycloplegia (loss of accommodation) by paralysing the ciliary muscle.

6. **Cardiovascular system:**
   - In small doses, there may be a brief bradycardia due to transient stimulation of vagal centre and blockade of presynaptic M_1 receptors on the postganglionic parasympathetic nerve supplying SA node. This is followed by tachycardia due to the blockade of vagus nerve on the heart.
   - In large dose, there may be rise in blood pressure due to stimulation of vasomotor centre.

- In very large doses, there may be cutaneous vasodilatation in face and neck (atropine flush) due to direct effect unrelated to cholinergic innervation.

7. **Central nervous system:**
   - In therapeutic dose (0.5 –1mg), atropine causes mild stimulation of respiratory centre, vagal centre and inhibition of tremor and rigidity of skeletal muscle in parkinsonism by reducing cholinergic over activity in basal ganglia.
   - However, larger doses produce marked central nervous system stimulation which may cause restlessness, irritability, excitement, agitation, disorientation, delirium and hallucination.
   - Death occurs due to respiratory failure and coma.

Pharmacokinetics: Being lipid soluble atropine is readily absorbed from the gut, mucous surfaces and from the intact skin. It can cross the blood–brain barrier, placental barrier and is secreted in milk and saliva. It is considerably bound to plasma proteins and partly metabolized in liver as glucuronide. About 50% is excreted unchanged and the rest as metabolites in the urine.

Side effects: The common side effects of atropine and other antimuscarinic drugs are dry mouth, visual disturbances (photophobia, and blurred vision), constipation, urinary retention, tachycardia and central nervous system effects.

In toxic doses, there also occurs difficulty in swallowing, hot and dry skin, rash on the face, neck and upper part of the trunk, weak and very rapid pulse, urinary urgency and difficulty in micturition.

Treatment of atropine poisoning consists of:
a. Gastric lavage
b. Physostigmine—0.5–2 mg i.v. bolous dose, repeated at 5–10 minutes till the clinical signs of poisoning disappear. It is preferred on neostigmine due to its central and peripheral effects.
c. Artificial respiration
d. Alcohol sponging to reduce fever.

Anticholinergic drugs are contraindicated in gluacoma, and should be given with care to elderly patients.

Semisynthetic and Synthetic Cholinergic Antagonists

According to their therapeutic uses, they have been classified into following groups:

1. **Mydriatic and cycloplegic drugs:** These drugs are used topically. They can be used in cases of intolerance to atropine. As against the atropine and hyoscine, these drugs have shorter duration of action and are devoid of systemic effects when instilled locally.
   Drugs: Homatropine, eucatropine, cyclopentolate, tropicamide.

2. **Antispasmodic drugs:** The common features of these drugs are:
   - Most of them are either quarternary compounds or tertiary amines.
   - Oral absorption is poor and unpredictable.
   - Duration of action is longer than atropine.
   - Do not cross blood–brain barrier and conjunctival barrier.
   - Their fate and excretion from the body are little known.
   - Mainly used to reduce secretions and spasm of gastrointestinal and genitourinary system
   - There occurs ganglion blockade in higher dose.
   - In still higher doses, neuromuscular blocked and respiratory paralysis may occur.

   Drugs:
   A. *Quarternary compounds:*
   i. Semisynthetic: Atropine methonitrate, homatropine methylbromide, and hyoscine methylbromide, hyoscine butylbromide, amprotropine, anisotropine.

ii. Synthetic: Propantheline, isopropamide, oxyphenonium, ipratropium bromide, clidinium, glycopyrrolate, mepenzolate, penthienate, pipenzolate. Although this group includes a large number of drugs, there is no much advantage of one compound over the other.

B. *Tertiary amines:* Synthetic: Dicyclomine, pirenzepine, telenzepine.

3. **Antiparkinsonian drugs:** These synthetic atropine substitutes cross blood–brain barrier. Acting on basal ganglia, they restore the balance between the neurotransmitters acetylcholine (excitatory) and dopamine (inhibitory) which is disturbed in parkinsonism.

Drugs:
- Benzhexol hydrochloride
- Benztropine
- Mesylate
- Biperidine hydrochloride
- Orphenadrine hydrochloride
- Procyclidine hydrochloride
- Promethazine hydrochloride

Therapeutic Uses of Cholinergic Antagonists

1. **Central nervous system conditions:**

   a. *Parkinsonism:* Anticholinergic drugs are less effective than levodopa. These are used in mild cases, in drug induced extrapyramidal syndrome and as helping drug to levodopa. Synthetic antimuscarinic drugs are more selective for this purpose.

   b. *Motion sickness:* Hyoscine hydrobromide is preferred due to its more sedative and central effects.

   c. *Twilight sleep:* Hyoscine plus meperidine are used during labour to produce amnesia, analgesia and a relaxed state.

   d. *Maniacal state* during withdrawal of alcohol in chronic alcoholics. Hyoscine is used because of its sedative effect.

2. **Eye conditions:**

   a. Atropine and its congeners (preferred due to shorter duration and minimal side effects) are used as an eyedrop or ointment to produce mydriasis and cycloplegia for examination of retina and measurement of refractive error.

   b. Atropine sulphate can be used alternating with a miotic to break the adhesions between the iris and lens in uveitis and iritis.

   c. Since atropine has long lasting mydriatic-cycloplegic and local anodyne action on cornea, it is very effective in the treatment of iritis, iridocyclitis, choroiditis, keratitis, corneal ulcer.

3. **Gastrointestinal conditions:**

   a. Synthetic atropine substitutes can be used as antispasmodics in:
   - Intestinal colic
   - Ulcerative colitis
   - Biliary colic
   - Traveler's diarrhoea

   b. Peptic ulcer: They are employed as adjuncts to antacids or H_2 receptor blockers.

   c. Irritable colon

   d. Gastritis, gastric hypermotility, nervous dyspepsia, pylorospasm.

4. Atropine and antimuscarinics are used as preanaesthetic medication:
   - To reduce bronchial and salivary secretions caused by irritant volatile and gasseous anaesthetics.
   - To prevent excessive vagal slowing of the heart.

5. Atropine is sometimes used to treat irregularities of the heart caused by partial block of the conducting tissue and also to treat bradycardia in myocardial infarction.

6. Atropine is used as an antidote in poisoning due to cholinesterase inhibitors.

7. Inhaled ipratropium bromide is useful in the management of asthmatic bronchitis and chronic obstructive pulmonary disease.

Points for Dental Students

1. Atropine is kept as one of the emergency drugs in dental clinic.
2. Adverse effects of many drugs are due to their anticholinergic actions. So the knowledge of basic principles of this system is important for dental students to understand such side effects and minimize those taking precautions.
3. Some anticholinergic drugs such as scopolamine, glycopyrrolate and propantheline are used in dental procedures to control excessive salivation. These are used to provide dry oral cavity during surgery. Out of the two, glycopyrrolate is preferred because it is a selective antisialagogue and has low incidence of tachycardia in therapeutic doses.

TO REMEMBER

1. Anticholinergic drugs selectively reduce or abolish the muscarinic receptor mediated effects of acetylcholine and parasympathetic stimulation. Nicotinic actions of acetylcholine are blocked by neuromuscular blocking (d-tubo-curarine) and ganglionic blocking (mecamylamine) agents.
2. Synthetic antimuscarinic drugs (benzhexol, benztropine, biperidine, orphenadrine, procyclidine and promethazine) are more selective for the treatment of parkinsonism.
3. Hyoscine is preferred in motion sickness due to its more sedative and central effects.
4. Hyoscine plus meperidine are used during labour to produce amnesia, analgesia and a relaxed state (twilight sleep).
5. Hyoscine is used to treat maniacal state during withdrawal of alcohol in chronic alcoholics due to its sedative effect.
6. To examine retina and measure refrective error, atropine congeners are preferred due to short duration and minimal side effects.
7. To break the adhesions between the iris and lens in uveitis and iritis, atropine sulphate can be used alternating with a miotic.
8. Atropine is used: (a) as an antidote in poisoning due to cholinesterase inhibitors, (b) to treat irregularities of the heart and (c) as preanaesthetic medication.
9. Synthetic atropine substitutes can be used as antispasmodics in intestinal colic, ulcerative colitis, biliary colic and traveller's diarrhoea.

Chapter 21

Adrenergic Agonists (Sympathomimetics)

Drugs which produce effects similar to those of adrenergic nerve stimulation or injection of epinephrine are known as sympathomimetics. Before considering these drugs, an account of the physiology of adrenergic nerves would be helpful.

Biosynthesis: The varicosities (terminal swollen areas) of the adrenergic neurons are the sites of synthesis of norepinephrine. L-tyrosine, an essential amino acid, is the precursor of norepinephrine. It is taken up from the extracellular fluid and oxidized to dihydroxy phenylalanine (DOPA) with the help of L-tyrosine hydroxylase enzyme. Dopa is further converted into dopamine by dopa decarboxylase enzyme. Finally, dopamine is acted upon by dopamine beta hydroxylase and transformed into norepinephrine (Fig. 21.1).

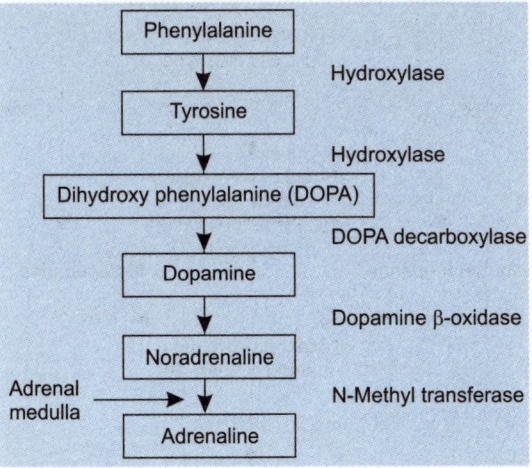

Fig. 21.1: Biosynthesis of catecholamines

In the chromaffin cells of the adrenal medulla, norepinephrine, in the presence of N-methyl transferase and S-adenosylme-thionin, is changed to epinephrine.

Storage of norepinephrine: Inside the nerve ending, there are two stores of norepinephrine: granular and cytoplasmic. The granular store consists of tiny granules or vesicles which are bound by distinct membranes. Within them, norepinephrine exists partly in free state and partly in combination with ATP in a ratio of 4:1. The complex with ATP is then absorbed on a specific protein called chromogranin. The uptake of norepinephrine from the cytoplasm into granules is an active process, which can be inhibited by reserpine. There is equilibrium between the granular and cytoplasmic store, and norepinephrine can pass from the former to the latter by passive diffusion.

The cytoplasmic store consists of free norepinephrine. Most of it is formed by intraneuronal biosynthesis, but some is absorbed from extracellular fluid through the axonal membrane by an active process which can be blocked by cocaine and reserpine. The size of the cytoplasmic store is probably regulated by mitochondrial monoamine oxidase (MAO).

Release of norepinephrine: When the impulse comes, there is localized depolarization of the postganglionic nerve terminal membrane. This results in an increased Ca^{++} permeability which causes fusion of storage vesicles to the inner surface of neuronal membrane and release of norepinephrine (along with ATP and neuropeptide Y) occurs by exocytosis into the synaptic cleft.

Actions on adrenergic receptors: On release in the synaptic cleft, norepinephrine acts on postsynaptic adrenoceptors on the effector organ or cell and produce appropriate action depending on the type of receptors activated. A part of norepinephrine, however, acts on:

a. Presynaptic alpha-2 adrenoceptors which exert a local inhibitory effect on the terminal from which it was released.

b. Presynaptic beta-2 adrenoceptors which facilitate the release of norepinephrine from the terminal.

Thus the neuronal release of norepinephrine is regulated through these presynaptic receptors according to the need of the body. Presynaptic receptors of dopamine, histamine, prostaglandins, angiotensin-II and enkephalin are also present on the adrenergic neurons and all of them also modulate the release of noradrenaline.

Fate of norepinephrine: 75–80% of norepinephrine released into the synaptic cleft is taken up back into nerve terminal by an active process against concentration gradient for reuse (uptake 1). This process is blocked by cocaine. Some of norepinephrine is removed from circulation at extraneuronal site (uptake 2). A small portion is excreted unchanged in urine, and another small portion combines with receptors to initiate the response. The remainder part of the neurotransmitter is metabolized by two enzymes, monoamine oxidase (MAO) and catechol-O-methyl transferase (COMT).

A portion of norepinephrine which leaks out from granules into cytoplasm as well as that taken up by axonal transport is probably first attacked by MAO within the neuron and converted into 3,4 dihydroxymendalic acid; subsequently outside the neuron, this is acted upon by COMT to form 3-methoxy 4-hydroxy mendalic acid (VMA or vanilomendalic acid). VMA is then excreted in the urine. The norepinephrine which diffuses into circulation is first converted by COMT to normetanephrine in liver and other tissues and subsequently by extraneuronal MAO to vanilomendalic acid which is excreted in urine. In case of epinephrine, it is first converted by COMT to metanephrine and subsequently to vanilomendalic acid by MAO (Fig. 21.2).

A normal individual excretes 4–8 mg of VMA and 50–100 µg of free epinephrine and norepinephrine in 24 hours. These values are considerably raised in pheochromocytoma, a tumor of the adrenal medulla.

Mechanism of Action of Adrenergic Drugs

1. Some adrenergic agents act directly on the adrenergic receptors located on the effector cells and initiate a pharmacological response such as epinephrine, norepinephrine, dopamine, isoproterenol and phenylephrine.

2. Others act indirectly by stimulating the release of norepinephrine from nerve endings such as amphetamine, ephedrine,

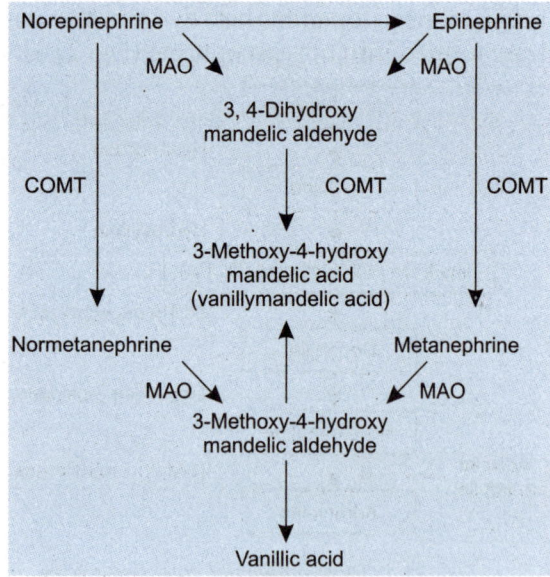

Fig. 21.2: Metabolism of norepinephrine and epinephrine

and tyramine. The continuous use or repeated administration of indirectly acting drugs produce progressive reduction in the response due to depletion of norepinephrine from nerve terminals. This diminished response over a period of time, is called tachyphylaxis.

All adrenoceptors are G-protein coupled receptors. These have seven transmembrane α-helical segments and show considerable molecular heterogenicity. Alpha-1 receptors are coupled to phospholipase C. They produce inositol 1, 4, 5,-triphosphate (IP3) and diacylglycerol (DAG) as second messengers and raise intracellular calcium. The alpha-2 receptors are negatively coupled to adenyl-cyclate cyclase. So their stimulation leads to decrease in cAMP formation. All three types of beta receptors, however, stimulate adenylate cyclase. So there occurs increase in cAMP formation.

Classification of Adrenergic Agonists

Directly Acting

1. Non-specific alpha and beta receptors agonists:
   - Epinephrine
   - Norepinephrine.
2. Non-specific beta-receptors agonist:
   - Isoprenaline
3. Alpha-1 agonists:
   - Phenylephrine
   - Oxymetazoline
   - Xylometazoline
   - Naphazoline
   - Phenylpropanolamine
   - Mephentramine
   - Methoxamine
   - Metraminol.
4. Alpha-2 agonists:
   - Clonidine
   - Alpha-methyldopa
   - Guanfacine
   - Gaunbenz

5. Beta-1 receptor agonists:
   - Dobutamine
   - Dopexamine
   - Xamoterol
6. Beta-2 receptor agonists:
   - Salbutamol
   - Terbutaline
   - Orciprenaline
   - Soxuprine
   - Ritodrine
   - Isoetharine
   - Fenoterol
   - Nylidrine
   - Salmeterol.
7. DA receptor agonist:
   - Dopaeoale.

Indirectly Acting

- Amphetamine
- Dexamphetamine
- Methamphetamine
- Hydroxy-amphetamine
- Phenametrazine

Pharmacology of Catecholamines

The term catecholamine is derived from the structure of the molecule, which consists of catechol (3, 4 dihydroxy benzene) and ethylamine side chain. Epinephrine, norepinephrine, isoproterenol and dopamine are catecholamines.

Effect on cardiovascular system: Acting on β_1 receptors, epinephrine increases the rate and force of contraction of heart and the cardiac output. Conduction across AV node is enhanced and ventricular arrhythmias may be produced.

Both epinephrine and norepinephrine produce powerful vasoconstriction of the blood vessels of the skin and mucous membrane which contain alpha-receptors. Being pure beta-receptor agonist, isoprenaline has no effect on the vasculature of these vessels. The blood vessels in the visceral organs including kidney contain mainly alpha-receptors. So epinephrine and norepinephrine cause vasoconstriction and decrease blood flow through these organs. Isoprenaline produces no effect or may cause a week vasodilatation in these organs where beta-receptors are present. Epinephrine has a complex action on the blood vessels of skeletal muscle which contain both alpha and beta-2 receptors. Low doses of epinephrine cause dilation of blood vessels whereas large doses will induce vasoconstriction. If large doses are used first, there occurs vasoconstriction followed by vasodilatation. The former effect is mediated by alpha-receptors and later is mediated by beta-2 receptors.

Blood pressure: On intravenous administration, blood pressure rises rapidly. Since systolic blood pressure is increased more than diastolic blood pressure, pulse pressure is also increased. As the concentration of epinephrine decreases in the blood, the mean blood pressure falls below normal before returning to control level. The increase in blood pressure is due to its direct effect on heart (positive inotropic and positive chronotropic effect) and vasoconstriction of blood vessels. Fall in blood pressure below normal is due to vasodilatation of blood vessels which is long lasting than vasoconstrictor effect. Norepinephrine increases systolic and diastolic blood pressure and total peripheral resistance. However, cardiac output is unchanged. Norepinephrine produces compensatory vagal reflex bradycardia. The coronary blood flow is enhanced by epinephrine and norepinephrine.

Effect on respiration: On intravenous administration, epinephrine produces brief apnea followed by short lived stimulation.

Effect on smooth muscles: Acting on β_2-adrenoceptors epinephrine and isoproterenol cause potent bronchodilation. Catecholamines relax smooth muscle of the gastrointestinal tract, reduce motility and contract sphincters. However, these effects are transient when catecholamines are used clinically. The effect of epinephrine on human uterus varies depending on different stages of pregnancy. During the last month of pregnancy, epinephrine inhibits uterine tone and contraction. More specific beta-receptor stimulants like albuterol and terbutaline may be useful in delaying premature labour.

Epinephrine and norepinephrine relax detrusor muscle (beta-receptor) and contract the trigone and sphincter muscles (alpha-receptor) of the urinary bladder. This may lead to hesitancy in urination and retention of urine.

Epinephrine and to a lesser extent norepinephrine cause mydriasis (dilation of pupil).

Metabolic effects: Norepinephrine has least metabolic effects. Acting on beta-receptors, epinephrine and isoproterenol increase oxygen consumption; stimulate hepatic and skeletal muscle glycogenolysis and release free fatty acids from adipose tissue.

Effect on central nervous system: There is no significant effect on central nervous system in therapeutic doses. Restlessness, apprehension, headache and tremor may be seen as a secondary effects due to the profound cardio-respiratory and peripheral metabolic effects of catecholamines.

Side effects: Fear, anxiety, restlessness, throbbing headache, tremor, weakness and palpitation appear as side effects. These effects disappear with rest, quiet and reassurance. Cardiac arrhythmias, hypertension, cerebral haemorrhage and acute pulmonary oedema occur with accidental overdose of catecholamines.

Preparation and Dosage

1. **Epinephrine (adrenaline):** It is available as 1 : 1000 sterile solutions in 1 ml ampules. It may be administered by subcutaneous, intramuscular or intracardiac routes. It is

also available for inhalation (1% aqueous solution) purpose. It is employed with local anaesthetics in concentrations of 1:1, 00,000 to 1:20,000 to prolong its effect.

2. **Norepinephrine (noradrenaline, levarterenol):** It is supplied as 1 mg/ml of levarterenol bitartrate. It is generally diluted with 1000 ml of 5% dextrose solution to give a final concentration of 4 µg/ml of levarterenol base. The solution is infused at a rate of 0.5 to 1 ml/minute.

3. **Isoproterenol (isoprenaline, isuprel):** It is available for parenteral use (1:5000), for inhalation (1:200; 1:100) and for sublingual (15–20 mg) administration. It may also be given by rectal route.

4. **Dopamine:** It is a naturally occurring catecholamine. It is the immediate precursor of the norepinephrine. Dopamine acts on alpha, beta and specific dopamine receptors. It also releases norepinephrine from storage vesicles. It produces a positive inotropic effect and increases systolic and pulse pressure. It has less prominent effect on heart rate. In low doses, it produces vasodilatation of renal and mesenteric blood vessels by acting on specific dopamine receptors. It is given by infusion at a rate of 20 µg/kg/min.

5. **Dobutamine:** It has structural resemblance with dopamine. It is a selective beta-1 adrenoceptor stimulant. It increases the force of contraction without increasing the heart rate. It does not act on the dopaminergic receptors in the renal vasculature. It is administered by intravenous infusion at a rate of 2.5–10 µg/kg/min.

6. **Dopexamine:** It is an inotropic agent which stimulates cardiac dopamine and peripheral beta-2 receptors. It is given by intravenous infusion via caval catheter in the dose of 0.5–1 µg/kg/min.

Therapeutic Uses

Epinephrine: Its important uses are:
- Allergic disorders (opposing the effects of histamine and other mediators of allergic reactions-physiological antagonist):
  a. Anaphylactic shock
  b. Urticaria
  c. Hay fever
  d. Angioneurotic oedema
  e. Serum sickness
- Bronchial asthma and status asthmaticus.
- To prolong the action of infiltration anaesthesia (with local anaesthetics).
- In ophthalmology for reducing intraocular pressure in cases of simple glaucoma.
- As expedient measure in insulin hypo-glycaemia.
- Epinepherine hydrochloride (1:1000) or phenylepherine hydrochloride (1:100) is used to control capillary bleeding during surgical procedure on gingival tissue.

The cardiovascular uses of epinephrine such as sudden cardiac arrest in healthy individuals and Stokes-Adam syndrome are limited as it can produce fatal cardiac arrhythmias.

Norepinephrine: It has been used in:
- States of shock by infusion. However, it is not used for the treatment of endotoxic or haemorrhagic shock where circulating catecholamine level is already very high.
- Partial or complete AV block to maintaine sufficient ventricular rate

Dopamine is useful in the treatment of:
- Shock, particularly cardiogenic or bacteremic shock
- Chronic cardiac decompensation as in congestive heart failure

Dobutamine: It is used in the treatment of heart failure associated with myocardial infarction.

Dopexamine: It is used in heart failure associated with cardiac surgery.

Pharmacology of Non-catecholamines

Although catecholamines are very powerful adrenergic drugs, they have certain disadvantages as under:

- They are inactive orally.
- They have a short duration of action being rapidly metabolized by MAO and COMT enzymes.
- They are generally non-selective, acting on both alpha and beta receptors.
- They do not cross blood–brain barrier.

To overcome these difficulties, a number of non-catecholamine compounds have been developed. These compounds have following properties:

- Some of them are orally effective, e.g. amphetamine, dexamphetamine.
- Some of these compounds (amphetamine, dexamphetamine, and ephedrine) cross blood–brain barrier due to lipid solubility and produce central effects.
- Some of these compounds (amphetamine and related drugs) resist degradation by MAO and COMT and have long duration of action.
- Many of the directly acting drugs of this group have receptor selectivity, e.g. phenylepherine (alpha-1 agonist), clonidine (alpha-2 agonist) and salbutamol (beta-2 agonist).

Phenylepherine: It is a potent alpha-receptor agonist with very little beta-activity. It causes rise in blood pressure by causing vasoconstriction of peripheral blood vessels. As a pressor agent, drug can be given intramuscularly or intravenously in a dose of 5 mg followed by 10 mg if necessary. It is also used as mydriatic and nasal decongestant (2.5 mg/ml).

Metaraminol: It is a directly acting sympathomimetic drug with similar actions as that of norepinephrine. However, it has longer duration of action as it is not metabolized by MAO enzyme. It is used mainly as a pressor agent for maintaining blood pressure during anaesthesia, haemorrhage and other hypotensive states. It is used intramuscularly in a dose of 2–10 mg. It can also be given by slow intravenous infusion.

Methoxamine: It acts almost exclusively on alpha-receptors and has no stimulant action on heart. It increases systolic and diastolic blood pressure. Reflex bradycardia is seen. It has a prolonged action (1–1.5 hr) as not metabolized by MAO or COMT enzymes. It is used to restore or maintain blood pressure during spinal anaesthesia or general anaesthesia. It is given by intramuscular or intravenous route (10–20 mg/ml).

Ephedrine: It is a naturally occurring alkaloid, obtained from plants of the genus Ephedra. It mainly acts by causing the release of norepinephrine (indirect effect) and also has some direct action on alpha-receptors. So ephedrine raises arterial blood pressure. It also has CNS stimulating property. Ephedrine is mainly used as bronchodilator in asthma (15–60 mg, given 3–4 times daily orally). It is also used as nasal decongestant (0.5% solution), mydriatic (2–5% solution) and in certain allergic disorders. Side effects are tachycardia, premature systoles, insomnia, nervousness, and emotional disturbances.

Amphetamine (dexedrine): It is an indirectly acting sympathomimetic amine. So its effect depends on the release of norepinephrine from adrenergic nerves. It has a potent CNS stimulant action. Its occasional uses are:

- Obesity (due to anorexia effect and CNS stimulant effect)
- Narcolepsy (sleep occurring in fits)
- Epilepsy to counteract sedation caused by antiepileptics
- Parkinsonism to improve mood and reduce rigidity(slight)
- Hyperkinetic children (attention deficit hyperkinetic disorder) to calm down these children

- Nocturnal enuresis in children and urinary incontinence due to its central action as well as its ability to increase tone of vesicle sphincter

Methamphetamine is very similar to amphetamine with even higher degree of CNS stimulant property.

Selective Beta-2 Adrenoceptor Stimulants

These drugs are selective agonists of β_2 receptors and produce relaxation of smooth muscles of bronchi, uteri, and gastrointestinal tract. Adverse effects are similar to those of isoprenaline though they are less severe. Amongst the β_2 agonists, salbutamol is widely used.

Salbutamol: It has long duration of action because it is not metabolized by MAO and COMT. It is almost completely devoid of cardiovascular effects. It can be given by all routes of administration. It is used in asthma (Oral: 2–4 mg TDS and inhalation: Dose 100–200 µg). It may be administered in a dose of 10–45 µg/min by slow intravenous infusion to inhibit uterine contraction (tocolytic action) to prevent delivery/birth prior to 37th week of gestation (preterm delivery/birth).

Terbutaline: It is chemically related to orciprenaline but has more selective action on β_2 receptors. It is used as a bronchodilator in asthma (Oral: 2.5 to 5 mg BD or TDS). Important side effects are nervousness, tremor, palpitation, drowsiness, nausea and vomiting. It is contraindicated in patients with hyperthyroidism and hypertension.

Salmeterol is a long acting (12 hours) β_2 adrenergic agonist. It is weaker agonist than salbutamol. Its onset of action is slow. It is used in the prevention of asthmatic attacks, especially the nocturnal ones and those induced by exercise. Its dose is 1–2 puffs (25 µg per puff) every 12 hours.

Isoetharine (30–40 mg/day), **rimiterol** (200 µg inhalation) and **fenoterol** (100–200 µg inhalation) are other β_2 selective agonists, which are used for the treatment of acute episodes of bronchoconstriction.

Ritodrine is a β_2 selective agonist which is administered in doses of 50 µg/min i.v. infusion in obstetrics as tocolytic agent.

Reproterol (0.5–1 mg by aerosol inhalation) is used in intermittent episodes and for prophylaxis in exercise-induced bronchospasm.

Other Sympathomimetics

- **Cocaine:** It is a local anaesthetic with a sympathomimetic action. It acts by inhibiting the neuronal reuptake of norepinephrine. It readily enters the brain and possesses potent CNS effects. It is widely abused (addicting) drug.
- **Tyramine:** It is found in many food products such as cheese, beer and wine. It has indirect sympathomimetic action. It is readily metabolized by MAO enzyme. Some of the food drug interactions are due to tyramine content of food.

Points for Dental Students

1. Concern often arises regarding the use of vasoconstrictor in patients with hypertension and heart disease. Vasoconstrictors enhance the depth and duration of local anaesthesia, thus reduces the anaesthetic dose and potential toxicity. If caution is used to avoid intravascular injection, lidocaine with 1:100,000 epinephrine (limited to a total of 0.036 mg epinephrine) can be used safely in those with controlled hypertension and stable coronary heart disease, arrhythmia, or congestive heart failure. Precaution should be taken with patients to tricyclic antidepressants and non-selective beta blockers, since these drugs may potentiate the effect of epinephrine.

2. Pressor agents may be required to maintain blood pressure during dental surgery. So a dental student must learn their pharmacodynamic and pharmacokinetic properties for safe use.

3. Adverse effects of many drugs are due to their action on adrenergic receptors (α or β). So it is important to learn the basic principles of this system. It will be useful to understand the side effects and minimize them.

4. Do not use terbutaline powder for inhalation in asthmatic patients because it may harm tooth enamel and cause tooth erosion due to its < 5.5 pH.

TO REMEMBER

1. Adrenergic agonists are drugs which produce effects similar to those of adrenergic nerve stimulation or injection of epinephrine.

2. Norepinephrine is synthesized in the varicosities of the adrenergic neuron. Inside the nerve ending, there are two stores of norepinephrine.

3. Norepinephrine and epinephrine are metabolized by catechol-O-methyl transferase and monoamine oxidase enzymes and excreted in urine as vanilomendalic acid.

4. Some adrenergic agonists (catecholamines) act directly on the adrenergic receptors located on the effector cells and initiate pharmacological response while others (non-catecholamines) act indirectly by stimulating the release of norepinephrine from nerve endings. Some may act by both the mechanisms.

5. Important uses of epinephrine are anaphylactic shock, urticaria, angioneurotic oedema, serum sickness, bronchial asthma, status asthmaticus and to prolong the action of infiltration anaesthesia.

6. Norepinephrine may be used in states of shock and partial or complete heart block.

7. Dopamine is used in the treatment of shock and congestive heart failure.

8. Dobutamine is employed in the treatment of heart failure associated with myocardial infarction by i.v. infusion.

9. Dopexamine stimulates cardiac dopamine and peripheral beta-2 receptors. It is used in heart failure associated with cardiac surgery.

10. Other pressor agents are phenylepherine, metraminol, and methoxamine. Phenylepherine is also used as mydriatic and nasal decongestant.

11. Ephedrine is used in bronchial asthma, as nasal decongestant, mydriatic and in certain allergic disorders.

12. Salbutamol, terbutaline, isoetharine and salmeterol are selective agonists of beta-2 receptors and produce relaxation of smooth muscles of bronchi, uteri, and gut. Amongst them, salbutamol is widely used in asthma and to inhibit uterine contraction.

Chapter 22

Adrenoceptor Blocking Agents

Adrenoceptor blocking agents or adrenoceptor antagonists are drugs that inhibit responses mediated by adrenoceptor activation caused by epinephrine and related drugs. They also block (less completely) effects of adrenergic nerve stimulation. On the other hand, adrenergic neurone blocking drugs act on adrenergic neuronal membrane or contents and block (more completely) the effects of adrenergic nerve stimulation. However, they do not block the effects of injected epinephrine; they actually may potentiate its effect.

Adrenoceptor antagonists are competitive antagonists at alpha or beta adrenergic receptors. So they are classified as alpha-adrenoceptor blocking agents and beta-adrenoceptor blocking agents.

ALPHA RECEPTOR BLOCKING DRUGS

These drugs inhibit adrenergic responses mediated through alpha-adrenergic receptors. They do not affect those responses mediated through beta-receptors.

Classification

I. **Selective alpha-adrenoceptor blockers**
   a. Alpha-1 blockers: Prazosin, alfuzosin, terazosin, doxazosin, trimazosin, indoramin.
   b. Alpha-2 blockers: Yohimbine, idazoxan.
   c. Selective alpha-1A blocker: Tamsulosin

II. **Non-selective alpha-adrenoceptor blocker**
   a. *Reversible*
      • Imidazoline: Tolazoline, phentolamine
      • Ergot alkaloids: Ergotamine, ergotoxine
      • Hydrogenated ergot alkaloids: Dihydroergotamine
      • Phenothiazine: Chlorpromazine.
   b. *Non-reversible*
      • Beta haloalkyl amine: Phenoxybenzamine, dibenamine.

General Effects of Alpha-adrenoceptor Blockers

1. These drugs cause fall in blood pressure by blocking alpha-vasoconstrictor receptors. So there occurs reduction in peripheral resistance and pooling of blood in capacitance vessels. Due to this, venous return and cardiac output are reduced and blood pressure is decreased. They also interfere with postural reflex; so there occurs marked hypotension on standing and individual suffers with dizziness and syncope. Hypovolemia accentuates the hypotension. Pressor and other actions of selective alpha-agonists (norepinephrine, phenylephrine) are also antagonized. They block pressor action of epinephrine by blocking alpha vasoconstrictor receptors.

167

So after their administration epinephrine causes fall in blood pressure due to beta mediated vasodilatation. This phenomenon is called vasomotor reversal of Dale.

2. Reflex tachycardia occurs due to fall in mean arterial pressure and increased release of noradrenaline due to blockage of presynaptic α_2-receptors.

3. They cause miosis and nasal stuffiness due to blockage of alpha-receptors in radial muscles of iris and in nasal blood vessels, respectively.

4. Diarrhoea may occur due to partial inhibition of relaxant sympathetic influences and increased intestinal motility.

5. They may cause sodium retention and increase in blood volume due to reduction in renal blood flow and glomerular filtration rate as a result of hypotension. So there occurs more complete reabsorption of Na^+ and water in the tubules.

6. Alpha-adrenoceptor blocking agents inhibit ejaculation and may lead to impotence.

Most of these common effects are manifested as side effects such as palpitation, postural hypotension, nasal stuffiness, diarrhoea, fluid retention, inhibition of ejaculation and impotence.

Imidazoline

Tolazoline: It is a competitive antagonist of alpha-adrenoceptors. It causes fall in blood pressure due to direct action on vascular smooth muscles and partly due to competitive blockade of alpha-adrenoceptors. It has histamine like action on gastrointestinal motility. In therapeutic doses, it causes cardiac stimulation. It is fairly well absorbed from gastrointestinal tract on oral administration and is excreted by kidney mostly unchanged. It is mainly used in Raynaud's disease, thromboangitis obliterance, frostbite, etc. Oral dose is 25 to 50 mg thrice a day.

Phentolamine: It is also a competitive antagonist of alpha-adrenoceptors. In normal therapeutic doses, it does not block other receptors. However, very large doses of phentolamine can block the action of 5-HT also. It has a quick onset of action and short duration of action. It produces vasodilatation and fall in blood pressure by blocking the alpha-adrenoceptors on the vascular smooth muscles.

It is mainly used as a preliminary test (Regitine test) in the diagnosis of pheochromocytoma. An intravenous injection of 5 mg phentolamine causes a sizeable fall in blood pressure, if it is high due to large quantities of catecholamines circulating in the blood. A fall of 35/25 mm Hg is diagnostic. False positive results do occur. Hence if the test is positive, further investigations like estimation of urinary VMA are necessary.

Ergot alkaloids: Ergot (*Claviceps purpurea*) is a fungus that grows on rye. The alkaloids of ergot are divided into two groups:

a. *Amino acid alkaloids:* Ergotamine and ergotoxine (mixture of ergocristine, ergokryptine, and ergocornine). Also called peptide alkaloids.

b. *Amine alkaloid:* Ergonovine.

Erogotamine and erogotoxin possess alpha-receptor blocking, oxytocic and partial agonistic activity on alpha-receptors. The vasoconstrictor action of these alkaloids is partly due to partial alpha-agonistic activity as well as also due to direct action on the vascular smooth muscles. So this action is opposite to the indirect alpha blocking action. The semisynthetic hydrogenated derivatives are dihydroergotamine and hydergine. They are devoid of oxytocic, partial alpha agonistic and direct vasoconstrictor actions and are primarily alpha-receptor blockers. Ergonovine (ergometrine), an amine alkaloid, is primarily an oxytocic and is used for the same purpose.

Ergotamine is a potent vasoconstrictor and it is, therefore, used in migraine headache. It is preferred to be given by subcutaneous or intramuscular routes because of the poor oral absorption (0.25–0.5 mg). It is also used by sublingual route (2–4 mg). Caffeine acts synergistically with ergotamine in controlling the pulsations of cranial arteries and in relieving migraine. Tablets composed of 1 mg ergotamine and 100 mg caffeine are often used.

Erogotamine and other ergot preparations cause nausea, vomiting, vascular insufficiency and gangrene (due to excessive use) of extremities.

Beta haloalkylamines are phenoxy-benzamine and dibenamine. They produce an irreversible competitive antagonism of alpha-adrenoceptors of long duration (14–48 hr). It is also called non-equilibrium type of blocked because in the later stages it is not altered by increasing the concentration of the catecholamines at the receptor sites. Out of the two, phenoxybenzamine is used because dibenamine is more toxic. Phenoxybenzamine can also block the responses of acetylcholine, histamine and 5-HT. It inhibits reuptake of released NA by presynaptic adrenergic nerve terminals. It causes more tachycardia, palpitation, and increase in cardiac output than prazocin because of its action on α_2 receptors and inhibition of NA reuptake.

It is mainly used in the treatment of pheochromocytoma. In addition to usual side effects, it causes sedation, fatigue and nausea because it crosses blood–brain barrier being lipid soluble.

Prazosin: It is an extremely potent and highly selective α_1 receptor blocker. It has no action on presynaptic α_2 receptors. A central effect decreasing sympathetic flow to heart has also been observed. It is more effective in the treatment of hypertension when given in combination with a diuretic which corrects retention of salt and fluid caused by prazocin.

Dose: 1 mg 2–3 times a day.

Terazosin: It is related to prazosin. Its plasma half-life is longer (12 hrs) than prazosin (3–4 hrs) as it undergoes very little first pass metabolism in liver.

Dose: 2–10 mg once daily.

Other long acting once daily administered selective α_1 blockers are trimazosin and doxazosin. Doxazosin is also used in benign prostate hyperplasia.

Indoramin is a selective, competitive α_1-antagonist. It also competitively antagonises H_1 and 5-HT receptors. It is used in hypertension and to decrease incidence of Raynaud's phenomenon. Sedation, dry mouth

Table 22.1: Important uses of alpha-blockers

Hypertension	Selective alpha-1 blockers like prazosin, terazosin, trimazosin, doxazosin are used
Secondary shock (Due to blood or fluid loss)	α-blocker with fluid replacement
Pheochromocytoma	a. Phenotolamine test for diagnosis b. Phenoxybenzamine for inoperable and malignant tumours c. Phenoxybenzamine for 1–2 weeks preoperatively and continue it during surgical removal of the tumour
Peripheral vascular diseases	For symptomatic relief, tolazoline, prazosin and phenoxybenzamine may be used
Benign hypertrophy of prostate	To increase urinary flow and complete emptying of bladder prazosin, terazosin or tamsulosin may be used
Congestive heart failure	Prazosin affords improvement for short period

and failure of ejaculation may occur as side effects.

Urapidil is a selective α_1 antagonist. It also has weak α_2-agonist and 5-HT_{1A}-agonistic actions. It is recommended for the treatment of hypertension. It is extensively metabolized. It has a half-life of 3 hours.

Tamsulosin has higher affinity for α_{1A} subtype of α_1 receptors. These receptors predominate in the bladder base and prostate. So it is an uroselective drug and used to relieve urinary symptoms of benign hyperplasia of prostate. Significant side effects are dizziness and retrograde ejaculation. Its modified release capsule is required to be given once daily.

Yohimbine: It is an indolealkylamine alkaloid obtained from a West African tree. It readily crosses the blood–brain barrier and selectively blocks α_2 receptors and facilitates the release of NA at the synaptic cleft. It is not used therapeutically.

BETA-ADRENOCEPTOR BLOCKING AGENTS

Beta-adrenoceptor blocking agents are synthetic analogues of isoprenaline. They selectively and competitively block the actions of catecholamines mediated through beta-receptor stimulation.

Classification

I. **Non-selective** ($\beta_1 + \beta_2$)
- Beta blocker with membrane stabilizing activity, e.g. propranolol
- Beta blockers with membrane stabilizing activity and intrinsic sympathomimetic property, e.g. oxprenolol, pindolol, alprenolol
- Specific beta blockers without intrinsic sympathomimetic activity, e.g. timolol, nadolol
- With additional alpha blocking property, e.g. labetalol, dilevalol

II. **Cardioselective** (β_1) blocker, e.g. metoprolol, atenolol, acebutolol, esmolol, betaxolol, bisoprolol, celiprolol, nabivolol

Pharmacokinetics: On oral administration, beta blockers are absorbed. In most of the cases, bioavailability is 30–50% except pindolol (90%). These drugs are metabolized in the liver and are excreted in urine. The plasma t½ of most of the beta blockers is between 3 and 6 hours. But nadolol has a t½ of 14–24 hours, atenolol 6–9 hours and esmolol only in minutes. So atenolol is given once a day and esmolol by i.v. infusion. Since propranolol has been thoroughly investigated and has been widely used, it will be discussed in detail as prototype of this group.

Propranolol

Although it exists in levo- and dextro-form, the commercial preparation is however, recemic. It is highly lipophilic. On oral administration, it is completely absorbed and is extensively metabolized (first-pass effect) in the liver. One of the metabolites (4-OH-propranolol) is biologically active. Its plasma half-life is 4–6 hours. It crosses the blood–brain barrier and 90% binds with plasma protein. The drug and its metabolites are excreted in urine.

Pharmacological Actions

Cardiovascular system: Its effects on cardiovascular system are dose dependent and can be antagonized by isoprenaline. It blocks cardiac β_1 receptors and produces bradycardia, decrease in cardiac contractility, automaticity and cardiac output; oxygen consumption is decreased and there is increase in exercise tolerance. It depresses the heart due to membrane stabilizing action. So it is not used in presence of congestive heart failure.

ECG shows prolongation of PR interval and slow AV conduction. Antiarrhythmic effect of propranolol is due to beta-blocking activity and not to membrane stabilization.

Blood pressure: Although propranolol has no effect on blood pressure of normotensive individuals, it produces slowly developing fall in blood pressure of hsypertensive patients. Its antihypertensive effect is due to:

- Bradycardia and decreased cardiac output which occur as a result of blockade of β_1 receptors in heart; with continued treatment total peripheral resistance decreases due to gradual adaptation of resistance vessels to chronically reduced cardiac output
- Blockade of presynaptic β_2 receptors (facilitatory to adrenergic neurons) leads to reduced norepinephrine release from sympathetic terminals
- Inhibition of release of renin from juxtaglomerular cells of kidney (β_1-mediated)
- Central action reducing sympathetic outflow by blocking presynaptic β receptors centrally
- Stimulation of prostacycline synthesis in vascular beds
- Increase in natriuretic peptide secretion caused by β-blockade

Respiratory system: Propranolol increases airway resistance, so it is contraindicated in patients of asthma and other forms of respiratory insufficiency.

Eye: Propranolol reduces formation of aqueous humour by decreasing cAMP formation and thus decreases intraocular pressure. It has local anaesthetic effect on conjunctiva, but not used for this purpose because of its irritant property.

Central nervous system: Propranolol produces sedation, lethargy, depression, disturbed sleep and increased dreaming because it crosses the blood–brain barrier. In a high dose (1–2 g), it produces antipsychotic effect by direct membrane stabilizing effect or antiserotonin action. Propranolol decreases anxiety in short-term stressful situations due to peripheral rather than a central action.

Metabolic effects: Propranolol antagonizes catecholamine induced glycogenolysis and lipolysis mediated by beta-receptors. It increases VLDL and lowers plasma HDL levels (undesirable effect). So it is better to be given along with prazosin in hypertensive patients because prazosin increases HDL levels.

Skeletal muscle: Propranolol blocks facilitatory presynaptic β_2 receptors and antagonizes adrenaline induced tremor.

Other Beta Blockers

The pharmacological actions of other beta blockers are similar to that of propranolol. The individual differences are due to pharmacokinetic peculiarities, receptor selectivity, membrane stabilizing and intrinsic sympathomimetic (partial agonistic) actions. Beta-blockers with partial agonistic activity can be used in the presence of congestive heart failure while those causing membrane stabilization are not indicated. Cardioselective β_1 blocker does not affect pulmonary ventilation and tissue perfusion, so it can be used with great caution in patients with bronchial asthma. They are also preferred in patients suffering from diabetes mellitus or peripheral vascular spasmodic diseases.

Pindolol is a potent beta blocker having prominent intrinsic sympathomimetic activity. It is useful to treat hypertensive patients who develop marked bradycardia with propranolol. Ouccrrence of withdrawal rebound hypertension is less. However, it has narrow effective dose range.

Oxprenolol and alprenolol have similar pharmacological profile as that of pindolol, but are less potent and short acting.

Timolol (non-selective beta blocker): Used as eyedrop in cases of wide angle glaucoma to decrease intraocular pressure. It has no effect on ciliary muscle and pupillary size.

Nadolol is a long acting beta blocker which is used to treat hypertension. It has less central side effects and is given once daily.

Metoprolol (cardioselective beta blocker): It is well absorbed on oral administration; undergoes first-pass metabolism in liver; protein binding is 12%; plasma half-life is 3–4 hours; and the metabolites are excreted by the kidney.

Dose: 100–200 mg.

Atenolol (potent β_1 blocker): It has no central action in therapeutic doses. On oral administration, 46–62% is absorbed; plasma half-life is 6–9 hours and is excreted mainly by kidney.

Dose: 50–100 mg per day.

Esmolol (selective β_1 blocker) is given by i.v. infusion because it has an ultrashort half-life of 10 minutes due to rapid hydrolysis of its ester linkage.

Bisoprolol is a cardioselective beta blocker without intrinsic sympathomimetic activity. It is used once daily in angina and hypertension

Celiprolol is a selective β_1 blocker with weak β_2 agonistic activity. It reduces vascular resistance and somewhat safe in asthmatics

Acebutolol is useful in patients with low cardiac reserve because it produces less myocardial depression and bradycardia due to partial beta agonistic activity. The abnormality in lipid profile is also less than with propranolol.

Nebivolol is a cardioselective β blocker and a nitric oxide (NO) donor. It produces vasodilatation and improves endothelial function.

Labetalol: It has both α_1 and β blocking activity. On oral administration, it is well absorbed and rapidly metabolized in liver. It reduces both systolic and diastolic blood pressure. It is useful in the treatment of hypertension, rebound hypertension after sudden withdrawal of clonidine and pheochromocytoma. Oral dose is 50 mg BD; increased up to 100–200 mg TDS.

Dilevalol is 3–4 times more potent in blocking β_1, β_2 receptors but 6 times less potent in blocking α_1 receptors than labetalol. Like labetalol it is an effective antihypertensive by oral route and can be injected i.v. to produce predictable hypotension during emergencies. Dose: 200–800 mg orally daily.

Carvedilol is also $\beta_1 + \beta_2 + \alpha_1$ adrenoceptor blocker. It produces vasodilatation due to α_1 blockade as well as direct action. It also has antioxidant action. It is used in hypertension and as cardioprotective in congestive heart failure.

Therapeutic Uses of Beta Blockers

1. **Essential hypertension:** Beta blockers are now considered as the first line drug in the treatment of essential hypertension. They are usually combined with diuretics which contribute to the hypotensive effect by a different mechanism and also prevent development of tolerance.

2. All beta blockers are used in the prophylaxis of angina pectoris of effort to reduce the number and severity of attacks. However, it is not effective in variant or unstable angina where vasospasm is the causative factor.

3. When beta blockers are used for several years in patients of myocardial ischaemia they decrease the incidence and recurrence of myocardial infarction due to beta blockade effect, prevention of platelet aggregation, promotion of fibrinolysis and prevention of sudden ventricular fibrillation at the second attack of myocardial infarction.

4. Propranolol is effective in all supraventricular tachycardias associated with high levels of circulating catecholamines, e.g. halothane or cyclopropane anaesthesia, thyrotoxicosis, pheochromocytoma and also in digitalis toxicity due to its ability to increase refractory period of AV node and direct membrane stabilizing action.

5. Since beta blockers increase the stroke volume as a result of slowing of heart, it is used to relieve congestion and dyspnoea associated with obstruction of ventricular outflow in the presence of hypertrophic cardiomyopathy, mitral stenosis with tachycardia, dissecting aortic aneurysm and Fallot's tetralogy.

6. Propranolol and nadolol are useful in portal hypertension to reduce bleeding from oesophageal varices and gastric erosion.

7. Propranolol is used to reduce tachycardia, tremor, cardiac irregularities, sweating nervousness and raised BMR in cases of thyrotoxicosis.

8. Pheochromocytoma: Beta blockers may be employed in combination with alpha adrenoceptor blocker in pheochromocytoma during removal of the tumour, to prevent excessive cardiac stimulation by catecholamines released from the tumour. Labetalol may also be used in this condition.

9. Glaucoma: Timolol (0.25–0.5%) is used as an eyedrop in cases of wide angle glaucoma to reduce intraocular tension.

10. Neurological disorders: Propranolol has been found to be useful in:
    a. Reducing the frequency and severity of migraine
    b. Reducing anxiety states by inhibiting somatic manifestations of anxiety such as palpitation, tachycardia, sweating and diarrhoea
    c. Reducing the central adrenergic over activity during alcohol withdrawal
    d. The treatment of essential tremor

Adverse reactions: Beta blockers may cause following adverse reactions:

- Extreme bradycardia and hypotension
- Precipitate or worsen congestive heart failure due to withdrawal of cardiac sympathetic derives.
- Precipitate or worsen bronchial asthma

- Propranolol may cause fatigue, depression, sleep disturbances and vivid dreams.
- Abrupt withdrawal of beta blockers may result in a rebound phenomenon (severe angina or myocardial infarction) and death may occur in patients of ischaemic heart disease.
- Beta-blockers potentiate the hypoglycaemic action of insulin and oral antidiabetic agents.

Contraindications: Beta blockers are contraindicated in:

- Mental depression
- Incipient heart failure and heart block
- Anaesthesia with cardiac depressant drugs.

In the following conditions, beta blockers are contraindicated except selective β_1 blockers which may be tried with care if needed the most:

- Bronchial asthma
- Peripheral vascular spasmodic diseases
- Insulin dependent diabetes mellitus.

Points for Dental Students

Beta adrenoceptor blocking agents are widely used drugs. So if a patient on beta blocker comes to a dentist, he should be careful prescribing other drugs due to important drug interactions. For example, the effect of beta blockers is increased by furosemide, cimetidine, hydralazine, etc. and decreased by phenytoin, rifampin, indomethacin and other NSAIDs, etc. Further, beta blockers enhance the hypoglycemic effects of insulin and oral hypoglycemic agents; sympathomimetics (non-selective) increase pressor response due to availability of unopposed functional vasopressor alpha-receptors. This is important in dental practice when adrenaline containing local anaesthetic solution is used to a patient on propranolol. If per chance adrenaline is absorbed in sufficient concentration there can occur serious rise in blood pressure leading to even hypertensive crisis.

To treat ventricular arrhythmias, xylocaine is infused i.v. in large doses in coronary care units. In such cases, coadministration of propranolol is contraindicated to avoid xylocaine toxicity which occur due to: (i) inhibition of oxidation of xylocaine and (ii) decreased hepatic blood flow leading to reduced delivery of xylocaine for metabolism.

TO REMEMBER

1. Alpha-receptor blocking drugs inhibit adrenergic responses mediated through alpha-adrenergic receptors.
2. Tolazoline is a competitive antagonist of alpha-adrenoceptors. It is used in Raynaud's disease, thromboangitis obliterance, frostbite, etc.
3. Phentolamine is used as a preliminary test (Regitine test) in the diagnosis of pheochromocytoma. A fall of blood pressure by 35/25 mm Hg is diagnostic.
4. Ergotamine is a potent vasoconstrictor which is used in migraine headache.
5. Phenoxybezamine causes irreversible competitive antagonism of alpha-adrenoceptors of long duration. It is mainly used in the treatment of pheochromocytoma.
6. Prazocin, terazocin, doxazocin, trimazocin, indormin and urapidil are extremely potent and highly selective α_1 receptor blocker which have no action on presynaptic α_2 receptors. They are used to treat hypertension along with a diuretic.
7. Beta-adrenoceptor blocking agents are synthetic analogues of isoprenaline. They selectively and competitively block the actions of catecholamines mediated through beta-receptor stimulation.
8. Beta-adrenoceptor blocking agents are used to treat essential hypertension, angina pectoris, myocardial ischaemia, supraventricular tachycardia, hypertrophic cardiomyopathy, portal hypertension, thyrotoxicosis, pheochromocytoma, glaucoma and neurological disorders.
9. Beta blockers are contraindicated in mental depression, incipient heart failure, heart block, bronchial asthma, peripheral vascular diseases, insulin dependent diabetes mellitus.
10. Important beta blockers other than propranolol are metoprolol (cardio-selective beta-blocker), atenolol (potent β_1 blocker), esmolol (selective β_1 blocker) and timolol (non-selective beta-blocker; used in wide angle glaucoma). Nebivolol is a cardioselective β blocker and a nitric oxide donor.
11. Acebutolol and pindolol are useful in patients with low cardiac reserve.
12. Labetalol, dilevalol, carvedilol have both α_1 and beta blocking activity. They are useful in the treatment of hypertension, rebound hypertension after sudden withdrawal of clonidine and pheochromocytoma.

Chapter 23

Ganglionic Blockers and Nicotine

Acetylcholine is the neurotransmitter in both sympathetic and parasympathetic ganglia. Transmission through autonomic ganglia is complex. Both types of cholinergic receptors are present at postganglionic neurone cell bodies. Acetylcholine, released from pregang-lionic fibres, produces a series of changes as follows:

The primary event is that acetylcholine acts on postsynaptic nicotinic (N_1) receptor and causes depolarization and propagation of excitatory postsynaptic potential (EPSP). Acetylcholine also releases noradrenaline and dopamine from interneurons which generate inhibitory postsynaptic potential (IPSP). Finally there develops late excitatory postsynaptic potential (late EPSP) due to release of number of cotransmitters such as peptides (neuropeptide Y, VIP, LHRH, angiotensin-II, enkephaline and substance P), amines (histamine, 5HT) and GABA. This is followed by hydrolysis of acetylcholine by cholinesterase and repolarization.

Ganglionic Stimulants

They are not used in therapeutics. But they are of considerable importance because of nicotine which has the ability to stimulate (in small doses)as well as block (in large doses) ganglionic receptors. The other ganglionic stimulants are lobeline,tetramethylammonium and 1, 1-dimethyl 1-4-phenyl piperazinium (DMPP).

Nicotine: It is an alkaloid obtained from the leaves of tobacco plant (*Nicotiana tobacum*). It is a brown liquid. It can easily penetrate intact skin and mucous membranes. On inhalation of nicotine, cigarette smoke (0.3 to 1 mg) may cause slight increase in heart rate, blood pressure and respiration. Skin temperature may decrease. Nicotine may cause tremors, convulsions, nausea, vomiting and release of antidiuretic hormone from pituitary.

Nicotine increases the gastric, salivary and bronchial secretions. Nicotine smoking causes an induction of metabolizing enzymes in the liver and intestine. Nicotine produces tolerance to its central effects rapidly. It also produces dependence and symptoms of withdrawal may appear within 24 hours. Clonidine has been found to be effective to reduce craving and insomnia.

Adverse reactions: Smoking is injurious to health. Chronic smoking may lead to :
a. Dyspnoea, wheezing, pain chest, and upper respiratory tract infection
b. Increased incidence of cancer of oral, laryngeal, oesophageal, duodenal, pancreatic lung and bladder
c. Increased incidence of hypertension, ischaemic heart disease and thrombo-angitis obliterance
d. Anxiety, insomnia, irritability and depression
e. Increased incidence of pre-eclampsia, abortion, low birth weight and fewer pregnancies

f. Toxic amblyopia may occur in smokers of strong tobacco and cheap cigarettes.

Ganglionic Blocking Agents

These drugs block the transmission across the autonomic ganglia. Once they were extensively used in the treatment of hypertension. However, now they have limited use because of the following reasons:

i. High incidence of undesirable side effects due to their non-specific nature of action, i.e. they block both sympathetic and parasympathetic autonomic ganglia.
ii. Development of tolerance to hypotensive effect rapidly.
iii. Unpredictable absorption from the gut.
iv. Advent of safer and equally potent hypotensive agents.

The ones which are still in use are mecamylamine and trimethaphan.

Mecamylamine: It is a secondary amine. On oral administration, it is almost completely absorbed and can also cross the blood–brain barrier. So it produces prominent central nervous system effects such as tremor, confusion, seizures, mania and depression. It is excreted unchanged by the kidney. On prolonged use, mecamylamine produces tolerance. The common adverse effects are postural hypotension (due to blockade of normal protective vasomotor reflexes mediated through baroreceptors and the sympathetic nervous system), drowsiness, dry mouth, impotence, paralytic ileus. Dose: Initial 2.5 mg twice daily; gradually increased up to 20–30 mg per day. It is used in the treatment of moderate to severe hypertension if other drugs are ineffective.

Trimethaphan (arfonad): It has a very short duration of action. It is only used as intravenous infusion (3–4 mg/min) to produce controlled hypotension in surgery. It should be carefully used in patients of allergy because it releases histamine.

Points for Dental Students

It is important to know whether a patient is a smoker or not because nicotine smoking causes an induction of metabolizing enzymes in the liver and intestine. It means the metabolism of number of drugs such as beta-adrenoceptor blocking agents, corticoids, calcium channel blockers, doxycycline, estrogens, itraconazole, ketoconazole, phenothiazines, quinidine, etc. is increased. So dosage adjustment is needed when one of these drugs is used clinically to have a desired therapeutic effect.

TO REMEMBER

1. Acetylcholine is the neurotransmitter in both sympathetic and parasympathetic ganglia.

2. Ganglionic stimulants are not used in therapeutics but they are of considerable importance because of nicotine abuse. Nicotine produces tolerance, and dependence and withdrawal may appear within 24 hours. Clonidine has been found to be effective to reduce craving and insomnia.

3. Ganglionic blocking agents block the transmission across the autonomic ganglia. They have limited use in hypertension because of high incidence of undesirable side effects, development of tolerance to hypotensive effect and unpredictable absorption from gut.

4. Mecamylamine is a secondary amine which is used in moderate to severe hypertension if other drugs are ineffective.

5. Trimetaphan (arfonad) is an ultrashort acting ganglionic blocking agent which is used to produce controlled hypotension in neurosurgery.

Drugs Acting on Peripheral (Somatic) Nervous System

Section 5

Drugs Acting on Peripheral (Somatic) Nervous System

24. Local Anaesthetics

25. Skeletal Muscle Relaxants

Chapter 24

Local Anaesthetics

Local anaesthetics (LA) are drugs which have following features:

1. Used for topical application or local injection.
2. Cause reversible loss of sensory perception in a restricted area of the body.
3. Prevent generation and propagation of nerve action potential at all parts of the neuron where they come in contact, without causing any structural damage.
4. They interrupt sensory as well as motor impulses in a mixed nerve and can lead to muscular paralysis and loss of autonomic control as well.
5. Do not alter consciousness.
6. Can be used safely for poor health patient also.
7. Useful only for minor surgery.

Chemistry and Classification

The clinically useful local anaesthetics are weak bases. They have amphiphilic property. They consist of a hydrophilic secondary or tertiary amine on one side and a lipophilic aromatic residue on the other side. Two are joined by an alkyl chain through an ester or amide linkage. So based on linkage they can be classified as:

I. Ester-linked local anaesthetics: Cocaine, procaine, chloroprocaine, tetracaine, cyclomethycaine, benzocaine, benoxinate.

II. Amide-linked local anaesthetics: Lidocaine, mepivacaine, bupivocaine, dibucaine. They differ from the former group as under:

- They bind to alpha-1 glycoprotein in plasma.
- Generally longer acting.
- Not hydrolyzed by plasma esterases.
- Hypersensitivity reactions are less frequent.
- No cross-sensitivity with ester-linked local anaesthetics.

Local anaesthetics can also be classified on the basis of type of local anaesthesia produced by them, as shown in the Table 24.1.

Mechanism of action: Local anaesthetics block nerve conduction by reducing entry of Na^+ through the voltage gated channels either by an effect on the membrane or by specifically plugging Na^+ channels. Due to this, they block the initiation and propagation of nerve impulse. They block nociceptive and sympathetic transmission first and motor nerves are blocked last.

Pharmacokinetics: Surface anaesthetics are rapidly absorbed from mucous membranes and abraded areas. However, procaine does not significantly penetrate mucous membranes. After oral administration, both procaine and lignocaine have high first pass metabolism in the liver. So for antiarrhythmic purpose, they are given parenterally.

Table 24.1: Classification of local anaesthetics based on type of local anaesthesia

Type of local anaesthesia	Local anaesthetics used	Method of induction of anaesthesia
Surface or topical	Lignocaine Tetracaine Cyclamethylcaine Dyclomine Proparacaine Benzocaine.	Local application on mucous membrane of nose, buccal cavity, tracheobronchi, oesophagus, rectum, anus, urethra, vagina, cutaneous or cornea.
Infiltration	Lignocaine Bupivacaine Prilocaine Procaine	Directly inject LA into tissues to paralyze sensory nerve endings and small cutaneous nerves.
Nerve block	Lignocaine Bupivacaine Prilocaine Procaine	Inject LA close to a nerve trunk like brachial plexus, sciatic nerve, cervical plexus, or intercostal nerves to induce anaesthesia distal to the injection site.
Spinal	Lignocaine Prilocaine Bupivacaine Procaine	Inject LA in subarachnoid space which contains cerebrospinal fluid.
Epidural	Lignocaine Prilocaine Bupivacaine Procaine	Inject LA into extradural space between dura and the bony spinal canal.

Most local anaesthetics are effective within 5 minutes. Their duration of action ranges between 1 and 1.5 hours. This can be increased to 2–3 hours by the addition of a vasoconstrictor like adrenaline or noradrenaline or a synthetic vasopressin, felypressin.

Ester-linked local anaesthetics are rapidly hydrolyzed by plasma pseudocholinesterase and the remaining amount by esterases in liver. Amide-linked local anaesthetics are metabolized in the liver by microsomal enzymes (dealkylation and hydrolysis).

Pharmacological Actions

Local: Clinically used local anaesthetics have no/minimal local irritant action. They block sensory nerve endings, nerve trunks, neuromuscular junction, ganglionic synapse and receptors (non-selectively). They also decrease release of acetylcholine from motor nerve endings. Local anaesthetics block nerve conduction in the following order:
- Small myelinated axons (sensory, autonomic)
- Non-myelinated axons
- Large myelinated axons (motor)

So, nociceptive and sympathetic transmission is blocked first and motor nerves are blocked last.

Systemic: Any local anaesthetic applied locally or injected is ultimately absorbed. Depending on its concentration in the plasma and tissues, it can produce systemic effects.

Central nervous system: All local anaesthetics are capable of producing a sequence of stimulation followed by depression. The basic effect of these drugs is neuronal inhibition. Initial apparent stimulation is due to inhibition of inhibitory neurons.

Cocaine is a powerful CNS stimulant. At safe clinical doses, procaine and other synthetic local anaesthetics produce little apparent CNS stimulation. However, in higher doses, they produce CNS stimulation followed by depression. At clinical doses, lidocaine causes drowsiness and lethargy but higher doses produce excitation followed by depression.

Cardiovascular system: No significant effect is observed on heart in conventional doses of local anaesthetics. At high doses, they decrease excitability, conductivity and contractility. Lignocaine has antiarrhythmic activity.

Hypotension is due to direct vasodilatation, ganglionic blockade, and inhibition of sympathetic system.

Adverse reactions: Excessive systemic absorption can result in light headedness, dizziness, auditory and visual disturbances, mental confusion, disorientation, shivering, twitching, tremors and finally convulsions and respiratory arrest. These adverse reactions can be prevented or treated by diazepam. There also occurs bradycardia, hypotension, cardiac arrhythmias and vascular collapse. Hypersensitivity reactions (such as skin rashes, bronchial asthma, and anaphylactic shock) are rare. Lignocaine and prilocaine can induce methaemoglobinaemia due to an aniline metabolite.

Drug Interactions

- Antibacterial action of sulfonamides is interfered because procaine releases para-aminobenzoic acid (PABA) on hydrolysis.
- Cimetidine increases the plasma levels of lignocaine and other amide type of local anaesthetic by inhibiting hepatic microsomal enzyme.
- Propranolol increases the plasma levels of amide type of local anaesthetics by decreasing hepatic blood flow.
- Phenobarbitone decreases plasma levels of amide local anaesthetics by hepatic enzyme induction.
- Lignocaine potentiates succinylcholine action.

Characteristic Features of Individual Local Anaesthetics

Lidocaine (Lignocaine, Xylocaine)

- Most widely used local anaesthetic including dental practice
- Onset of action—quick
- Duration of action—long (1.5 hours when used with epinephrine)
- Metabolized in liver by mixed function oxidases
- Safely administered to patients who are sensitive to procaine
- Xyliclide is its active metabolite with local anaesthetic activity
- Also used i.v. to treat ventricular arrhythmias

Procaine

- As potent LA as lidocaine
- Duration of action short
- Not effective for surface anaesthesia due to poor absorption from the mucous membranes
- Poor analgesic
- Readily hydrolyzed by plasma cholinesterase into para-amino benzoic acid

Cocaine

- It is a drug of abuse
- Never injected due to central nervous system toxicity
- Causes cardiac depression in hypersensitive patients
- Onset of action—quick
- Duration of action—long
- Not used along with epinephrine as cocaine potentiates the action of epinephrine

Mepivacaine

- Chemically and pharmacologically related to lidocaine
- Not effective topically
- Used for infiltration, nerve block, and epidural anaesthesia
- Generally used in dentistry

Bupivacaine

- Onset of action—slow
- Duration of action—long (8 hours)
- Mainly used in:
  - a. Spinal anaesthesia
  - b. Lumbar blockade
  - c. During labour for analgesia

Prilocaine

- As effective as lidocaine
- Can cause methaemoglobinaemia
- Used for infiltration, nerve block and dental anaesthesia

Amethocaine

- Used topically to venous puncture or venous cannulation.
- Should not be applied to inflamed, traumatized or highly vascular surfaces.

Benzocaine

- Useful in surface anaesthesia
- Used in dusting powder
- Used in throat lozenges

Ropivacaine

- Used for surface anaesthesia.

Spinal and Epidural Anaesthesia

Spinal anaesthesia is a safer alternative of general anaesthesia in patients in whom general anaesthetics are contraindicated. It is mainly used for surgical procedures carried out on lower abdomen, perineum and lower limbs. Its advantages on general anaesthesia are :

- It is safe.
- Produces good analgesia and muscle relaxation without loss of consciousness.
- Cardiac, pulmonary, renal disease and diabetes pose fewer problems.

However, it can induce some complications, such as:

- Respiratory depression. It is rare. It occurs in lower level spinal anaesthesia. It is mainly due to intercostal muscle paralysis. So breathing is maintained by diaphragm which is supplied by phrenic nerve.
- Hypotension may occur due to sympathetic blockage. It can be treated with vasopressor agents like mephentramine.
- Headache occurs due to leakage of cerebrospinal fluid. It can be corrected by the use of aspirin.
- Cauda equina syndrome may occur due to spinal cord injury.
- Septic meningitis may occur very rarely due to introduction of infection during lumbar puncture.
- Nausea and vomiting after abdominal operation.

Contraindications

- Uncooperative or mentally ill patient.
- Infants and children because control of level is difficult.
- Hypotension and hypovolemia.
- Vertebral abnormalities, e.g. kyphosis lordosis.
- Sepsis at injection site.

The clinical use of epidural anaesthesia is similar to spinal anaesthesia. It may be thoraxic, lumbar or caudal depending on the site of its administration. Technically, it is a more difficult procedure and large amount of anaesthetic agent is required to be used which may induce systemic toxicity. However, the side effects of spinal anaesthesia are rarely noted in this type of local anaesthesia or are less severe.

Biological Toxins with Local Anaesthetic like Actions

The following biological toxins cause blockade of Na^+ conductance through the voltage-gated channels. So they inhibit action potential generation and propagation in all excitable tissues, including the heart, neuromuscular junction and nerves.

a. Tetrodotoxin (pufferfish)
b. Saxitoxin (marine shellfish)
c. Cignatoxin (marine fish)

The following biological toxins act by increasing Na^+ conductance through the voltage-gated channels. So they cause persistent depolarization of excitable cells and lead to their inactivation.

a. Batrachotoxin (South American frog)
b. Scorpion venom
c. Sea anemone

Use of Vasoconstrictors along with Local Anaesthetic Agents

All clinically effective injectable local anaes-thetics possess some degree of vasodilating activity. The degree of vasodilatation varies. It is significant in case of procaine while minimal with prilocaine and mepivacaine. It also may vary with both injection site and individual patient response. The blood vessels are dilated after injection of local anaesthetic into tissues. This results in an increased perfusion at the site and leads to the following reactions:

- Rate of absorption of the local anaesthetic into the circulation is increased. So this removes it from the injection site (redistribution).
- Increased risk of toxicity due to higher plasma levels of the local anaesthetic.
- Decreased depth of anaesthesia and a decreased duration of action due to rapid diffusion of local anaesthetic away from injection site.
- Increased bleeding at the site of treatment due to increased perfusion.

Vasoconstrictors are drugs that constrict blood vessels and thereby control tissue perfusion. They are added to local anaesthetic solutions to oppose their vasodilatory effects. The vasoconstrictors are, therefore, important additions to a local anaesthetic solution for the following reasons:

- Vasoconstrictors reduce blood flow (perfusion) to the site of administration by constricting blood vessels.
- Absorption of local anaesthetic into circulation is slowed and results in lower anaesthetic plasma levels. Hence the risk of local anaesthetic toxicity is minimized.
- Increased amount of the local anaesthetic remains in and around the nerve for longer periods. Due to this, vasoconstrictor increases (in some cases significantly, in others minimally) the duration of action of most local anaesthetics.
- Vasoconstrictors decrease bleeding at the site of administration. They are, therefore, useful when increased bleeding is anticipated, e.g. during surgical procedures.

Commonly used vasoconstrictors in conjunction with local anaesthetics are following sympatho-mimetics:

- **Epinephrine:** It is most potent and widely used vasoconstrictor in dentistry. Least concentrated solution that produces effective pain control should be used. Lidocaine is available with two dilutions of epinephrine—1: 50,000 and 1: 100,000.

Epinepherine prevents or minimizes blood loss during surgical procedures effectively. However, it also produces a rebound vasodilatory effect as the tissue level of epinephrine declines. This leads to possible bleeding postoperatively, which potentially interferes with wound healing. Epinephrine possesses both α and β actions. It produces vasoconstriction through it's α effects. Used in 1:50,000 concentration and even at 1:100,000 (but to a lesser extent), epinephrine induces a definite rebound β-effect once the α-induced vasoconstriction has ceased. This is responsible for increased postoperative blood loss, which if significant (usually in dentistry it is not), could compromise a patient's cardio-vascular status.

- Levonordefrin is used as a vasoconstrictor with mepivacaine in a 1:20,000 dilution. For all patients, the maximum dose should be 1 mg per appointment; 20 ml of a 1:20,000 dilution (11 cartridges).
- Felypressin (a synthetic vasopressin) is employed in a dilution of 0.03 IU/ml with 3% prilocaine. Felypressin containing solutions are not used when hemostasis is necessary. This is because of their predominant effect on the venous rather than the arterial circulation. The maximum recommended dose is 0.27 IU/ml; 9 ml of 0.03 IU/ml for patients with clinically significant cardiovascular impairment. It has the advantage that it does not affect the heart rate and blood pressure.

Points for Dental Students

1. Commonly used local anaesthetics in dentistry are xylocaine, mepivacaine, bupivacaine and prilocaine. So thorough knowledge of local anaesthetics is required by dental students for their judicious and safe use.
2. Nerve block anaesthesias are to be avoided in aplastic anaemia because of the risk of thrombocytopenia and the bleeding tendency. However, intraligamental anaesthesia can be used safely in these cases.
3. For all patients and for some in particular, the benefits and risks of including vasopressor in local anaesthetic solution must be weighed against the benefits and risks of using a 'plain' anaesthetic solution. In general these groups are:
   - Patients with more significant cardiovascular diseases (ASA III and IV group)
   - Patients with certain non-cardiovascular diseases, e.g. thyroid dysfunction, diabetes and sulfite sensitivity
   - Patients receiving MAOI, tricyclic antidepressants and phenothiazines

However, it may be stated that local anaesthetic with vasoconstrictors are not absolutely contraindicated for patients whose medical condition has been diagnosed and is under control through medical or surgical means and if the vasoconstrictor is administered slowly in minimal doses, after regular routine aspiration has been ensured.

4. Local anaesthetic should be carefully given in small children (up to 6 years) because maximum dose limits are quickly reached. Local anaesthetic with opioid sedation may increase the risk of developing local anaesthetic overdose. So this should be particularly taken care of during pedodontic surgery in children to avoid fatalities.

   Recently a useful non-invasive method has been developed to produce local anaesthesia in pedodontic procedures by using EMLA (Eutectic mixture of local anaesthetics) cream consisting of 2.5% xylocaine + 2.5% prilocaine.
5. Monitoring preoperative vital signs specially the blood pressure, heart rate and rhythm is strongly recommended for all patients but is especially in patients receiving β-blockers. Re-recording of these vital signs at 5–10 minutes after the administration of a vasoconstrictor is strongly recommended.
6. Little higher dose of xylocaine + adrenaline combination is needed for proper local anaesthetic effect in patients with acute alcohol intoxication because much of the vasoconstrictor effects of adrenaline are rather neutralized by the cutaneous vasodilatory effects.
7. Take special care while injecting xylocaine + adrenaline to a patient of cardiac failure on digoxin to avoid developing cardiac arrhythmias which occur if vasoconstrictor

enters intravascularly. Similarly in digitalized patients use haemostatic retraction cords impregnated with astringents in place of local anaesthetic + adrenaline.

8. Avoid use of local anaesthetic + adrenaline in Parkinson's patients taking l-dopa as cardiac arrhythmia may be precipitated due to stimulation of cardiac β_1 receptors by dopamine formed peripherally from l-dopa.

9. Modest increase in plasma concentration of local anaesthetic by erythromycin due to hepatic enzyme inhibition.

10. Large doses of xylocaine are usually i.v. infused to treat ventricular arrhythmias in coronary care units. In such cases, co-administration of propranolol can lead to xylocaine toxicity due to:
    • Inhibition of metabolic oxidation of xylocaine
    • Decreased hepatic blood flow (responsible for diminished delivery of xylocaine in liver).

11. Local anaesthetic + adrenaline can lead to serious rise in blood pressure and cardiac arrhythmia in hypertensive patients on prolonged use of guanethidine which induces super-sensitivity of adrenoceptor receptors to exogenously administered adrenaline.

TO REMEMBER

1. **Local anaesthetics:** Used locally to abolish sensation in a limited region of the body. Generation and propagation of nerve impulse action potential are prevented by them.

2. **Types of local anaesthesia:** Surface, infiltration, nerve block, spinal and epidural.

3. **Status of local anaesthetics:**
   • *Lidocaine:* Most popular local anaesthetic. Used to induce all types of local anaesthesia.
   • *Bupivacaine:* Used as a surface anaesthetic and occasionally for spinal anaesthesia.
   • *Benzocaine and butylaminobenzoate:* Being not systemically absorbed they are used as lozenges/dusting powder /ointment and suppository for local applications.
   • *Oxethazine:* Used in anaesthetizing gastric mucosa being a very potent topical anaesthetic and unique in ionizing to a very small extent even at low pH.
   • *Tetracaine:* Use is restricted to topical application.
   • *Procaine:* Rarely used after the introduction of lidocaine.
   • *Cocaine:* Use not warranted because it is protoplasmic poison; produces psychological drug dependence and ocular toxicity.

Chapter 25

Skeletal Muscle Relaxants

Skeletal muscle relaxants reduce muscle tone and/or cause paralysis. To achieve this, they may act peripherally at the neuromuscular junction/muscle fibre itself or centrally in the cerebrospinal axis. Drugs, that block transmission of impulses at the skeletal neuromuscular junction, are called neuromuscular blocking agents. These blockers act mainly at the post-junctional level. On the basis of their mechanism of action, they are classified as:

1. Non-depolarising or competitive blockers
   - D-tubocurarine
   - Pancuronium
   - Gallamine
   - Alcuronium
   - Atracurium
   - Mivacurium
   - Doxacurium
   - Rocuronium
   - Vecuronium
2. Depolarizing blockers:
   - Succinylcholine
   - Decamethonium
3. Dual action blocker:
   - Benzoquinonium
4. Directly acting neuromuscular blocking agents:
   - Dantrolene sodium
   - Quinine

Neuromuscular Blocking Agents

Non-depolarizing agents: These agents competitively block acetylcholine receptors on the motor end plate. The blockage can be overcome or reversed by increasing the concentration of acetylcholine at the receptor site. The salient features of pharmacokinetics of these agents are:

- Being quarternary compounds, these are not absorbed on oral administration; usually given i.v.
- Except gallamine, none of these drugs cross blood–brain barrier. These drugs do not cross placental barrier (can be given during caesarean).
- Route of administration plays an important role to determine their duration of action such as:
  a. Longer duration of action with drugs excreted by kidney
  b. Intermediate to short duration of action with drugs eliminated by liver
  c. Shorter duration of action with drugs which are inactivated by plasma cholinesterase
  d. Intermediate action with some isoquinoline derivatives (atracurium and cisatracurium) which are inactivated spontaneously by Hofmann elimination (rupture of the ester containing bridge joining the two isoquinoline moieties)
- Steroidal neuromuscular blocking drugs, primarily metabolized in liver (e.g. vecuranium, rocuranium, and rapacuranium), may accumulate on prolonged administration.

- Duration of action of atracurium is reduced during respiratory alkalosis caused by hyperventilation because it is chemically unstable at alkaline pH.
- These drugs do not show pharmacogenetic variation in metabolism/response.

Curare: It is the generic name for various South American arrow poisons. It is obtained from strychnos toxifera, chondrodendron tomentosum and related plants. The active principles of curare are d-tubocurarine, toxiferins, etc. Since absorption is irregular and poor from the gastrointestinal tract, d-tubocurarine is given by parenteral route. Neuromuscular blockage occurs in 3–4 minutes and lasts up to 30 minutes. The muscle relaxation is of progressive flaccid paralysis type. Hypothermia decreases its effect while neuromuscular blocking drugs such as ether and aminoglycoside antibiotics potentiate it. Neostigmine antagonizes its effect on neuromuscular junction. Hypotension is its major side effect which is due to histamine release and ganglionic blockage. It is a dose related phenomenon. Histamine release is also responsible for an erythematous rash on the chest and neck as well as for bronchospasm. Its dose depends on the type of anaesthesia used. Usually adult dose is 0.2 to 0.7 mg/kg intravenously.

Dimethyl tubocurarine iodide is three times as potent as d-tubocurarine. However, it may be avoided in patients sensitive to iodides.

Pancuronium: It has a steroid nucleus. Its onset of action is quick (40–50 seconds). It is more potent than d-tubocurarine and causes full (100%) muscle relaxation. Histamine release is not significant. It does not cause significant change in blood pressure and is devoid of ganglionic blocking property. Increase in heart rate and cardiac output are its modest side effects which can be abolished by prior administration of atropine. It is given intravenously in a dose of 60–100 µg/kg for initial intubation and then 30–40 µg/kg for muscle relaxation.

Gallamine: Its onset of action is rapid but duration of action is short than d-tubocurarine. Histamine release is insignificant and acetylcholine esterase inhibitors reverse its effect less readily. It causes tachycardia by depressing the vagus nerve. Since it crosses placental barrier, it should be used with great care during caesarean sections. It is employed intravenously in doses of 80–120 mg.

Alcuronium: It has no advantage on tubocurarine or pancuronium. It is given intravenously in a dose of 10–15 mg. Other short acting neuromuscular blocking agents are vecuronium and atracurium.

Atracurium and its congeners: Atracurium is a bis-quarternary compound. It is unstable at physiological pH but indefinitely stable at an acidic pH. Its duration of action is short. Its ester moiety is hydrolysed by plasma pseudo-cholinesterases. It is also degraded by spontaneous or Hofmann degradation. It can be safely given to patients with renal and hepatic impairments because its metabolism is not affected in these two conditions.

Mivacurium and doxacurium are new congeners of atracurium. Mivacurium has short duration of action (onset 2–4 minutes; duration of action: 12–18 minutes) because it is rapidly catalyzed by cholinesterases. On the other hand, doxacurium has longer duration of action (onset 4–6 minutes; duration of action 90–120 minutes) because it is not significantly affected by cholinesterases.

Rocuronium is a new agent. Its onset of action is very quick like succinylcholine, but duration of action is long (30–40 minutes). So it can be used as an alternative to succinylcholine to facilitate tracheal intubation (relaxes laryngeal and jaw muscles).

Depolarizing agents: These agents mimic acetylcholine like action at neuromuscular junction but cause blockage by producing prolonged depolarization, i.e. dissociation of the drug from the receptor site and subsequent breakdown is slower than acetylcholine. There occurs rapid, complete and predictable paralysis and the recovery is spontaneous. Muscle fasciculations occur prior to the development of paralysis. There may occur prolonged paralysis leading to apnoea in patients with atypical plasma pseudocholinesterase enzyme. Succinylcholine belongs to this group.

Succinylcholine: It is ultrashort acting skeletal muscle relaxant. Its action occurs with in 15 seconds and is reversed on cessation of its administration because it is rapidly metabolized by plasma pseudocholinesterase enzyme. It causes initial fasciculations followed by flaccid paralysis. Hypothermia and neostigmine potentiate its relaxant effect. It causes negligible histamine release. It produces bradycardia in children which can be overcome by prior use of atropine. Postoperative muscle pain is common in patients who show muscle fasciculations. It stimulates cardiac muscarinic receptors and causes bradycardia in low doses. However, in large doses, it causes tachycardia. Other side effects are nausea, vomiting, hyperkalaemia and raised intraocular pressure. In presence of abnormal pseudocholinesterase enzyme, there occurs prolongation of its effect leading to apnoea. Another pharmacogenetic toxicity is occurrence of malignant hyperthermia. It should not be used in severe liver disease and in burn patients. According to the patient's need, it is given intravenously in a dose of 30–100 mg. Blocking action of succinylcholine can be prolonged by hexafluorenium which is a selective inhibitor of plasma pseudocholinesterase.

Toxicity and treatment: There occurs paralysis of the diaphragm muscle and respiratory paralysis leading to death when an excessive dose of tubocurarine and related drugs are administered. Certain general anaesthetics (ether in particular) and aminoglycoside antibiotics potentiate the action of these agents. The treatment consists of insertion of endotracheal tube and artificial respiration with oxygen. Neostigmine or edrophonium may be given intravenously to overcome muscle paralysis. However, they may worsen the hypotension and bronchospasm produced by d-tubocurarine. To counter muscarinic stimulation, atropine or glycopyrrolate is administered.

Uses of neuromuscular blocking agents:

1. Used as adjunct to general anaesthesia to have adequate muscle relaxation.
2. Succinylcholine is used for brief procedures, e.g. endotracheal intubation, laryngoscopy, bronchoscopy, oesophagoscopy, reduction of fractures and dislocations.
3. Succinylcholine is also used to avoid convulsions and trauma from electroconvulsive therapy.
4. If diazepam and other drugs do not control severe cases of tetanus and status epilepticus, a neuromuscular blocker (repeated doses of competitive blocker) may be used to induce paralysis and maintain on intermittent positive pressure respiration.

Directly Acting Muscle Relaxants

Dantrolene: It acts directly on the contractile machinery of skeletal muscle. It causes uncoupling of excitation from contraction in the muscle and reduces the depolarization-induced Ca^{++} release into sarcoplasm caused by conducted muscle action potential. It has little effect on smooth and cardiac muscles. It is given in doses of 25 mg orally daily. Important side effects are gastrointestinal disturbances, drowsiness, weakness, fatigue and mental disturbances. It is used in the treatment of spasticity due to stroke, spinal, cerebral and multiple sclerosis.

Quinine: It decreases the muscle tone by increasing the refractory period and decreasing the excitability of motor end-plates. It is used in myotonia congenita and nocturnal leg cramps (200–300 mg).

Centrally Acting Muscle Relaxants

These drugs do not alter consciousness. They decrease muscle tone by selectively depressing spinal and supraspinal polysynaptic reflexes. They do not affect monosynaptically mediated stretch reflex significantly and do not block transmission of impulses at the neuromuscular junction. They are classified as:

i. **Mephenesin group:**
  • Mephenesin
  • Meprobamate
  • Carisoprodol
  • Chlorzoxazone
  • Chlormezanone
  • Methocarbamol

ii. **Benzodiazepines:**
  • Diazepam and others
  • GABA derivatives (baclofen).

Mephenesin: It is the first centrally acting muscle relaxant. At present it is not used for this purpose systemically because it causes thrombophlebitis, haemolysis, marked fall in blood pressure, strong gastric irritation and has short duration of action. However, it has been included in counter irritant ointments.

Meprobamate: It is a mephenesin congener. It is seldom used now because of having low muscle relaxant: sedative ratio and drug dependence liability like barbiturates.

Carisoprodol: It is a useful centrally acting muscle relaxant with weak analgesic, antipyretic and anticholinergic actions.

Chlorzoxazone: Its pharmacological actions are similar to mephenesin. However, it has longer duration of action and better tolerated orally.

Chlormezanone: It is an antianxiety and hypnotic drug which is used for tension associated with muscle spasm.

Methocarbamol: It is a better muscle relaxant than mephenesin because it is less sedative, longer acting, available by oral route and does not produce thrombophlebitis and haemolysis on intravenous administration.

Note: Clinical usefulness of none of the above drugs as centrally acting skeletal muscle relaxant is well established.

Diazepam: It is a benzodiazepine derivative which enhances GABAergic transmission in the brain on specific receptors. It is a popular anxiolytic-sedative and is used for reducing tone.

Baclofen: It is a GABA (gamma-amino-butyric acid—an inhibitory transmitter) derivative. It is potent neuronal depressant. It mainly acts in the spinal cord on presynaptic mechanism rather than postsynaptic GABA-B receptors. It reduces the release of excitatory transmitters. It is lipophilic and crosses the blood–brain barrier with much ease. On oral administration, it is rapidly absorbed and is excreted unchanged in urine. The recommended daily dose is 5 mg 3 times a day to be increased every 3–4 days up to a maximum of 80 mg per day. Drowsiness, lassitude, and mental disturbances may appear as side effects.

Uses of Centrally Acting Muscle Relaxants

1. Mephenesin like and benzodiazepine muscle relaxants are often combined with analgesics and are used in the treatment of acute muscle spasms, torticollis, lumbago, backache, and neuralgias. However, efficacy of these drugs is not impressive.

2. Diazepam group of drugs and chlormezanone are used to treat increased tone of muscle associated with anxiety and tension.

3. Baclofen, diazepam and dantrolene have beneficial effect in the treatment of hemiplegia, paraplegia, spinal injuries, multiple sclerosis, and cerebral palsy. However, therapy of these disorders is far from satisfactory.

4. Diazepam or methocarbamol is used to treat tetanus, to reduce intensity of convulsions during electro-convulsive therapy and at the time of orthopedic manipulations. For this purpose, they are given intravenously.

5. Centrally acting muscle relaxants are used in myofacial pain of temporomandibular disorder in dental practice.

Points for Dental Students

1. Skeletal muscle relaxants are used as adjuncts to general anaesthetic for adequate muscle relaxation. Initially succinyl choline is used for endotracheal intubation. This is followed by an administration of non-depolarizing drug such as pancuranium or vecuronium. Such a procedure will prolong the action of non-depolarizing drug; so lower doses of drug can be used.

2. Centrally acting muscle relaxants such as chlorzoxazone plus an antianxiolytic drug alprazolam are used in myofacial pain of temporomandibular disorder in dental practice.

3. For setting mandibular fractures, neuromuscular blockers can be used in dental practice. For this purpose short acting non-depolarizing agents (mivacurium or rapocurium) are preferred. Although short acting succinyl choline can also be used but not preferred because it causes muscle fasciculations which may aggravate the fracture associated injury.

4. Succinyl choline is used to prevent laryngospasm in certain dental procedures.

TO REMEMBER

1. Peripherally acting muscle relaxants cause paralysis of skeletal muscles with loss of voluntary movements. They are practically always given i.v. for short-term purposes (as adjunct to surgical anaesthesia). They act by blocking the neuromuscular transmission and has no effect on central nervous system.

2. Centrally acting muscle relaxants act by selectively inhibiting polysynaptic reflexes in central nervous system. They decrease muscle tone without reducing voluntary power. However, they cause some central nervous system depression. They can be given orally as well as some times parenterally. Although they have been used in chronic spastic conditions, acute muscle spasms, tetanus, etc. efficacy of these drugs is not impressive.

Section 6

Cardiovascular System

Chapter 26

Cardiac Electrophysiology, Sodium, Potassium and Calcium Channels

Heart is a vital organ. It works as a pump to maintain an effective circulation through the blood vessels. The functional integrity of the blood vessels is necessary for circulatory homeostasis. The blood carries oxygen and other nutrients and circulates through various tissues of the body.

Cardiac rhythmicity: Automaticity means that the pacemaker cells (SA node) have the inherent property to depolarize spontaneously during diastole. The automaticity can be acquired by AV node, Purkinje fibres and even myocardial cells under exceptional or pathological states. The excitability of the cells is determined by the level of the membrane potential at which the cardiac cell can generate an action potential.

Electrophysiology of Cardiac Cell

A lipoprotein membrane bounds the cardiac cell. The membrane has receptor channels (ion-selective membrane-spanning proteins) crossing it. These channels permit passive movement of ions(Na^+, K^+, Ca^{++}, and Cl^-) down their electrochemical gradients. The movement of ions occurs during the open but not during the closed state of the channels. The sodium channels are fast channels. They are present in the myocytes of the atria, ventricles, and the His-Purkinje tissue. They are absent from the SA node and the AV node. The other ion channels are present in all the cardiac tissues. The cardiac cell has high concentration of Na^+ outside and K^+ inside. It has a resting membrane potential of 80 to 90 mV. On excitation, the depolarization of the cardiac tissues, in which sodium channels are present, is due to inward movement of the Na^+ ions. However, in case of SA node and AV node the depolarization occurs due to inward movement of Ca^{++} through the 'slow' calcium channels. On the other hand, repolarization in all the cardiac tissues is due to outward movement of K^+. Further, the cardiac myocytes also have two energy requiring exchange pumps:

a. **Na^+ and K^+ exchange pump:** It is unidirectional 'adenosine triphosphatase (ATPase) energized membrane pump. It pumps Na^+ into the exterior of the cell and K^+ into the interior of the cell. For every three Na^+ ions pushed out of the cell, the pump pushes two K^+ ions into the cell. Thus this pump is electronegative. This pump operates continuously. It does not switch on and off during the action potential of the cardiac cells.

b. **Na^+-Ca^{++} exchange pump:** It is bidirectional but mainly pumps Ca^{++} from inside the cell to the exterior. Such extrusion depends on the activity of the Na^+- K^+ pump and diminishes when the latter becomes inoperative.

The action potential of cardiac cells is divided into five phases:

- *Phase zero* (rapid depolarization): It is due to rapid entry of Na^+ through Na^+ specific channels (fast channel). However, in case of pacemaker cells, phase 'O' is not of rapid depolarization. There it is a slow process due to slow inward Ca^{++} current.
- *Phase 1* (rapid partial repolarization) is due to a gradual inactivation of the rapid inward Na^+ current and an activation of short lived inward Ca^{++} current.
- *Phase 2* (plateau phase) is due to entry of Ca^{++} into the cell through voltage operated slow channel and activates contractile machinery, which is inhibited by Ca^{++} channel blockers.
- *Phase 3* (rapid repolarization) is due to an outward positive current. Na^+ K^+ and ATPase pump takes part in restoring the intra- and extracellular concentration of these cations to their pre-excitation level.
- *Phase 4* (slow diastolic spontaneous depolarization) is a result of inward positive current carried by Na^+.

During depolarization process, the myocardial cell remains refractory to other stimuli. Absolute refractory period extends from phase 'O' to mid-phase 3 and during this period cardiac cell does not respond to any stimulus. Relative refractory period is at the last part of phase 3. During this period, the cardiac cell responds to strong stimulus. The sum of absolute and relative refractory periods is called effective refractory period.

Electrocardiogram (ECG): It tells about the electrical events within the heart. With each beat of the heart, the action potentials of cardiac muscle fibres are propagated throughout the heart. These currents produce voltage differences at the body surface. So they can be detected by electrodes placed at different sites on the body. A typical normal ECG is recorded as the potential difference between the right and left wrists. The first wave 'P' represents atrial depolarization. The second 'QRS' complex occurs approximately 0.1 to 0.2 seconds later. It represents ventricular depolarization. The ventricular repolarization is represented by the final 'T' wave.

Sodium Channels

There occurs an inward current of Na^+ ions on activation of Na^+ channel and causes generation of action potential in all the excitable cells of nerves and heart (depolarization of membrane). DDT, aconitine, veratridine, etc. activate Na^+ channels and in case of heart they induce extrasystoles and cardiac arrhythmias. Many drugs such as local anaesthetics (procaine, lignocaine), antiarrhythmic agents (quinidine, procainamide) and neurotoxins block voltage sensitive Na^+ channels and make it more difficult for an action potential to be produced. They are called Na^+ channel blockers or membrane stabilizers.

Potassium Channels

Resting membrane potential is controlled by K^+ ions. Membrane hyperpolarization occurs on opening of K^+ channels which produce outward flow of K^+ because intracellular concentration of K^+ is much higher (150 mM) compared to extracellular (4.5 mM). This opposes the opening of voltage-gated Ca^{++}

Voltage sensitive receptor channels of cells of lipoprotein membrane	
Channel	Tissue of clinical importance
Sodium	Heart and central nervous system
Potassium	Blood vessels, heart and smooth muscles
Calcium	Blood vessels, heart and smooth muscles

channels which need depolarization above a certain threshold membrane potential for activation.

So there occurs reduction of cellular contractile activity at the myocardial and vascular level as a result of fall of cytosolic Ca^{++} concentration.

There are three types of K^+ channels:

- **Voltage-gated K^+ channels** are opened when the cell is depolarized and help in the process of repolarization. They are mainly present in the blood vessels, heart, and smooth muscles. Diazoxide, minoxidil, pinacidil, etc. open these K^+ channels and cause hyperpolarization of membrane resulting in vasodilatation and plain muscle relaxation.
- **ATP-sensitive K^+ channels** are present in cardiac muscle and beta cells of islet of Langerhans of pancreas. These channels are closed when intracellular ATP is increased and there occurs depolarization of cells. So K^+ channel openers act by antagonizing the actions of intracellular ATP on these channels. There occurs hyperpolarization and relaxation of cardiac muscle on opening of these channels. Diazoxide or benzo-thiadiazine diuretics open these channels of beta cells of Langerhans and cause decreased secretion of insulin. Blockade of these channels by sulfonylurea causes depolarization of beta cells of Langerhans which stimulates insulin release.
- **Calcium-activated K^+ channels** are opened by an increase in intracellular Ca^{++} concentration during phase-2 of action potential. Due to this, entry of K^+ is facilitated and the cell is repolarized. These channels are sensitive to a number of neurotransmitters such as 5-HT, ACh, and NE.

Several other types of K^+ channels have also been identified, viz. receptor operated Na^+ activated and cell volume sensitive K^+ channels. They serve diverse functions and differ towards their sensitivities to different drugs.

Therapeutic Uses of K⁺ Channel Openers

- Hypertension (Drugs: diazoxide, minoxidil, pinacidil)
- Angina pectoris (Drug: nicroandil)
- Myocardial infarction : Cardioprotective by decreasing infarct size and ischaemia induced fibrillation.
- Other uses:
  a. Cerebral vasospasm
  b. Peripheral vascular diseases (cromo-kalim and pinacidil)
  c. Anticonvulsant and antineurotoxin agent
  d. Bronchial asthma, irritable bladder syndrome, and as intestinal antispasmodic
  e. Skeletal muscle fatigue and paralysis.
  f. Impotence
  g. To induce hair growth of male type

Potassium Channel Blockers

They primarily delay re-entry of K^+ during the action potential. They, therefore, prolong action potential duration and increase the refractory period. The potassium channel blockers are:

- Sulphonylureas block ATP-sensitive K^+ channels of beta cells of islet of Langerhans and they cause depolarization of cell membrane. So Ca^{++} enters in beta cells and there occurs release of insulin.
- Antiarrhythmic agents (amiodarone, bretylium)
- Non-selective K^+ channel blockers such as tetraethylammonium (TEA) and 4-amino-pyridine
- Polypeptide toxins: Apamin (from bee venom) and charybdotoxin (from scorpion venom) block Ca^{++}-activated K^+ channels while voltage-activated K^+ channel is blocked by dendrotoxin (from green mamba snake venom).

Calcium Channels

Calcium plays an important role in various biological processes. In case of cardiac and smooth muscles, entry of extracellular Ca^{++} is important for muscle contraction. In skeletal muscles, Ca^{++} is intracellular; so calcium channel blockers are ineffective on skeletal muscle.

Calcium Channel Blockers (Antagonists)

Calcium channel blockers block voltage operated slow Ca^{++} channels of cardiac and vascular smooth muscles. Thus they decrease the availability of intracellular Ca^{++}. Calcium channel blockers act on T-(transient) and L-(long lasting) type channels. Therapeutically important calcium channel blockers act on L-type of channels.

Classification (L-Type Calcium Channel Blockers)

- Benzyl-isoquinoline compounds (papaverine derivative): Verapamil, gallopamil.
- Dihydropyridine compounds: Nifedipine, nimodipine, nicardipine, felodipine, amlodipine.
- Benzothiazepine compounds (diphenylalkylamines): Cinnarazine, lidoflazine, flunarizine.

Pharmacokinetics

Verapamil, diltiazem and nifedipine are described here because they are most commonly used drugs. On oral administration, they are rapidly and completely absorbed. However, their bioavailability is low, specially of verapamil and diltiazem due to first-pass hepatic metabolism. Nifedipine can also be used sublingually because it is rapidly absorbed being lipid soluble. They are highly bound to plasma proteins (80–90%) and plasma half-like is 3–6 hours. Verapamil and nifedipine are primarily excreted in urine and diltiazem in the faeces.

Pharmacological Actions

1. **Heart:** Verapamil has main effect on heart while nifedipine exerts greater effect on smooth muscles. Diltiazem is intermediate in action. Verapamil causes:
   - Negative chronotropic and negative dromotropic actions;
   - Prolongation of effective refractory period of AV node
   - Depression of excitability of Purkinje's fibres.

   Verapamil is commonly used as antiarrhythmic agent because of its above cited properties as well as its ability to decrease oxygen consumption. Reflex tachycardia occurs due to hypotensive effect of nifedipine.

2. **Blood vessels:** Vascular smooth muscle is very sensitive to calcium channel blockers. So they cause:
   - Reduction in vascular resistance
   - Coronary vasodilatation
   - Inhibition of platelet aggregation
   - Prevention of deposition of calcium in atherosclerotic plaques
   - Inhibition of phospholipases (antioxidant action) so they have protective effect in myocardial ischaemia.

   Calcium channel blockers (especially nifedipine group) cause fall in blood pressure due to peripheral vasodilatation of resistance arteriolar vessels more than veins. So postural hypotension is not a real problem. Among the dihydropyridines, nifedipine has stronger effect on coronary and peripheral blood vessels, nimodipine on cerebral blood vessels.

3. **Plain muscles:** The resting tone and contractile responses of all types of smooth muscles are dependent on transmembrane Ca^{++} influx. Calcium channel blockers cause relaxation of smooth muscles. So they have antispasmodic effect on uterus, oesophageal sphincter, bronchi and urinary bladder.

Therapeutic Uses

1. **Cardiovascular conditions:**
   - Essential hypertension
   - *Angina pectoris and myocardial ischaemia:* They are more useful in variant angina or prinzmetal angina than glyceryl trinitrate. This is because calcium channel antagonists dilate large and small branches of coronary blood vessels while glyceryl trinitrate dilates only the big branches.
   - Cardiac arrhythmias
   - *Hypertrophic cardiomyopathy:* Verapamil is most suitable. It reduces myoplasmic calcium and leads to improvement of ventricular relaxation and reduction of the obstruction to the left ventricular outflow.
   - *Congestive cardiac failure:* Nifedipine produces a reduction in the after load and an increase in cardiac output. So it may be used in congestive cardiac failure with hypertension. Verapamil and diltiazem are not suitable for this condition due to their negative inotropic actions.
   - Peripheral vascular diseases.
   - *Cerebrovascular conditions:* Nimodipine, flunarizine and gallopamil can cross the blood–brain barrier. So they effectively reduce cerebral vasospasm and ischaemia associated with subarachnoid haemorrhage, cerebrovascular accidents and during intracranial surgery.
   - Nifedipine is used to decrease the progress of atheromatous lesions in coronary and other blood vessels by reducing accumulation of Ca^{++} in arterial wall and prevention of platelet aggregation.

2. **Neurological conditions:**
   - Migraine (drugs used—flunarizine, nimodipine)
   - Vertigo, associated with Meniere's disease, cervical spondylosis and vestibular neuronitis (drug—cinnarizine).
   - Grandmal epilepsy (drug—flunarizine)
   - Pschiatric disorders such as manic depressive psychosis, depression, schizophrenia, AIDS, dementia, and tremor (drug—verapamil)

3. **Non-vascular smooth muscles:** Nifedipine has been found useful in the following conditions:
   - Bronchial asthma
   - Gynecological disorders such as primary dysmenorrhoea, premature uterine contractions and hypertension with pregnancy.
   - Gastrointestinal disorders such as hiccup diffuse oesophageal spasm and achalasia.
   - Urinary incontinence due to nerve injury.

4. **Other uses:** Verapamil has been found to:
   - Improve the antineoplastic action of drugs like vincristine, daunorubicin, and adriamycin.
   - Have beneficial effects in chloroquine-resistant malaria by increasing the intracellular accumulation of chloroquine.

Adverse Effects

- Constipation, nausea.
- Cardiac effects (mainly with verapamil): Bradycardia, hypotension, cardiac arrest and congestive heart failure.
- Vascular (mainly with nifedipine): Flushing, palpitation due to reflex tachycardia, dizziness, headache, peripheral oedema, weight gain, and occasionally worsening of angina.

Drug Interactions

- Verapamil increases plasma concentration of digoxin.
- Propranolol prevents reflex tachycardia of nifedipine but may potentiate myocardial depressant action of verapamil.

TO REMEMBER

1. Heart is a vital organ which works as a pump to maintain an effective circulation through the blood vessels.

2. Aconitine, veratridine and DDT induce extrasystoles and cardiac arrhythmias by activating Na^+ channels of the heart. Na^+ channel blockers or membrane stabilizers are procaine, lidocaine, quinidine, and procainamide.

3. Diazoxide and minoxidil open voltage-gated K^+ channels of smooth muscles of blood vessels and cause hyperpolarization of membrane resulting in vasodilatation. They are useful in hypertension, angina pectoris and as cardioprotective. Amiadarone and bretylium are antiarrhythmic agents which act as K^+ channel blockers.

4. Calcium channel blockers block voltage operated slow Ca^{++} channels of cardiac and vascular smooth muscles.

5. Nifedipine is used to treat congestive cardiac failure while verapamil and diltiazem are not suitable because of their negative ionotropic actions.

6. Nimodipine, flunarizine and gallopamil effectively reduce cerebral vasospasm and ischaemia because they can cross the blood–brain barrier.

7. Nifedipine is used to decrease the progress of atheromatous lesions in coronary and other blood vessels.

8. Calcium channel blockers have also been used to treat migraine (flunarizine and nimodipine), vertigo (cinnarizine), grandmal epilepsy (flunarizine), and psychiatric disorders (verapamil).

9. Nifedipine has been found useful in bronchial asthma, gynecological and gastrointestinal disorders.

10. Verapamil improves the antineoplastic action of drugs and has beneficial effects in chloroquine resistant malaria.

Chapter 27

Antihypertensive Drugs

Hypertension

Clinically hypertension is persistently raised arterial pressure which is primarily due to increased vascular resistance in the systemic circulation. In due course of time, heart undergoes hypertrophy and subsequently failure because it has to work against a permanently increased after load. If the condition remains untreated and uncontrolled for a long period, there occurs irrepairable damage to other vital organs of the body such as brain, heart, kidney and eyes. In essential or primary hypertension (90%), the underlying cause is not known. In 10% of the cases, hypertension is secondary to some recognizable pathological condition and can be treated by removing or treating that condition. On the other hand, essential hypertension is treated by antihypertensive drugs.

Classification of Antihypertensive Drugs

Based on the mode of action, the antihypertensive drugs can be classified as follows:

1. **Diuretics:** Hydrochlorothiazide, chlorthalidone, frusemide.
2. **Drugs which lower sympathetic tone:**
   - *Centrally acting:* Clonidine, alpha-methyldopa, guanfacine, moxonidine
   - *Autonomic ganglionic blockers:* Trimetaphen
   - *Postganglionic adrenergic neuron blockers:* Guanethidine, guanadrel, bethanidine, debrisoquin, reserpine

   - *Beta-adrenoceptor blockers:* Propranolol, atenolol, metoprolol, labetalol
   - *Alpha-adrenoceptor blockers:* Prazosin, terazosin, indoramin
   - *Mixed adrenoceptor blockers:* Labetalol, carvediol
3. **Vasodilators:**
   - *Smooth muscle relaxant:*
     i. Arteriolar: Hydralazine, indapamide, zipamide
     ii. Arteriolar-venular: Sodium nitroprusside
   - *Calcium channel blockers:* Verapamil, diltiazem, nifedipine, felodipine, amlodipine, nitrendipine, lacidipine
   - *Potassium channel openers:* Minoxidil, pinacidil, diazoxide
4. **Inhibitors of renin-angiotensin system:**
   - *ACE-inhibitors:* Captopril, enalapril, lisinopril, ramipril, perindopril
   - *Angiotensin II subtype-1 (AT_1) receptor blocker:* Saralasin, losartan

1. Diuretics

Mechanism of action: Initially diuretics cause slight fall in blood pressure due to increased elimination of sodium and water which reduces blood volume and cardiac output. However, blood volume returns to normal on continuing treatment for 6 to 8 weeks but the antihypertensive effect persists by a slowly developing reduction in total peripheral vascular resistance. The later effect may be due to:

a. Lowering of electrolyte and water content of vascular smooth muscle which may decrease stiffness of vessel wall, increase their compliance, and reduction in their responsiveness to effects of noradrenaline and angiotensin-II

b. Increased production of PGI_2 in selected vascular beds to cause reduction of vascular resistance.

Diuretics also potentiate the action of most of the antihypertensive drugs on combined use.

Thiazide diuretics: These drugs are the first line of treatment in mild or moderate hypertension either alone or in combination with sympatholytic and vasodilator drugs. They can be given to patients of respiratory insufficiency, congestive heart failure, and insulin dependent diabetes mellitus while alpha-blockers cannot be used in presence of these diseases.

- *Hydrochlorothiazide:* 25–50 mg once or twice daily.
- *Chlorthiazide:* 25–100 mg per day.

Frusemide (high efficacy (loop) diuretic). It is not indicated in mild or moderate hypertension because it causes severe reduction of blood volume and electrolyte imbalance. However, it is indicated in hypertensive emergency, congestive cardiac failure and renal insufficiency.

Potassium sparing diuretics are usually employed in combination with thiazide diuretics to avoid excessive depletion of potassium and magnesium.

2. Antihypertensive Drugs which act by Lowering Sympathetic Tone

Centrally acting drugs: Clonidine and alpha-methyldopa, stimulate alpha-2 receptors on the vasomotor centre of the brain and thus decrease sympathetic outflow from the CNS to the peripheral vessels. Due to this, there occurs decrease in cardiac output and heart rate and thus fall in blood pressure. Clonidine acts as such while alpha-methyldopa gets converted intraneuronally into methyl noradrenaline which is responsible for antihypertensive effect. Abrupt withdrawal of both drugs may lead to severe rebound hypertension. These drugs are used in moderate hypertension. When used alone there occurs tolerance to their anti-hypertensive effect due to retention of sodium and increase in plasma volume. This can be overcome by simultaneous administration of a diuretic.

Clonidine: It is well absorbed on oral administration. It is mostly excreted in urine as unchanged drug. Important side effects are dry mouth, drowsiness, constipation, gastric upset and impotence. It should not be given to patients who are at risk of depression. The antihypertensive effect of clonidine is blocked on concomitant treatment with tricyclic antidepressants.

The usual oral dose of clonidine is 0.1 mg twice a day. The dose may be increased up to 0.6 mg 3 times a day.

Alpha-methyldopa: The antihypertensive action to methyl dopa develops slowly. On oral administration, peak effect on blood pressure is seen after 2–6 hours. It is excreted in urine both as an unchanged drug and a conjugated metabolite. Important side effects are sedation, drowsiness, nasal congestion, orthostatic hypotension and impotence.

Dose: 250 mg 2 to 3 times a day. In hypertensive emergencies, it is given i.v. (250–500 mg).

Guanfacine is related to clonidine and has actions similar to clonidine. However, its duration of action is prolonged.

Moxonidine: It is a selective imidazole receptor (I_1 receptor) agonist. It stimulates I_1 receptor in the medulla. So it reduces central sympathetic drive and peripheral vascular resistance. Concentrations of catecholamines and rennin in plasma are decreased. Due to these actions, it produces fall in blood pressure. It is particularly beneficial in obese hypertensive patients with co-existing glucose intolerance and/or dyslipidemia due to its ability:

- To have beneficial effect on lipid and carbohydrate metabolism
- To improve insulin-mediated glucose disposal in obese patients

Ganglion blocking agents: Except trimetaphan, other ganglion blocking agents are no more used as antihypertensive drugs being non-selective. Trimetaphan is a rapidly acting drug. It is given i.v. for hypertensive emergencies and to induce controlled hypotension for neurosurgery.

Adrenergic neuron blocking agents: Guanethidine and **reserpine** lower blood pressure by interfering with the release of adrenergic transmitters from postganglionic sympathetic neurons and other tissues. Guanethidine is a synthetic compound. It is incompletely absorbed from the gut, and does not cross blood–brain barrier. It is slowly excreted from the body and produces cumulative effect. Like noradrenaline, it is taken up from the plasma by the adrenergic neurons and causes adrenergic blockade. So it causes:

- Inhibition of release of norepinephrine at the sympathetic nerve endings
- Blockade of re-uptake of norepinephrine by the sympathetic nerve endings
- Depletion of norepinephrine stores at the sympathetic nerve endings and tissues. Cocaine and tricyclic antidepressants prevent the neuronal uptake of guanethidine by competing for the same uptake mechanism.

Guanethidine is given orally in severe hypertension, usually in combination with diuretic and vasodilators. Important adverse effects are orthostatic hypotension, nasal stuffiness, parotid tenderness, diarrhoea, muscle pain, supersensitivity of adrenergic receptors and retention of water and electrolytes.

Guanadrel, bethanidine, and debrisoquin are related to guanethidine and have similar mechanism of action.

Reserpine: It is an alkaloid. It is obtained from the roots of *Rauwolfia serpentina*. It is readily absorbed on oral administration. It slowly depletes catecholamines and serotonin from brain, adrenergic neurons and all other tissues. This results in loss of transmitter and fall in arterial pressure. However, it is no more used because of its toxicity related to CNS and gut and availability of more selective and less toxic drugs.

Beta-adrenoceptor blockers: Many clinicians consider that beta-adrenoceptor blockers are the drugs of first choice for the treatment of essential hypertension. Several mechanisms are involved in their hypotensive effect. Their hypotensive effect, therefore, is due to following reasons:

- On prolonged administration, blood pressure gradually falls in hypertensives but not in normotensives. Initially, total peripheral resistance (t.p.r.) is increased due to blockade of β_2-mediated vasodilatation and cardiac out put is reduced due to blocked of β_1-receptors of the heart. So there occurs little change in blood pressure. However, with continued treatment, resistance vessels gradually adapt to chronically reduced cardiac output so that t.p.r. decreases and both systolic and diastolic blood pressure falls.
- Reduction of sympathetic out flow from central nervous system due to blocked of presynaptic β-receptors centrally to peripheral blood vessels.
- Blocked of peripheral facilitatory presynaptic β_2-receptors to reduce sympathetic vasoconstrictor nerve activity.

- Reduction of renin release due to blocked of β_1 receptors of the juxtaglomerular cells of the renal cortex.
- An increase in biosynthesis of prostacycline in vascular beds.
- Increase in natriuretric peptide secretion caused by beta blockers.

Propranolol is contraindicated in bronchial asthma and diabetes mellitus being a non-selective beta blocker. Further, it is to be given 2–3 times a day.

Atenolol: It is a selective beta blocker. It can, therefore, be given to patients suffering from bronchial asthma and diabetes mellitus. Since the drug is given once a day the patient compliance is better.

Metoprolol is a cardio-selective β_1-receptor blocker. So it is given to hypertensive patients with diabetes.

Alpha-adrenoceptor blocker: Prazosin is an alpha-adrenoceptor blocker. Its antihypertensive effect is due to its ability to selectively block α_1 receptors. It allows nor-adrenaline to continue to act on α_2 receptors and inhibit its own release. So it causes less tachycardia than the non-selective alpha-blockers. Renal blood flow is not impaired and it increases HDL level in blood. Initially it is given 1 mg 3 times a day. The dose is gradually increased up to 20–30 mg a day. The first dose is given at bedtime because fainting or syncopal attack may occur after the first dose due to precipitous fall in blood pressure while standing. This does not occur in long-term treatment with prazosin.

Terazosin and doxazosin are the analogues of prazosin which are used as antihypertensives. They are preferred over prazosin because of their longer duration of action. They are either used alone in mild hypertension or in combination with other drugs.

3. Vasodilators

Smooth muscle relaxants: These drugs act directly and dilate the blood vessels. Due to this, there occurs fall in blood pressure. Their action is independent of the innervations of the vascular smooth muscle and is not mediated by adrenergic, cholinergic or histaminergic receptors.

Hydralazine, indapamide and xipamide are effective orally whereas sodium nitroprusside is administered by intravenous route. Important side effects are headache, flushing, nasal congestion, tachycardia and palpitation. On prolonged administration in high doses, hydralazine produces reversible lupus-like syndrome.

Hydralazine: It is a synthetic drug. It is used in a dose of 100–200 mg per day. It acts directly on arteriolar smooth muscle and not on veins. It is used to treat moderate to severe hypertension and is also used in chronic congestive cardiac failure. It is given in combination with a diuretic (to prevent sodium and water retention) or a beta blocker (to prevent tachycardia and increased renin secretion due to reflex sympathetic stimulation).

Indapamide and xipamide: They are related to chlorthalidone diuretic. They are given in single sub-diuretic doses in mild to moderate hypertension. They should be avoided in pregnancy, severe renal or hepatic insufficiency and in combination with diuretics.

Sodium nitroprusside: It is a very potent vasodilator. It acts directly on arterioles and venules. The onset of action is instantaneous and the effect lasts for 5–10 min. So it is given by continuous i.v. infusion at a rate of 0.001 mg/kg/min for the treatment of hypertensive emergencies.

Excessive hypotension, arrhythmias and accumulation of cyanide are reported as side effects.

Calcium channel blockers: These drugs block voltage operated slow L-type Ca^{++} channels of vascular smooth muscles. So they reduce the frequency of their opening in response to depolarization. This results in a marked decrease in transmembrane Ca^{++} current in vascular smooth muscle. They, therefore, dilate peripheral arterioles by inhibiting calcium influx in the arteriolar smooth muscle and reduce total peripheral resistance and blood pressure. Important side effects are headache, hypotension and dizziness.

Among the three prototype drugs, verapamil is relatively cardioselective, nifidipine is relatively vascular smooth muscle selective, while diltiazem exhibits intermediate selectivity. So for the treatment of hypertension, nifedipine and its analogues are preferred over the other two groups. The other important features of nifedipine group (dihydropyridines) are:

- These drugs block Ca^{++} channels of vascular smooth muscle at a concentration b e l o w that required for cardiac depressant effects. So these are less cardiac depressant than verapamil and diltiazem.
- However, reflex tachycardia with nifedipine (though to a lesser degree with long acting dihydropyridines such as felodipine and amlodipine) in therapeutic doses is more common as compared to diltiazem and verapamil due to their direct negative chronotropic effect.

Calcium channel blockers are among first choice antihypertensives because of:

- Convenient dosage schedule
- Better patient compliance
- Stroke preventing benefits

These are very useful in patients with low renin hypertension and in geriatric people with stiff blood vessels.

Nifedipine is used in a dose of 10–20 mg in hypertension, hypertensive emergencies and hypertension associated with pregnancy, diabetes mellitus and renal impairment.

Felodipine is administered in doses of 5 to 10 mg once daily. Amlodipine is given in doses of 5 to 10 mg once daily.

> **Action, effect and main uses of various types of vasodilators**
> - Vasodilators act:
>   - To increase local tissue blood flow
>   - To reduce arterial pressure
>   - To reduce central venous pressure
> - Net effect is reduction of:
>   - Cardiac preload (reduced filling pressure)
>   - Cardiac after-load (reduced vascular resistance)
>   - Cardiac work
> - Main uses are:
>   - Hypertension (e.g. ACEI and α_1 antagonists)
>   - Angina pectoris (e.g. calcium channel blockers)
>   - Cardiac failure (e.g. ACEI)

Potassium channel openers: They cause vasodilatation by opening voltage-gated K^+ channels of blood vessel and membrane hyperpolarization. They dilate arterioles with no effect on venules.

Minoxidil: It is given orally in a dose of 5 mg 1 to 2 times a day. The dose may be increased up to 50 mg per day. It is used to treat moderate to severe hypertension which are refractory or do not respond to conventional drug therapy. It is usually given in combination with a beta-blocker and a loop diuretic to minimize the dose of the drug, tachycardia, and retention of water and electrolytes. It causes serious side effects such as pericardial effusion, hirsutism, fatigue, tachycardia, angina pectoris, and retention of fluid.

Diazoxide: It has structural resemblance with thiazide diuretic, but it causes retention of sodium and water instead of diuresis. It is a K^+ channel opener. Oral absorption is erratic, so it is given rapidly i.v. It causes fall in blood pressure within 3–5 minutes and the effect lasts for 8–12 hours. It promptly decreases the tone of resistance vessels without an effect on capacitance vessels. It is used in the treatment of hypertensive emergencies. Reflex tachycardia can be prevented by beta blocker. It is also used to treat hypoglycaemia secondary to insulinoma because it inhibits insulin release from the pancrease.

Pinacidil and cromakalim are also K^+ channel openers which are being tried in hypertension.

4. Renin-angiotensin System Inhibitors

High plasma renin activity leads to:
- Increased formation of angiotensin-II (potent arteriolar vasoconstrictor)
- Stimulation of aldosterone secretion (promotes retention of Na^+ and water)
- Release of catecholamines

All these factors cause increase in the total peripheral resistance and ultimately essential hypertension. Renal ischaemia, adrenergic over activity and hyponatraemia may stimulate renin release.

Angiotensin converting enzyme (ACE) inhibitors: These drugs competitively inhibit ACE and thereby reduce the synthesis of angiotensin-II. Since ACE metabolizes bradykinin, they also preserve the concentration of bradykinin (potent vasodilator). So they reduce peripheral vascular resistance and lower the blood pressure. The other factors responsible for hypotensive effect may be via prostaglandin synthesis and reduction in adrenergic activity. These drugs can be used safely in patients with ischaemic heart disease because they do not change significantly heart rate and cardiac output. Further, they also reduce both preload and after load without the side effects of other hypotensive drugs.

Captopril: It is given 25 mg 3 times a day orally one to two hours before food. The dose may be increased at 1–2 week intervals to 150 mg per day.

Enalapril: It is a prodrug. Food does not interfere with its absorption from gastrointestinal tract. On oral administration 70% of the drug is absorbed. In the liver, it is converted into the active drug enalaprilat (half life 11 hours). It is given in doses of 10–20 mg once daily.

Lisinopril: It is a lysine derivative of enalaprilat which is given in doses of 10–80 mg once daily orally. It is slowly absorbed and its half-life is 12 hours.

Ramipril and perindopril are the other ACE inhibitors in use. They are given orally once a day.

Therapeutic uses:
- Mild to moderate hypertension with or without high plasma renin activity. The drug can be used alone or with a thiazide diuretic.
- Malignant hypertension.
- Congestive cardiac failure.

Adverse reactions are uncommon, but may be serious in some cases such as:
- Hypotension after the first dose in sodium depleted patients.
- Bone marrow depression and proteinuria.
- Minor side effects are cough, headache, dizziness, fatigue, allergic skin rash, drug fever, alteration in taste sensation.

They are contraindicated in patients with bilateral renal artery stenosis because they may precipitate acute renal failure.

Angiotensin receptor blocker: Saralasin is an analogue of angiotensin-II. It is a competitive inhibitor of angiotensin-II at vascular receptor site. However, it also has significant partial agonist property. It is used to diagnose renal cause of hypertension by blocking the pressor effects of circulating angiotensin-II and lowering the blood pressure in high renin states. It is given by i.v. infusion at a rate of 20 mg/kg/min because it has a very short half-life (4 min).

Losartan: It is phenyl tetrazone substituted imidazole compound. It is selective angiotensin-II receptor type-1(AT_1) antagonist. Unlike saralasin, it does not have intrinsic agonist property. Its side effects are skin rashes and neuropsychiatric disturbances(insomnia, confusion, nightmare, agitation and depression). It is useful in the treatment of essential hypertension.

Valasarten, irbesartan and candesartan are the newer analogues of losartan.

At present, clinical uses of angiotensin-II subtype 1 (AT_1) receptor antagonists are kept reserved by many clinicians for patients with hypertension in whom ACE inhibitor is indicated, but who are unable to tolerate this because of dry cough. This side effect is not caused by AT_1 antagonists.

Other possible indication is heart failure which is currently being explored in clinical trials.

PRESENT DAY STATUS OF ANTIHYPERTENSIVE DRUGS

- Drug treatment of hypertension is carried out with those drugs which have proven benefit and least likely to produce side effects. At present, ganglion blockers, adrenergic neuron blockers, and reserpine are no more used because they produce fearsome array of adverse effects.
- Thiazide diuretic or β-adrenoceptor blockers are commonly used as starting points for the treatment of mild hypertension. They abolish the excess risk of stroke and reduce the risk of myocardial infarction. There adverse effects are much less severe in comparison to methyldopa or guanethidine.
- To control moderate or severe hypertension without causing side effects, use combination of low doses of different drugs with complementary mechanism of action, e.g. diuretic with angiotensin converting enzyme inhibitor(ACEI). The efficacy of diuretic is limited by the increased plasma rennin activity that it causes.

This side effect is controlled by ACEI. Further, high doses of antihypertensive drugs are often not very effective in chronic administration due to homeostatic mechanisms and they cause side effects also.

- ACEI and calcium channel blockers are used alone or in combination to control moderate or severe hypertension. AT_1 receptor antagonist is especially indicated if patient is unable to tolerate ACEI because of cough.

One of the following drugs is added(in case of severe hypertension) or substituted (in case of moderate hypertension) if the above mentioned treatment is not sufficient to control the blood pressure. In both groups, when target blood pressure (140/ 85 mm Hg) is reached and consistently maintained, try to step down the antihypertensive drug treatment to the initial drugs.

- During pregnancy, toxaemic hypertension may develop. It is associated with a hyper-adrenergic state, decrease in plasma volume (despite oedema) and increase in vascular resistance. Selection of antihypertensive should be made from the following drugs:
  a. Hydrallazine
  b. Methyldopa
  c. Dihydropyridine calcium channel blockers
  d. Cardio-selective β-blockers and those with sympathomimetic activity
  e. Prazocin and clonidine-provided postural hypotension can be avoided.
- In hypertensive emergencies, one of the following drugs is used:
  a. Sodium nitroprusside by i.v. infusion
  b. Nitroglycerine-5–20 µg/minute i.v. infusion
  c. Diazoxide fractional i.v. bolous injection
- In hypertensive urgencies, one of the following drugs can be used:
  a. Nifedipine 10 mg, chewed and swallowed, repeated 1/2 to 1 hour
  b. Clonidine 100 µg oral or i.m. every 1–2 hours

c. Captopril 25 mg oral, repeated as needed
d. Hydrallazine 10–20 mg i.m. or i.v. (slowly), repeated every 2 hours.

Points for Dental Students

During history taking, find out whether patient is suffering from hypertension. If so dentist must be aware of medications which are being administered to the patient due to following reasons:

1. This is important because these drugs have drug interactions with other drugs which may be prescribed by the dentist, e.g.
   - The effect of beta adrenoceptor blocker agents may be decreased by indomethacin and other NSAIDs.
   - Beta blockers increase pressor response of sympathomimetics. This is particularly important when local anaesthetic with sympathomimetics is used in dental practice. If per chance sympathomimetic agent is absorbed in such cases, the blood pressure may be increased due to unopposed action of α-receptors.
   - Beta blockers potentiate the hypoglycemic effect of insulin and oral antidiabetics. This is important if patient is also suffering from diabetes and receiving one of these drugs.
   - The effect of ACE inhibitors is decreased by NSAIDs.
   - The metabolism of calcium channel blockers is decreased by itraconazole and ketoconazole while is increased by rifampin, phenytoin. On the other hand, calcium channel blockers decrease the metabolism of carbamazepine and cyclosporin.

2. If blood pressure in hypertensive patient is fluctuating, use a local anaesthetic without a sympathomimetic.

3. Commonly used antihypertensive agents may have intraoral changes that are of importance to the provision of dental care such as:
   - Diuretics produce oral dryness.
   - Adrenergic inhibitors may cause oral dryness and oral ulceration.
   - Calcium channel blockers may induce gingival overgrowth.
   - Angiotensin converting enzyme inhibitors induce lichenoid reactions of the oral mucosa. These drugs also produce cough and loss of taste that may be of importance during dental procedures.

4. Before initiating dental care, assess hypertension and determine presence of target organ disease. Dental treatment for patients with elevated blood pressure is determined as under:
   - Asymptomatic, BP < 159/99 mm Hg, no target organ disease: No dental modifications are needed and such cases can be treated in a dental outpatient setting.
   - Asymptomatic, BP = 160–179/100–109 mm Hg, no history of target organ disease; assess on individual basis with regard to type of dental procedure.

Treatment of hypertension

1. Non-pharmacologic measures:
   - Increased exercise
   - Reduced dietary salt
   - Reduced saturated fat
   - Increased fruit and fibre
   - Reduction in weight and alcohol intake
2. Pharmacologic measures:
   - Mild hypertension: Thiazide diuretic or β-adrenoceptor blocker
   - Moderate or sever hypertension: Use combination of low doses of different drugs with complementary mechanism of action such as diuretic + ACEI or ACEI and calcium channel blockers (alone or in combination)

- BP ≥ 180/110 mm Hg, no history of target organ disease; do not carry elective dental procedures.
- Target organ disease or poorly controlled diabetes mellitus: Elective dental care is carried out only when BP is controlled preferably < 140/90 mm Hg.

5. Sometime syncope may be precipitated due to anxiety during dental procedures. It is defined as a transient loss of consciousness and postural tone due to inadequate cerebral blood flow. This is mediated by the Bezold-Jarisch reflex. It is usually triggered by a reduction in venous return due to a stressful and painful experience. Concomitant sympathetic activation then leads to vigorous contraction of the relatively under filled ventricles. In turn this leads to the reflex by stimulating ventricular mechanoreceptors. This reflex produces parasympathetic (vagal) activation and sympathetic withdrawal causing bradycardia, vasodilatation or both. Premonitory symptoms such as nausea, diaphoresis, tachycardia, and pallor are usual. Episode can be aborted by head-up-tilt method. It involves asking the patient to lie down on a table that is then tilted to an angle of 70° for up to 45 minutes. Drug treatment is often un-necessary but in severe cases β-blockers (which inhibit the initial sympathetic activation) or disopyramide (a vagolytic agent) may be helpful.

6. Some antihypertensive drugs (e.g. prazosin, terazosin, labetalol, guanethidine, etc.) cause postural hypotension. So a patient on these antihypertensive drugs should not stand suddenly upright on being in a supine position for some time on a dental chair to avoid postural hypotension.

TO REMEMBER

1. Clinically, hypertension is persistently raised arterial pressure which is primarily due to increased vascular resistance in the systemic circulation.
2. Hydrochlorothiazide is commonly used to treat mild or moderate hypertension either alone or in combination with sympatholytic and/or vasodilator drugs.
3. Frusemide causes severe reduction of blood volume and electrolyte imbalance, so it is not used in routine. It is indicated in hypertensive emergency, congestive cardiac failure and renal insufficiency.
4. Clonidine and alpha methyldopa cause fall in blood pressure by stimulating alpha-2 receptors on the vasomotor centre of the brain and thus decreasing sympathetic outflow from central nervous system to the peripheral vessels.
5. Except trimetaphan, being non-selective, other ganglionic blocking agents are no more used. Trimetaphan is used i.v. for hypertensive emergencies and to induce controlled hypotension for neurosurgery.
6. Because of frequent and disturbing side effects, guanethidine has practically gone out of use now.
7. Because of frequent side effects and limited efficacy, reserpine is seldom used now.
8. To treat mild hypertension, a thiazide or a beta blocker is used initially. Combined (2-drug) therapy may be given if response is not satisfactory.
9. To treat moderate or severe hypertension, use ACEI or calcium channel blockers alone or in combination. Add or substitute additional antihypertensive drugs, if patient is not responding to therapy.
10. To treat hypertension emergency, sodium nitroprusside or diazoxide is used parenterally. Alternatively, nifedipine sublingually or parenterally or hydralazine parenterally may be used.

Chapter 28

Antianginal Drugs

Heart supplies blood to all parts of the body. However, it gets its own supply of blood through the coronary arteries (4% of cardiac output; oxygen extraction 75% in comparison to 25% in the systemic circulation). The coronary flow of blood occurs during the diastole only.

Angina pectoris is a clinical condition which occurs due to the imbalance between the oxygen supply and oxygen demand. It is manifested as a severe, pressing retrosternal (substernal) pain which radiates to the chest, left shoulder, upper arm and neck. There occurs accumulation of acidic metabolites due to ischaemic changes during obstruction in coronary flow. These metabolites stimulate myocardial pain mediating nerve endings.

In *angina of effort (or exertional or classical angina)*, the pain appears on exercise, exertion, emotion or meals. It lasts for several seconds and subsides on rest. It occurs due to an increase in oxygen demand which cannot be met due to atherosclerosis of larger coronary arteries.

In *variant (Prinzmetal's) angina*, on the other hand, the pain appears even during rest. It is usually unrelated to exercise. It occurs either due to coronary spasm or to platelet emboli causing reduction in coronary flow.

The *unstable (crescendo or preinfarction) angina* is characterized by recurrent attacks of angina. It occurs with minimal exertion. It is precipitated due to combination of athero-sclerotic plaque, platelet aggregation at ruptured plaque and vasospasm.

Antianginal Drugs

1. Organic Nitrites and Nitrates

Traditionally, both nitrites and nitrates are referred as nitrates. Based on their onset and duration of action, they are classified into two groups:

  i. Rapid onset and short duration of action:
   • Glyceryl trinitrate (nitroglycerine)
   • Amylnitrite
  ii. Slow onset and long duration of action:
   • Pentaerythritol tetranitrate
   • Isosorbide dinitrate
   • Isosorbide mononitrate

Mechanism of action (Fig. 28.1): Organic nitrates enter smooth muscle cells and relax all types of vessels but the post-capillary vessels (venules and veins) are particularly sensitive. Inside the smooth muscle cells, they are rapidly denitrated to release reactive free radical nitric oxide (NO). In turn, nitric oxide is converted into a reactive nitrosothiol intermediate (R-S NO) which activates guanylyl cyclase and stimulates formation of cGMP. cGMP activates protein kinase and leads to relaxation. Further, raised intracellular cGMP may also reduce Ca^{++} entry which also contributes to relaxation.

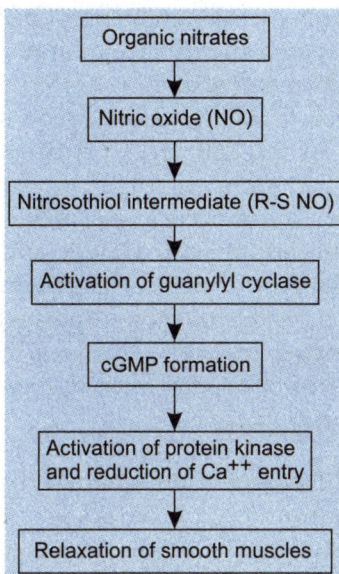

Fig. 28.1: Mechanism of action of nitrates

Pharmacological Actions

- Nitrates cause relaxation of smooth muscles directly (bronchi, ureter, sphincter of Oddi and blood vessels).
- Cardiovascular system: Nitrates cause dilatation of both arterioles and venules but in low doses venodilatation is more marked than the arteriolar dilatation. Due to generalized venodilatation, blood tends to pool in the vein leading to fall in the venous return and fall in left ventricular end diastolic pressure (preload). The oxygen demand is also reduced due to diminished wall tension. There also occurs reduction in external cardiac work and oxygen demand due to lowering of arterial pressure by nitrites.
- Nitrates cause selective vasodilatation of large epicardial vessels and help in redistribution of coronary blood flow to ischaemic subendocardial vessels by opening up of collaterals, without increasing the total flow. So the beneficial effect on heart is secondary to the vascular action of nitrate. However, in very large doses nitrates depress myocardium.

Side effects: Throbbing headache (due to dilatation of meningeal vessels), flushing (due to dilatation of cutaneous vessels), rise in intraocular tension (due to dilatation of retinal vessels), dizziness, postural hypotension and tachycardia are commonly seen. Tolerance to headache and antianginal effect may develop on prolonged use.

Pharmacokinetics: Organic nitrates are absorbed well from gastrointestinal tract being lipid soluble. Glyceryl trinitrate, however, undergoes first pass metabolism and is ineffective orally. It is administered sublingually or as skin patch. Its metabolites (di- and mononitrates) are active. Other nitrates are given orally. The nitrates are metabolized by glutathione-organic nitrate reductase enzyme in liver. The metabolites are eliminated.

Therapeutic Uses

1. **Angina pectoris:** Nitrites and organic nitrates are used as prophylaxis and for treatment of classical as well as variant angina pectoris.
2. Nitroglycerine may be tried in biliary colic due to its spasmolytic effect.
3. Isosorbide dinitrate is being increasingly used to reduce the preload in intractable congestive cardiac failure and left ventricular failure patients, not responding to diuretic therapy.
4. Amyl nitrite inhalation or sodium nitrite (0.3–0.5 gm in 10 ml) i.v. may be used to treat cyanide poisoning, followed by administration of sodium thiosulphate (25%–50 ml i.v.).
5. Glyceryl trinitrate is used as an adjunct to dilate coronaries during percutaneous coronary angioplasty and thrombolytic therapy of myocardial infarction.
6. Sublingual administration of nitroglycerine quickly relieves pain of oesophageal spasm. If given before a meal, it facilitates feeding in oesophageal achalasia by reducing oesophageal tone.

Contraindications

- Acute myocardial infarction because nitrates aggravate stroke by further reducing blood pressure.
- Severe anaemia because nitrates increase oxygen debt and hypoxia by forming methaemoglobinemia.

2. Beta-adrenoceptor Blockers

Propranolol, atenolol and metoprolol are commonly used drugs in angina pectoris (stable angina). They increase exercise tolerance by diminishing the cardiac response to sympathoadrenal activity, decreasing the emotion or exercise-induced increase in heart rate and force of contraction. They also decrease work load on the heart by causing bradycardia and reduction in cardiac contractility. Thus they significantly reduce myocardial oxygen demand, the frequency and severity of anginal attacks and prevent ECG changes. Nearly 85% of the patients do not get attacks of angina if propranolol with nitroglycerine is used judiciously. If this combination is used for several years, there occurs significant decrease in the incidence of myocardial infarction and death.

3. Calcium Channel Blockers

Verapamil and diltiazem decrease myocardial contractile force, cardiac rate and oxygen demand. Nifedipine inhibits coronary arterial spasm, dilates arterioles and increases oxygen supply to myocardium in patients of variant angina. Nifedipine also diminishes workload of myocardium by reducing after-load because it causes peripheral vasodilatation. These drugs also have antiplatelet aggregatory effect which contributes to their beneficial effects in variant angina. These drugs are useful in the treatment of both angina of effort and variant angina.

Nifedipine can be used in AV conduction defects because it acts mainly on arterioles and does not decrease AV conduction. On the other hand, verapamil and diltiazem cannot be used due to their negative inotropic effect on heart. Nicardipine, felodipine, amlodipine, nitrendipine are other dihydropyridines. Their pharmacodynamic profile is similar to nifedipine. There occurs less reflex sympathetic stimulation with slower and longer acting dihydropyridines. At present, these drugs are preferred over nifedipine which has been reported to have increased mortality among post-myocardial infarction patients.

4. Potassium Channel Openers

Nicorandil is a new antianginal drug with nitrate like moiety. Its arterial vasodilator effect is due to its ability to activate ATP sensitive K^+ channels leading to hyperpolarization of vascular smooth muscle. On the other hand, its venodilator effect is due to nitrate like activity, i.e. donating nitric oxide (NO) which leads to relaxation of blood vessels by increasing cGMP. However, unlike nitrates tolerance does not develop to its effects. It increases coronary blood flow without causing coronary steal phenomenon and without producing significant cardiac effects. It is as effective antianginal agent as nitrates, beta blockers, Ca^{++} channel blockers. Its side effects are flushing, palpitation, headache, dizziness, stomatitis, nausea and vomiting. It is contraindicated in presence of cardiogenic shock, left ventricular failure with low filling pressure and hypotension.

5. Antiplatelet Drugs

i. Aspirin is used in low doses to reduce the incidence of ischaemia in patients of coronary artery disease. Recently, it is shown that aspirin blunts the vasodilator effect of ACE inhibitors, probably due to reduction in bradykinin mediated vasodilatory prostaglandin synthesis by aspirin.

ii. Ticlopidine and clopidogrel are anti-platelet drugs. They do not appear to interfere with prostaglandin synthesis. They reduce platelet aggregation by inhibiting binding of adenosine diphosphate (ADP) to its receptors irreversibly. Clopidogrel is safer drug than ticlopidine (lesser thrombocytopenia and leucopenia). Like aspirin, it is used:
   • In the secondary prevention of stroke.
   • For unstable angina.
   • To prevent thrombosis in patients undergoing coronary bypass surgery.
iii. Dipyridamol is a potent coronary dilator and also inhibits platelet aggregation. It has minimal effect on blood pressure and cardiac output because it does not reduce venous return. It inhibits adenosine deaminase and phosphodiesterase enzymes. So there occurs accumulation of adenosine and cAMP respectively that then inhibit platelet aggregation and may also stimulate release of prostaglandin I_2.

It is not useful as an antianginal drug because by dilating resistance vessels in the non-ischaemic zones, it diverts the already reduced blood flow away from ischaemic zone where it is most needed (coronary steal "phenomenon"). However, it is used:
   • For prophylaxis of coronary and cerebral thrombosis in post-myocardial infarction and post-stroke patients.
   • To prevent thrombosis in patients with prosthetic heart valves along with warfarin.
   • To prevent platelet activation by extra-corporeal bypass pump, two days prior to open heart surgery.

Important side effects are exacerbation of angina, headache, tachycardia and gastro-intestinal distress.

6. Cytoprotective Drugs

i. Trimetazidine is a calcium channel blocker. It has cytoprotective effect on myocardium metabolism in the presence of ischemia. However, it has no effect in the presence of normal oxygen supply to myocardium. It has been found useful in angina of effort and in patients with stable angina in doses of 20 mg orally three times a day.
ii. Dilazep is a new but weaker calcium channel blocker. It also has cytoprotective effect on myocardium metabolism in the presence of ischaemia. It is used for stable angina and for symptomatic relief in coronary artery spasm. Its side effects are gastrointestinal distress, headache, stomatitis and allergy.

Drugs of lesser importance are lidoflazine, oxyfedrine and pentoxiphylline. Their brief description is as under:
   • Lidoflazine is another Ca^{++} channel blocker. It reduces AV conduction. It is not a popular drug to decrease frequency of anginal attacks. Altered taste sensation occurs as side effect.
   • Oxyfedrine improves myocardial metabolism to sustain stress due to hypoxia. It has beta-agonist action in low doses but β-blocking properties in high doses. Its therapeutic potential is questionable in angina and myocardial infarction.
   • Pentoxiphylline (oxypentifylline) is a theobromine analogue. It reduces blood viscosity and improves blood flow in ischaemic area through microcirculation by inhibiting phosphodiesterase enzyme. It is used to treat transient ischaemic attacks.

Its other uses are:
   • Non-haemorrhagic stroke
   • Chronic cerebrovascular insufficiency
   • To improve symptoms like vertigo and memory defects
   • Trophic leg ulcers
   • Obstructive circulatory disturbances of retina

- To improve sperm motility
- Diabetic neuropathy
- In AIDS patients with increased TNF to inhibit production of tumor necrosis factor

Many other drugs such as papaverine, cyclandelate, nicotinyl xanthinate, nicotinic acid, theophylline, prenylamine, kheline, MAO inhibitors and alcohol are practically of no value in angina pectoris.

Doses and Mode of Administration of commonly used Antianginal Drugs

1. **For acute attack of angina:**
   - Nitroglycerine 0.5 mg sublingually; if not relieved repeat every 5 minutes; maximum 3 doses; spit out tablet after relief.
   - Isosorbide dinitrate 5–10 mg sublingual; as an alternative of nitroglycerine.
2. **For prophylaxis:**
   i. *Beta blockers:*
      - Propranolol 20–80 mg oral, three times a day; gradually increase doses if required.
      - Atenolol 50–100 mg oral, once daily.
      - Metoprolol 50–100 mg oral, twice a day.
   ii. *Organic nitrates:*
      - Isosorbide dinitrate 5–10 mg oral, four times a day.
      - Isosorbide mononitrate 10–20 mg oral, thrice a day.
      - Pentaerythritol tetranitrate 10–20 mg oral, three times a day.
      - Nitroglycerine transdermal ointment (2%) or patch (5–10 mg)/24 hr.
   iii. *Calcium channel blockers:*
      - Verapamil 40–80 mg oral, three times a day.
      - Diltiazem 30–60 mg oral, three times a day.
      - Nifedipine 5–10 mg oral, three times a day.
      - Nicardipine 20–40 mg oral, three times a day.
      - Felodipine 5–10 mg oral, once daily.
      - Amlodipine 5–10 mg oral, once daily.
      - Nitrendipine 5–20 mg oral, once daily.
   iv. *Potassium channel openers:*
      - Nicorandil 5–20 mg oral, twice a day.
3. **For prophylaxis against myocardial infarction:**
   - Dipyridamole (75 mg) + aspirin (60–100 mg) one tablet three times a day.

Useful Antianginal Combinations

- The combined use of beta blocker and organic nitrate is very effective in the treatment of classical exertional angina. Their additive effect is due to the fact that one drug blocks the adverse effects of the other on net myocardial oxygen consumption.
- The combination of nitrates with calcium channel blockers may be valuable in variant angina because nitrates decrease preload while calcium channel blockers decrease after load. Hence their combined use may decrease cardiac work to an extent not possible by either drug alone.
- A combination of amlodipine (causes tachycardia) and atenolol (causes bradycardia) may be useful to patients of exertional angina.
- In severe and resistant cases of classical angina, all the three group of drugs, viz. organic nitrates (decrease preload) + beta blocker (decreases cardiac work) + calcium channel blocker (decreases after load) can be used. However, combination of verapamil or diltiazem with a beta blocker increases the risk of conduction defects and left ventricular dysfunction. Hence they should be used with great care.

Points for Dental Students

1. Several considerations need to be addressed when treating dental patients with coronary artery disease (CAD) to prevent recurrence of angina or infarction.
2. The determination of vital signs such as blood pressure, pulse rate and rhythm prior to dental care is essential.
3. Patients with CAD are at increased risk of demand-related ischemia with increased heart rate and blood pressure. Anxiety can increase the heart rate and blood pressure and can provoke angina or ischaemia. So a dentist must take care of following points:
   - In patients with CAD, dental care should be provided in the late morning or the early afternoon due to the influence of cicardian variation on the triggering of acute coronary events between 6 AM and noon. This may be due to sympathetic nervous system activation and an increased coagulative state. Medications designed to prevent these events, such as beta blockers, aspirin, and antihypertensives should be continued.
   - Patients of angina pectoris must be advised to keep sublingual tablet of nitroglycerine or isosorbide mononitrate with him so that same may be used to abort the acute attack if precipitated.
   - Fortunately risk is low during out patient dental procedures. Depending on level of anticipated stress premedication with antianxiety drugs (benzodiazepines) and/or inhalation nitrous oxide may be employed to reduce the anxiety.
4. The use of xylocaine+ adrenaline injection or adrenaline-impregnated gingival retraction cord is contraindicated in patients taking propranolol as an antianginal drug.
5. Elective dental procedures especially those requiring general anaesthesia should be avoided for at least 4 weeks following an acute myocardial infarction as there is small risk of recurrent events.
6. Since beta blockers and calcium channel blockers are used for prophylaxis of angina pectoris, all those precautions should be taken as mentioned in chapter 27 for these drugs under points for dental students on prescribing other drugs concomitantly.

TO REMEMBER

1. Angina pectoris is a clinical condition. It occurs due to imbalance between the oxygen supply and oxygen demand. It may be angina of effort (or exertional or classical angina), variant (Prinzmetal's) angina (occurs even during rest), and unstable (crescendo or preinfarction) angina (occurs with minimal exertion).
2. To abort or terminate an acute attack of classical or variant angina, sublingual glyceryl trinitrate or isosorbide dinitrate is taken on 'as and when' required basis.
3. For chronic prophylaxis, generally one agent from beta blocker or nitrates or calcium channel blocker group is used initially. When it fails to provide adequate relief in tolerated doses, two or three drugs may be tried concurrently.
4. For chronic prophylaxis of classical angina, a beta blocker may be combined either with nitrate or dihydropyridine (nifedipine). The advantages of such a combination are:
   a. Blocking of nitrate induced tachycardia by beta blocker or dihydropyridine
   b. Counteracting the tendency of beta blocker to cause ventricular dilatation by nitrate or dihydropyridine and

c. Opposing the tendency of beta blocker to reduce total coronary flow by nitrate or dihydropyridine.

5. For chronic prophylaxis of severe variant angina, nitrates are used in combination with calcium channel blockers. Such combination may decrease cardiac work to an extent not possible with either drug alone.

6. For chronic prophylaxis of most severe and resistant cases of classical angina, combined use of all the three classes is indicated. Such a combination will lead to supradditive effect due to difference in their primary mechanism of action.

7. Beta blockers are not used in combination with verapamil or diltiazem because such a combination will have marked depressant effects on SA and AV node.

8. Nitrates primarily decrease preload.

9. Calcium channel blockers mainly reduce after load.

10. Due to direct action on heart, beta blockers decrease cardiac work.

Chapter 29

Cardiac Glycosides and other Drugs for Congestive Heart Failure

Before discussing the drugs of this system, it is pertinent to deal with certain aspects of physiological parameters of normal cardiac circulation.

Left atrium receives oxygenated blood from lungs through pulmonary veins. It pumps blood to left ventricle which pumps blood to systemic circulation through aorta and systemic arteries. In systemic circulation, blood is deoxygenated (supplies O_2 to various tissues and receives CO_2). In turn, deoxygenated blood reaches to right atrium through superior vena cava, inferior vena cava, and coronary sinus. Right atrium pumps blood to right ventricle which sends blood to lungs, through pulmonary arteries. In the lungs, the blood is oxygenated and the cycle starts once again. During normal cardiac circulation, the following features are important because they will be helpful in understanding the drug therapy of heart failure.

- The right side of the heart (right atrium and right ventricle) pumps blood to lungs but does not to other organs. On the other hand, the left side of the heart (left atrium and left ventricle) pumps oxygenated blood into the systemic circulation except for lungs.
- The end of the atrial systole (contraction) is also the end of the ventricular diastole (relaxation). Thus each ventricle contains about 130 ml of blood at the end of diastole (relaxation). This blood volume is called the end diastolic volume (EDV).

- The left ventricle ejects about 70 ml of blood into aorta and the right ventricle ejects the same amount of blood into the pulmonary artery. That means at the end of every systole, the remaining amount of blood in each ventricle is 130–70 = 60 ml. This is called end systolic volume (ESV). It means the volume of blood ejected per beat after the systole from each ventricle is 70 ml. This is called stroke volume (SV). That means SV= EDV–ESV (130–60 = 70 ml).
- Cardiac output (CO) is the volume of blood ejected from left ventricle into the aorta or from right ventricle into the pulmonary trunk. So CO (ml/min) = SV (ml/beat) × HR (beat/min). Normally SV = 70 ml /beat and HR = 72 beats/min. So CO = 70 × 72 = 5040 ml or about 5 litre/min. This is close to total blood volume. Thus, entire blood volume flows through lungs and body organs each minute. Factors which increase stroke volume or heart rate will also increase cardiac output.
- Three factors regulate the stroke volume (SV) to ensure that the left and right ventricles should pump equal volume of blood to the aorta and pulmonary trunk. These are: (a) preload; (b) after load; and (c) force of contraction of each ventricle.
- Preload: Preload is proportional to EDV (i.e. if more blood fills the ventricles at the end of diastole, more is preload on the heart). This will happen if either venous return

215

(volume of blood returning to right ventricle) increases, or when the duration of ventricular diastole increases. The stretch of cardiac muscle becomes more if preload increases. Due to this, the force of contraction during next systole also increases, i.e. next contraction is more forceful. According to Frank-Starling law, the heart keeps equal volume of blood flowing to pulmonary circulation from right ventricle and to systemic circulation from the left ventricle. If per chance, the left ventricle pumps out a little more blood to systemic circulation as compared to right ventricle, the volume of blood returning to the right ventricle (venous return) also increases. This increased EDV of right ventricle (preload) will make it to contract more forcefully on the next beat (systole) to bring the output of both the sides back to normal.

- **After load:** It refers to the resistance against which the ventricles must pump the blood. It increases if total peripheral resistance increases. If after load increases, stroke volume (amount of blood ejected per beat) decreases. So more blood would remain in the ventricle at the end of systole (ESV).
- **Cardiac contractility:** It is the strength of contraction at any given preload. Positive inotropic drugs increase the force of contraction while negative inotropic drugs decrease the force of contraction.

Cardiac Glycosides

Cardiac glycosides are valuable drugs in the treatment of congestive cardiac failure and supraventricular tachycardias, especially atrial fibrillation. Dried leaves of *Digitalis purpura* are the source of cardiac glycosides. Clinically used main glycosides are digoxin, digitoxin and ouabain. Cardiac glycosides are steroidal glycosides. Chemically, these glycosides have three structural components—a sugar moiety,

steroid nucleus and 5 member lactone ring. The steroid nucleus with the lactone ring forms the aglycone part and is responsible for the pharmacological activity. The sugar moiety determines the water solubility, cell penetration and so the pharmacokinetics of the glycoside.

Pharmacokinetics: There is no fundamental difference in the effects of cardiac glycosides on the heart. They differ from each other quantitatively regarding to their lipid solubility, rapidity and degree of absorption, protein binding, metabolic pathway and excretion. They are administered orally or i.v. They are not given subcutaneously or intramuscularly because the absorption from these sites is unreliable and they may produce local irritation, tenderness, swelling and abscess. The most commonly used cardiac glycosides are digoxin, digitoxin and ouabaine.

Lanatoside C is obtained from *Digitalis lanata*. It is poorly absorbed on oral administration. Deslanoside is its deacetyl derivative which is more soluble and is given intravenously. Its maximum effect is reached in 3 hours and the effect lasts for 5 days; plasma half-life is 36 hours.

Mechanism of action: Most of the cardiac actions of digitalis are more evident in a decompensated heart than in a normal heart. The primary action of digitalis on the heart is twofold. Firstly it has a positive inotropic effect, i.e. directly it increases the contractility of the myocardium, without any significant extra consumption of oxygen. This is the pharmacological basis of use of digitalis in congestive heart failure. The increase in force of contraction of heart muscle leads to:

- Increased cardiac output
- Decreased heart size
- Decreased venous pressure
- Decreased blood volume
- Shorter duration of systole, giving greater time for ventricular filling and rest to the heart

- Improved perfusion of kidneys due to increased cardiac output; so there occurs diuretic action leading to relief of oedema. The most likely mechanism of glycosides to modify force of contraction is as follows:
- Glycosides inhibit the Na^+/K^+ pump.
- Increased {Na^+} slows extrusion of Ca^{++} via the Na^+/Ca^{++} exchange transport. Increasing {Na^+}$_1$ reduces the inwardly directed gradient for Na^+; the smaller this gradient the slower is extrusion of Ca^{++} by Na^+/Ca^{++} exchange.
- Increased {Ca^{++}} is stored in the sarcoplasmic reticulum, thus increases the amount of Ca^{++} released by each action potential.

In other words, the stimulant action on the heart is mediated through Na^+/K^+ ATPase enzyme (digitalis receptor). Digitalis inhibits this enzyme by binding to a site on the extracellular aspect of the $\pm$ subunit of the Na^+/K^+ATPase and increases movement of free intracellular calcium ions responsible for the stimulant action on the heart.

Secondly, digitalis both directly and indirectly (increasing the vagal tone by sensitizing the baroreceptor) modifies the formation and conduction of electrical impulses in the myocardium, resulting in bradycardia and reduction in conduction rate. These effects of digitalis are important both therapeutically and toxicologically. This property is particularly useful for the treatment of cardiac supraventricular arrhythmias.

Digoxin: It is the glycoside of choice due to its quick onset and short duration of action. A dose of 0.25 mg twice a day for over a week can produce complete digitalization in patients with congestive cardiac failure. The maintenance dose depends on the clinical response and ventricular rate which should not be permitted to fall below 60 beats per minute. Generally, the maintenance dose is 0.25–0.5 mg daily. It has a plasma half-life of 36 hours.

Side effects: These are due to extracardiac effects of digitalis. Nausea and vomiting are common with digitalis preparation due to stimulation of the chemoreceptor trigger zone in the medulla. Anorexia, diarrhoea and abdominal discomforts are equally common.

Hypokalaemia (depletion or loss of potassium stores) caused by digitalis predisposes the patient to cardiac toxicity. Thiazide diuretics also cause potassium depletion. So they may precipitate digitalis toxicity if both the drugs are given together.

Visual disturbances (blurring of vision, photophobia, a dark spot in centre of vision, disturbances of colour vision) and psychic symptoms along with confusion may occur due to its central effects.

Cardiac toxicity includes ventricular extrasystoles, paroxysmal atrial tachycardia, with heart block. Heart block may be treated with intravenous atropine and ventricular tachycardia is treated with intravenous phenytoin (100 mg by slow i.v. infusion). The other measures include withdrawal of the drug and oral administration of potassium chloride.

Dose:
- **Digoxin:** Orally in a dose of 0.25 mg twice daily during digitalization, then 0.25–0.5 mg daily.
- **Digitoxin:** Orally 0.05 to 0.2 mg daily.
- **Deslanoside:** 1–1.5 mg given initially by intramuscular or intravenous route which is then followed by 0.25 mg every 6 hours until the patient is completely digitalized.
- **Ouabaine:** Initially 0.25–0.5 mg by slow intravenous injection followed by 0.1 mg every hour or digoxin orally until the patient is digitalized.
- **Beta methyl digoxin:** Initially 0.2 mg twice daily for 3 to 5 days followed by 0.2–0.3 mg daily as maintenance dose.

Therapeutic uses:

1. In congestive cardiac failure, digitalis preparation (digoxin) is taken alone or in combination with diuretics. It is used in patients who remain symptomatic despite optimal use of diuretic and angiotensin converting enzyme inhibitors.

2. Digitalis is used in the management of supraventricular tachyarrhythmias (atrial flutter and atrial fibrillation) with or without congestive cardiac failure. Digitalis protects the ventricle from the continuous bombardment by irregular impulses originating from ectopic foci in the atrium by prolonging the refractory period of the AV node. Thus digitalis is used to improve ventricular function (reduces ventricular rate and increases cardiac output) without curing the arrhythmias. Digitalis corrects paroxysmal atrial tachycardia due to reflex vagal stimulation.

Digitalization: The effective administration of digitalis preparation until the signs and symptoms of congestive cardiac failure have disappeared is called digitalization. After the loading dose, the maintenance dose is worked out depending upon the renal elimination of the drug. Digitalization procedure could be rapid or slow depending on the patient's requirement.

Other Drugs used in Congestive Cardiac Failure

1. Cardiotonic Agents

Selective β₁ agonists (dobutamine, elopexamine, xamateral and dopamine): Dobutamine seems to be best in this group. They are useful in CCF because they have positive inotropic action in appropriate doses with very little positive chronotropic activity or increase in peripheral resistance. However, these drugs have only limited use because they have some alpha-agonistic action and they tend to increase myocardial oxygen consumption. So they are used to treat acute but potentially reversible heart failure(e.g. following cardiac surgery or in some cases of cardiogenic or septic shock) on the basis of their positive ionotropic action. Dobutamine, for reasons that are not well understood, produces less tachycardia than other β₁-agonists. It is administered i.v.

Amrinone and milrinone (pipyridines): They are used in the treatment of refractory cases of severe CCF. They enhance myocardial contractility with little chronotropic effect by inhibiting specific enzyme subtype(type III) of phosphodiesterase and thereby increasing cAMP. They also reduce pulmonary and systemic resistance by vasodilatation. No doubt they improve haemodynamic indices in patients with heart failure but paradoxically worsen survival, presumably because of their postdysrhythmic effect.

Amrinone is given i.v. and milrinone orally. Amrinone produces a dose related reversible thrombocytopenia in 20% of patients. Gastrointestinal upsets may also occur.

Glucagon (polypeptide hormone): It is very useful in treating CCF induced by or complicated by beta adrenergic blockage by activating adenylyl cyclase, and thus increasing synthesis of cAMP.

2. Reduction of Preload

Diuretics: These drugs reduce oedema, pulmonary congestion and preload. Thiazides are very useful in mild CCF while frusemide is useful in acute heart failure (cardiac asthma).

Nitrates: These drugs relax venous capacitance vessels and thus reduce venous return and workload on heart. Long acting nitrates (isosorbide di- or mononitrate) may be used.

3. Reduction of After Load

Hydralazine: It reduces work load on heart by decreasing peripheral resistance due to arteriolar dilatation.

Beta-2 selective agonists (albuterol and pirbuterol)are being investigated in patients of CCF.

4. Reduction of Preload and After Load

Angiotensin converting enzyme inhibitors reduce:

* After load by inhibiting vasoconstrictor action of angiotensin
* Preload by decreasing aldosterone secretion. However, treatment with these drugs (enalapril) must be initiated carefully with small doses to prevent marked fall in blood pressure.

Congestive cardiac failure (CCF) means failure of the heart as a pump. Usually left ventricle fails more often than and earlier than right ventricle. Due to this, cardiac out put is inadequate to meet the metabolic demands of the body during exercise and ultimately also at rest. If the left ventricle fails first, it cannot pump out all the blood it receives from the lungs. As a result, blood backs up in the lungs causing pulmonary oedema. If the right ventricle fails first, it cannot pump all the blood it receives from systemic circulation. So there occurs peripheral oedema (more noticeable in feet and ankles) due to:

* Increased venous pressure, leading to increased formation of tissue fluids
* Reduced renal blood flow which activates the renin-angiotensin-aldosterone system, causing Na^+ and water retention.

Important causes of CCF are:

* Ischaemic heart disease
* Volume overload due to leaky valves or atriovenous shunts caused by congenital defects
* Pressure overload due to hypertension or stenosed narrowed valves.

Heart failure is called low output cardiac failure when the metabolic demands of the body are within normal limits but the heart is unable to meet them. It is called high output cardiac failure when the metabolic demands of the body are so increased as in case of hyperthyroidism or anaemia that even an increased cardiac output is insufficient to meet them. So the high output cardiac failure can be corrected by treating the underlying cause.

Some compensatory mechanisms start operating when the pumping mechanism of the heart is failing. These are:

* Increased in sympathetic activity
* Activation of renin angiotensin system
* Cardiac remodelling (means cardiomegaly or dilatation)

If the compensatory mechanisms can restore the cardiac output then the heart is said to be compensated. Ultimately these mechanisms worsen the heart failure and become self-defeating. The heart failure is now called decompensated. The decompensated heart is characterized by:

* Pulmonary and peripheral oedema
* Dyspnoea with cyanosis
* Hepatomegaly (due to hepatic congestion)
* Cardiomegaly (due to cardiac remodelling)
* Decreased urine formation (renal congestion)
* Decreased exercise tolerance (due to decreased cardiac output)

Important events in congestive cardiac failure

* Decreased cardiac output
* Decreased renal blood flow
* Activation of renin-angiotensin-aldosterone system
* Na^+/water retention and oedema
* Increased central venous pressure due to Na^+/water retention and oedema
* Increased preload due to increased central venous pressure
* Increased after load due to formation of angiotensin-II

Drugs used in congestive cardiac failure

- *Loop diuretics (frusemide):* To promote sodium excretion
- *Angiotensin-converting enzyme inhibitors (e.g. captopril, enalapril):* To reduce neuro-humoral activation
- *β-adrenoceptor antagonists (e.g. metoprolol):* To reduce neurohumoral activation
- *Organic nitrates (e.g. isosorbid mononitrate):* To reduce preload central venous pressure
- *Hydralazine:* To reduce after load
- *Spironolactone:* To antagonize aldosterone
- *Digoxin:* To reduce ventricular wall stress

Points for Dental Students

1. No specific dental modifications are necessary for well-compensated patients with heart failure, unless the underlying causes for the heart failure require modifications.
2. In uncompensated heart failure, it is important to enquire about the patient's ability to be placed in supine position because severe dyspnoea may develop while lying down in a dental chair.
3. Avoid use of gingival retraction cord impregnated with adrenaline in digitalized patients to prevent development of cardiac arrhythmias. In such patients, use haemostatic retraction cords impregnated with astringents.

TO REMEMBER

1. Congestive heart failure develops when cardiac output is insufficient to meet the demands of tissue perfusion. Severe anaemia, thyrotoxicosis, left-right or arteriovenous shunt causes high output failure which responds poorly to digitalis because scope of further increasing cardiac output is limited. Increased impedence to ventricular outflow (due to hypertension, post-rheumatic valvular defects or congenital heart disease) or lowered myocardial work capacity (due to ischaemic heart disease, myocarditis, cardiomyopathies, or arrhythmias) may lead to low output failure which responds beneficially to digitalis.
2. Digoxin is the glycoside of choice due to its quick onset and short duration of action. A person is considered to be digitalised when pulse rate becomes 60 per minute or there occurs nausea and vomiting. Afterwards the effect is maintained by a maintenance dose.
3. By prolonging the refractory period of the AV node, digitalis protects the ventricle from the continuous bombardment by irregular impulses originating from ectopic foci in atrium in the presence of atrial flutter and atrial fibrillation.
4. Other drugs used in congestive heart failure are:
   a. Cardiotonic agents (selective beta 1 agonists, pipyridines and glucagone)
   b. Those which cause reduction of preload (diuretics and nitrates)
   c. Those which cause reduction of after load (hydralazine beta 2 selective agonists) and
   d. Those which cause reduction of preload and after load (angiotensin converting enzyme inhibitors).
5. Glucagone is very useful in treating congestive cardiac failure induced by or complicated by beta adrenergic blockage by activating adenylate cyclase.

Chapter 30

Antiarrhythmic Drugs

Cardiac arrhythmia is a disturbance of normal rhythm of the heart due to heart disease or toxic action of some drugs. Arrhythmia may occur either due to defect in the impulse generation (abnormal impulse formation, ectopic) or due to abnormal propagation of impulse generation (conduction defect, circus or re-entry mechanism). Sometimes a combination of both these factors may be responsible for arrhythmia. Depending upon the disorders of impulse generation, these arrhythmias are classified as under:

i. Extrasystole (premature contraction): they originate in atria or ventricle (ectopic)
ii. Paroxysmal supraventricular tachycardia
iii. Atrial flutter (heart rate 250–350 per minute)
iv. Atrial fibrillation (heart rate 500 per minute and irregular)
v. Ventricular tachycardia and fibrillation.

Classification of Antiarrhythmic Drugs

On the basis of mechanism of action, these drugs are divided into the following classes:

Class-I: These drugs act by blocking voltage sensitive myocardial Na^+ channels. They are also called membrane stabilizing agents. They decrease inflow of sodium during phase O, excitability, conduction velocity and auto-maticity. They are further subdivided into the following three subclasses:

a. Those which prolong refractory period and cause moderate depression of conduction such as quinidine, procainamide, diso-

pyramide and imipramine. These are used in supraventricular and ventricular arrhythmias.

b. Those that shorten refractory period and cause minimal depression of conduction such as lignocaine, phenytoin, tocainide, mexiletine, and moricizine. These are used in ventricular arrhythmia.

c. Those having negligible effect on refractory period but caused marked depression of conduction, e.g. flecainide, encainide, propafenone, and indecainide. These are used in supraventricular and ventricular arrhythmias.

Class-II: Beta-adrenoceptor antagonists such as propranolol, esmolol, and metoprolol.

Class-III: Those drugs which prolong effective refractory period and block K^+ channels, e.g. amiodarone, bretylium and sotalol.

Class-IV: Calcium channel blockers, e.g. verapamil, diltiazem and betridil.

Following are the antiarrhythmic drugs which are unclassified in the above system of classification:

Drug	Use
• Adenosine	Supraventricular tachycardia
• Adrenaline	Cardiac arrest
• Atropine	Sinus bradycardia
• Calcium Chloride	Ventricular tachycardia due to hyperkalaemia
• Digoxin	Rapid atrial fibrillation
• Isoprenaline	Heart block
• Magnesium	Ventricular fibrillation

221

Following are the important features of selected commonly used drugs.

1. Quinidine

It is an alkaloid which is isolated from cinchona bark. It is d-isomer of quinine. It is rapidly absorbed on oral administration and peak effect is seen in 1–3 hours. Its duration of action is 6–8 hours. It is primarily eliminated by hepatic metabolism. Although like quinine, it has antimalarial and antipyretic activity, but the most predominant action of quinidine is on the heart. It directly depresses the heart. It increases the refractory period, depresses contractility and excitability. It slows conduction in the heart muscle. It has prominent anticholinergic effect on vagus.

Important side effects are AV block and syncope in over dose; cinchonism characterized by visual disturbances, ringing in the ears, nausea, headache, diarrhoea and cramps. Hypersensitivity reactions such as thrombocytopenic purpura may occur. It is absolutely contraindicated in complete heart block.

Dose: 100–200 mg 3 times a day orally.

Therapeutic uses:

i. Supraventricular tachycardia
ii. Ventricular arrhythmias.

Uses of class I antiarrhythmic drugs
- Class I a (e.g. disopyramide):
  - Ventricular arrhythmias
  - Prevention of recurrent paroxysmal atrial fibrillation triggered by vagal over activity
- Class I b (intravenous lidocaine):
  - Treatment and prevention of ventricular tachycardia and fibrillation during and immediately after myocardial infarction
- Class I c (e.g. flecainide)
  - To prevent paroxysmal atrial fibrillation, Wolff-Parkinson-White (flecainide) syndrome

Uses of class II antiarrhythmic drugs (e.g. propranolol)
- To reduce mortality following myocardial infarction
- To prevent recurrence of paroxysmal atrial fibrillation provoked by sympathetic overactivity.

2. Procainamide

It is an amide of procaine. It does not undergo enzymatic hydrolysis and is devoid of central nervous system effects. It is rapidly and completely absorbed from oral route and is acetylated in liver. Peak effect is seen in 1 hour and duration of action is 3–4 hours. Its cardiac actions are similar to quinidine. However, it is less potent myocardial depressant. It is used in ventricular arrhythmias in doses of 250–500 mg four times a day orally. Important side effects are anorexia, nausea, bitter taste, diarrhoea, rashes, fever, lupus erythematosus like effects.

3. Phenytoin

It is an important antiepileptic agent. However, it is also used for the treatment of ventricular arrhythmias, particularly digitalis induced cardiac arrhythmias. The electro-physiological properties of phenytoin are similar to procainamide. It also depresses the automaticity of the heart. Its important side effects are hypotension, bradycardia and confusion. It is administered by slow intravenous infusion at the rate of 50 mg/min (total dose up to 700–1000 mg). The drug may

Uses of class III antiarrhythmic drugs
- Amiodarone is used to treat tachycardia associated with the Wolff-Parkinson syndrome and wide range of other supraventricular and ventricular tachyarrhythmia
- Racemic sotalol is used in paroxysmal supraventricular arrhythmias and suppresses ventricular ectopic beats and short runs of ventricular tachycardia.

Uses of class IV antiarrhythmic drugs
- Verapamil is used:
  - To prevent recurrence of paroxysmal supraventricular tachycardia (SVT)
  - To reduce the ventricular rate in patients with atrial fibrillation, provided they do no have Wolff-Parkinson-White syndrome
- Adenosine is used in SVT.

be repeated if required so. When the arrhythmia is brought under control the patient is kept on oral maintenance dose of 1 gm per day which is given in divided doses.

4. Lignocaine

It is an important local anaesthetic agent. It is a very useful drug to treat ventricular arrhythmias associated with acute myocardial infarction, digitalis intoxication and cardiac surgery because of its rapid direct action on the heart muscle, easy reversibility of action and short duration of action. Common side effects are confusion, drowsiness, and convulsions. It may some time cause numbness of lips and tongue and speech disturbances. It is given intravenously in doses of 50–100 mg; repeated if required within 5–10 minutes. Maintenance dose is given at a rate of 1–4 mg/min by intravenous infusion.

5. Tocainide and Mexiletine

These drugs are related to lidocaine and are effective on oral administration. Their pharmacological actions and therapeutic uses are similar to lidocaine. Tocainide is used in a dose of 400–600 mg three times a day while mexiletine in a dose of 200–300 mg three times a day.

6. Flecainide and Encainide

Flecainide and encainide are fluorinated analogs of procainamide. These are used only to treat life-threatening ventricular arrhythmias without coronary artery disease due

to their proarrhythmogenic effect even in normal doses.

7. Propafenone

It has structural resemblance with propranolol and has some β-blocking action; so is contraindicated in CHF and bronchial asthma. It also has proarrhythmogenic effect; so is used in life threatening ventricular arrhythmias.

8. Moricizine

It prolongs QRS interval. It has a lower incidence of proarrhythmogenic effects. It is used to treat refractory life-threatening ventricular arrhythmias.

9. Propranolol

Propranolol and other beta blockers are used as antiarrhythmic agents due to their beta-blocking property and the myocardial depressant effect. Bradycardia, hypotension, heart failure and bronchospasm are their important side effects. Propranolol is given in a dose of 30–600 mg daily orally. It can also be given by intravenous injection in a dose of 0.5–5 mg. It is mainly used to treat paroxysmal supraventricular tachycardia and digitalis induced arrhythmias.

10. Bretylium

It is an adrenergic neuron blocking agent. It is indicated in life-threatening ventricular tachyarrhythmias and digitalis-induced arrhythmias not responding to procainamide or lignocaine. It is administered in a dose of 5 mg/kg intramuscularly or intravenously; may be repeated in 6–8 hours if needed. Nausea and hypotension may occur as side effects.

11. Disopyramide

Its actions are similar to quinidine. It is also used to treat ventricular arrhythmias in a dose of 100–150 mg 4 times in a day orally. Dryness of mouth, blurred vision, myocardial depression, hypotension and urinary retention may occur as side effects.

12. Verapamil

It is a calcium channel blocker. It produces antiarrhythmic effect by reducing the movement of calcium across cardiac membrane. It depresses myocardial contractility and slows SA and AV nodal conduction. Since both verapamil and diltiazem depress nodal conduction, they are indicated in cardiac arrhythmias. They are contraindicated in heart block. Bradycardia, hypotension, nausea and vomiting may occur as side effects. Verapamil is used to treat supraventricular arrhythmias and in angina verapamil is given orally in a dose of 40–80 mg three times a day. It may also be administered by slow intravenous route in a dose of 5 mg and maximum up to 100 mg per day.

13. Amiodarone

Being a toxic drug, it is used as a last resort in treatment of life-threatening ventricular arrhythmias and Wolff-Parkinson-White syndrome refractory to conventional therapy. It has following several peculiarities that complicate its use:

- A very long elimination half-life (10–100 days).
- Extensively bound in tissues
- Accumulation in the body during repeated use
- Development of action takes days or weeks
- Important and numerous adverse effects such as corneal microdeposits, peripheral neuropathy and disturbed thyroid function are reported as side effects.

Because of above mentioned pharmacokinetic features, a loading dose is used, and for life-threatening arrhythmias this is given i.v. via a central vein (it causes phlebitis if given into a peripheral vessel).

14. Sotalol

Unlike other β-adrenoceptor blockers, it prolongs the cardiac action potential and the QT interval by delaying the slow onward K⁺ current. Racemic sotalol (the form prescribed) appears to be some what less effective than amiodarone in preventing chronic malignant ventricular arrhythmias.

15. Adenosine

It acts on A_1-receptors which are linked to the cardiac K⁺ channel (KACh) and hyperpolarizes cardiac conducting tissue and slows the rate of rise of the pacemaker potential accordingly. It is administered i.v. to terminate supraventricular tachycardia. It has largely replaced verapamil for this purpose because it is safer due to its short lived effect (20–30 seconds). Once supraventricular tachycardia is terminated, the patient usually remains in sinus rhythm even though adenosine is no longer present in plasma.

TO REMEMBER

1. For vasovagal syndrome, atropine sulphate is the choice of drug.
2. For partial heart block, sympathomimetics are used. Alternative drug is atropine sulphate.
3. In case of atrial ectopics, reassurance is the choice of treatment along with the removal of the precipitating cause, e.g. tobacco.
4. For treatment of paroxysmal atrial tachycardia, vagotonic maneuvers is the first choice while rapid digitalization is the second choice. Alternative treatment includes cardioversion, use of quinidine/sotalol.
5. Cardioversion is the first choice of treatment for atrial flutter and rapid digitalization is the second choice. Alternative for long-term use of drugs are verapamil/amiodarone/propranolol. Same treatment is carried out for atrial fibrillation except in alternative treatment quinidine is used in place of amiodarone.

6. To treat ventricular ectopics, lignocaine (i.v.) is the first choice and procainamide is the second choice. Quinidine/diso-pyramide/amiodarone are the alternative drugs.

7. Cardioversion is the first choice for treating ventricular tachycardia and fibrillation while use of lignocaine (i.v.) is the second choice. Alternative drugs are procainamide for ventricular tachycardia and bretylium (i.v.) for ventricular fibrillation.

8. To treat digitalized induced tachycardia, phenytoin (i.v.) is the first choice while lignocaine (i.v.) is the second choice.

9. Sotalol is the first choice for the treatment of Wolff-Parkinson's-White syndrome and amiodarone is the second choice.

10. Artificial pacemaker is used for complete heart block.

Section 7

Haemopoietic System

Chapter 31

Haematinics

Anaemia is due to deficient numbers of circulating red blood cells or reduction in hemoglobin content per unit of blood volume. Important causes of anaemia are blood loss, nutritional deficiency or complex hereditary deficiencies. Aplastic anaemia occurs due to failure of bone marrow to produce red blood cells. Haematinics or antianaemics are the agents which are required for the proliferation and maturation of red blood cells. They are iron, folic acid and vitamin B_{12}. Anaemia may develop as a result of deficiency of any of these haematinics. Further, some haemopoietic growth factors also play very special function.

The rational treatment of anaemias depends on proper diagnosis of the type so that specific therapy can be given. Indiscriminate use of blood transfusion should be avoided.

Nutritional anaemias occur due to inadequate ingestion, or absorption or utilization, or increased excretion or increased requirement of iron. These anaemias can be treated by giving the deficient nutrient such as iron, vitamin B_{12}, folic acid or vitamin C in appropriate form and dosage.

Iron Deficiency Anaemia (Hypochromic-Microcytic Anaemia)

Iron

Total body iron is about 4.5 g in adult males and 2.5 g in adult females. It is stored in the reticuloendothelial system cells in liver, spleen, and bone marrow. It is also stored in hepatocytes, myocytes and intestinal mucosa as ferritin and haemosiderin. Haemosiderin is aggregated ferric hydroxide crystals with a partial envelope of apoferritin. Iron is indicated in case of demonstrable iron deficiency. Daily iron requirements range between 1 to 2.5 mg per day. However, during growth, menstruation, pregnancy and pathological bleeding, iron requirements are greatly increased (up to 60 mg or more per day in iron deficiency anaemia). Iron is present in a wide variety of foods. Dietary sources of iron are:

- **Rich:** Egg yolk, dry beans, dry fruits, liver, wheat germ, yeast.
- **Medium:** Apple, banana, chicken, fish, meat, oyster, spinach.
- **Poor:** Milk and its products, root vegetables.

About 10 to 50% of dietary iron is absorbed depending on the need of body. Ferrous form (Fe^{++}) of iron is easily absorbed than the ferric form (Fe^{+++}). Ferric form needs to be converted into ferrous form before absorption. Conversion to Fe^{++} form occurs readily in presence of ascorbic acid, and thio- or other reducing groups. Iron is normally absorbed in the duodenum and proximal jejunum where the acid medium enhances solubility. Other parts of small intestine can also absorb iron, if necessary. A number of factors influence absorption of iron are which are shown in Table 31.1.

Table 31.1: Factors influencing absorption of iron

Factors facilitating iron absorption	Factors impeding iron absorption
• Acid	• Alkalies (antacids)
• Ascorbic acid	• Phosphates
• SH-containing amino acids	• Phytates
• Meat	• Tetracyclines
	• Food in the stomach

Orally administered iron passes directly into the bloodstream. In the blood, it immediately gets attached to transferrin (β_1-globulin) which helps in the transport of iron from the site of absorption to areas of utilization.

Iron is excreted after removal from iron-containing cells from the bowel, skin, urine and sweat. In normal individual, a total iron excretion (loss) is 0.5 mg/day. It is doubled during menstruation.

Oral iron therapy: It is initiated with dried ferrous sulphate which is given in doses of 100–200 mg after food to minimize gastric irritation. Iron liquid preparations are available especially for children but tablet is the preparation of choice for adults. Nausea, epigastric pain and diarrhoea may occur as side effects. However, in some persons, it may cause constipation on continuous adminis-tration. Rarely acute iron intoxication may occur from ingestion of more than 50 g of iron preparation. It is characterized by abdominal pain, vomiting, acidosis, cardiovascular collapse followed by coma and death in 6–24 hours. The treatment consists of gastric lavage, and intravenous administration of iron binding chelates (desferrioxamine); fluid and electrolyte replacement.

Preparation and dose:

1. *Ferrous sulphate dried:* 200–300 mg daily up to 1 year.
2. *Ferrous gluconate:* 1.2–1.8 g in divided daily doses.
3. *Ferrous fumarate:* 200–400 mg in divided daily doses.
4. *Ferrous succinate:* 200–400 mg in divided daily doses.
5. *Colloidal iron:* 200–400 mg daily.
6. *Ferric ammonium citrate:* 200–400 mg daily.
7. *Sodium iron-edetate:* 150 mg daily.

Iron and folic acid (containing equivalent of 100 mg of ferrous iron and 200 µg of folic acid) are prescribed for prevention of iron and folic acid deficiencies in pregnancy.

Parenteral iron therapy: It is indicated when oral iron therapy fails to recover iron deficiency anaemia. Deep intramuscular injections of following preparations are given.

1. Iron dextran injection (imferon 50 mg/ml of elemental iron): Dose: 2–5 ml daily for 15 days.
2. Iron sorbital injection (50 mg/ml of iron): Dose: 2 ml daily for 15 days.

Iron dextran can also be given by i.v. infusion over 1–2 hours after diluting in saline. However, test should be done for any allergic reactions before i.v. administration.

Therapeutic use: Iron deficiency anaemia, which can be caused by:
- Chronic blood loss, e.g. with colon cancer, hook worm and menorrhagia.
- Inadequate absorption, e.g. following gastrectomy.
- Inadequate dietary intake.
- Increased demand, e.g. in pregnancy and early infancy.

Chronic iron toxicity (haemochromatosis or haemosiderosis): It occurs when body is unable to excrete an excess of iron, which is deposited in the heart, liver, pancreas and other organs. It leads to organ failure and death. It may be an inherited disorder due to excess iron absorption or following repeated blood transfusions as in the case of thalas-saemia. The treatment consists of intermittent phlebotomy (removal of iron every week). If procedure is not sufficient, desferrioxamine is given parenterally along with it. The drug is much less effective, more expensive and hazardous. Recently deferiprone has been introduced. It is orally absorbable iron chelator which is given in doses of 75 mg/kg /24 hours in divided doses. It is administered in patient with thalassaemia major, in whom desferrioxamine is contraindicated or not tolerated.

Vitamin B$_{12}$ or Folic Acid Deficiency Anaemia (Megaloblastic-Macrocytic Anaemia)

Vitamin B$_{12}$ and folic acid are required for the formation of erythrocytes because they are essential for DNA synthesis and, consequently, for cell proliferation. In the absence of B-complex vitamins, megaloblastic anaemia occurs due to failure of maturation of the large, nucleated erythrocyte-precursor blood cells (megaloblasts). Vitamin B$_{12}$ deficiency also causes important disorders of nerves which are not corrected by treatment with folic acid. On the contrary, folic acid may even make them worse. Deficiency of vitamin B$_{12}$ can be either due to absence of intrinsic factor (pernicious anaemia, gastrectomy) or malabsorption from distal ileum. In folic acid deficiency anaemia, the neurological signs are absent.

Vitamin B$_{12}$ (Cyanocobalamin)

It is synthesized by certain micro-organisms in the intestine lumen. It is not synthesized by animal or plants. Liver, kidney, heart, egg yolk and milk are rich sources of vitamin B$_{12}$. Commercial source of vitamin B$_{12}$ is from streptomyces greseus. The daily nutritional requirements are 3–5 μg, which must be obtained from animal by-products in the diet. Parietal cells of the stomach secrete intrinsic factor (a specific glycoprotein) which forms a complex with vitamin B$_{12}$ (extrinsic factor). This complex is absorbed in the distal ileum by a highly specific receptor-mediated transport system. In blood, vitamin B$_{12}$ is transported with a specific plasma globulin (transcobalamin). Some vitamin B$_{12}$ (3–7 μg) is excreted in bile every day, but most of it is reabsorbed (enterohepatic circulation). Excess amount of vitamin B$_{12}$ remains in free form and excreted in urine. Vitamin B$_{12}$ is available as injectable as well as for oral administration. Its absorption by oral route is not reliable in absence of or deficiency of intrinsic factor.

Cyanocobalamin is given by deep intramuscular or deep subcutaneous injection. It is available in combination with other minerals and vitamins for oral administration.

In human beings, two main biochemical reactions require vitamin B$_{12}$:
- The conversion of methyl-tetrahydrofolate (FH4), inactive form of FH4, to active formyl-FH4 which after polyglutamation, is a cofactor in the synthesis of purines and pyrimidines.
- Isomerisation of methyl malonyl-CoA to succinyl CoA.

Hydroxocobalamin is now the form of vitamin B$_{12}$ of choice. Since it is more protein bound, it is retained for longer time in the body. A single dose can maintain plasma vitamin B$_{12}$ concentration in the normal range for up to 3 months. It may, however, produce antibodies to the vitamin complex.

Dose: Cyanocobalamin up to 30 μg is administered by intramuscular route.

Hydroxocobalamin is given in a dose of 1 mg initially which may be repeated every 2–3 days.

Liver preparations containing vitamin B$_{12}$ activity are also available.

Therapeutic uses:
- Vitamin B$_{12}$ deficiency
- Pernicious anaemia
- In degeneration of spinal cord
- Prophylactically after surgical removal of stomach (site of production of intrinsic factor)or the terminal ileum (site of vitamin B$_{12}$ absorption).

Folic Acid (Pteroylglutamic Acid)

It is composed of pteridine heterocycle ring, para-aminobenzoic acid (PABA) and glutamic acid. In the body, folic acid is converted into dihydrofolic acid (H_2-folate) by dihydrofolate synthetase enzyme which is then further converted into tetrahydrofolic acid (H_4-folate) by dihydrofolate reductase enzyme. H_4-folate can subsequently be transformed to folate cofactors possessing 1-carbon units for donation at various levels of oxidation. H_4-folate and folate cofactors are inconvertible. So H_4-folate is recycled. Folates are required for the conversion of deoxyuridylate monophosphate. This is rate limiting in mammalian DNA synthesis. It is catalysed by thymidylate synthetase with folate acting as methyl donor.

Folic acid is present in almost all foods. Highest content is in liver, yeast and green vegetables. The normal daily requirement of folic acid is 50 µg. It is mainly absorbed from the small intestine and is distributed to all tissues. Excess amount is excreted in the urine. Mostly it is stored in liver and is non-toxic.

Dose: 10–20 mg daily orally for 14 days or until haematological picture is improved. Daily maintenance dose is 5 mg. Folic acid preparations are available alone or in combination with other vitamins and minerals.

Therapeutic uses:

1. Megaloblastic anaemia, which can be caused by:
   - Poor diet (common in alcoholics)
   - Malabsorption syndromes
   - Drugs, e.g. phenytoin
2. Prophylactically in individuals who can develop folate deficiency, e.g. pregnant women, premature infants, patients with severe haemolytic anaemia.
3. Treatment or prevention of toxicity from methotrexate.

Haemopoietic Growth Factors

These factors are necessary for maintenance of haemopoiesis. They direct the division and maturation of the progeny of these cells.

1. **Erythropoietin:** It is produced in juxtatubular cells in the kidney and also in macrophages. It stimulates committed erythroid progenitor cells to proliferate and generate erythrocytes. Two forms of recombinant human erythropoietin, epoietin alfa and epoietin beta, are available. Clinically, they are indistinguishable. So they are simply referred as epoietin. Important features of erythropoietin are:
   - It regulates red blood cell production.
   - It is given i.v., s.c., i.p.
   - It can cause transient "flu-like" symptoms, hypertension, iron deficiency and increased blood viscosity.
   - Clinically epoietin is used to treat anaemia due to:
     – Chronic renal failure
     – Chemotherapy for cancer
     – AIDS
     – Chronic inflammatory conditions such as rheumatoid arthritis
   - Epoitin is also used to prevent anaemia of premature infants and to increase yield of autogenous blood before donation.
2. **Granulocyte colony-stimulating factor (G-CSF):** It is produced mainly by monocytes, fibroblasts, and endothelial cells. It primarily controls the development of neutrophils. It is available as filgrastim. It is given i.v., or s.c.
3. **Granulocyte macrophage colony-stimulating factor (GM-CSF):** It stimulates development of progenitor cells. It is available as molgramostim. It is given i.v.or s.c. Side effects are fever, rashes, bone pain, hypotension, gastrointestinal symptoms, and arterial oxygen desaturation.

Colony-stimulating factors are used in specialized centres:

- To reduce the severity and duration of the neutropenia induced by cytotoxic drugs
- To stimulate release into the circulation of progenitor cells
- To expand the number of harvest progenitor cells ex-vivo before infusing them
- For persistent neutropenia in advanced HIV infection
- In treatment of aplastic anaemia

Points for Dental Students

1. Elective oral surgical or periodontal procedures should not be performed on patients with marked anaemia because of the potential for increased bleeding, risk of bacterial infection (particularly with anaerobic bacteria, due to tissue hypoxia) and impaired wound healing. General anaesthesia should not be administered unless the hemoglobin is at least 10 g/dL. Such patients should never be treated with iron until the cause of the microcytic hypochromic anaemia is found and corrected or until a thorough search for the cause has proved fruitless.

2. The severity of anaemia owing to hemolysis (G6PD def.) and its correction should be evaluated before major dental interventions because the decline in haemoglobin (Hb) can reach 3–4 g/dL during haemolytic episodes. Blood transfusion may be used prior to dental treatment in severe cases. Drugs that might induce hemolysis, such as dapsone, sulfasalazine and phenacetin should be avoided. However, non-narcotic analgesics and antibiotics can be given safely in therapeutic doses.

3. Elective dental procedures involving the soft tissues should not be performed in with poorly controlled sickle cell disease unless absolutely necessary because of increased risk of complications secondary to chronic anaemia and delayed wound healing.

4. The two most common oral manifestations of cyclic neutropenia are oral mucosal ulcers and periodontal disease (marginal gingivitis) to rapidly advancing periodontal bone loss caused by bacterial infection of the dental supporting structures. The use of colony stimulating factors has reduced oral ulcers and periodontal disease in these patients.

5. Avoid use of narcotic analgesics in presence of anaemia because there will occur grave side effects of respiratory depression.

TO REMEMBER

1. Total body iron is about 4.5 g in adult males and 2.5 g in adult females. Deficiency of iron will lead to iron deficiency anaemia (hypochromic-microcytic anaemia).

2. Absorption of iron is facilitated by gastric juice, reducing substances such ascorbic acid and SH-containing amino acids and is decreased by antacids, phosphates, maize, wheat and tetracyclines.

3. Vitamin B_{12} and folic acid are required for the maturation of the large, nucleated erythrocyte-precursor blood cells (megaloblasts). So deficiency of these substances will lead to megaloblastic-macrocytic anaemia. When deficiency of vitamin B_{12} is due to absence of intrinsic factor, it is called pernicious anaemia.

4. Of the two therapeutically used cobalamins, hydroxy cobalamin is more protein bound, and therefore better retained than cobalamin.

5. In case of vitamin B_{12} deficiency, administration of folic acid alone is contraindicated because neurological manifestations appear or aggravated.

Chapter 32

Coagulation, Anticoagulants and Coagulants

To keep the blood in a fluid state, the coagulating as well as anticoagulant factors are delicately balanced in the circulating blood. There may occur spontaneous bleeding or intravascular thrombosis due to any disturbance in this delicately balanced system. Blood coagulation means the conversion of blood to a solid gel or clot. The clotting system consists of a cascade of proteolytic enzymes and cofactors which are present in blood as inactive precursors (zymogens). These coagulation factors are:

Factor I (fibrinogen), II (prothrombin), III (thromboplastin or tissue factor; TF), IV (Ca++), V (accelerator globulin or proaccelerin), VI (proconvertin or serum prothrombin conversion accelertor; SPCA), VII (antihaemophilic factor-A), VIII (christmas factor or plasma thromboplastin component [PTC] or antihemophilic factor-B), IX (stuart factor or thrombokinase), X (plasma thromboplastin antecedent [PTA], or antihaemphilic factor-C), XI (hageman factor or contact factor), XII (fibrin stabilizing factor or fibrinase).

Inactive precursors are activated in series. In this process each one gives rise to more of the next. The last enzyme is thrombin which is derived from prothrombin (II). This enzyme converts soluble fibrinogen (I) to an insoluble meshwork of fibrin in which cells are trapped and thus a clot is formed.

There are two pathways in the cascade which result in activation of factor X which then converts prothrombin to thrombin. These pathways are:
- The extrinsic pathway which operates in vivo. It needs a tissue factor (a lipoprotein-called tissue thromboplastin) which is released from damaged tissue into the circulating blood. In this system, factor Xa is formed within seconds due to one step reaction.
- The intrinsic or contact pathway, which operates in vitro. It requires all the factors for coagulation which are present in circulating blood. In this system factor Xa takes several minutes for formation.

Calcium ions and a negatively charged phospholipid (PL) are essential for three steps, namely the action of:
- Factor IXa on X
- Factor VIIa on X
- Factor Xa on II

Negatively charged phospholipid (PL) is provided by activated platelets adhering to the damaged vessel. Some factors promote coagulation by binding to PL and a serine protease factor, e.g. factor Va in the activation of II by Xa; VIIIa in the activation of X by IXa (Fig. 32.1).

ANTICOAGULANTS

They are classified as under:
1. **Parenteral:** Heparin, danaparoid, lepirudin, bivalirudin, and argatroban

234

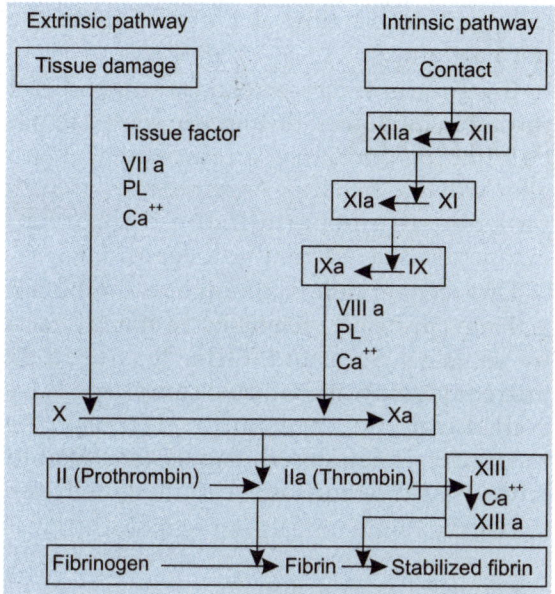

Extrinsic pathway   Intrinsic pathway

Fig. 32.1: The coagulation cascade

2. **Oral:**
   a. *Coumarin derivatives:* Dicoumarol, tromexan, warfarin, phenprocoumon, acenocoumarol and nicoumalone
   b. *Indandione derivatives:* Phenindione, diphenadione, anisindione and bromindione out of all these compounds, warfarin is the most important and most widely used. Other important oral anticoagulants are acenocoumarol and phenindione.
3. **In vitro anticoagulants:** Sodium citrate, sodium oxalate, and sodium edetate.

Parenteral Anticoagulants

Heparin

Heparin is a mixture of sulphated muco-polysaccharides (MW 3000–40,000). It has strong electronegative charge. It is present in mast cells, intimal layers of blood vessels and granules of basophils. Lungs, liver and intestinal mucosa are the richest sources of heparin. For commercial use, it is extracted from porcine intestinal mucosa and bovine lung. Circulating blood contains no heparin except when the mast cells are disrupted. Its physiological role is to maintain blood in fluid state. It does not affect other organs of the body even in large doses. It also has a lipaemia - clearing effect.

Mechanism of action: Heparin is effective both in vitro and in vivo. It is a powerful immediately acting anticoagulant. Heparin accelerates the action of antithrombin III which prevents the conversion of fibrinogen into fibrin by inhibiting the activated clotting factors. In this process, heparin acts as catalyst. Besides, it also slows down the conversion of prothrombin to thrombin and stabilizes platelets against dumping and disintegrating.

Heparin is of two types:
- High molecular weight (HMW) heparin
- Low molecular weight (LMW) heparin.

Former is a strong anticoagulant while later is a weak anticoagulant.

Pharmacokinetics: Heparin is not effective by oral route because it is precipitated by gastric juice, and digested by enzymes. So it is administered parenterally (i.v. or s.c.). It has a dose dependent action. Since heparin does not cross the placental barrier and also not secreted in mother's milk it may be given during pregnancy and lactation. It does not affect bleeding time in therapeutic doses. Heparin is metabolized (up to 50%) in the liver by heparinase and the rest of the drug is excreted in urine as unchanged drug.

Haemorrhage, haematuria and gastro-intestinal bleeding are common side effects. Prolonged use of heparin (for 6 months) may lead to osteoporosis and spontaneous fractures.

Heparin is contraindicated in:
- Haemophilia
- Peptic ulcer
- Severe hypertension

- Bacterial endocarditis
- Active tuberculosis
- Threatened abortion
- Other haemorrhagic disorders

Dose: Heparin sodium contains 120 units per mg. A loading dose of 5000 units of heparin is followed by continuous intravenous infusion up to 40,000 units in 24 hours. It may be given by subcutaneous route (5000 units) but intramuscular injections are painful and may have the risk of haematoma formation at the site of injection.

Therapeutic uses:

- Deep vein thrombosis
- Intravascular coagulation
- To prevent postoperative thrombosis

Protamine sulphate is used up to a maximum dose of 50 mg i.v. as heparin antagonist to counteract over dosage of heparin. One mg neutralizes 100 units of heparin.

Other Parenteral Anticoagulants

Danaparoid: It is a mixture of heparin-like glycosaminoglycans (84% heparin sulphate, 12% dermatan sulphate, and 4% chondroitin sulphate). It is isolated from porcine intestinal mucosa. It is used:

- For prophylaxis of deep vein thrombosis (750 antifactor Xa units, s.c. twice daily)
- As anticoagulant for patients with heparin induced thrombocytopenia (750 antifactor Xa units, i.v. twice daily)
- For postoperative deep vein thrombosis following active hip replacement surgery

It acts mainly by promoting inhibition of factor Xa by antithrombin III.

Lepirudin: It is recombinant derivative of hirudin. It is a 65-amino acid polypeptide. It directly inhibits thrombin by binding tightly to both catalytic and exosite I sites of thrombin. It is used as anticoagulant in patients with heparin induced thrombocytopenia. It is administered i.v. at a dose adjusted to maintain the prothrombin time at 1.5 to 2.5 times the normal value.

Bivalirudin and argatroban are other direct thrombin inhibitors. Bivalirudin is used in per cutaneous coronary angioplasty as an alternative to heparin. Argatroban is used in patients with heparin-induced thrombo-cytopenia as an alternative to lepirudin.

Drotrecogin alfa is a human recombinant activated protein-C. It inhibits thrombin effects by inhibiting Va and VIIIa. It is used as anticoagulant. It is also employed by continuous i.v. infusion to decrease the mortality from severe sepsis (associated with organ dysfunction) in adults at high risk death.

ORAL ANTICOAGULANTS

Oral anticoagulants are chemically related to vitamin K. So they act by competitively antagonizing the actions of vitamin K. Thus they inhibit the synthesis of vitamin K dependent clotting factors. It takes about 36–48 hours for the anticoagulant effect to develop. Unlike heparin, they are not active in vitro.

Pharmacokinetics

Warfarin and the other oral anticoagulants are readily absorbed on oral administration. These drugs cross the placental barrier and are also secreted in the mother's milk. These drugs are extensively bound to plasma albumin. So these drugs have:

- Very low volume distribution
- No urinary excretion
- Long plasma half-life
- Several displacement drug interactions

Warfarin is metabolized in the liver into inactive metabolite which is excreted in the urine.

The main side effect of all oral anticoagulants is haemorrhage (2–4%). Anorexia, nausea, vomiting and diarrhoea are other minor side effects. These are contraindicated in:

- Peptic ulcer
- During first trimester of pregnancy
- Colitis

Drug Interactions

1. **Action of warfarin is potentiated due to:**
   - Inhibition of its metabolism by cimetidine, metronidazole, cotrimoxazole, erythromycin, ciprofloxacin, disulfiram, chloramphenicol.
   - Displacement from plasma protein by phenylbutazone, ethacrynic acid and sulphinpyrazone.
   - Inhibition of platelet functions by nonsteroidal anti-inflammatory drugs.
   - Inhibition of intestinal vitamin K synthesis by tetracyclines, cephalosporins (3rd generation).
   - Enhanced catabolism of clotting factors by d-thyroxin, hyperthyroidism, and fever.
   - Decreased synthesis of clotting factors by hepatic disease.
2. **Action of warfarin is decreased due to:**
   - Enzyme induction by barbiturates, rifampicin, carbamazepine.
   - Inhibition of intestinal absorption by sucralfate and cholestyramine.
   - Increased clotting factors by vitamin K and oestrogen.
   - Reduced catabolism of clotting factors by hypothyroidism.
   - Hereditary resistance.

Doses are adjusted according to requirements and tests. The doses of commonly used oral anticoagulants are:

Warfarin sodium: 10 mg daily.
Acenocoumarol: 2–10 mg daily.
Phenindione: 50–150 mg daily.

Therapeutic uses:

- Deep vein thrombosis
- To prevent development of emboli on the heart valves.

COAGULANTS

Coagulants promote coagulation. They are indicated in haemorrhagic state. For immediate effects, whole blood or plasma is the best because it supplies all the endogenous coagulating factors. To restore haemostasis, following are the other drugs.

Systemic Coagulants

Vitamin K

It is a fat soluble coagulation vitamin. It is present in leafy vegetables (as vitamin K_1, phytonadione) and intestinal bacterial flora also synthesizes vitamin K (K_2, menaquinone). Bile salts are required for the absorption of vitamin K_1 and K_2 from intestine. However, a water-soluble synthetic vitamin K_3 has also been developed which does not require bile salts for its oral absorption. Daily requirement of vitamin K is 50–100 µg/day.

Vitamin K acts as a cofactor in the synthesis of prothrombin, factors VII, IX and X. Deficiency of vitamin K occurs due to obstructive jaundice, liver disease, malabsorption, long-term antimicrobial therapy which alter intestinal flora. It is manifested by bleeding tendency such as haematuria, bleeding from gut, nose and ecchymoses.

Vitamin K is employed:

- In prophylaxis and treatment of bleeding (Vitamin K_3 orally or K_1 parenterally).
- As specific antidote for over dosage of oral anticoagulants. Vitamin K_1 oxide is given i.m. due to its fast onset in comparison to vitamin K_3 because of its delayed onset (24 hrs.).
- To treat vitamin deficiency in adults.

Rapid i.v. injection of emulsified vitamin K produces fall in blood pressure, flushing, breathlessness and a sense of constriction in the chest.

Fibrinogen

It is a fraction of human plasma. It is used to control bleeding in haemophilia, antiha-emophilic globulin (AHG) deficiency and acute afibrinogenemic states. It is given in a dose of 0.5 g by i.v. infusion.

Antihaemophilic factor is a concentrated human antihaemophilic globulin. It is prepared from pooled human plasma. It is used to control bleeding episodes due to haemophilia and AHG deficiency. It is given by i.v. infusion in a dose of 5–10 µg/kg every 6–12 hours.

Fibrinolytic Inhibitors

Aminocaproic acid and its analogue tranexamic acid: They competitively inhibit activation of plasminogen and are used in hyperplasminaemic state.

Aprotinin inhibits plasmin, kallikrein and platelet activation. It is used for hyperplas-minaemia caused by fibrinolytic drug overdose and to prevent blood loss during cardiac surgery.

Local haemostatics (styptics) are particularly effective on oozing surfaces, e.g. tooth sockets, open wounds, etc. They act by providing a network of fibrin which promotes coagulation.

The preparations include:

- **Human or bovine thrombin:** It is applied as dry powder or freshly prepared solution on the oozing surfaces. It is employed in haemophilia, neurosurgery, skin grafting, etc.
- **Fibrin foam/sheets:** Prepared from human plasma. Dried fibrin sheets or foam are used to cover or pack bleeding surfaces from where it gets absorbed in the body.
- **Gelatin sponge:** It is used for packing wounds after moistening with saline or thrombin solution.

- **Russell's viper venom:** Applied locally to stop external bleeding in haemophiliacs. It acts as a thromboplastin.
- **Adrenaline:** It is a vasoconstrictor. 1% solution of adrenaline is used for this purpose. Sterile cotton gauze, soaked in this solution, is packed to stop epistaxis or other similar bleeding.
- **Adrenochrome monosemicarbazone**
- **Ethamsylate:** It reduces capillary bleeding and improves capillary wall stability. It has antihyaluronidase action. It inhibits PGI_2 production and corrects abnormal platelet function. It is used for the prevention and treatment of capillary bleeding, e.g. epistaxis, after tooth extraction and abortion.
- **Tannic acid** (20% in glycerine): It is an astringent which is used for bleeding gums and bleeding piles.

Points for Dental Students

1. Topical treatment to stop gingival bleeding includes the use of absorbable gelatin or collagen sponges, topical thrombin or the placement of microfibrillator collagen held in place by packing or splints.
2. Another way of management of gingival bleeding is with oral rinses of antifi-brinolytic agents such as tranexamic acid or ε-aminocaproic acid.
3. If these local measures are not successful in stopping significantly gingival haemorrhage, platelet transfusions are necessary.
4. Tranexamic acid or ε-aminocaproic acid oral rinse is effective in preventing post-extraction bleeding in haemophiliacs A and B with fewer side effects.
5. Fibrin sealants or fibrin glue has been effective as an adjunct with adhesive and haemostatic effects to control bleeding at

wound or surgical sites. Its use has allowed reduction in factor concentrate replacement levels in hemophiliacs undergoing dental surgeries when used in combination with antifibrinolytics. Extemporaneous fibrin sealant can be made by combining cryoprecipitate with a combination of 10, 000 units topical thrombin powder diluted in 10 ml saline and 10 ml calcium chloride. When dispensed over the wound simultaneously from separate syringes, the cryoprecipitate and calcium chloride precipitate simultaneously to form a clear gelatinous adhesive.

6. If warfarin anticoagulation is maintained within the therapeutic range currently recommended for prevention of venous thrombosis, arterial fibrillation, or mechanical heart valve, the patients undergoing tooth extraction or alveolar and gingival surgery rarely experience uncontrolled bleeding. While the risk of bleeding is low, embolic complications and death have been reported during subtherapeutic anticoagulation. So therapeutic anticoagulation should be confirmed before and continued through the procedure. Similarly, low dose aspirin (e.g. 81 to 325 mg) can be safely continued. Bleeding is controlled with local pressure (e.g. gauze), suturing, topical thrombin, or tranexamic acid mouth wash.

TO REMEMBER

1. Heparin is a mixture of sulphated mucopolysaccharides and has strong electronegative charge. It exists as high molecular weight (strong anticoagulant) and low molecular weight (weak anticoagulant) heparin. It is effective both in vitro and in vivo.

2. Heparin is a powerful immediately acting anticoagulant which is always administered parenterally.

3. Protamine sulphate is used as heparin antagonist.

4. Oral anticoagulants act by competitively antagonizing the actions of vitamin K and inhibit the synthesis of vitamin K dependent clotting factors. So vitamin K_1 is used as oral anticoagulant antagonist.

5. Oral anticoagulants are not effective in vitro and take 36–48 hours for the anticoagulant effect to develop.

6. Coagulants promote coagulation. They are used in haemorrhagic state.

7. Important coagulants are vitamin K, fibrinogen, antihaemophilic factor, aminocaproic and tranexamic acids.

8. Vitamin K is employed in prophylaxis and treatment of bleeding.

9. Fibrinogen and antihaemophilic factor are used to control bleeding episodes due to haemophilia and antihaemophilic globulin deficiency.

10. Aminocaproic acid and tranexamic acid are fibrinolytic inhibitors and are used in hyperplasminaemic state.

11. Local haemostatics are called styptics and are particularly effective on oozing surfaces. These are used in dental practice to control bleeding during various dental procedures.

Chapter 33
Antiplatelet Drugs, Thrombolytic Agents, Antihyperlipidaemic Agents, Blood Substitutes and Plasma Expanders

ANTIPLATELET DRUGS

The flow of blood may be reduced, if a thrombus (clot) is formed in a blood vessel. Thrombosis may decrease or block the flow of blood to vital organs like brain, lung, heart or kidney and the condition may be fatal. Each thrombus consists of white thrombus (platelets) surrounded by red thrombus (fibrin and cellular elements). Antiplatelet drugs are more useful in the prevention of arterial thrombosis while anticoagulants are more useful in venous thrombosis.

Important antiplatelet drugs are:

I. Drugs whose Effect is Prostaglandin Mediated

1. **Aspirin:** It is used as a prophylaxis of myocardial infarction in high-risk cases and also as a prophylaxis against secondary myocardial infarction in low doses (75–150 mg/24 hr). It acts by causing irreversible acetylation of platelet cyclo-oxygenase. In low doses, the effect of aspirin on vascular cyclo-oxygenase is nominal and transient. Thus low-dose aspirin significantly reduces the incidence of non-fatal myocardial infarction and reinfarction.

2. **Epoprostenol (PGI$_2$):** It is a potent inhibitor of platelet aggregation. However, its use is precluded due to its very short t½. It may be used during renal dialysis or cardiac bypass surgery in patients in whom heparin is contraindicated.

II. Other Drugs

1. **Dipyridamole:** It is a coronary vasodilator and inhibits platelet adhesion to thrombogenic surfaces by increasing platelet cAMP due to inhibition of phosphodiesterase. It may also release PG precursors from vascular endothelium. It is used with anticoagulants to prevent thrombus formation on prosthetic heart valves or in rheumatic valvular disease in doses of 100 mg, 3 to 4 times a day.

2. **Ticlopidine:** It is thienopyridine. Acting on surface receptors on platelets, it inhibits ADP-dependent platelet aggregation. Its onset of action is slow (3–7 days) and it acts through an active metabolite. It is used to reduce the incidence of non-fatal myocardial infarction and reinfarction. Dose: 250 mg twice a day with meals.

3. **Clopidogrel:** It is a new congener of ticlopidine. It also inhibits ADP-induced platelet aggregation through an active metabolite. Its therapeutic efficacy is similar to ticlopidine, but it appears to be better tolerated. Dose: 75 mg once a day.

4. **Abciximab** is the Fab fragment of a chimeric monoclonal antibody against GPIIb/IIIa. It is recommended to be given along with aspirin + heparin in high-risk patients undergoing coronary angioplasty.

5. **Eptifibatide and tirofiban** are cyclic peptide GPIIb/IIIa receptor antagonists, which are developed as alternative to absciximab.

Therapeutic Uses of Antiplatelet Drugs

The main drug is aspirin. Other drugs with different mechanism of action (e.g. dipyridamol, clopidogrel) can be used as adjunct.

1. To reduce mortality and prevention of reinfarction, low dose aspirin is started immediately after myocardial infarction.
2. To prevent reocclusion after thrombolytic therapy.
3. To reduce the risk of myocardial infarction and sudden death, aspirin is used in patients with unstable angina.
4. For primary and secondary prevention of myocardial infarction.
5. To reduce the incidence of transient ischaemic attacks (TIAs) and stroke in patients with TIAs or persistent atrial fibrillation and in those with past history of stroke.
6. To maintain the patency of implanted bypass vessel.
7. To prevent formation of micro-thrombi on prosthetic heart valves and embolism.
8. To increase the life of atrioventricular shunt used for haemodialysis.

FIBRINOLYTIC (THROMBOLYTIC) AGENTS

Fibrinolytic drugs are used to dissolve clot in vivo. To break thrombi, these drugs degrade fibrin by activating plasminogen to form plasmin.

1. **Streptokinase:** It is a protein and is synthesized by beta-haemolytic streptococci. It is employed in the treatment of life-threatening venous thrombosis and in pulmonary embolism. It is given by intravenous infusion as a loading dose (2,50,000 units in 30 minutes) followed by 1,00,000 units per hour for 24–72 hours. During therapy, thrombin time should be closely monitored. Intracoronary administration of streptokinase within 6 hours of an acute coronary thrombosis can restore flow in occluded artery and may reduce mortality.

2. **Urokinase:** It is a proteolytic enzyme. It is derived from the human kidney and is present in urine. It is now prepared from tissue cultures of human renal cells. So it is non-antigenic. It directly converts plasminogen into plasmin. It is given intravenously as a loading dose (3, 00,000 units) followed by 3, 00,000 units per hour for 12 hours. Recently a new recombinant pro-urokinase has been produced by recombinant DNA technology. It is more fibrin-selective because it is converted to urokinase on binding to fibrin. It is used in thrombosed arteriovenous shunts and for thrombolysis in the eye.

3. **Alteplase (tissue plasminogen activator; TPA):** It is also fibrinoselective and avoids systemic activation. It has been obtained from cultured human melanoma cells and by recombinant DNA technology. It is given in a dose of 100 mg intravenously in 3 hours.

4. **Anisolylated plasminogen-streptokinase activator** is a complex of human plasminogen and streptokinase which has been made inactive by the introduction of p-anisolyl group. In the blood, anisolyl group is removed by a hydrolytic deacylation process. It is given as a single injection intravenously over 4–5 minutes and the fibrinolytic activity is sustained for 4–6 hours.

Therapeutic Uses

  i. Multiple pulmonary emboli
 ii. Central deep vein thrombosis
iii. Acute coronary thrombosis
 iv. Peripheral arterial occlusion

Adverse Drug Reactions

- Bleeding
- Multiple micro-emboli from disintegrating the pre-existing thrombus
- Mild allergic reactions may occur with drugs containing streptokinase.
  Contraindications: These drugs should not be used in the following conditions:
- Conditions having risk of bleeding
- Vascular aneurysm
- Endocardial thrombi
- Allergy to streptokinase

ANTIHYPERLIPIDAEMIC AGENTS

Lipids are heterogenous group of compounds. These are related to fatty acids. These are insoluble in water. However, these are soluble in ether and chloroform. These are of three types:

a. **Simple lipids:** These are esters of alcohol and fatty acids. The fatty acids, present in diet, may be:
  - Saturated fatty acids such as lauric and palmitic acids.
  - Monounsaturated fatty acids such as oleic acid and palmitoleic acids.
  - Polyunsaturated fatty acids such as linolenic acid and arachidonic acid; abundant in corn oil and safflower oil; have hypolipidaemic effect.

b. **Compound lipids:** These are also esters of alcohol and fatty acids but certain other groups are also present in their structure, e.g. sulfolipids and phospholipids.

c. **Neutral lipids:** These are non-polar lipids such as glycerides, cholesterol and cholesterol esters. Triglycerides are composed of three fatty acids which are linked to 3-atom containing alcohol or glycerol. Cholesterol is a lipid that chemically is a sterol but not a fat.

Lipoproteins are spherical particles. They transport triglycerides and cholesterol esters through the plasma. Both are non-polar hydrophobic lipids. They form the core of the lipoprotein, which is surrounded by a hydrophilic surface coat of phospholipids, unesterified cholesterol and apoproteins. Due to hydrophilic surface coat, the lipoprotein becomes soluble in plasma and acts as an interface between the plasma and the core components. Apoproteins also help in lipoprotein metabolism as well as in the regulation of lipid transport/exchange. Lipoproteins have been classified on the basis of their densities as under:

- Chylomicrons
- Very low density lipoproteins (VLDL)
- Intermediate density lipoproteins (IDL)
- Low density lipoproteins (LDL)
- High density lipoproteins (HDL)
- Lipoprotein-A [LP (a)]; similar to LDL with additional apoprotein-A besides apoprotein-B 100. It is a homologue of plasminogen but does not have plasminogen's enzymatic activity. It is a competitive inhibitor of plasminogen and has tendency to increase thrombosis due to its preferential deposition in atherosclerotic tissues.

Apoproteins (Apos) are the surface proteins of various lipoproteins. They provide structural stability to the lipoproteins and play an important role in determining the metabolic fate of the lipoproteins on which they reside. There are 9 types of Apos, viz. Apo-A-1, Apo-A-II, Apo-A-IV, Apo-B-48, Apo-B-100, Apo-C-I, Apo-C-II, Apo-C-III, and Apo-E.

Transport of exogenous (dietary) lipids: In the intestinal mucosa, dietary triglycerides and cholesterol are incorporated into the core of chylomicrons. The surface coat of chylomicrons is composed of phospholipids, free cholesterol and various apoproteins. The chylomicron is then transported to the circulation via the thoracic duct. Finally dietary triglycerides are delivered to fat and muscle cells (as fatty acids) and dietary cholesterol is taken up by the liver. The fatty acids leave the cells, ionize in plasma (pH 7.4), combine with albumin and are known as free fatty acids (FFAs). These then reach other cells where they are oxidized by β-oxidation to provide energy.

Cholesterol is not used for energy. It serves as a structural component of all cell membranes, as a precursor for adrenal and gonadal steroids and as precursor of hepatic bile acids. In liver, it may be stored, oxidized to bile acids or alternatively incorporated into HDL or VLDL and resecreted as lipoprotein-cholesterol back into circulation.

Dietary cholesterol regulates endogenous hepatic cholesterol synthesis. In liver, the cholesterol is synthesized from mevalonic acid which is obtained from reduction of acetyl coenzyme-A by 3-hydroxy-3-methyglutaryl-coenzyme-A reductase (HMG-CoA reductase) enzyme. A small amount of cholesterol is also absorbed from the gut which is also taken up by hepatocytes. The total intracellular cholesterol in hepatocytes provide a negative feedback for cholesterol synthesis by inhibiting HMG-CoA reductase. Due to this, synthesis of cholesterol by the liver is decreased.

Transport of endogenous lipids: Lipids (triglycerides, cholesterol, and cholesterol esters) are transported from liver to the peripheral tissues and back to the liver by the endogenous lipid transport system. The atherogenic Apo-B 100 lipoprotein guided system transports VLDL, IDL and LDL while antiatherogenic Apo-AI governed lipoprotein system transports HDL.

When concentrations of cholesterol or triglycerides or both in plasma are very high, the condition is called hyperlipidaemia or hyperlipoproteinemias. Medical attention is required, if the level of cholesterol is above 250 mg/100 ml and triglycerides is above 150 mg/100 ml.

Atherosclerosis (hardening of arteries due to deposition of lipoid material in the intimal layers of the arteries) occurs due to elevated level of plasma lipoproteins and can lead to coronary thrombosis and infarction. Drugs used for the treatment of hyperlipidaemia are called hypolipidemic agents. The aim of the treatment is to lower the concentration of VLDL and LDL and raise HDL.

1. Drugs which Primarily Reduce Plasma Triglycerides

i. **Nicotinic acid (niacin, B$_3$):** It is a water soluble vitamin. It lowers plasma triglyceride levels. Vitamin B$_3$ reduces the levels of circulating FFAs by strongly inhibiting lipolysis in adipose tissue. It acts by inhibiting the hepatic triglyceride production and VLDL secretion due to decreased supply of FFAs which act as a major precursor for triglyceride. So it reduces LDL levels indirectly because it is derived from VLDL in plasma. HDL is increased modestly. It stimulates secretion of tissue plasminogen activator and lowers plasma fibrinogen. Due to this, it reverses some of the hypa ercholesterolaemic associated endothelial cell dysfunction contributing to thrombosis. It is contra-indicated in pregnancy. Important side effects are flushing, dizziness and palpitation. It is used to treat several types of hyperlipidaemias in combination with a bile acid-binding resin (colestipol or chloestyramine). In hypercholestero-laemia, it has been given in combination with lovastatin (decreases cholesterol synthesis) or neomycin (decreases cholesterol absorption). The usual dosage of nicotinic acid is 2–8 g daily.

ii. **Fibric acid derivatives (fibrates):** Fibrates include clofibrate, gemfibrozil, benzafi-brate and fenofibrate.

They lower the plasma concentrations of cholesterol and triglyceride. These drugs have marked effect in lowering the VLDL, and hence triglycerides, with a modest (approximately 10%) reduction in LDL and an approximately 10% increase in HDL. These drugs act:

- By stimulating lipase (LPA) activity due to activation of a nuclear receptor (transcription factor) termed peroxisomal proliferation activated receptor factor (PPAR-α).
- By stimulating hydrolysis of triglycerides in the plasma.
- By reducing the incorporation of fatty acids into VLDL in the liver. So they inhibit the synthesis and secretion of VLDL.

The fibrates are absorbed orally, partly metabolized in the liver and excreted in urine. They are contraindicated in the presence of severe hepatic or renal dysfunctions, and in pregnant woman. Side effects are relatively low and mild. Nausea, diarrhoea, abdominal discomfort, skin rash and impotence are reported.

They are used in hyperlipidaemias. Fenofibrate also has uricosuric effect. So it is used where hyperuricaemia coexists with hyperlipidaemia.

iii. **Guggulipid:** It is a mixture of sterones. It is obtained from an ayurvedic herb *Commiphora mukul*. It is a useful drug for the treatment of mild hyperlipidaemia, atherosclerosis, and obesity. It decreases cholesterol biosynthesis and also increases excretion of cholesterol through the gut. It also stimulates thyroid activity and reduces platelet aggregation. Although it is claimed to be free from toxicity, special precaution, however, is needed while using in patients with hepatic disease, dysentery or diarrhoea.

iv. **Omega-3 marine triglycerides:** These are derived from some marine fish oils. They may induce profound lowering of plasma triglycerides, but increase plasma cholesterol.

2. Drugs which Primarily Reduce Plasma Cholesterol

i. **Anion-exchange resins (colestipol, and cholestyramine):** These are quarternary ammonium ion-exchange resins. They are insoluble in water and have a very high molecular weight. One gram of the drug can bind about 100 mg of bile salts. They enhance the excretion of bile salts in the faeces by sequestering bile acids in the intestine and preventing their reabsorption and entrohepatic circulation. So there occurs decreased absorption of exogenous cholesterol and increased metabolism of endogenous cholesterol into bile acids in the liver. This leads to increased expression of LDL receptors on the liver cells and increased removal of LDL from blood to liver. They are, therefore, mainly useful when high blood cholesterol is due to raised LDL concentration. They are neither absorbed nor metabolized in liver. Important side effects are nausea, abdominal discomfort, indigestion and constipation. They may interfere with the absorption of fat soluble vitamins A, D, E, and K from the intestine. They may also interfere with the absorption of several drugs. So other drugs may be taken 1 hour before or 4 hours after the administration of these drugs. These drugs are used for treating hypercholesterolaemia.

ii. **Neomycin:** It is an aminoglycoside antibiotic which is poorly absorbed from gut. It inhibits reabsorption of cholesterol and bile acids. It is not a safe drug because intestinal sterilization may give rise to superinfection and gastrointestinal symptoms.

iii. **Plant sterols (beta-sitosterols):** Beta-sitosterol and a new synthetic drug ezetimibe block uptake of cholesterol in the intestine by competition for its absorption sites, without themselves getting absorbed. Due to this, they reduce total cholesterol, LDL cholesterol, triglycerides and APO-B while increase HDL cholesterol. They are used to treat familial hypercholesterolaemia, familial combined hyperlipidaemia and hyperlipo-proteinaemias.

iv. **Cholesterol synthesis inhibitors (statins):** The important members of this group are atorvastatin, lovastatin, mevastatin, simvastatin, pravastatin, fluvastatin and rosuvastatin.

Cholesterol is synthesized in liver from mevalonic acid. Statins act by competitively inhibiting the conversion of acetyl coenzyme-A to mevalonic acid by HMG-CoA reductase enzyme. So there occurs depletion of hepatic intracellular supply of cholesterol which is compensated by liver by increasing the uptake of plasma LDL by increasing number of LDL receptors. Due to this, plasma LDL level is decreased. Statins also produce a moderate lowering of triglycerides level due to reduction of VLDL secretion by the liver and increased uptake of IDL and VLDL remnants by LDL receptors. However, there occurs slight increase in HDL-cholesterol.

One of the limiting factors in the use of Statins is diminished effect after prolonged use even with increased dosages. This ceiling-dose effect is due to "feedback compensatory induction" of HMG-CoA reductase enzyme which tends to increase cholesterol biosynthesis.

Different statins differ in their potency. Plasma half-lives of these drugs range from 1–3 hours, except for atorvastatin (14 hrs.) and rosuvastatin (19 hrs.). So with the exception of these two drugs, other HMG-CoA reductase inhibitors are administered at night because cholesterol biosynthesis takes place predominantly at night. They are used to treat elevated plasma low density lipoproteins and cholesterol in familial or multi-factorial hypercholes-terolaemia or combined familial hyper-lipidaemia either alone or in combination with niacin or bile-acid-binding resins.

Recently, it is suggested that statins may lower the risk of stroke, dementia, Alzheimer's disease and may improve bone density in postmenopausal women due to their combined cholesterol lowering, antiproliferative, anti-inflam-matory or antioxidant properties.

These drugs may cause hepatotoxicity, myositis and lenticular opacity. They are contraindicated in pregnancy, lactation, children and liver diseases.

v. **Probucol:** It causes a moderate fall in plasma cholesterol levels. It probably acts by inhibiting sterol synthesis and improves transport of cholesterol from the periphery to liver. At present, it is no more used as an antihyperlipidaemic drug because it reduces HDL cholesterol levels and LDL cholesterol levels only marginally. It also has antioxidant action and has been shown to inhibit athero-genesis because it directly prevents the oxidation of LDL. It, thus, exerts an antia-therogenic effect because macrophages consume LDL in oxidized form. Important side effects are nausea, vomiting, flatulence, diarrhoea, abdominal pain. Rarely angioneurotic oedema and hypersensitivity reactions are reported. It is given in a dose of 500 mg twice daily with food.

Combination Drug Therapy

It is very useful in the treatment of severe hyperlipoproteinemia (HLP) and familial hypercholesterolaemia (F-HC) in whom satisfactory plasma levels of LDL-C are not achieved with single drug. Commonly used drug combinations shown in Table 33.1.

Table 33.1: Commonly used drug combinations

Drug combination	Disease	Remarks
1. Bile acid binding resin + statins	Familial hypercholesterolaemia	Give statins 1 hr. before or 4 hrs. after the resin to ensure proper absorption
2. Bile acid binding resin + niacin + statin	Severe cases of familial hypercholesterolaemia and familial combined hyperlipidaemia	Complimentary action; reduced doses; sustained effect with minimal toxicities
3. Bile acid binding resin + fibrates	Familial combined hyperlipidaemia	Increased risk of cholelethiasis
4. Bile acid binding resin + niacin	Familial combined hyperlipidaemia and familial hypercholesterolaemia	Resin reduces niacin-induced gastric irritation
5. Statins + ezetimibe	Primary and familial hypercholesterolaemia	Synergistic combination
6. Niacin + statin	Familial combined hyperlipidaemia and familial hypercholesterolaemia	Synergistic combination

BLOOD SUBSTITUTES AND PLASMA EXPANDERS

Shock is a state of acute circulatory failure. It is mainly due to reduced blood volume (hypovolemia). It is, therefore, essential to restore the intravascular blood volume as quickly as possible by intravenous fluid therapy. The various types of fluids used for replacement are:

1. Whole blood and plasma
2. Plasma substitutes:
   a. Colloidal such as dextran, hydroxyethyl starches, polyvinyl pyrrolidone, oxypolygelatin.
   b. Crystalline, e.g. normal sodium chloride and dextrose solution.

Plasma expanders are substances of relatively high molecular weight. On infusion, they remain long enough to augment the volume of circulating fluid by increasing the osmotic pressure.

1. **Dextran:** It is originally isolated from beet sugar. In therapeutics, dextran having different molecular weight is used.
   Dextran 40 (MW 40 million): 10% in dextrose or in sodium chloride intravenous infusion.
   Dose: Initial dose 500–1000 ml; the first 500 ml may be given in 30 minutes which may be followed by 100 ml by continuous infusion for 2–3 days. Be careful in patients with renal impairment, congestive heart failure or polycythaemia.
   Dextran 70 (MW 70, 000) and dextran 110 (MW 110, 000): 6% in dextrose or in sodium chloride intravenous infusion. They are used for the management of hypovolemic or haemorrhagic shock.
   Dextrans are probably almost ideal plasma expanders because they can be easily sterilized and can be stored for long time. However, rarely allergic reactions to these preparations may occur.

2. **Polyvinylpyrrolidone:** It is a synthetic water soluble preparation. It has average molecular weight of 35,000–40,000. It is sterile 40% solution in buffered physiological saline. It has a tendency to bind with insulin and penicillin.

3. **Gelatin:** Commercially available gelatin has molecular weight of 30,000. It is given intravenously, 500–1000 ml of 3.5–4% solution, in low blood volume.

4. **Electrolyte and water replacement:** To meet normal fluid and electrolyte requirement, normal saline (sodium chloride, 0.9% w/v) is the most widely used intravenous preparation. It is indicated in fluid losses which are

accompanied by sodium depletion as in severe diarrhoea, diabetic ketosis, in order to provide water and sodium ions in physiologically comparable amounts.

To replenish major fluid losses or to meet the daily water requirements dextrose intravenous infusion (5% w/v) is used. Its energy content is low. So it makes only a minimal contribution to the body's requirement.

Points for Dental Students

1. The most commonly used antiplatelet drug is aspirin. It is used chronically in very low doses (40 to 325 mg per day) to prevent cardiovascular and cerebrovascular events. It irreversibly decreases platelet aggregation and consequently increases the bleeding time. At these doses, anticipated effect will have little impact on bleeding after oral surgical procedures.

2. However, if the patient has other underlying medical conditions that predispose to impaired haemostasis (such as uremia or liver disease), takes other anticoagulants (including non-aspirin NSAIDs) or abuses alcohol, aspirin should be discontinued 3 to 7 days prior to surgery.

3. If emergency surgery needs to be performed and the patient's bleeding time is higher than 15 to 20 minutes, 1-desamino-8-D-arginine vasopressin (DDAVP) can be used to improve haemostasis within 1 hour of surgery.

TO REMEMBER

1. Antiplatelet drugs are more useful in the prevention of arterial thrombosis.
2. Aspirin with/without dipyridamol is used to prevent arterial thrombosis in high risk patients and during coronary artery bypass as well as to prevent attacks of secondary myocardial infarction.

3. To prevent arterial thrombosis, aspirin is used during haemodialysis and aspirin + warfarin is employed after using prosthetic heart valve.

4. To treat acute myocardial infarction fibrinolytic therapy is started within 6 hours which is followed by aspirin with/without dipyridamol.

5. Fibrinolytic therapy is also indicated in acute peripheral arterial thrombosis.

6. Aminocaproic acid and tranxamic acid inhibit activation of plasminogen to plasmin which breaks down fibrin in vivo.

7. Nicotinic acid, fibrates (clofibrate, gemfibrozil, benzafibrate), guggulipid, and omega-3-marine triglycerides primarily decrease plasma triglycerides.

8. Anion exchange resins, neomycin, betasitosterols, statins, probucol, d-thyroxine primarily reduce plasma cholesterol.

9. Since low density lipoproteins and very low density lipoproteins are both raised and single agent is ineffective in reducing low density lipoproteins, drug combinations are used in hyperlipidaemia, e.g. bile acid binding resin + fibrates to treat familial combined hyperlipaedimia; bile acid-binding resin + niacin to treat familial hypercholesterolaemia and familial combined hyperlipaemia; bile acid-binding resin+statin to treat familial hypercholesterolaemia; and niacin + statin + bile acid-binding resin to treat patients with severe disorders involving elevated low density lipoproteins levels.

10. To correct hypovolemia in shock, either whole blood and plasma or plasma substitutes are used as quickly as possible to avoid generalized impairment of cellular function.

Drugs Acting on Kidney

Section 8

Drugs Acting on Kidney

Diuretics

Chapter 34

Diuretics

The diuretics are drugs which increase the rate of urine formation. They promote a net loss of water and sodium from the body.

Classification and Mechanism of Action

1. **High efficacy diuretics:** They are also called high ceiling or loop diuretics. Their main site of action is thick ascending limb of loop of Henle (Table 34.1). They exert inhibitory effect on sodium, potassium and chloride carrier system and inhibit the reabsorption of both sodium and chloride. The drugs belonging to this group are:
   i. *Sulphonamides:* Frusemide, bumetanide, piretanide
   ii. *Non-sulphonamides:* Ethacrynic acid, ticrynafen, indacrynic acid
   Most widely used drug in this group is frusemide.
2. **Moderate efficacy diuretics:** They act on cortical diluting segment and early portion of distal convoluted tubule (Table 34.1). They act by inhibiting sodium chloride cotransport system. The important drugs are:

   i. *Thiazides:* Hydrochlorothiazide, bendroflumazide, polythiazide, cyclopenthiazide.
   ii. *Other compounds with different chemical structure:* Chlorthalidone, metolazone, indapamide, xipamide.
   Hydrochlorothiazide is the most commonly used drug of this group.
3. **Low efficacy diuretics:**
   i. *Potassium sparing diuretics:* They act on distal collecting tubule and duct.

   Examples are:
   * *Spironolactone:* It acts by blocking aldosterone receptor.
   * *Triamterene and amiloride:* They act by blocking sodium channels controlled by aldosterone (sodium-potassium exchange).
   ii. *Osmotic diuretics:* Their main site of action is proximal convoluted tubule; also act on descending limb of loop of Henle and collecting tubules. By osmotic action, they retain water in filtrate. Important members of this group are mannitol, glycerol and urea.

Table 34.1: Main site of action of diuretics

High efficacy diuretics	Thick ascending limb of the loop of Henle
Moderate efficacy diuretics	Cortical diluting segment and early portion of distal convoluted tubule
Low efficacy diuretics	
a. Potassium sparing diuretics	Distal collecting tubule and duct
b. Osmotic diuretics	Proximal and distal convoluted tubules
Carbonic anhydrase inhibitors and mercurial diuretics	Proximal and distal convoluted tubules

4. **Miscellaneous:**

   i. *Carbonic anhydrase inhibitors:* Main site of actions are proximal and distal tubules.

   They act by inhibiting carbonic anhydrase enzyme, so that H^+ is not available for H^+/Na^+ exchange. The drugs in this group include acetazolamide, ethoxzolamide, methazolamide and dichlorphenamide.

   ii. *Mercurial diuretics:* The main sites of action are proximal and distal convoluted tubules. They depress reabsorption of Na^+ and Cl^- due to their affinity for SH group of enzymes of renal tubules. They are no more used because of their toxicity.

   iii. *Xanthine diuretics* (caffeine, theophylline and theobromine): These are weak diuretics. These act by increasing renal blood flow and by inhibiting reabsorption of sodium and water in the proximal convoluted tubule. They are now rarely used as a diuretic; used as bronchodilators only.

   iv. *Acidifying salts* (ammonium chloride): It is rarely used as diuretic because of its base saving mechanism.

High Ceiling (Loop) Diuretics

These drugs are called high ceiling diuretics because of highest efficacy. They are also known as loop diuretics due to their action on the thick ascending limb of the loop of Henle. The urinary excretion of Na^+ and Cl^- is profoundly increased by blocking $Na^+K^+2Cl^-$ cotransport. Potassium and calcium loss is also increased.

The onset of action of these diuretics is quick (30 min. after oral and 5 min. after intravenous injection). These agents show peak diuresis in about 2 hours and the total duration of action is 6 to 8 hours.

Side Effects

- **Related to renal actions:** Hypokalaemia, metabolic hypochloraemic alkalosis, depletion of calcium and magnesium, hypovolaemia (hypotension), and hyperuricaemia.
- **Others:** Gastrointestinal disturbances, hyperglycaemia, skin rash, pancreatitis. Deafness may appear rarely with ethacrynic acid (ototoxicity).

Therapeutic Uses

i. Acute pulmonary oedema (acute left ventricular failure, following myocardial infarction)

ii. Refractory oedema associated with congestive heart failure

iii. Along with normal saline infusion in hypercalcaemia and hyperkalaemia

iv. Forced diuresis in poisoning by barbiturates and halides

v. To reduce intracranial tension.

vi. Along with blood transfusion in severe anaemia to prevent vascular overload

vii. In hypertension only in presence of congestive heart failure, renal insufficiency and resistant hypertensive emergencies

Doses: Frusemide: 20–80 mg daily.

Ethacrynic acid: 25–100 mg daily.

Bumetanide: 1–5 mg daily.

Moderate Efficacy Diuretics

Thiazide diuretics lead to increased excretion of Na^+, Cl^- and water due to:

- Inhibition of the Na^+/Cl^- cotransport system in the distal convoluted tubule
- Blocking the active reabsorption of Na^+ and Cl^- with water in distal tubule. They also increase K^+ loss and reduce Ca^{++} loss.

Orally administered thiazides are rapidly absorbed. Diuretic effect is seen in 1 hour and their duration lasts up to 12–24 hours.

Chlorthalidone has longer duration of action. These agents are bound to plasma proteins to varying degrees and this has no correlation to their half-life.

Side Effects

Hypokalaemia, hyperuricaemia, hyperglycaemia are reported as the main side effects. Less common side effects are skin rashes and thrombocytopenia.

Therapeutic Uses

• Thiazide diuretics are used alone or in combination with other drugs in the management of hypertension on long-term basis.
• They are often used for short-term therapy in controlling oedema associated with congestive heart failure, cirrhosis and premenstrual tension.
• Rarely thiazides are employed in diabetes insipidus (DI). This is a paradoxical use. They are effective in DI of pituitary origin (neurogenic) as well as of DI of renal origin (nephrogenic). The mechanism of action is not well understood. The possible explanations are:
  a. More complete reabsorption of glomerular filtrate iso-osmotically due to a state of thiadzide induced sustained electrolyte depletion.
  b. Presence of smaller volume of less dilute urine to the collecting duct due to reduced salt absorption in the cortical diluting segment and same is passed out.
  c. Thiazides reduce glomerular filtration rate and thus fluid load on the tubules.

Doses: Chlorothiazide and hydrochlorothiazide are used in a dose of 0.5–1 g and 25–100 mg daily, respectively. The long acting thiazides are bendroflumathiazide (2–5 mg/day), chlorthalidone (25–100 mg/day) and polythiazide (4–8 mg/day). Newer compounds related to thiazide diuretics are indapamide (2.5 mg/day) and xipamide (20–40 mg/day).

Potassium Sparing Diuretics

1. **Spironolactone:** It competitively inhibits the actions of aldosterone on the distal tubule, so aldosterone mediated sodium reabsorption. It is used in a dose of 50–100 mg daily. Spironolactone is used during primary (Conn's syndrome) or secondary (due to congestive cardiac failure, hepatic cirrhosis, nephrotic syndrome) hyperaldosteronism in combination with other diuretics.
2. **Amiloride and triamterene:** Acting on the distal tubule they prevent the reabsorption of sodium by blocking sodium channels controlled by aldosterone.

Doses: Amiloride: 5–20 mg daily and triamterene 100–200 mg daily. They are used for the treatment of hypertension in combination with other diuretics, as this combination augments the excretion of sodium while diminishing excretion of potassium.

Side Effects

Hyperkalaemia, gastrointestinal upsets, drowsiness and mental confusion. Spironolactone may cause gynaecomastia and impotence by interfering with other steroid receptors in males and menstrual irregularities and hirsutism in females.

Triamterene when given with indomethacin may result in acute renal failure.

Osmotic Diuretics

These substances are water soluble. They are pharmacologically inert and poorly reabsorbable non-electrolytes. The extent of diuresis produced is proportional to the quantity of osmotic diuretic used. They do not cause marked loss of electrolytes. Diuretic effect of osmotic diuretics is due to:

• Increased glomerular filtration rate and inhibition of renin release because they expand extracellular fluid volume

- Reduction in passive salt reabsorption because of disappearance of cortico-medullary osmotic gradient as a result of increased renal blood flow
- Retention of water iso-osmotically in proximal tubule which dilutes luminal fluid and opposes sodium chloride reabsorption
- Inhibition of transport processes in the thick ascending loop of Henle

Mannitol is most widely used osmotic diuretic. It is a sugar alcohol. It is employed to induce forced diuresis in cases of drug overdose and in cerebral oedema. Other uses are prophylaxis of acute renal failure, cardiovascular operations, severe traumatic injury, operation in the presence of severe jaundice and management of haemolytic transfusion reaction. In each of these conditions, there is a precipitous fall in the flow of urine. Mannitol is given by intravenous infusion, 50–200 g over a period of 24 hours. It is available in concentration of 5–25% solution for intravenous administration. It is contraindicated in congestive heart failure in order to avoid expansion of blood volume because mannitol is rapidly distributed in the intravascular compartment and extracts water from cells. So prior to the diuresis, this leads to expansion of the extracellular volume of hyponatremia. This effect can complicate heart failure and may produce florid pulmonary edema

Points for Dental Students

A dental student must learn the precautions to be taken in prescribing other drugs to a patient who is already taking a diuretic. It is possible if the student learns and keeps the following drug interactions in mind.

1. Chance of thrombocytopenia increases if cotrimoxazole is administered with loop diuretics.

2. The action of high ceiling diuretics is diminished by indomethacin and other non-steroidal anti-inflammatory drugs because they inhibit synthesis of PGI_2 and PGE_2 which also contribute to Na^+ and K^+ excretion to some extent. This is particularly important in patients of hepatic cirrhosis and nephrotic syndrome.
3. Loop diuretics and aminoglycoside antibiotics have additive ototoxicity; so they should not be administered together.
4. Loop and thiazide diuretics may increase digitalis toxicity and precipitate cardiac irregulatories due to hypokalaemia.
5. Loop and thiazide diuretics may cause rise in serum lithium by increasing its absorption from proximal tubule.
6. Probenecid competitively inhibits tubular secretion of furosemide and thiazides at proximal tubule and therefore decreases their activity.
7. Potassium sparing diuretics cause hyperkalaemia. Hence they should not be administered with potassium supplements and ACE inhibitors to avoid exacerbation of hperkalaemia.
8. Amiloride should not be given with indomethacin because the combination can lead to fatal acute renal failure.
9. Amiloride with quinidine may increase the risk of arrhythmias.

TO REMEMBER

1. Frusemide and ethacrynic acid are diuretic of choice for acute pulmonary oedema, and severe congestive cardiac failure. To treat less severe congestive cardiac failure thiazide/chlorthalidone + potassium sparing diuretic is preferred.
2. Thiazides/chlorthalidone + potassium sparing diuretic are diuretic of choice for the treatment of essential hypertension.

3. Cerebral oedema is treated with mannitol or glycerol diuretics + glucocorticoids.

4. Nephrotic syndrome requires frusemide + spironolactone + high protein diet salt restriction.

5. Mannitol and frusemide are diuretic of choice for acute oliguric renal failure, while frusemide, in large doses, is employed to treat chronic renal failure.

6. Thiazides are used to treat diabetes insipidus and idiopathic hypercalciuria and renal calculi.

7. Hepatic cirrhosis with ascites is treated with potassium sparing diuretic+ thiazide/frusemide.

8. Frusemide (with i.v. saline) is diuretic of choice to treat hypercalcaemia and hyperkalaemia while indacrinone/ ticrynafen is used to treat hyper-uricaemia.

9. Acetazolamide is diuretic of choice to treat hypokalaemic periodic paralysis, resistant epilepsy, acute mountain sickness and hyperphosphataemia.

10. Thiazides with K^+ supplements will be required to treat iatrogenic oedema due to corticosteroids or oral contraceptives.

11. Mannitol is the diuretic of choice for glaucoma and during intraocular surgery.

12. In salicylate, halide, or barbiturate poisoning frusemide (with plenty of i.v. saline) will be employed and aceta-zolamide is used to alkalinize the urine.

Section 9

Respiratory System

Section 9

Respiratory System

35. Drugs for Bronchial Asthma

36. Antitussive Agents, Expectorants, Mucolytic Agents and Nasal Decongestants

Chapter 35

Drugs for Bronchial Asthma

Asthma is a chronic disease. It is characterized by:

- Difficulty in breathing (dyspnoea)
- Intermittent wheeze or cough
- Production of mucoid sputum.

It is primarily an inflammatory condition, which is due to underlying hyper-reactivity. Only in 10% patients there is an allergic basis for the disease. In rest of the cases, a variety of trigger factors (infection, irritants, pollution, exercise, exposure to cold air, psychogenic) may be involved. Asthma is of two types:

- Extrinsic asthma: It is mostly episodic and is less prone to status asthmaticus.
- Intrinsic asthma: It is usually perennial and is more prone to status asthmaticus.

Mast cells are present in lungs. They release mediators (histamine, LTC_4 and D_4, TXA_2, PAF, etc.) which constrict bronchial smooth muscle and cause mucosal oedema and viscid secretions. Thus they cause reversible airway obstruction and difficulty in breathing.

Other factors, implicated in the etiology of bronchial asthma are:

- Imbalance between constrictor (PGF_2-α) and dilator (PGE_2) prostaglandins
- Imbalance between alpha and beta adreno-ceptors
- Imbalance between sympathetic and parasympathetic influences

The primary drugs that are used in asthma are:

- a. Bronchodilators
- b. Corticosteroids
- c. Prophylactics

Bronchodilators

Commonly used bronchodilators are:

- **Xanthine derivatives:** Theophylline
- **Sympathomimetic amines:** Epinephrine, isoprenaline, and beta-2 adrenoceptor stimulants
- **Anticholinergics:** They are rarely used at present due to unpleasant side effects.

Bronchodilators, when given by appropriate route, cause the relaxation of the bronchial smooth muscle and improve pulmonary function. Thus they relieve symptoms of asthma and improve breathing.

Theophylline

To treat severe attacks of asthma, theophylline and its more soluble salt, aminophylline are the bronchodilators of choice. Theophylline is an alkaloid that occurs in varying proportion in coffee beans, tea leaves and cocoa seeds. Tea leaves contain the highest concentration of theophylline. By inhibiting the enzyme phosphodiesterase, theophylline increases the intracellular accumulation of cAMP in bronchial smooth muscle due to prevention of the hydrolytic breakdown of cyclic adenosine monophosphate (cAMP). In addition, it also inhibits the release of histamine and slow reacting substance of anaphylaxis (SRS-A). So theophylline removes obstruction and improves pulmonary function in asthmatics by causing relaxation of bronchial smooth muscle. Further, it also causes central nervous system excitation and cardiac stimulation. Nausea, vomiting, tachycardia and palpitation are most common side effects.

Aminophylline (theophylline ethylene-diamine) can be given by slow intravenous injection (250–500 mg); oral dose is 100–300 mg 3–4 times a day. On rapid intravenous administration, it may cause convulsions.

Sympathomimetic Amines

Aerosol administration of sympathomimetic amines can rapidly relieve mild to moderate attacks of asthma. Non-selective sympatho-mimetics like adrenaline, ephedrine or isoprenaline have higher incidence of side effects than the selective β_2 adrenoceptor stimulants (salbutamol, terbutaline). So selective β_2 adrenoceptor stimulants are preferred over non-selective sympathomimetics.

Adrenaline is given by subcutaneous or intramuscular injection (1:1000). It may also be given by inhalation of nebulised solution in concentration of 200–500 µg.

Isoprenaline is administered by sublingual route (10–20 mg), by aerosol inhalation (1–2 mg) or by inhalation spray (0.5–3%).

Orciprenaline is a derivative of isoprenaline. It is given by oral route (20 mg).

Ephedrine is given orally in doses of 30–60 mg.

The selective β_2 adrenoceptor agonists are the first line of drugs in the treatment of asthma. Their main features are:

- They dilate the bronchi by directly acting on the β_2 adrenoceptors of the bronchial smooth muscles.
- They are the physiological antagonists of spasmogenic mediators.
- They may inhibit the vagal tone.
- Acting on the cilia, they increase mucous clearance.
- Usually these drugs are administered by inhalation of aerosol, powder or nebulised solution. However, some of them may be given orally or by injection. For purpose of

inhalation, a metered-dose inhaler is used. Children and old persons may find difficult to use inhaler, in such cases 'spacer' devices can be used.

Commonly used β_2 adrenoceptor stimulants in asthma are salbutamol and terbutaline (short acting) and salmeterol (long acting). Salbutamol (asthaline) and terbutaline (bricanyl) are given by oral route (1–5 mg), subcutaneously (250–500 µg) or by aerosol inhalation (100–300 µg). Terbutaline has long duration (4–6 hr) of action on oral administration. Onset of action of salmeterol is slow. It is given on twice daily schedule for maintenance therapy and for nocturnal asthma (25 µg per metered dose inhaler). It is not used for acute asthma. Tachycardia, tremor, headache and insomnia are common side effects of sympathomimetics. These effects are relatively less when these drugs are given by inhalation. In patients of ischaemic heart disease and hyperthyroidism, these drugs should be employed with caution. The β_2 agonists (e.g. terbutaline) are also used to control premature labour by intravenous infusion. However, they may produce tachycardia, pulmonary oedema in mother and hypoglycaemia in the newborn.

Anticholinergic

Ipratropium of this group is used for treatment of asthma. Its important features are:

- Relaxes the bronchial constriction caused by increased parasympathetic tone.
- Not effective against allergen challenge.
- Inhibits the augmentation of mucous secretion associated with asthma.
- Increases mucociliary clearance of bronchial secretion.
- Has few side effects and is safe and well tolerated.

Corticosteroids

Corticosteroids are indicated when other drugs fail to relieve the symptoms of asthma. They improve pulmonary airway function due to their anti-inflammatory property. They do not cause bronchodilatation. Their onset of action is slow. So on chronic administration, the corticosteroids improve pulmonary function and reduce frequency and severity of acute asthma attacks. For this purpose prednisone, prednisolone, beclomethasone, and hydrocortisone are commonly used. Their doses are selected on the basis of severity of asthma. Hydrocortisone is used in a dose of 4 mg/kg every 4 to 6 hours in severe acute attack whereas prednisone or prednisolone are started with 30–60 mg/day orally. Beclomethasone diproponate (bedate inhaler) is available as aerosol inhalation (100 µg). By this route, the systemic effects of corticosteroid are minimized. Adrenal atrophy, peptic ulcer, diabetes and Cushing's syndrome may occur as side effects. They are contraindicated in systemic fungal infection.

Sodium cromoglycate: Its important features are:
- It is not a bronchodilator.
- It prevents the release of chemical mediators, responsible for the asthma attack by stabilizing cell membranes.
- This drug is beneficial, if asthma occurs due to allergy.
- It is only effective when given by inhalation (20 mg 4 times a day).
- Throat irritation and transient broncho-spasm are the commonest side effects.
- It has only prophylactic value in the management of asthma.

Budesonide: It is a non-halogenated gluco-corticoid. It has better activity in asthmatic patients than beclomethasone. Dose: 200–800 µg/day.

Mucolytic agents have limited role in asthma. They liquefy the sputum and facilitate expectoration. However, in sensitive individuals, these agents may cause bronchospasm. Inhalation of steam is more effective for liquefying the sputum.

Nedocromil is similar to sodium cromo-glycate. It has a greater inhibitory action on lung mast cells.

Ketotifen: Its important features are:
- It has antihistaminic (H_1) as well as sertonergic antagonist effect.
- It is neither a bronchodilator nor an anti-inflammatory agent.
- It inhibits stimulation of immunogenic and inflammatory cells.
- It is an orally effective prophylactic drug for bronchial asthma and allergic disorders. So it resembles in its action to sodium chromoglycate.
- It induces some sedation.
- Its dose is 1–2 mg twice a day.

Leukotriene modulators: Leukotrienes are powerful mediators of inflammation. They cause leukocyte recruitment, broncho-constriction, and mucous secretion, decreased mucociliary clearance and increased capillary permeability leading to pulmonary oedema. Cysteinyl leukotrienes (LTC_4, LTD_4 and LTE_4) activate leukotriene receptor (LT-recep-tor) to cause bronchoconstriction. Hence following leukotriene modulators have been developed.

Zileuton acts by inhibiting the synthesis of leukotrienes by blocking the 5-lipoxygenase enzyme of metabolic pathway of arachidonic acid. Since it causes hepatotoxicity, it is rarely used.

Zafirlukast, montelukast, iralukast and pranlukast act by blocking the action of leukotrienes and LT-receptors. These are used as adjunct with inhaled corticosteroids in poorly responding patients. They reduce the doses of β adrenergic agonists as well as inhaled corticoids for maintenance.

Commonly used leukotriene modulator is montelukast which is given once daily, usually in the evening. It is quite safe. Iralukast is similar to montelukast. Pranlukast is a newer addition and considered to be safest.

Monoclonal anti-IgE antibody: Omalizumab is a recombinant humanized monoclonal antibody. It acts by:

• Inhibiting the binding of IgE to mast cells and basophils
• Inhibiting the activation of IgE already bound to mast cells and thus prevents their degranulation
• Downregulating FCεR-1 (Fc epsilon R-1) receptors present on mast cells and basophils.

In short, omalizumab neutralizes the free IgE in circulation by forming a high affinity IgE-omalizumab complex. It is given in doses that inhibit 90% of circulating free IgE. It is indicated for asthmatic patients who are not adequately controlled by inhaled corticoids and who demonstrate sensitivity to aero-allergens. It is not suitable for acute attacks including status asthmaticus.

Status Asthmaticus

In this condition, the patient has continued attack of asthma and has marked dyspnoea, cynosis and dehydration. It is a serious medical emergency. It requires the administration of corticosteroids. Generally hydrocortisone is used (100–200 mg) parenterally and the dose may be repeated every 2–4 hours.

Oxygen therapy, rehydration, and the use of antibiotics to overcome associated infection are other measures which must be initiated.

Points for Dental Students

Dental treatment for asthmatic patients requires special attention to the oral manifestations of this condition, as well as its potential underlying systemic complications. So a dentist must address the following recommendations during dental care to asthmatic patients:

1. If patient is using theophylline avoid using erythromycin, clarithromycin, and quino-lone antibiotics because they decrease the metabolism of theophylline.
2. Avoid using non-selective non-steroidal analgesics for control of pain. Etodolac, selective COX-2 inhibitor may be used as analgesic drug.
3. Tetracyclines have accentuated side effects if used with theophylline.
4. Stress usually precipitates an acute attack of asthma. So during dental procedure factor of stress may precipitate acute attack of asthma. Hence patient must be asked to bring salbutamol/beclomethasone dipropoate inhaler inorder to meet with the emergency situation.
5. If required, use stress reducing techniques such as nitrous oxide can be used for this purpose. However, it should be avoided in severe asthmatic patients because it may irritate the airways.
6. Schedule dental care in asthmatic patients during late morning or later in the day inorder to minimize the risk of an attack of asthma.
7. Institute fluoride supplements for all asthmatic patients, particularly those taking β agonists.
8. Reinforce oral hygiene to reduce the incidence of gingivitis and periodontitis.
9. Instruct the patient to rinse the mouth after using inhaler.
10. Avoid dental material that may precipitate an attack, e.g. dental material with methyl methacrylate.
11. Cure acrylic appliances prior to insertion.
12. Usually local anaesthetics containing epinephrine are not contraindicated. However, sodium metabisulfite preservative may exacerbate asthma in susceptible patients. Further, interactions between epinephrine and β_2 agonists may result in synergistic effect, producing increased blood pressure and arrhythmias.

13. Administer antifungal drugs if needed; this is particularly required in patients who are taking inhaled corticoids.
14. Use steroid prophylaxis in patients who are taking long-term systemic corticoids.
15. Carefully position suction tips to avoid cough reflex.
16. During acute attack of asthma, discontinue the dental procedure. Remove all intraoral devices; place the patient in a comfortable position; make sure the airway is opened and administer β_2 agonist and oxygen. If no improvement, administer epinepherine s.c. (1:1000 concentration—0.01 mg/kg up to a maximum of 0.3 mg) and alert emergency medical assistance.

TO REMEMBER

1. Asthma is a chronic inflammatory condition, which is due to hyper-reactivity. It may be extrinsic or intrinsic asthma. Later is more prone to status asthmaticus.
2. Theophylline and aminophylline are the bronchodilators of choice to treat severe attacks of asthma.

3. Among sympathomimetic broncho-dilators, selective β_2 adrenoceptors (salbutamol, terbutaline) are preferred over non-selective sympathomimetics (adrenaline, ephedrine, isoprenaline) because of less incidence of side effects.
4. Corticoids are indicated when other drugs fail to relieve the symptoms of asthma. Becolomethasone dipropionate is available as aerosol inhalation. By this route, the systemic effects of corticosteroids are minimized.
5. By stabilizing cell membranes, sodium cromoglycate prevents release of chemical mediators responsible for asthma. It is given by inhalation only and is effective in asthma which occurs due to allergy.
6. Status asthmaticus is a serious medical emergency in which hydrocortisone is used parenterally in doses of 100–200 mg and the dose may be repeated every 2–4 hours. Other measures are oxygen therapy, rehydration and the use of antibiotics.

Chapter 36

Antitussive Agents, Expectorants, Mucolytic Agents and Nasal Decongestants

Cough is a protective reflex. It helps in the expulsion of respiratory secretion or foreign particles from air passages. Stimulation of mechano- or chemoreceptors in throat, respiratory passages or stretch receptors in the lungs leads to cough.

Antitussives

Cough suppressant agents are called antitussives. These drugs act:

- By raising the threshold of cough centre in the central nervous system
- By reducing tussal impulses in the respiratory tract peripherally
- By both peripheral and central action

They are employed to depress the cough reflex in acute bronchitis, pneumonia, chronic bronchitis and bronchiectasis. They induce symptomatic relief of cough. They do not cure the underlying pathology. In fact they are not needed if antibacterial therapy is started promptly. Clinically used antitussive agents are:

- **Opioids:** Codeine(10–30 mg) and pholcodeine(10 mg)
- **Non-opioids:** Dextromethorphan (10–20 mg), noscapine (15–30 mg), carbetapentane (30 mg), chlophedianol (20–40 mg) and pipazethate (40–80 mg)

Codeine is the most widely used narcotic antitussive. Dextromethorphen, pholcodeine, noscapine and methadone are other narcotic antitussive agents. They are used as linctus 3 to 4 times daily. They are useful in dry cough. Dextromethorphan is not an analgesic and causes less drowsiness and constipation than codeine.

Expectorants (Mucokinetics)

These are used to expel the mucous from the air passage by increasing bronchial secretion or reducing its viscosity. Ammonium chloride (0.3 to 1 g), ipecauanha (25–100 mg), potassium iodide (0.3 g) and squill (0.3 to 2 ml), tolu balsum (0.3–0.6 g), vasaka syrup (2–4 ml), terpin hydrate (0.1–0.3 ml), guaiacol (100–200 mg) sodium and potassium citrate or acetate (0.3–1 g) are commonly used expectorants. Although expectorants do not have any useful role, several combinations of expectorants, cough suppressants and sedatives are marketed. Expectorants are useful in children and in bronchial asthma.

Mucolytic Agents

To liquefy sputum and facilitate expectoration mucolytic agents are employed. Bromhexine, acetylcysteine, methylcysteine, and carbocysteine are commonly used mucolytics. However, simple inhalation of steam can be more effective to liquefy the sputum. Acetylcysteine (10–20%) is used as an inhalation. It may cause nausea, fever, stomatitis and bronchospasm in certain individuals. Although bromhexine can be given orally, intravenously or by inhalation, it is usually administered orally in a dose of 8–16 mg 3 times daily.

Nasal Decongestants

Allergic rhinitis, hay fever and sinusitis cause mucosal congestion, which can be relieved by nasal decongestants. Sympathomimetics are generally used for this purpose. They give relief to the nasal obstruction by producing vasoconstriction of mucosal blood vessels and decreasing the thickness of the swollen nasal mucosa. However, there occurs rebound 'after congestion' with most of the sympathomimetic agents. So they cause chronic rhinitis on prolonged use. Some of them may show systemic effects and local irritation. They are contraindicated in young children.

Naphazoline, oxymetazoline, phenylephrine and xylometazoline are commonly used nasal decongestants. They are more potent, have long duration of action and likely to cause less rebound nasal congestion than ephedrine, which is also used as nasal decongestant. Xylometazoline and oxymetazoline are less liable to induce tolerance. These agents are used in 0.5% (ephedrine), 0.1% (xylometazoline) solution as nasal drops. Ephedrine and pseudoephedrine are also given orally as nasal decongestants.

They are often combined with antihistaminics, antipyretics, analgesics, and antitussives for the relief of cold and other upper respiratory conditions. However, these preparations are of doubtful value.

TO REMEMBER

1. Antitussives (cough suppressants) induce symptomatic relief of cough by depressing the cough reflex in acute bronchitis, pneumonia, chronic bronchitis, and bronchiectasis.
2. Codeine (most widely used), dextromethorphen, pholcodeine, noscapine and methadone are narcotic antitussives while benzonatate is non-narcotic antitussive.
3. Ammonium chloride, ipecauanha, potassium iodide and squill are expectorants which are used to expel the mucous from the air passage.
4. Bromhexine, acetylcysteine, methylcysteine and carbocysteine are commonly used mucolytics which liquefy sputum and facilitate expectoration.
5. As nasal drops, nasal decongestants (naphazoline, oxymetazoline, phenylephrine and xylometazoline) relieve the nasal obstruction by producing vasoconstriction of mucosal blood vessels and decreasing the thickness of swollen nasal mucosa. Ephedrine and pseudoephedrine are also given orally as nasal decongestants. Disadvantage with these preparations is rebound after congestion.

Section 10

Antacids and Related Drugs

Histamine, 5-Hydroxytryptamine and their Antagonists

Eicosanoids

Chapter 37

Histamine, 5-Hydroxytryptamine and their Antagonists

Local hormones are substances which occur naturally in body and possess potent biological actions. They are also called tissue factors or autacoids (auto meaning self) because of their self-regulation. They are different from hormones because they are produced in the tissue and not by the endocrine glands. Autacoids are involved in a number of physiological and pathological processes, and even serve as transmitters or modulators in the nervous system. Important autacoids are histamine, 5-hydroxytryptamine (serotonin), prostaglandins, angiotensin, bradykinin, kallidin, leukotrienes, and platelet activating factor.

Histamine

Histamine is widely distributed in almost all body tissues. Tissues rich in histamine are skin, gastric and intestinal mucosa, lungs, liver and placenta. In the presence of histidine decarboxylase enzyme, histamine is synthesized from the amino acid histidine. Histamine is stored in the granules of mast cells, basophils, mucosal layer of the gastrointestinal tract and in the central nervous system. In the mast cells and basophils, it is present in a complex along with heparin and an acid protein. Non-mast cell histamine occurs in 'histaminocytes' in the stomach and in histaminergic neurons in the brain. Turnover of mast cell histamine is slow while that of non-mast cell histamine is fast. It

is released from the mast cells both by exocytotic and non-exocytotic process. Histamine release from the mast cells occurs by specific antigen in the presence of hypersensitivity reaction. Histamine is metabolized by histaminase and/or by the methylating enzyme imidazole N-methyl transferase. So far H_1, H_2 and H_3 histamine receptors have been described. H_1 receptors are present in the bronchi and intestinal smooth muscles; H_2 receptors are present in cardiac tissue and control gastric acid secretory actions of histamine; H_3 receptors occur at presynaptic sites and serve as an autoreceptor controlling histamine release from neurons in brain.

H_1-receptors are linked to transduction system which increases intracellular Ca^{++}. These receptors are blocked by mepyramine. H_2-receptors are linked to transduction systems which involve the activation of adenylate cyclase and increased cAMP. These receptors are blocked by H_2 antagonists e.g. cimetidine. H_3-receptors are blocked by thioperamide.

Intradermal injection of histamine produces typical triple response consisting of:
- *Redspot:* due to intense capillary dilatation.
- *Wheal:* due to exudation of fluid from capillaries and venules.
- *Flare:* i.e. redness in the surrounding area due to arteriolar dilatation mediated by axon reflex.

Histamine receptor		Tissue site
• H_1	–	Bronchi
	–	Interstitial smooth muscles
• H_2	–	Cardiac tissue
	–	Oxyntic cells
• H_3	–	Neurons in brain

Other prominent effects of histamine are:

1. Histamine causes fall in blood pressure due to dilatation of arterioles, capillaries and venules. Individuals experience throbbing headache due to dilatation of brain arterioles.

2. Histamine causes the contraction of bronchial and intestinal smooth muscles. Asthmatics are more sensitive to the action of histamine.

3. Histamine induces gastric acid and pepsin release.

4. Histamine acts as one of the mediators in hypersensitivity reactions.

5. Histamine is the afferent transmitter which is responsible for the sensation of itch and pain at sensory nerve endings. It appears to act as transmitter in brain, specially in hypothalamus and midbrain.

6. Histamine may act as a mediator of vasodilatation and other changes that occur during inflammation. It has been suggested to play an essential role in the process of growth and repair.

Histamine has no therapeutic use. Histamine (0.01 mg/kg) or its analogue betazole (0.5 mg/kg) is used for diagnosis of hypochlorhydria and achlorhydria.

Antihistaminics

There are two types of histamine antagonists namely H_1 receptor antagonists (classical type) and H_2 receptor antagonists (used in peptic ulcer). Only H_1 receptor antagonists are described below and H_2 receptor antagonists will be discussed along with other drugs used for the treatment of peptic ulcer.

H_1 histamine antagonists act by competitively blocking the histamine receptors. They do not control the release of histamine. They block the triple response and antagonise the smooth muscle effects of histamine. They do not block the gastric secretory and cardiac stimulant actions of histamine.

Some of the actions of these drugs may not be related to blockade of H_1-receptors. They may be as a result of their effects at other receptors such as 5-HT receptors, α_1-adrenoceptors, and acetylcholine muscarinic receptors, both peripherally and in the central nervous system. So the other actions of H_1-receptor antagonists are:

• The older antihistamines produce variable degree of sedation. This depends on their ability to cross blood-brain barrier and their affinity for the central H_1-receptors.

• Certain H_1-antihistamines (e.g. promethazine, diphenhydramine, dimenhydrinate, cyclizine, and meclizine) possess antimotion sickness properties.

• Promethazine also controls vomiting of pregnancy and other causes.

• Promethazine and few other antihistaminics reduce tremors, rigidity, and sialorrhoea of Parkinsonism due to their anticholinergic and sedative properties.

• Some of the antihistamines such as chlorpheniramine, diphenhydramine, and promethazine are also effective anitussives.

• Many H_1-blockers antagonize muscarinic actions of acetylcholine. So they enhance the anticholinergic actions of atropine or its congeners, phenothiazines, tricyclic antidepressants and disopyramide.

• Some H_1-blockers such as mepyramine and antazoline have strong membrane stabilizing property while others have weak action. Due to this, antazoline may be used as antiarrhythmic agent. However, they are not used as local anaesthetics because they cause irritation when injected s.c.

- On i.v. injection, most of the antihistamines cause a fall in blood pressure.
- Many H_1-blockers inhibit neuronal uptake of noradrenaline.

The newer long acting and least sedative H_1-blockers are astemazole, ceterizine, loratadine, desloratadine, terfenadine, fexofenadine, azelastine, mizolastine, ebastine. At present, the use of astemazole and terfenadine has been stopped because they induce potentially fatal arrhythmia and torsades de pointes. Currently loratadine, desloratadine and fexofenadine of this class are used because they are devoid of the above mentioned side effects. New azelastine has good topical activity. So it is used for seasonal and perennial allergic rhinitis by nasal spray to provide quick symptomatic relief which lasts for 12 hours.

On oral administration, antihistaminics are rapidly absorbed and the peak effect is observed in one hour. The duration of action is for 4 hours in case of old antihistaminics. They are metabolized in liver and excreted in the urine. The important side effects are drowsiness, dry mouth, and blurring of vision. They also potentiate the action of other central nervous system depressants.

Preparations, Doses and Route of Administration

A. Highly sedative

Diphenhydramine	25–50 mg oral
Dimenhydrinate	25–50 mg oral, i.m.
Promethazine	25–50 mg oral, i.m. (1 mg/kg).
Doxylamine	15–25 mg oral
Hydroxyzine	25–50 mg oral

B. Moderately sedative

Antazoline	50–100 mg oral, i.m.
Buclizine	25–50 mg oral
Cyproheptadine	4 mg oral
Carbinoxamine (clistin)	4–8 mg oral
Clemastine	2–6 mg oral
Meclizine	25–50 mg oral
Pheniramine	20–50 mg oral
Pyrilamine	25–50 mg oral
Tripelenamine	25–50 mg oral

C. Mild sedative

Chlorpheniramine	4–8 mg oral
Cyclizine	50 mg oral
Mepyramine	25–50 mg oral, i.m.
Dexchlorpheniramine	4–6 mg oral
Tripolidine	2.5–5 mg

D. Long acting and least sedative

Astemazole	10 mg oral
Cetirizine	10 mg oral
Levocetirizine	5 mg oral
Loratadine	10 mg oral
Desloratadine	5 mg oral
Terfenadine	60 mg oral
Azelastine	4 mg oral
Mizolastine	10 mg oral
Ebastine	10 mg oral
Fexofenadine	60 mg oral

E. Antivertigo drug

Cinnarizine	25–50 mg oral

Uses

- They are extensively used to prevent allergic reactions or to treat their symptoms such as allergic rhinitis, hay fever and urticaria.
- Promethazine is used as antiemetic agent.
- Diphenhydramine, dimenhydrinate, buclizine, cyclizine and meclizine are used for the prevention and treatment of motion sickness. However, their use in nausea and vomiting (morning sickness) of pregnancy is controversial.
- Antihistamines with central nervous system depressant action such as pyrilamine and diphenhydramine have been used as sedative and to induce sleep, specially in children.

- They are also employed in the management of cardiac arrhythmia, parkinsonism, idiopathic pruritus, cough, vertigo and acute muscle dystonia caused by antiemetic antipsychotic drugs.
- Antihistamine with antimuscarinic effects, e.g. dimenhydrinate (50–100 mg oral), meclizine (25–50 mg oral) or promethazine (25 mg oral) are used for short control of salivation (as in occlusal adjustment or impression making in dentistry) 30 min before these procedures. These are used when patient is taking calcium carbonate containing antacid which decreases the absorption of scopolamine, glycopyrrolate and propantheline used to control excessive salivation in dentistry in routine.

Serotonin and its Antagonists

Serotonin is also known as 5-hydroxytryptamine (5-HT). About 90% of body's 5-HT content is found in the enterochromaffin cells of the intestinal wall and rest in the blood platelets and in the central nervous system. It is formed from the amino acid tryptophan. It is metabolized by monoamine-oxidase enzyme to 5- hydroxyindole acetic acid (5-HIAA). Physiologically, it is believed to act as a putative neurotransmitter in central nervous system and plays an important role in the peristalsis of gastrointestinal tract. Although the serotonin receptors (5-HT$_1$, 5-HT$_2$, 5-HT$_3$ and 5-HT$_4$ subtypes of 5-HT receptors) have been extensively studied in the recent years for the development of receptor specific 5-HT antagonists and agonists for clinical use, serotonin as such has no clinical use as a drug.

Cyproheptadine (periactin): It is a serotonin antagonist which has additional H$_1$ antihistaminic, mild anticholinergic and sedative properties. It has been used in allergy and as antipruritic due to its antihistaminic property. Its anti-5-HT activity is utilized in controlling intestinal manifestations of carcinoid and postgastrectomy dumping syndrome. Besides, it is also useful as prophylactic in migraine headache. Its dose is 4 mg 3–4 times a day. Side effects are drowsiness, dry mouth, confusion, ataxia and weight gain.

Methysergide: It is a potent serotonin (5-HT$_2$) antagonist which is chemically related to ergot alkaloids. It blocks the vasoconstrictor, pressor and smooth muscle effects of serotonin. It is useful for migrain prophylaxis, carcinoid and postgastrectomy dumping syndrome. Its dose is 2 mg twice or thrice daily. Important side effects are drowsiness, weakness, heart burn, diarrhoea, nausea, vomiting, hallucination and euphoria.

Ketanserin: It has selective 5-HT$_{2A}$ receptor blocking property with negligible action on 5-HT$_1$ and 5-HT$_3$ receptors. It is devoid of partial agonistic activity. It has additional weak α_1, H$_1$ and dopaminergic blocking activities. It is useful in the treatment of migraine, carcinoid syndrome and peripheral vascular diseases. Dizziness, tiredness, nausea and dry mouth may occur as side effects.

Mianserin: It has similar actions and uses as that of ketanserin.

Ondansetron: It is a potent 5-HT$_3$ receptor antagonist. It is very effective antiemetic agent, particularly for patients receiving cancer chemotherapy. It is also effective in migrain when given during the headache phase. In case of chemotherapy-induced emesis, it is given i.v. (0.1–0.2 mg/kg) 30 minutes before chemotherapy. Oral dose is 4–8 mg. Other clinically used 5-HT$_3$ blockers are granisetron (0.1 mg/kg, i.v.) and dolasetron (0.6–3 mg/kg, i.v.). Minor side effects are diarrhea and headache.

Buspirone: It is 5-HT$_{1A}$ agonist. It has antianxiety effects. It is devoid of tolerance and dependence liability. It is useful for generalized anxiety, phobia and panic attacks. Its beneficial effects appear after days or weeks and that is the disadvantage over benzodiazepines. Dizziness, restlessness, nausea and headache are side effects. It is given in doses of 20–30 mg orally daily.

Ipsapiron: It has similar actions and uses as that of buspirone.

Sumatriptan: It is 5-HT$_1$ agonist which is effective in the treatment of migrain and anxiety. A single dose of 100–200 mg aborts the attack of migraine within 2 hours.

Fluprazine and **ethoprazine** are other 5-HT$_1$ agonists, which have been marked for antiaggressive activities. They do not significantly affect cognitive, motor and behavioural functions.

Cisapride and **renzapride** are selective 5-HT$_4$ agonists.

TO REMEMBER

1. Autacoids (auto means self) or tissue factors are local hormones which occur naturally in the body and possess potent biological actions.

2. Histamine is widely distributed in almost all body tissues. So far H$_1$ (smooth muscles of bronchi and intestine), H$_2$ (cardiac and gastrointestinal tract) and H$_3$ (neurons in brain) histamine receptors have been described.

3. Although histamine has no therapeutic use, it is used to diagnose hypochlorhydria and achlorhydria.

4. H$_1$ histamine antagonists act by competitively blocking the H$_1$ receptors and are extensively used to prevent allergic reactions or to treat their symptoms, viz. allergic rhinitis, hay fever and urticaria.

5. Promethazine, diphenhydramine, dimenhydrinate, buclizine, cyclizine, and meclizine are used for the prevention and treatment of motion sickness. Promethazine is also useful antiemetic agent.

6. Pyrilamine and diphenhydramine have been used as sedative and hypnotic, especially in children.

7. Long-acting non-sedative antihistaminics (loratadine and cetirizine can be used in allergic asthma and as an adjunct to the standard treatment of bronchial asthma.

8. Serotonin (5-hydroxytryptamine) is believed to act as a putative neurotransmitter in central nervous system and plays an important role in the peristalsis of gastrointestinal tract. However, serotonin as such has no clinical use as a drug.

9. Cyproheptadine is a serotonin antagonist with additional H$_1$ antihistaminic, mild anticholinergic and sedative properties. It is used in allergy, pruritus, carcinoid tumor, postgastrectomy dumping syndrome and migraine headache prophylaxis.

10. Methysergide is useful for migraine prophylaxis, carcinoid tumor and postgastrectomy dumping syndrome.

11. Ketanserin and mianserin are useful in the treatment of migraine, carcinoid syndrome and peripheral vascular diseases.

12. Ondansetron is very effective antiemetic agent.

13. Buspirone and ipsapiron are useful for generalized anxiety, phobia and panic attacks.

14. Sumatriptan is effective in migrain and anxiety.

Chapter 38

Eicosanoids

Prostaglandins, thromboxanes, prostacycline, hydroperoxyeicosatertraenoic acids (HPETEs), hydroxyeicosatekraenoic acids (HETEs) and the leukotrienes are derived from arachidonic acid which is an important constituent of phospholipids of the cell membranes of all tissues. They are now called eicosanoids because they are derived from the same eicosanoic (Eicosa-20 carbon; enoic-containing double bonds) acid precursors.

Prostaglandins

Prostaglandins are unsaturated fatty acids. Since they were originally obtained from prostate gland and were present in semen they were termed as prostaglandins. They have cyclopentane ring and two aliphatic side chains in a 20-carbon skeleton. Two cyclo-oxygenase enzymes (COX-1 and COX-2) convert arachidonic acid into different prostaglandins. Both enzymes promote oxygenation and cyclization of arachidonic acid and lead to formation of PGG_2. The later is then rapidly converted to PGH_2 by peroxidation, mediated by PGH synthase enzyme. Both endoperoxides (PGG_2 and PGH_2) are highly unstable. These are quickly converted to:

- Prostaglandins (PGE_2, $PGF_2\alpha$ and PGD_2) by PGE synthetase (isomerases) enzyme
- Prostaglandin (PGI_2) by PGI synthase enzyme

- Thromboxane A_2 (TXA_2) by thromboxane synthase enzyme.

Thus this pathway leads to:

- TXA_2 in platelets
- PGI_2 in vascular endothelium
- PGD_2 in mast cells
- PGE_2 in vasculature, gastrointestinal tract, lungs and other tissues
- $PGF_2\alpha$ in smooth muscles of gastrointestinal tract, bronchi, uterus and blood vessels

Prostaglandins are widely distributed in body tissues. All prostanoid receptors are G-protein coupled receptors. They utilize IP_3/DAG or cAMP transducer mechanisms. They are released in response to inflammation, pain, trauma, bacterial attack and allergic reaction. So large number of physiological roles has been assigned to them. However, the most important effect is on the reproductive system, platelets and gut. Some of the prostaglandins (PGD_2) modulate the release of hypothalamic and pituitary hormones. Since naturally occurring prostaglandins are quickly metabolized, prostaglandin analogues have been synthesized. They are more stable and are orally effective.

Therapeutic uses of prostanoids and their analogues

1. PGE_2, PGF_2 and their analogues are used to terminate pregnancy and to induce cervical ripening in pregnancy during first

and second trimester abortion. Commonly used analogues are:

- Dinoprostone (derivative of PGE_2)
- Misoprostol (PGE_1 derivative); used with mefepristone (an antiprogestin) or with methotrexate to induce abortion in first weeks of pregnancy

2. Oral PGE_2 is superior to oral oxytocin analogues and is equally effective as i.v. oxytocin in augmenting labour and to check postpartum haemorrhage. Carboprost is used to control postpartum haemorrhage when oxytocin or methyl ergonovine is not effective.

3. Misoprostol (a stable PGE_2 analogue) is used to treat peptic ulcer. This and enprostil (PGE_2 analogue are used for healing of NSAIDs induced ulcers.

4. Epoprostenol (PGI_2 derivative) is used to prevent platelet aggregation in extracorporeal circulation such as renal dialysis and cardiopulmonary bypass.

5. PGI_2 and PGE_1 can be used in smaller amounts for storage of platelets for transfusion.

6. Epoprostenol (PGI_2) and treprostinil (PGI_2 derivative) have been used to treat pulmonary hypertension by i.v. infusion due to their ability to lower peripheral, pulmonary and coronary resistance.

7. Alprostadil (PGE_1) or epoprostenol (PGI_2 prepration) is given by i.v. infusion to maintaine the patency of foetal ductus arteriosus.

8. PGE_1 or PGI_2 i.v. infusion and beraprost (stable oral PGI_2 derivative) are used to promote ulcer healing in intermittent claudication.

9. Ocular drops of latanoprost (a stable and long acting $PGF_2\alpha$ derivative) are as effective as timolol in reducing intraocular pressure in glaucoma. Newer additions in this series include bimatoprost, travaprost, and unoprostone. Side effects are blurring of vision, iris pigmentation and dryness of eyes.

10. Miscellaneous uses are male impotence (alprostadil-PGE_1), to reduce infarct size (iloprost) and bronchial asthma (areoosolised PGE_2).

Adverse effects: Abortifacient PGs may cause chills, fever, nausea, vomiting, diarrhoea, bronchoconstriction, syncope, dizziness and flushing. Intra-amniotic injection of carboprost ($PGF_2\alpha$ derivative) may cause anaphylactic shock and cardiovascular collapse. Misoprostol and enprostil usually cause gastrointestinal discomfort and diarrhoea.

HPETE, HETE and Leukotrienes

Leukotrienes are the products of lipo-oxygenase pathway. Lipo-oxygenases are soluble enzymes that are located in cytosol of lungs, platelets, mast cells and white blood cells. 5-lipo-oxygenase is the main enzyme which is responsible for the synthesis of leukotrienes. As a first step, this enzyme adds a hydroperoxy group at C-5 in arachidonic acid to give 5-hydroperoxy eicosatetraenoic acid (HPETE) and hydroxy eicosatetraenoic acid (HETE). They are chemotactic factors. They attract granulosites to the site of inflammation. They are potent inhibitors of prostacycline formations in the vascular tissues. Leukotrienes (LTs) are formed from 5-HPETE which is converted to LTA_4 leading to the formation of either LTB_4 or a series of peptidoleukotrienes (LTC_4, LTD_4 and LTE_4). LTB_4 are cysteinyl leukotrienes which are produced by macrophages. LTC_4 and LTD_4 are potent bronchoconstrictors. These are primary component of the slow releasing substance of anaphylaxis (SRS-A), that is secreted in asthma and anaphylaxis. So these are important mediators of bronchial asthma. They are released in the lung during anaphylaxis (called

SRS-A) and produce a slow long lasting contraction of smooth muscle of bronchus, gut, and uterus, increase vascular permeability and cause coronary vasoconstriction but dilatation of most vessels and increase capillary permeability. Leukotrienes act on specific receptors for which selective antagonists have now been synthesized. Aspirin and other NSAIDs inhibit cyclooxygenase pathway. So they may enhance formation of LTs (SRS-A) and precipitate bronchial asthma or anaphylaxis in sensitive individuals.

Platelet Activating Factor (PAF)

Platelet activating factor (PAF) is an important mediator in acute and chronic inflammation, arterial thrombosis and endotoxic shock. It also plays an important role in inducing bronchial hyper-responsiveness and in the delayed phase of bronchial asthma. It is released from many inflammatory cells (neutrophils, basophils, macrophages, platelets and eosinophils) when they are stimulated. Phospholipase-A_2 produces lysoglyceryl-phosphoryl choline from cell membrane phospholipids. It is the precursor of platelet activating factor. Its release is inhibited by glucocorticoids by suppressing phospholipase A_2. PAF is also produced by foetus at final term and may be involved in progression of labour. PAF is most potent peptic ulcerogen.

Isoprostanes are produced by peroxidation of arachidonic acid by free radicals. These are stored as part of membrane constituents. It is believed that they play some role in the hepatorenal syndrome where renal dysfunction occurs without renal pathology. This syndrome is produced by a combination of decreased renal perfusion and hyperaldosteronism that is secondary to liver disease.

Cytokines: They are peptides. They are released from various types of cells and are important regulators of inflammation and immune reactions.

TO REMEMBER

1. Eicosanoids are derived from the same eicosanoic acid precursors.
2. Among the prostaglandins, only PGE and PGF series are of biological interest.
3. Prostaglandins and their analogues have been used in the treatment of peptic ulcer (PGE_1, PGE_2 and their synthetic analogues); for induction of labour and therapeutic abortion ($PGF_2\alpha$, and their analogues); postpartum haemorrhage; to prevent platelet aggregation and perivascular diseases (PGI_2 or PGE_2); and to maintain patency of the foetal ductus arteriosus (PGI_2).
4. HPETE and HETE are chemotactic factors which attract granulosites to the site of inflammation.
5. Leukotrienes (LTs) are formed from 5-HPETE and are important mediators of bronchial asthma. Aspirin and other NSAIDs inhibit cyclooxygenase pathway and may enhance formation of LTs (SRS-A) which precipitate bronchial asthma or anaphylaxis in sensitive individuals.
6. Platelet activating factor (PAF) is an important mediator in both acute and chronic inflammation, arterial thrombosis and endotoxic shock.
7. Cytokines are important regulators of inflammation and immune reactions.

Section 11

Hormones and Related Drugs

Chapter 39

Hormones of Hypothalamus, Anterior and Posterior Pituitary

There are both neural and vascular communications between hypothalamus and anterior pituitary. Several peptide hormones are secreted by hypothalamus. These hormones pass through the hypophyseal portal vessels to the anterior pituitary and influence its secretions. The hypothalamic hormones with their actions are given in Table 39.1.

In addition, the release of melanocyte stimulating hormone (MSH) is also under the control of hypothalamic stimulating or inhibiting factors. Although hypothalamic hormones are not used clinically, they play an important role of mediators of physiological feedback system of anterior pituitary hormones.

ANTERIOR PITUITARY (ADENOHYPOPHYSIS)

Hormones of the anterior pituitary can be divided into two groups:

I. Those hormones which regulate the functions of other endocrines:

- Adrenocorticotropic hormone: It controls the function of adrenal cortex.
- Thyroid stimulating hormone: It controls the secretion of thyroid gland.
- Follicular stimulating hormone and luteinizing hormones: They control the functions of ovary.

II. Those hormones which act directly on target organs:

- Growth hormone: It regulates the growth of the body as well as cellular metabolism in a variety of tissues.
- Prolactin: It helps in the preparation of mammary gland for lactation and maintenance of lactation once the secretory process has been initiated. Although prolactin is also found in man but its physiological role in man is not clear. However, several drugs like antipsychotics, antianxiety drugs influence the secretion of prolactin.
- Melanocyte stimulating hormone (MSH): Three types of MSH, alpha, beta

Table 39.1: Hypothalamic hormones and their actions

Hypothalamic hormone/factor	Action on anterior pituitary
1. Corticotropin releasing factor (CRF)	Stimulates secretion of corticotropin (ACTH)
2. Thyrotropin releasing hormones (TRH)	Stimulates secretion of thyrotropin (TSH)
3. Growth hormone releasing factor (GHRF)	Stimulates secretion of growth hormone (GH)
4. Growth hormone release inhibiting factor (GHRIF) (somatostatin) (STN)	Inhibits secretion of growth hormone (GH) and thyrotropin
5. Gonadotropin releasing factor (GRF)	Stimulates secretion of gonadotropins (FSH and LH)
6. Prolactin releasing factor (PRF)	Stimulates secretion of prolactin
7. Prolactin release inhibiting factor (dopamine) (PRIF)	Inhibits release of prolactin.

and gamma are secreted by the anterior pituitary. Its function in man is not known.

Clinical Uses of Anterior Pituitary Hormones

- **Growth hormone:** Used to treat pituitary dwarfism
- **Prolactin:** No clinical indication
- **Gonadotropins:**
  – Amenorrhoea and infertility due to decreased production of gonadotropins by pituitary
  – Hypogonadotrophic hypogonadism in males
  – Cryptorchism
  – To aid in vitro fertilization
- **Thyrotropin:** Used to differentiate myxoedema due to pituitary dysfunction from primary thyroid disease
- **Adrenocorticotropic hormone:** Used for the diagnosis of disorders of pituitary adrenal axis (plasma cortisol increases if adrenals are functional)

POSTERIOR PITUITARY (NEUROHYPOPHYSIS)

The hormones of the posterior pituitary are antidiuretic hormone (ADH) and oxytocin. They are synthesized in hypothalamus and pass down the hypothalamohypophyseal tract to get stored in the posterior pituitary for eventual release.

Oxytocin

It is a polypeptide hormone. It is released from posterior pituitary. It stimulates the cells of the glandular system of the mammary gland and helps in milk ejection. It is released during lactation in response to suckling stimulus. However, the role of oxytocin in non-pregnant non-lactating women is not known. It also has pronounced effects on uterine contraction. So

it is used clinically to induce labour. The sensitivity of the uterus to oxytocin increases rapidly during the last trimester of the pregnancy. Oxytocin stimulates slow long-lasting rhythmic contractions of the upper segment of the uterus with the relaxation of the cervix. Oxytocin (pitocin) is available for intravenous or intramuscular administration (10 units per ml). It is also available for nasal and sublingual routes of administration. Oxytocin is the drug of choice for the induction of labour at term in majority of cases as well as for the treatment of uterine inertia. It is preferred over ergotamine due to following reasons:

- Because of its short biological half-life and slow i.v. infusion, intensity of action can be controlled and action can be quickly terminated.
- Fetal oxygenation is maintained due to normal relaxation in between contractions because of low concentration used.
- Fetal descent is not compromised because lower segment of uterus is not contracted.

Antidiuretic Hormone (Vasopressin)

It is an octapeptide. It produces its effect by acting on G-protein coupled cell membrane vasopressin receptors. Antidiuretic hormone (ADH) enhances the reabsorption of water by distal convoluted tubule and collecting tubule of the kidney by increasing the permeability of tubular epithelium to water. The water along with some sodium and urea moves from the lumen into the interstitial fluid. The secretion of ADH occurs in response to increase in plasma osmolarity (during dehydration) while it is decreased in response to a decrease in plasma osmolarity (during hydration). A number of drugs influence ADH secretion. The secretion of ADH is inhibited by alcohol, atropine, corticosteroids and phenytoin while it is stimulated by nicotine, chlorpropamide, and anaesthetics.

ADH (pitressin) is available for intra-muscular injection. It produces antidiuresis for a period of 48–72 hours. The usual dose is 1.25 to 5 units every 2 to 3 days.

Uses

* Its primary therapeutic use is in the management of diabetes insipidus, which is characterized by polyurea, polydipsia and dehydration due to reduced secretion of ADH. It is effective only in neurogenic diabetes insipidus. It is ineffective in renal(nephrogenic) diabetes insipidus
* Bed wetting in children
* Bleeding oesophageal varices
* Haemophilia von Willebrand's disease
* Before abdominal radiography to expel gasses from bowel

It is available as:

* Aqueous vasopressin
* Lypressin: a synthetic lysine-vasopressin (less potent)
* Desmopressin: synthetic analogue(12 times more potent)

Other drugs used for diabetes insipidus are:

i. **Thiazides:** They paradoxically exert an antidiuretic effect in both, pituitary origin as well as renal diabetes insipidus. Probable mechanism of action is:
   * More complete reabsorption of glomerular filtrate iso-osmotically in proximal tubule due to a state of sustained electrolyte depletion.
   * Presentation of smaller volume of less dilute urine to the collecting ducts due to reduced salt absorption in the cortical diluting segment.
   * Reduction of fluid load on the tubules by reducing glomerular filtration rate.
   Commonly used drug is hydrochloro-thiazide in doses of 25–50 mg three times a day along with potassium supplement.
ii. **Amiloride:** It is a drug of choice for lithium induced nephrogenic diabetes insipidus. It acts by blocking entry of

lithium through sodium channels in the collecting duct cells.
iii. **Chlorpropamide** reduces urine volume in diabetes insipidus of pituitary origin only because it sensitizes the kidney to antidiuretic hormone action; so its effect depends on small amounts of the circulating hormone.
iv. **Carbamazepine** is effective in diabetes insipidus of pituitary origin, probably by increasing efficiency of V_2-ADH receptor transduction in collecting duct cells.

TO REMEMBER

1. Although hypothalamic hormones are not used clinically, they play an important role of mediators of physiological feedback system of anterior pituitary hormones.
2. Adrenocorticotropic hormone, thyroid stimulating hormone, follicular stimulating hormone and luteinizing hormone are the hormones of anterior pituitary which regulate the functions of other endocrines.
3. Growth hormone, prolactin, melanocyte stimulating hormones are secreted by anterior pituitary and act directly on target organs.
4. Oxytocin is a polypeptide hormone which is released from posterior pituitary. It is the drug of choice for the induction of labour at term in majority of cases.
5. Antidiuretic hormone (ADH) of posterior pituitary is used to treat diabetes insipidus. Other drugs used for the treatment of diabetes insipidus are thiazides, amiloride, chlorpropamide, and carbamazepine.
6. Secretion of ADH is inhibited by alcohol, atropine, corticosteroids and phenytoin while it is stimulated by nicotine, chlorpropamide and anaesthetics.

Chapter 40

Thyroid Hormones and Antithyroid Drugs

THYROID HORMONES

Thyroid gland secretes L-thyroxine (T_4 or tetraiodo-L-thyronine) and liothyronine (T_3 or tri-iodo-L-thyronine). T_3 is the major physiologically active natural thyroid hormone. It is three to five times more potent than T_4.

The basic unit of thyroid is follicle. It is a sphere of the epithelial follicular cells that surround a semifluid material called colloid. The colloid consists of thyroglobulin which is a high molecular glycoprotein. Glycoprotein contains about 115 tyrosine residues. In the biosynthesis of T_3 and T_4, the iodination of these tyrosine residues play an important role. There are parafollicular cells or C (clear) cells that lie embedded between the follicles and produce calcitonin, a hormone that influences Ca^{++} homeostasis. Another important feature of thyroid gland is that it stores T_3 and T_4 in large amount sufficient for nearly 100 days supply. On the other hand, other hormones are synthesized on demand and supply.

Iodine is utilized for the synthesis of thyroid hormones. In the first step, iodide is concentrated in the thyroid epithelial cells. This step is called 'iodide trap'. Thyroid stimulating hormone (TSH) stimulates iodide trapping process. The trapped iodide is then oxidized to iodine and iodine is concentrated almost 100 times in the thyroid cells. Iodination of tyrosine residues in thyroglobulin takes place by thyroid peroxidase enzyme to form monoiodotyrosine (MIT) and di-iodotyrosine (DIT). This process is called 'iodide organification'. Tri-iodthyronine is formed by coupling of mono- and di-iodotyrosine and tetraiodothyronine (thyroxine) is formed by coupling of two molecules of di-iodotyrosine. The process of coupling takes place in the thyroglobulin and both T_3 and T_4 are stored in the colloid of thyroid follicles as part of thyroglobulin. Release of thyroid hormones from thyroglobulin occurs by exocytosis and proteolysis at colloid border of the thyroid follicle. Thyroxine, T_3, MIT, DIT are released from the hydrolyzed thyroglobulin. Since the ratio of T_4 and T_3 within thyroglobulin is approximately 5:1 most of the hormone, released, is thyroxine. There occurs deiodination of MIT and DIT. The iodine, thus released, again enters the same cycle. In plasma, T_4 and T_3 are mainly reversibly bound to thyroxin binding globulin (TBG). However, small fractions of these hormones are also bound to albumin. Half-life of thyroxin is 6–7 days in normal individuals. There occurs considerable increase in its half-life in patients with hypothyroidism and decrease in patients with hyperthyroidism.

Thyroid hormones play an important role in the body by affecting some of the fundamental processes such as:

*   Oxygen consumption
*   Heat production

282

- Metabolism of carbohydrates, proteins and fats. Thyroid hormones (T_3 and T_4) regulate metabolic levels in most of the tissues of the body to maintain metabolic homeostasis.

Excessive secretion of these hormones will lead to hyperthyroidism which is characterized by:
- Tachycardia
- Cardiac arrhythmias
- Angina pain
- Tremors
- Nervousness
- Insomnia
- Weight loss
- Diarrhoea

Similarly, a deficiency in thyroid hormones causes hypothyroidism which is manifested by:
- Bradycardia
- Decreased reflexes
- Weight gain
- Constipation
- Menstrual abnormalities

Therapeutic Uses

1. Severe hypothyroidism is called myxedema in adult patients and cretinism in children. Thyroid hormone replacement therapy is indicated in hypothyroidism and simple goiter. Thyroxine sodium therapy is the treatment of choice for maintenance therapy. Initially 50–100 µg is given orally daily in patients of myxedema. The dose may be increased at intervals of 2 to 4 weeks by 25 to 50 µg till symptoms subside. The maintenance dose is 100–200 µg daily. In infants below one year of age, L-thyroxine is given initially in the dose of 25 µg, with increments of 12.5 to 25 µg every 6 months and maintenance dose is 6–8 µg/kg/day. Children above one year of age require a higher initial dose (50 µg).

Liothyronine sodium is not advocated for prolonged routine use in hypothyroidism because of high potency and incidence of cardiac side effects.

2. Hypothyroid coma is an emergency. If available, i.v. L-thyroxine (500 µg) is given followed by a daily maintenance dose after one week. Alternatively, liothyronine is administered i.v. in doses of 100 µg followed by 25 µg 6 hourly. It has a quick action than thyroxine. Corticosteroids may be given prophylactically to prevent unmasking of concurrently existing adrenal insufficiency due to restoration of thyroid status.

3. Papillary carcinoma of thyroid is often responsive to TSH. Temporary regression may be induced by giving full doses of thyroxine which suppresses TSH production.

4. Sometimes thyroxine is used in the following conditions without any rational and its response is unpredictable:
   - Refractory anaemia
   - Menstrual disorders, infertility not corrected by usual treatment
   - Carcinoma/non-healing ulcers
   - Obstinate constipation

Cardiac palpitation, arrhythmias, anginal pain, cramps in skeletal muscles, headache, restlessness, flushing, weight loss and insomnia are adverse effects of thyroid hormone.

They are contraindicated in acute myocardial infarction and other cardiovascular disorders.

Antithyroid Drugs

There are several types of hyperthyroidism. Hyperthyroidism occurs due to over production of T_3 and T_4 by the thyroid gland itself. This responds to drug treatment or by radioactive iodine or by surgical ablation of the gland. Thyrotoxicosis results from ingestion of excessive quantities of thyroid hormones, e.g. while treating hypothyroidism. This can be treated either reducing the dose or withholding it for several days. The two main causes of hyperthyroidism are Graves' disease (diffuse toxic goiter) and toxic nodular goiter. Graves' disease is an organ specific autoimmune disease. It is caused by thyroid stimulating immunoglobulin which is directed at the thyrotrophin receptor. In this condition, there occurs protrusion of the eyeballs and increased sensitivity to catecholamines.

Toxic nodular goiter is due to a benign neoplasm or adenoma. It produces thyroid hormone independent of TSH. It mostly supervenes on old non-toxic goiter.

The drugs used in hyperthyroidism are:

1. **Thionamides (carbimazole, methimazole, and propylthiouracil):** These drugs bind to thyroid peroxidase and prevent oxidation of iodide and/or iodotyrosyl residues. So these drugs reduce the synthesis of thyroid hormones by inhibiting iodination of tyrosine and coupling of iodotyrosine to form T_3 and T_4 in thyroglobulin. In addition, propylthiouracil inhibits peripheral conversion of T_4 to T_3. These drugs also suppress the synthesis of autoantibodies implicated in the aetiology of Graves' disease. These drugs are well absorbed from the gastrointestinal tract and they take several weeks before their action is noticed because existing hormone stores have to be depleted. They are rapidly excreted in the urine. Skin rash, myalgia, arthralgia, jaundice, drug fever and agranulocytosis may occur as side effects. Prolonged use may lead to goiter formation. They are to be used cautiously in pregnancy because they cross the placental barrier and are concentrated by the fetal thyroid.

Preparation and doses:
- *Propylthiouracil:* 300–400 mg daily.
- *Methylthiouracil:* 50 mg 4 times daily.
- *Carbimazole (neomarcazole):* 10–15 mg daily.
- *Methimazole:* 15–16 mg daily.

2. **Iodides:** Although exact mechanism of action is not clear, it is suggested that they interfere with iodination of tyrosine. Large doses of iodides inhibit secretion of thyroid hormones, induce involution and decrease vascularity of the gland. They have a rapid onset of action and the basal metabolic rate is decreased very quickly. Unfortunately, iodide therapy does not completely control the manifestations of hyperthyroidism and after certain time (2–8 weeks) beneficial effects disappear. So they are not used alone. Iodine in the form of potassium iodide (500 mg per day) or Lugol's iodine (5% iodine and 10% potassium iodide) is used in the management of thyrotoxicosis and hyperthyroidism prior to thyroidectomy. It is also used as a part of treatment of severe thyrotoxic crisis (thyroid storm).

3. **Radioactive iodine (I^{131}):** It is effective and safe for the management of thyrotoxicosis. It has a half-life of 8 days and emits both beta and gamma rays. It is available as radioactive sodium iodide which is administered orally in the dose of 5–8 m Curie. The dose depends upon:
- The size of thyroid gland
- The iodine uptake of the gland
- The rate of release of radioactive iodine from the gland subsequent to its deposition in the colloid.

The gland will shrink in size and the patient will become euthyroid after 6–12 weeks of its administration. I^{131} exerts its therapeutic effect primarily through beta-particles emission which have a short range and act on thyroid tissue without injuring surrounding areas including parathyroid gland. The major disadvantage of radioiodine therapy is the possibility of increased incidence of hypothyroidism.

4. **Ionic inhibitors (thiocyanates, perchlorates, nitrates):** They act by inhibiting iodide uptake. These drugs are no more used due to toxicity.

5. **Iodinated contrast media:** The iodinated contrast media are:
   - Oral: (a) Ipodate and (b) Ipanoic acid
   - Intravenous: Diatrizoate

   They prevent the conversion of T_4 to T_3 in the liver, kidney, pituitary gland and brain by inhibiting 5'-deiodinase enzymes. Due to this, they lead to dramatic improvement in signs and symptoms of hyperthyroidism. These are less toxic because iodine is covalently bound and are given at a lower dose than used in radiography. These are used with antithyroid drugs as short-term treatment for rapid control of elevated plasma T_3 concentrations in patients with severe thyrotoxicosis and significant morbidity (e.g. myocardial infarction or stroke) only because of development of resistance with time.

6. **Propranolol:** Although not strictly an antithyroid agent, propranolol alleviates many symptoms and signs of hyperthyroidism of the thyrotoxicosis such as palpitation, tachycardia, tremor, sweating, anxiety and thyrotoxic periodic paralysis. So it is employed:
   - In thyroid crisis
   - As adjunct in thyrotoxicosis
   - Prior to thyroid surgery
   - Hyperthyroid state during thyroiditis.

7. **Gaunethidine:** It is an adrenergic neuron blocking agent. It is used as eyedrops to ameliorate the exophthalmos of hyperthyroidism. Exophthalmos is not relieved by antithyroid drugs. Guanethidine relaxes the sympathetically inervated smooth muscle that causes retraction of eyelid. Sometimes ophthalmic Graves' disease may require glucocorticoids and surgical decompression.

Thyroid Storm

It is an extreme manifestation of thyrotoxicosis. It is invariably fatal. It is usually seen in patients with Graves' disease or with toxic multinodular goiter. It is precipitated abruptly in patients whose pre-existing thyrotoxicosis has been treated either incompletely or not at all. It is related to cytokine release and also to acute immunological disturbances precipitated by trauma, surgery, diabetic ketoacidosis and toxemia of pregnancy. The clinical picture shows severe hyper-metabolism with fever, profuse sweating, tachycardia, arrhythmias, diarrhoea and marked delirium. If crisis is not treated properly, there may develop pulmonary oedema, congestive heart failure, stupor and coma followed by death. It is managed as under:

- Propylthiouracil is administered in doses of 250 mg four times a day to block hormone synthesis and conversion of T_4 to T_3 at periphery.
- Collosal iodine (saturated KI solution) is given in doses of >6 mg daily orally or sodium ipodate in doses of 1 gm orally daily to reduce release of thyroid hormone from the gland and block the conversion of peripheral T_4 to T_3.
- Propranolol is given in doses of 40 to 80 mg four times a day or 1–2 mg slowly i.v. to control increased sympathetic activity and associated cardiovascular system manifestations.
- Hydrocortisone is administered in doses of 50 mg i.v. four times a day to protect patient against shock and block peripheral conversion of T_4 to T_3.

- Diltiazem is given in doses of 90–120 mg three or four times a day to treat asthma or heart failure complications.
- Plasmapheresis is done to remove large amount of protein bound thyroid hormones, if above measures fail.

Points for Dental Students

The dental practitioner must be knowledgeable about thyroid pathophysiology and the treatment of thyroid conditions because of following reasons:

1. Many signs and symptoms of thyroid disease are observable during examination of orofacial complex such as enlargement of the tongue, lingual thyroid tissue, difficulty in swallowing and a hoarse voice in hypothyroid state. Iodides are used along with other drugs in the management of thyrotoxic crisis. Prolonged use of iodides may lead to enlargement of parotid and submandibular glands due to its high concentration in salivary glands.
2. Under or over activity of thyroid gland can cause life-threatening cardiac events. A patient of hyperthyroidism may have increased blood pressure and heart rate due to effects of thyroid hormone on sympathetic nervous system (up regulation of β_1 receptors of cardiac muscle due to higher levels of T_3 and T_4). In such cases, a longer duration of local pressure is required to stop bleeding during dental procedures. Similarly local pressure for an extended time will be needed to control the small vessel bleeding in patients with long standing hypothyroidism because in such patients the ability of small vessels to constrict is decreased due to pressure of excess subcutaneous mucopolysaccharides whose degradation is reduced.
3. Thyrotoxicosis and higher doses of thyroxin may lead to osteoporosis of the alveolar bone and high incidence of dental caries and periodontal diseases.
4. The requirement of insulin in diabetic patients is increased during thyroid hormone therapy.
5. Thyroid hormone increases the metabolism of vitamin K dependant clotting factors. So the doses of anticoagulants have to be reduced during concomitant therapy.
6. A patient of myxoedema is usually sensitive to certain drugs like opioids, barbiturates and general anaesthetics due to low BMR.
7. In presence of myxoedema, stressful conditions such as infection or dental surgical procedures may precipitate myxoedematous coma.
8. Certain drugs like lithium, thioamides, iodides and amiodarone, etc. can precipitate hypothyroidism.

TO REMEMBER

1. Thyroid hormones (thyroxine and liothyronine) play an important role in the body by affecting oxygen consumption, heat production and metabolism of carbohydrate, proteins and fats.
2. Thyroid hormones replacement therapy is indicated in severe hypothyroidism (myxedema/cretinism) and simple goitre.
3. Thyroid hormones are contraindicated in acute myocardial infarction and other cardiovascular disorders because they cause sensitization of cardiac beta-receptors.
4. Thionamides (carbimazole, methimazole, and propyl thiouracil) are used in hyperthyroidism. Their beneficial effect is seen after several weeks of treatment because existing hormone stores have to be depleted.
5. Unfortunately iodide therapy does not completely control the manifestations of

hyperthyroidism and after certain time beneficial effects disappear, so it is used only in the management of thyrotoxicosis and hyperthyroidism prior to thyroidectomy.

6. Radioactive iodine (I^{131}) is effective and safe for the management of thyrotoxicosis.

7. Iodinated contrast media such as ipodate (oral), ipanoic acid (oral) and diatriozate (i.v.) prevent conversion of T_4 to T_3 in liver, kidney, pituitary and brain by inhibiting 5'-deiodinase enzyme.

8. Propranolol, although not strictly an antithyroid drug, induces symptomatic relief in patients of thyrotoxicosis.

9. Guanethidine drops are put in eye to treat ophthalmos of hyperthyroidism.

10. Thyroid crisis (thyroid storm) occurs suddenly due to aggravation of thyrotoxic state. This emergency is treated by administering:
   a. Propranolol (40–80 mg 6 hourly orally or 1–2 mg slowly i.v.),
   b. Collosal iodine (saturated KI solution),
   c. Propylthiouracil (250 mg 6 hourly through orogastric tube),
   d. Hydrocortisone (50 mg i.v. 6 hourly),
   e. Diltiazem (90–120 mg 6 or 8 hourly) and
   f. Plasmapheresis is performed, if above measures fail.

Chapter 41

Parathyroid Hormone, Calcitonin and Vitamin D

Parathyroid hormone, calcitonin and vitamin D are the main agents that control the homeostatic regulation of extracellular calcium, inorganic phosphate and bone growth (mineral metabolism). In the human adult, about 98% of the calcium and 85% of phosphorus are present in the bones. So the bones are the principal reservoir of these minerals. There occur cellular dysfunctions due to abnormalities in bone mineral homeostasis. Parathyroid hormone and vitamin D are the principal or primary regulators of calcium and phosphorus homeostasis. Besides these minerals, metabolism is also influenced by thyroid hormones (such as calcitonin), growth hormone, androgens, oestrogens, and Glucocorticoids, which are called as secondary regulators.

Parathyroid Hormone (PTH)

It is a polypeptide. It consists of 84 amino acids. It is secreted from the parathyroid gland. Its secretion is controlled by the plasma concentration of calcium. When the plasma levels of calcium are decreased (hypo-calcaemia) parathormone increases plasma calcium by:

- Transfer of calcium from bone to blood
- Absorption of calcium from the intestines
- Reabsorption of calcium from the kidney

Further, it lowers plasma phosphate levels. The release of calcitonin is inhibited during hypocalcaemia. Vitamin D helps in the absorption of calcium. The opposite effects are seen when serum calcium level is high (hypercalcaemia). Since hypoparathyroidism is best treated by vitamin D and calcium supplements, the clinical use of parathormone is very limited.

Vitamin D

Vitamin D occurs in two related forms:

a. **Cholecalciferol (vit. D_3):** It is produced in the skin from 7-dehydrocholesterol by the action of ultraviolet light from the sun rays.

b. **Ergocalciferol (vit. D_2; calciferol):** It is obtained from vegetable source. It is the form which is used in commercial vitamin formulations and in dairy products.

Vitamin D_3 is a prohormone and is not biologically active. It is first hydroxylated in the endoplasmic reticulum of liver to form to active calcifediol (25 (OH) D_3). This metabolite is then α-hydroxylated by the mitochondrial P-450 in the kidney to the major active metabolite calcitriol (1, 25 (OH)$_2$ D_3). This step is modulated by parathyroid hormone.

Vitamin D_3 and its metabolites circulate in plasma after tightly binding with alfa-globulin. Excess vitamin is stored in fat and adipose tissues.

Actions of Vitamin D on Target Tissues

1. Calcitriol stimulates calcium and phosphorus absorption from intestine.

2. Calcitriol has antirachitic effect due to its ability to increase osteoblast mediated activation of osteoclasts. It also promotes differentiation of osteoclast precursors which is facilitated by parathyroid hormone.
3. Both calcitriol and calcifediol increase reabsorption of calcium ions and phosphorus from proximal tubules. However, this action is weaker and less marked compared to PTH.
4. Vitamin D regulates secretion of PTH.
5. Vitamin D has some immunoregulatory properties because it enhances lymphokine production.

The net effect of vitamin D_3 is to raise both serum calcium and phosphorus levels. Their high levels reduce the rate of production of calcitriol by the kidney. Calcitriol itself inhibits PTH secretion. Thus there are negative feedback loops which control secretion of calcitriol and PTH.

Preparations of Vitamin D

- Cholecalciferol (1 µg vitamin D_3 = 40 IU of vitamin D): Daily requirement to prevent the deficiency symptoms is 200–400 IU/day.
- Ergocalciferol (calciferol, vitamin D_2) is derived from yeast and fungal sterol.
- Calcitriol (active vitamin D_2) is available for oral as well as parenteral use.
- Alfa calcidol (1-α-hydroxy cholecalciferol) and dihydrotachysterol are synthetic prodrugs which are rapidly hydroxylated to calcitriol in liver. These are used to treat renal rickets, vitamin dependent rickets and hypoparathyroidism.
- Calcipotriol (calcipotriene), doxercalciferol (1-α-hydroxy-D_2) and paricalcitol are calcitriol analogues. Their clearance is faster because they are poorly bound with alfaglobulin. So there is less risk of causing hypercalcaemia and hypercalciuria.

Therefore, they are useful in other conditions like psoriasis and secondary hyperthyroidism with chronic renal disease.

Vitamin D Deficiency

- In children, it causes rickets due to deficient calcification of osteoid tissue. So there occurs bony deformities like bow legs, enlarged skull, spinal curvature, chest deformities and hepatosplenomegaly.
- In adults, osteomalacia occurs due to decalcification and demineralization of bones. It is characterized by bone tenderness with pain and loss of bone density.

Hypervitaminosis D

Hypervitaminosis D develops after chronic administration of more than 15,000 IU/day of vitamin D_3. So there occurs increased plasma calcium levels and its ectopic deposition in blood vessels, parenchymal organs and soft tissues. It is characterized by weakness, fatigue, vomiting, diarrhoea, polyuria, renal stones, and hypertension and growth retardation (in children). Treatment consists of stopping vitamin intake and keeping the patient on low calcium diet. However, recovery may not be complete and may take longer time.

Drug Interactions

- Liquid paraffin reduces vitamin D absorption
- Phenytoin and phenobarbitone on prolonged use enhance metabolism of vitamin D by enzyme induction

Calcitonin

Calcitonin is synthesized and released from the parafollicular 'C' cells of the thyroid gland and both the processes are under the control of plasma levels of calcaemia. Hypercalcaemia stimulates the synthesis and release of calcitonin. Besides, the release of calcitonin is also stimulated by several compounds such as glucagon, prolactin, thyroxine, adrenergic drugs, gastrin and serotonin. Generally blood calcitonin levels are very low. It is a paradox that two antagonistic hormones, parathyroid hormone and calcitonin induce opposite biological response with a common target organ. The absorption or excretion of calcium by the kidney would depend on which hormone is present in more concentrations at a given time. Calcitonin may be used s.c. or i.m. in doses of 5 μg/kg to lower serum calcium concentration in patients with hypercalcaemia such as in tumour or in Paget's disease. Clinically, synthetic Salmon calcium is used because it is more potent than human calcitonin.

Glucocorticoids modify bone mineral homeostasis by:
• Antagonizing vitamin D-stimulated intestinal calcium transport
• Stimulating renal calcium excretion
• Blocking bone collagen synthesis
• Increasing PTH stimulated bone resorption
It is used:
• To treat hypercalcaemia
• As diagnostic test for determining the cause of hypercalcaemia

It should not be used for prolonged period because it will cause osteoporosis in adults and poor skeletal development in children.

Oestrogens are used for the prevention and/or treatment of postmenopausal osteoporosis because they reduce the bone resorbing action of PTH.

Non-hormonal Agents

Biphosphonates: These are analogues of pyrophosphonate. These are:
• Etridronate sodium
• Alendronate   } Given orally
• Risedronate
• Pamidronate sodium—given i.v.

They inhibit bone resorption but do not affect mineralization and growth. They act by:
• Slowing formation and dissolution of hydroxyapatite crystals in mineralized bone matrix
• Inhibiting osteoclasts because they get incorporated into them during bone resorption.

They have poor intestinal absorption which is further reduced if the drug is given with calcium or iron. These agents are therefore never given at meal times or with diary products. They should be given with full glass of plain water in the morning at least half to one hour before breakfast.

Uses
• Paget's disease
• Hypercalcaemia associated with :
  a. Malignancy osteoporosis
  b. Syndromes of ectopic calcification
• Multiple myeloma
• Bony metastasis
• Postmenopausal women at high risk of osteoporosis who forego hormonal replacement therapy
• Men with osteoporosis and all those individuals receiving high dose corticosteroid therapy

Side Effects
• Gastrointestinal upsets
• Oesophagitis and oesophageal ulceration
• Electrolyte imbalance; so use cautiously if renal function is impaired.
  Pilcamycin is a cytotoxic antibiotic. It is used in Paget's disease and hypercalcaemia.
  Thiazides: They increase the efficacy of PTH in stimulating calcium reabsorption in distal convoluted tubule. So they decrease renal calcium excretion. They are useful:
• In reducing hypercalciuria
• Incidence of stone formation in subjects with idiopathic hypercalciuria.

TO REMEMBER

1. The secretion of parathormone from parathyroid gland is increased during hypocalcaemia and decreased at hypercalcaemia. Its clinical use is very limited because hypoparathyroidism is best treated by vitamin-D and calcium supplements.

2. The secretion of calcitonin from parafollicular C cells of the thyroid gland is increased during hypercalcaemia and decreased during hypocalcaemia.

3. Therapeutic benefit of calcitonin is transient due to development of antibodies and down regulation of specific receptors.

4. Vitamin-D is used: (a) to prevent and cure rickets and osteomalacia; (b) in hypoparathyroidism; (c) in osteoporosis; (d) in Fanconi's syndrome; and (e) in vitamin D deficiency secondary to malabsorption, liver disease, and chronic renal diseases.

5. Glucocorticoids are used for a short period for the treatment of hyper-calcaemia and to determine the cause of hypercalcaemia.

6. Oestrogens are used for the prevention and/or treatment of postmenopausal osteoporosis.

7. Biphosphonates, pilcamycin and thiazides are non-hormonal agents which affect bone mineral homeostasis. Biphosphonates and pilcamycin are used in Paget's disease and to treat hypercalcaemia. Thiazides are used in reducing hypercalciuria and incidence of stone formation.

Chapter 42

Corticotropin and Adrenal Corticosteroids

CORTICOTROPIN (ADRENOCORTI-COTROPIC HORMONE)

Adrenocorticotropic hormone (ACTH) is a polypeptide. It consists of 39 amino acids. It is secreted by the anterior pituitary. The synthesis and secretion of ACTH is under the control of the hypothalamic corticotropin releasing factor (CRF), which is a polypeptide. CRF is released in response to stress, emotion, trauma, and diurnal rhythms. Synthetic preparations of CRF are available. CRF acts synergistically with antidiuretic hormone. CRF is mainly used in diagnostic tests to assess:

- The ability of the pituitary to secret ACTH
- Whether a deficiency of ACTH is caused by a pituitary or hypothalamic defect
- Hypothalamic pituitary function after therapy for Cushing's syndrome

The release of ACTH is also stimulated by vasopressin, and catecholamines. Gluco-corticoids inhibit the release of ACTH, either directly or through inhibition of CRF release. The former is called as the short negative feedback loop, whereas the latter is known as the long negative feedback loop.

ACTH stimulates the human adrenal cortex to secrete cortisol, corticosterone, aldosterone, and number of weakly androgenic substances by stimulating cAMP formation in cortical cells through specific cell surface G-protein coupled receptors. It is believed that ACTH also controls the synthesis of the enzymes responsible for the stepwise synthesis of steroid. Adrenocortical insufficiency occurs due to suppression of ACTH and prolonged suppression will lead to adrenocortical atrophy. On the contrary, adrenocortical hyper-secretion and relative hypertrophy occur due to increased ACTH secretion.

Uses

- **Diagnostic:** It is employed to distinguish primary adrenal insufficiency (Addison's disease) from secondary adrenal insufficiency due to pituitary cause. Administration of ACTH (25 IU i.v.) or tetracosactide (cosyntropin-0.25 mg i.v. infusion) will stimulate plasma cortisol levels in the later case only.

- **Therapeutic:** It has limited use in stimulating suppressed adrenal function following prolonged illness or severe traumatic stress and in rheumatoid arthritis, particularly in children. Since ACTH is less predictable and nonspecific as it stimulates secretion of mineralocorticoids and, therefore, may cause acute retention of salt and water, its synthetic analogue, tetracosactide is preferred for this purpose.

Tetracosactide (cosyntropin): It contains the first 24 amino acids sequence of ACTH. So it retains the physiological activity of ACTH, but has minimal immunogenicity. It is available as depot slow release formulation and administered i.m. twice weekly in dose of 0.5–1 mg to stimulate suppressed adrenal function.

ADRENAL CORTICOSTEROIDS

The mammalian adrenal cortex is divided into three concentric zones—the zona glomerulosa, zona fasciculata and zona reticularis.

- The zona glomerulosa produces aldosterone that is responsible for regulating salt and water metabolism;
- Zona fasciculata is responsible for secretion of glucocorticoids and
- Zona reticularis secretes the adrenal androgens.
- ACTH controls the secretions of zona fasciculata and reticularis while the renin-angiotensin system regulates the aldosterone secretion by the zona glomerulosa.

The glucocorticoids influence carbohydrate and protein metabolism whereas the mineralocorticoids affect water and electrolyte balance. Hydrocortisone (cortisol) is the most potent naturally occurring glucocorticoid. Both hydrocortisone and corticosterone have some mineralocorticoid activities also.

Aldosterone is the most potent naturally occurring mineralocorticoid.

Functions of corticosteroids: They play an important role in homeostasis. They are released during stressful situations and help the individuals to resist environmental changes. They have important regulatory effects on carbohydrate, protein, fat, purine metabolism and on electrolyte and water balance. The normal functions of many organs and systems such as lymphoid tissue, skeletal muscle, kidney, the cardiovascular system and the nervous system are also influenced.

Mechanism of action: Glucocorticoids enter target cells by diffusion and bind to specific receptors present in the cell nucleus. Thus they regulate protein synthesis by stimulating messenger RNA formation. Partly the metabolic effects of glucocorticoids may be due to increased synthesis of cAMP dependent kinase. Certain glucocorticoids stabilize lysosomal membranes and thereby inhibit the release of inflammatory mediators like eicosanoids, histamine, and cytosine or increase the generation of anti-inflammatory mediators. Steroids also depress prostaglandin synthesis by decreasing the release of arachidonic acid from phospholipids.

Pharmacological Actions
Metabolic Effects

- They may cause hyperglycemia by increasing gluconeogenesis and decreasing the peripheral utilization of glucose.
- They cause negative nitrogen balance and wasting of skeletal muscle by increasing protein catabolism and decreasing protein anabolism.
- They increase lipolysis due to a permissive effect on lipolytic hormones. They cause redistribution of fat, as in Cushing's syndrome.
- They induce negative calcium balance by decreasing its intestinal absorption and increasing renal excretion.
- Long-term administration can lead to osteoporosis because it increases osteoclastic activity and decreases osteoblastic activity.

Regulatory Actions

- Glucocorticoids have a negative feedback action on hypothalamus and anterior pituitary. Due to this, the release of endogenous glucocorticoids is reduced.
- Glucocorticoids reduce vasodilatation and decrease fluid exudation.
- They cause decreased influx and activity of leucocytes in areas of acute inflammation.
- There occurs decreased activity of mononuclear cells, decreased proliferation of blood vessels and less fibrosis in areas of chronic inflammation.

- In lymphoid areas, glucocorticoids decrease clonal expansion of T and B cells and decrease action of cytokine secreting T cells.
- Glucocorticoids have significant effect on inflammatory and immune mediators such as:
  — Decreased production and action of cytokines including many interleukins, tumor necrosis factor-r, and granulocyte-macrophage colony-stimulating factor.
  — Reduced generation of eicosanoids
  — Decreased generation of IgG
  — Decreased in compliment components in the blood.
- So the overall effects of glucocorticoids are reduction in chronic inflammation and autoimmune reactions. However, they also cause decreased healing and diminution in the protective aspects of the inflammatory response.

Other Effects

- They inhibit growth and cell division.
- They increase haemoglobulin synthesis.
- Euphoria occurs commonly. Sometimes there will be increased motor activity, insomnia, anxiety, or depression. Some patients treated with glucocorticoids become anxious, depressed or overtly psychotic.
- Glucocorticoids play a vital role in adaptation to stress.
- They cause feedback inhibition of CRF, ACTH and TSH while secretion of growth hormone is increased.

Disorders of corticosteroid secretion: Adrenocortical insufficiency leads to Addison's disease and hypoaldosteronism.

Similarly adrenocortical hypersecretion leads to Cushing's syndrome and hyperaldosteronism.

Synthetic analogues of corticosteroids are betamethasone, dexamethasone, prednisolone, prednisone, and triamcinolone. All of them have more potent glucocorticoid activity. Fludrocortisone is the most potent mineralocorticoid.

Therapeutic Uses

1. **Replacement therapy:** Addison's disease and hypopituitarism are treated by hydrocortisone which has some mineralocorticoid activity or by a combination of a synthetic glucocorticoid with fludrocortisone. Deoxycorticosterone (DOCA) is also occasionally used as a replacement therapy for aldosterone deficiency.
2. **Glucocorticoids** are very useful in the treatment of rheumatoid arthritis, osteoarthritis, and other form of chronic arthritis.
3. **Collagen diseases:** Glucocorticoid therapy may prove life saving in diseases like systemic lupus erythematosus, polyarteritis nodosa, dermatomyositis, and nephrotic syndrome.
4. **Hypersensitivity and allergic disorders:** Glucocorticoids are very useful in the treatment of anaphylactic shock, angioneurotic oedema, and serum sickness. Beclomethasone and budesonide are available as inhalation aerosol preparations. They are employed in chronic obstructive pulmonary disease including chronic bronchial asthma in order to minimize systemic adverse effects of glucocorticoids.
5. **Glucocorticoids** are also used to treat diseases having autoimmune aetiology such as haemolytic anaemia, idiopathic thrombocytopenia, ulcerative colitis and myasthenia gravis.
6. **Ocular conditions:** Glucocorticoids are used topically in the treatment of conjunctivitis, iritis, iridocyclitis, and keratitis. Retrobulbar or systemic therapy is employed for retinitis, uveitis and optic neuritis.

7. **Clobetasol** (a glucocorticoid) is used topically in pruritic skin conditions, active acute dermatoses and chronic dermatitis. To treat pemphigus, exfoliative dermatitis and Stevens-Johnson syndrome glucocorticoids are given systemically.

8. Since glucocorticoids cause lympholysis, they are used to treat acute lymphatic leukemia, lymphomas and Hodgkin's disease.

9. **Other uses:** They are also used in the treatment of:
   - Cerebral oedema
   - Rheumatic fever (not responding to salicylates)
   - Acute gout (intolerant to colchicine)
   - Acute/chronic hepatitis
   - Sarcoidosis
   - Mountain sickness

10. **Diagnostic uses:**
    a. Dexamethasone suppression test: If dexamethasone fails to decrease cortisol release (+ve test), the patient is having Cushing's syndrome due to anterior pituitary cause. Test is negative (decreases cortisol release), if patient is suffering from adrenocortical tumours.
    b. This test is also used to diagnose endogenous depression.

11. **Uses of steroids in dentistry:** The steroids are used to treat following diseases:
    - Oral ulceration and oral mucosal lesions: For this they may be used topically or systemically depending on need, e.g. (a) use of short course of systemic corticoids in moderate to severe erythema multiformis; (b) use of a high potency topical steroid preparation such as fluocinonide, betamethasone, or clobetasol in severe cases of recurrent aphthous stomatitis; (c) use of systemic corticosteroid therapy in oral manifestation of pemphigus; (d) use of topical medication with 0.05% fluocinonide and 0.05% clobetasol in oral lichen planus; (e) rarely use of systemic corticosteroid for brief treatment of severe exacerbations or for short period of treatment of recalcitrant cases of oral lichen planus that fail to respond to topical steroids (prednisolone 40–50 mg. daily for 10 days without tapering). For topical application, steroids are used in the form of paste so that they adhere to mucosa for a longer duration to have greater benefit.
    - Pulp inflammation: A combination of triamcinolone plus tetracycline is used locally over exposed dental pulp. This will reduce the pain and hypersensitivity of pulp.
    - Tempormandibular joint pain is treated by giving intra-articular injection of hydrocortisone or prednisolone.
    - Bell's palsy: Administer prednisolone systemically.
    - Postoperative pain and swelling after surgery, e.g. after removal of impacted third molar and after orthognathic surgery. So give i.m. injection of methyl prednisolone or betamethasone just before surgery.
    - For prophylactic purpose, hydrocortisone is used before any operative dental procedure in patients who are taking steroids for a month or more or who have taken them for a month or more during the previous year in order to avoid precipitation of adrenal crisis—a state of profound shock.
    - A preoperative antibiotic may be indicated during dental procedures in patients on large doses of glucocorticoids for longer periods because such patients are liable to have delayed wound healing and a decreased resistance to infections.

Toxic effects: These effects are seen on prolonged use or with overdose of corticosteroids. They are exaggerated physiological actions. Important toxic effects are:

- Hypertension
- Sodium retention
- Potassium loss
- Muscle weakness
- Diabetes mellitus
- Peptic ulcer and perforation
- Mental disturbances (depression or euphoria)
- Acute psychotic episodes
- Osteoporosis
- Pituitary adrenal suppression
- Posterior subcapsular cataract

Contraindications (relative)

- Congestive cardiac failure
- Diabetes mellitus
- Epilepsy
- Hypertension
- Osteoporosis
- Peptic ulcer
- Psychosis
- Pregnancy (risk of fetal defects)
- Renal failure
- Tuberculosis
- Other infections

The absolute contraindications are:

- Cushing's syndrome
- Herpes ocular infection

High doses of corticosteroids may cause Cushing's syndrome (moon face, striae and acne) which is reversible on stoppage of therapy.

Corticosteroid therapy should not be discontinued abruptly. Abrupt withdrawal will lead to signs of adrenocortical insufficiency. So its dosage should be reduced gradually.

The indiscriminate use of corticosteroids should be discouraged as it does more harm than good to patients.

Preparation and Doses

1. **Cortisone:** 25 mg/day orally in divided doses.

2. **Hydrocortisone (cortisol):**
   a. 20–30 mg/day orally
   b. 100–500 mg i.m., i.v.
   c. 0.2–2.5% ointment.
   d. 0.125–2.5% lotion

3. **Prednisolone (deltacortril):**
   a. 30 mg/day orally.
   b. 100 mg i.m. or i.v.
   c. 0.25% ointment
   d. 0.125–1% solution.

4. **Prednisone:** 30 mg/day orally

5. **Betamethasone (betnesol):**
   a. 5 mg/day orally.
   b. 4–20 mg i.m., i.v.
   c. 0.1% ointment
   d. 0.1% solution

6. **Dexamethasone (decadron):**
   a. 0.5–2 mg/day orally.
   b. 0.5–20 mg i.m., i.v.
   c. 0.05% ointment
   d. 0.1% solution.

7. **Triamcinolone (ledercort):**
   a. 24 mg/day orally.
   b. 40 mg i.m.
   c. 0.025–0.5% ointment
   d. 0.025–0.5% lotion.

8. **Methylprednisolone:**
   a. 16 mg/day orally
   b. 120 mg i.m., i.v.

9. **Fludrocortisone:** 0.1 mg/day orally.

Adrenocorticosteroid Biosynthesis Inhibitor

- Mitotane (O,P'-DDD)
- Metyrapone
- Trilostane
- Aminoglutethimide
- Ketonazole

Metyrapone, aminoglutethimide, and ketonazole act by inhibiting cytochrome P-450 enzymes which are involved in adrenocorticosteroid biosynthesis. Trilostane is a competitive inhibitor of the conversion of pregnenolone to progesterone, a reaction catalyzed by 3β-hydroxysteroid dehydrogenase. All these drugs must be used in appropriate doses and the status of the patient's hypothalamic-pituitary-adrenal (HPA) axis must be carefully monitored in order to avoid the precipitation of acute adrenal insufficiency. These drugs are used to treat:

- Cushing's syndrome secondary to autonomous adrenal tumours
- Hypersecretion associated with ectopic production of ACTH

Glucocorticoid Antagonist

Mifepristone is an antiprogestagen. At higher doses, it inhibits the glucocorticoid receptor by blocking feedback regulation of the HPA axis. So secondarily, it increases endogenous ACTH and cortisol levels. It is used in patients with hypercorticism.

Points for Dental Students

Glucocorticoid therapy will cause adrenal suppression. This affects adrenal function for up to 12 months. However, the patient's stress response will return within 14 to 30 days. So a dentist should take care of following points during dental procedures:

1. There is no need for replacement therapy for dental treatment in patients who have not taken glucocorticoids during the preceding 30 days.
2. Patients who are receiving alternate day therapy can be treated on an "off'" day without supplementation if they have been on the alternate day regimen for at least 2 weeks.
3. Patients who are receiving daily low dose corticoid therapy (< 30 mg hydrocortisone equivalent) will not need replacement therapy.
4. Patients who are receiving daily high-dose corticoid therapy (> 30 mg hydrocortisone

equivalent) should be treated as if they were completely adrenally suppressed and were without a normal stress response. The dose will need to be doubled on the day of treatment. The patient's primary care physician should be consulted if replacement dosage is uncertain or when highly stressful procedures are to be done (e.g. general anaesthesia).

TO REMEMBER

1. ACTH and its synthetic analogue tetracosactide are used to distinguish primary adrenal insufficiency (Addison's disease) from secondary adrenal insufficiency due to pituitary cause.
2. Tetracosactide is also used to stimulate suppressed adrenal function in doses of 0.5–1 mg i.m. twice weekly.
3. Corticosteroids play an important role in homeostasis during stressful situations and help the individuals to resist environmental changes.
4. Hydrocortisone is used for replacement therapy and in emergencies.
5. Fludrocortisone is used for Addison's disease.
6. Prednisolone, triamcinolone, betamethasone and dexamethasone are used for non-endocrine indications.
7. Corticosteroid therapy should not be discontinued abruptly because abrupt withdrawal will lead to signs of adrenocortical insufficiency. So it should be withdrawn gradually.
8. Teratogenicity of glucocorticoids, especially fluorinated agents, is well established. They can commonly cause cleft lip and palate.
9. Glucocorticoids should be used with caution in patients of diabetes mellitus, hypertension, congestive cardiac failure, epilepsy, peptic ulcer and during infections (particularly viral infection).

Chapter 43

Insulin and Oral Hypoglycaemic Agents

Diabetes mellitus is a very common chronic metabolic disease. It is characterized by hyperglycaemia, glycosuria, polyuria and polydipsia. It is induced by insulin deficiency. Excess of other hormones like growth hormone, glucocorticoids and glucagons may also be involved. The diabetes mellitus is classified into two major types:

1. **Type I or juvenile onset (insulin-dependent) diabetes:** Type I diabetes is commonly seen in juveniles in whom pancreatic beta cells are markedly decreased. So there is profound decrease in circulating insulin in plasma. Administration of insulin is essential in type I diabetes. It has an autoimmune aetiology and may have a genetic trait. Beta cells degeneration has been observed in viral infection and free radical. These patients are prone to ketoacidosis.

2. **Type II or maturity onset (non-insulin-dependent) diabetes:** Type II is a milder form of diabetes. It occurs predominantly in adults. There occurs varying degree of insulin deficiency or resistance to insulin. The latter is believed to be due to decrease in peripheral insulin receptors or defect in post-receptor insulin response. Dietary control and use of oral hypoglycaemic agents usually help to control type-II diabetes. These patients are not prone to ketoacidosis.

INSULIN

Insulin is a polypeptide. It is made up of two amino acid chains joined together by disulfide bonds. It is synthesized from proinsulin in the beta cells of the islets of Langerhans by proteolytic cleavage of a connecting peptide, C-peptide and is stored in secretory granules together with the associated C-peptide from where it is constantly being secreted into circulation. The insulin release is promoted by chemical (glucose, amino acids, fatty acids and ketone bodies), hormonal (glucagons) and neuronal (β_2-agonists, cholinergic drugs and vagal stimulation) mechanisms. Its release is inhibited by stomatostatin, PGE, α_2 adrenergic receptor agonists.

The principal factor, which controls the synthesis and secretion of insulin is the blood glucose concentration. The β cells respond to both the actual glucose concentration and also the rate of change of blood glucose. ATP-sensitive K^+ channels determine the resting membrane potential in the β cells. The intracellular concentration of ATP is increased by glucose metabolism which in turn blocks the K^+ channels causing depolarization. Due to this voltage-dependent Ca^{++} channels are opened up and lead to Ca^{++} influx. So insulin secretion is increased by exocytosis due to increased intracellular Ca^{++}. Insulin secretion is stimulated by high circulating levels of glucose.

Sulphonylurea hypoglycemic drugs also block ATP-dependent K^+ channels, depolarize the membrane and cause release of insulin by above explained mechanisms. Insulin receptors are present on cell membranes. Insulin receptors complex enters the cell where insulin is released. When insulin concentration is high these receptors are down regulated (number reduced), whereas in presence of low insulin concentrations, these receptors are up-regulated (number increased), leading to reduced and increased responsiveness respectively to insulin.

Physiological Actions of Insulin

- Insulin promotes the transport of glucose across cell membranes including muscle, hepatic and adipose cells. In the cell, it is transformed to fat or glycogen or oxidized to CO_2.
- Insulin increases the conversion of glucose to glycogen in skeletal muscle by enhancing the activity of enzyme, glycogen synthetase.
- Insulin inhibits the conversion of glucose from fat, proteins and amino acids.
- Insulin decreases glycogenolysis and gluconeogenesis in the liver and thus reduces blood glucose levels by reducing hepatic output of glucose.
- Insulin promotes the entry of amino acids and potassium into cells.
- Insulin promotes protein synthesis and inhibits breakdown of lipids.

Mechanism of Action of Insulin

Insulin acts by binding to a specific receptor on the surface of its target cells. The receptor is a large transmembrane glycoprotein complex which consists of two α- and two β-subunits. The α-subunits are entirely extracellular. Each α-subunit carries an insulin binding site. Insulin binds to alpha subunit and the insulin receptor complex is internalized.

The beta subunits are transmembrane proteins which have tyrosine kinase activity. By binding to beta subunits, insulin stimulates action of kinase on other target proteins.

Effects of Insulin Deficiency

- Hyperglycaemia occurs due decreased peripheral utilization of glucose, increased glycogenolysis, and augmented glucogenesis. Partly unopposed actions of the diabetogenic hormones, namely, glucagon, glucocorticoids, growth hormone and adrenaline may lead to these effects.
- Hyperlipaemia and ketoacidosis occur due to increased breakdown of lipids and increase in plasma free fatty acid levels, which in turn leads to increased levels of ketones, acetoacetate and beta-hydroxy-butyrate in blood.
- Protein metabolism is stimulated and is accompanied by increased gluconeogenesis.

Clinical Uses

1. **Diabetes mellitus:** It is used in type-I diabetes as well as in some types of type-II diabetic patients where dieting has failed.
2. Diabetic ketoacidosis.
3. Hyperosmolar non-ketotic diabetic coma. This may occur in type-II diabetics.
4. **Hyperkalaemia:** Insulin (1 unit/3 gm glucose) is administered i.v. with 300–500 ml 20% glucose to promote intracellular influx of potassium.
5. Insulin is used for anterior pituitary function (increase in growth hormone and ACTH), and completeness of vagotomy (decreased gastric acid response).

Preparations

Insulin is given by subcutaneous route. In case of diabetic coma, it is given by intravenous or intramuscular route. There are three main types of insulin preparations available.

Rapid Action Insulin Preparations

- Crystalline zinc insulin (regular, neutral, soluble insulin): Obtained from bovine, porcine, and human sources; onset of action—rapid; duration of action—short (6–8 hours on s.c. administration and 3–4 hours on i.v. administration).
- Semilente insulin (micro-amorphous crystalline insulin suspension): Onset of action: 1–2 hours; duration of action: 12–16 hours; administered s.c. only.

Intermediate Action Insulin Preparations

- Isophane (neutral protamine Hagedorn, NPH insulin). Onset of action 2 hours; duration of action: 12–24 hours; administered s.c. only.
- Lente insulin (insulin zinc suspension, amorphous): It is a mixture of 30% semilente insulin with 70% ultralente insulin. Onset of action: 2 hours; duration of action: 12–24 hours.

Prolonged Action Insulin Preparations

- Protamine zinc insulin: Onset of action 5–7 hours; duration of action 24–36 hours; administered s.c.
- Ultralente insulin Onset of action 5–7 hours; duration of action 24–36 hours.

Ultrashort acting (rapid acting):

- Insulin lispro: It is a recently introduced insulin analogue in which a lysine and proline residue are switched. Its onset of action is 15–20 minutes and its duration of action is 3–4 hours. It can be injected by the patient himself soon before the start of meal. Semisynthetic human insulins are prepared by modifying porcine insulin to human insulin amino acid structure employing enzymatic techniques. Biosynthetic human insulin is obtained by DNA recombinant technique.

Human insulin is less antigenic than animal insulins.

The type of insulin used, its dose, and frequency of administration depend on the needs of the patient. Diabetics with moderate to severe insulin deficiency are treated with isophane insulin.

Undesirable Reactions

- **Hypoglycaemia:** It occurs due to overdose and is characterized by sweating, headache, tachycardia, blurred vision, diplopia, mental confusion, coma and convulsions.

Treatment consists of:

a. Administration of glucose orally or i.v. depending upon severity.
b. Glucagon and diazoxide i.m. may also be used.
  - **Lipodystrophy** may occur at the s.c. injection site. So rotate the injection site.
  - **Hypersensitivity** is rare. It can be overcome by changing insulin preparation or using single component insulin.
  - **Insulin resistance:** A diabetic patient is said to be insulin resistant when the daily dose of insulin exceeds 200 units in the absence of infection or ketoacidosis. Insulin binding antibodies may be formed in these patients.

The potency of insulin is expressed in units. One milligram of insulin contains 22 units of insulin. Newer and more pure insulin preparations contain 26–30 units/mg.

Insulin is used as replacement therapy in insulin dependent diabetes. A total diabetic usually requires 30–50 units of insulin and in others the dose is adjusted according to patient's needs.

Insulin requirement is increased:

- By drugs (glucocorticoids, adrenaline, growth hormone, oral contraceptives, thiazides, frusemide, colchicine, thyroxine, vinblastine, and diazoxide)

- Stress (anxiety, pregnancy, infection, trauma)
- Obesity.

Insulin requirement is decreased:
- By exercise
- Drugs (sulphonamides and anticoagulants-release insulin).

Recently newer routes of delivery of insulin are being tried such as oral, nasal, rectal, s.c. pellet plantation, insulin pump-open or closed circuit, i.p. devices, closed loop artificial pancreas, islet cell and pancreatic transplantation and gene therapy.

ORAL HYPOGLYCAEMIC AGENTS

There are two major groups of drugs (sulphonylureas and biguanides) that can reduce hyperglycaemia. Unlike insulin, these drugs are effective by oral route of administration. They are mainly used in type-II diabetes mellitus.

Sulphonylureas

Tolbutamide and chlorpropamide are the older sulphonylureas while glibenclamide, glipizide, gliclazide, gliquidone, glibornuride and tolazamide are the newer members of this group. Sulphonylureas stimulate the beta cells of islet to secrete insulin. They cause degranulation of beta cells. They are effective only in patients who have residual insulin in their pancreatic beta cells. They are ineffective in insulin-dependent diabetic subjects. It has been shown that glibenclamide and glipizide increase the number of beta cells in the pancreas. They also potentiate the activity of peripheral intracellular receptors and reduce glucagon secretion. They are readily absorbed from gastrointestinal tract. They are strongly bound to plasma proteins. So their hypoglycaemic effect is increased by drugs that displace them from plasma proteins. Their biological half lives vary from 6 hours (tolbutamide, acetohexamide) to 36 hours (chlorpropamide). Most of these drugs are excreted in urine after hepatic metabolism. They cross placental barrier and may induce neonatal hypoglycaemia.

They are used in type-II diabetes along with dietary control. For better euglycaemic control, sulphonylureas are combined with a suboptimal dose of insulin.

Chlorpropamide has been used in diabetes insipidus.

Side Effects

Nausea, vomiting, epigastric discomfort, weakness, paraesthesia, hypersensitive reactions such as fever, rash, jaundice and antabuse like reaction with alcohol have been observed. More severe side effects are

Drug	Daily dose	No. of doses per day	Duration of action (hrs.)
Sulphonylureas			
Tolbutamide	0.5–3 g	2–3	6–8
Chlorpropamide	0.1–0.5 g	1	36–48
Glibenclamide	5–15 mg	1–2	18–24
Glipizide	50–20 mg	1–2	12
Gliclazide	40–240 mg	1–2	12–18
Glimepiride	1–4 mg	1	12–24
Biguanides			
Phenformin	25–150 mg	1–3	8–12
Metformin	0.5–2 g	2–4	6–8

hypoglycaemia and cardiovascular disturbances on prolonged use.

Hypoglycaemic effect of sulphonylureas may be potentiated by salicylates, phenylbutazone, propranolol, chloramphenicol and alcohol. They are contraindicated in pregnancy, severe infection, renal and hepatic impairment.

Doses

- Tolbutamide is relatively short acting drug. It is given in a dose of 0.5 to 1.5 gm per day.
- Chlorpropamide has slow onset of action. It is used in a dose of 0.5 gm daily.
- Acetohexamide has some uricosuric action. It is given in a dose of 0.25 to 1.5 gm daily.
- Glibenclamide is a potent drug. Its duration of action is between tolbutamide and chlorpropamide. It is used in a dose of 5 mg daily.
- Glipizide: Its half-life is 2–4 hours but the hypoglycaemic effect may last for 24 hours. It is used in a dose of 5 mg per day.

Biguanides

These drugs have limited therapeutic use than sulfonylureas. Phenformin has been withdrawn from market because of toxicity (fatal lactic acidosis). Metformin continues to be used. Its important features are:

- It does not lower normal fasting blood glucose but does lower the postprandial blood glucose. So some times it is called 'euglycemic' agent.
- Metformin is effective in the absence of functioning pancreatic beta cells or the residual insulin.
- It has the advantage of not inducing hypoglycaemia.
- It inhibits glucose absorption from gut.
- It inhibits hepatic gluconeogenesis.
- It accelerates peripheral uptake of glucose provided insulin is present.
- It increases insulin binding to its receptors.

- It causes reduction of plasma glucagons levels.
- It directly stimulates glycolysis in peripheral tissues, with increased glucose removal from blood.

Metformin rarely causes ketonuria and acidosis. Vitamin B_{12} deficiency occurs on prolonged use due to its reduced absorption. Diarrhoea and metallic taste in mouth may also occur.

It is used in type-II diabetes mellitus along with sulphonylureas. It is given in a dose of 1.5–2 gm daily.

Newer Antidiabetic Agents

1. **Aldose reductase inhibitors:** Aldose reductase is an enzyme. It converts sugars into polyols which are probably responsible for thickening of retinal capillaries and diabetic retinopathy. Tolerstat is an aldose reductase inhibitor. It has been tried in the treatment of diabetic neuropathy and retinopathy due to its ability to reduce the glucose toxicity in tissues such as eye, kidney, and nerve trunks.

2. **Thiazolidinedione derivatives are:**
   - Rosiglitazone: 4–8 mg per day.
   - Pioglitazone: 15–45 mg per day.
   - Troglitazone: 200–600 mg per day.

   They do not cause any increase in insulin release. They act primarily by:
   - Increasing the target tissue sensitivity to insulin
   - Potentiating the action of insulin to increase glucose uptake and glucose oxidation in both muscle and adipose tissues
   - Reducing hepatic glucose output by inhibiting hepatic gluconeogenesis
   - Inhibiting lipid-synthesis in muscle and fat cells

   These drugs are used to lower insulin resistance in diabetic type-II patients who require high doses of insulin (>100 U/day). If glitazone is to be added to the diabetic regimen, the dosage of sulfonylureas or of insulin should be reduced to compensate for any enhanced insulin sensitivity.

3. **α-Glucoside inhibitors:** The important features of these drugs are:
   - These drugs inhibit the action of intestinal brush border α-glucoside and thus reduce intestinal absorption of starch, dextrin, and disaccharides.
   - Postprandial increase in blood glucose is decreased due to inhibition of α-glucoside enzyme that is responsible for the absorption of carbohydrates.
   - They reduce plasma glucose levels in both insulin-dependent as well as non-insulin-dependent diabetes mellitus.
   - They do not cause hypoglycaemia because they do not stimulate insulin release.
   - They are used in combination with other oral antidiabetics and/or insulin.
   - Flatulence, diarrhea, abdominal pain and bloating are a few side effects.
   - Acarbose and miglitol belong to this group.

   These are administered at the start of meal in doses of 25 mg initially. The doses may be increased at interval of 4 to 8 weeks up to 75 mg before each meal.

4. **Insulin secretagogues are:**
   - Repaglinide(prandin): initial dose—0.5–1 mg before meals; may be increased gradually up to 16 mg per day.
   - Nateglinide(starlix): 120 mg before meals.

   Important features of these drugs are:
   - They stimulate insulin release by closing ATP dependent K^+ channels in pancreatic β cells
   - They are orally effective
   - They should be cautiously used in patients with hepatic insufficiency

because they are metabolized primarily in liver
   - Major side effect of repaglinide is hypoglycaemia
   - Nateglinide produces fewer episodes of hypoglycaemia

5. **Pramlintide:** It is a synthetic analogue of amylin. It suppresses glucagon release, delays gastric emptying and has central nervous system mediated anorectic effects. It is administered s.c. in the abdomen and thigh in doses range from 15 to 120 µg; arm administration is less reliable. It is rapidly absorbed; peak level occurs within 20 minutes and duration of action is 2 hours and 30 minutes. It is administered in addition to insulin in those individuals who are unable to achieve their target postprandial blood sugar immediately before eating. Because of risk of hypoglycaemia, meal time insulin doses should be decreased by 50% or more. Adverse effects are hypoglycaemia and GIT disturbances.

6. **Exenatide:** It is a synthetic analog of glucagon like polypeptide-1. It causes potentiation of glucose mediated insulin secretion, suppression of postprandial glucagons release, slowed gastric emptying and central loss of appetite. It is used as adjunct to metformin or sulfonylureas in patients who have suboptimal glycemic control. It is injected s.c. within 60 minutes before a meal in doses of 5 µg twice a day, with a maximum dosage of 10 µg twice a day. Peak concentration occurs at 2 hours and duration of action is up to 10 hours. It is excreted through kidney. Reduce doses of pre-existing sulfonylurea therapy to avoid hypoglycaemia. Major adverse effects are nausea, vomiting and diarrhoea.

7. **Sitagliptine phosphate:** It is an orally active, potent and highly selective inhibitor of the dipeptidyl peptidase

4 (DPP-4) enzyme. It is recommended in the treatment of type 2 diabetes. The DPP-4 enzyme inhibitors act as incretin enhancers. So it increases the levels of two known active incretin hormones, glucagon like peptide-1 (GLP-1) and glucose dependent insulinotropic polypeptide (GIP). Incretins play an important role in the physiological regulation of glucose homeostasis. GLP-1 and GIP increase synthesis and release of insulin from pancreatic beta cells when blood glucose concentrations are normal or elevated. GLP-1 also reduces hepatic glucose production by lowering glucagon secretion from pancreatic alpha cells. Thus it differs from sulfonylureas which cause insulin release even when glucose levels are low and can precipitate hypoglycaemia in patients with type 2 diabetes and in normal subjects.

It is used to improve glycemic control in type 2 diabetes mellitus: (a) as an adjunct to diet and exercise; (b) in combination with metformin, or sulfonylurea or thiazolidinediones when single agent alone does not provide adequate glycemic control; (c) in combination with metformin and a sulfonylurea dual therapy that fails to provide adequate glycemic control. It is administered in doses of 100 mg once daily. On oral administration, it is readily absorbed. It is primarily eliminated unchanged in urine (79%) and rest in the form of metabolites (10%). Approximately, 13% is eliminated in faeces. The drug is considered quite safe. However, rarely hypersensitivity reactions have been reported. They usually occur within 3 months of its use. It should not be used during pregnancy and in lactating mothers. It is contraindicated in patients with type-1 diabetes or for the treatment of diabetic ketoacidosis.

Drugs used in Hypoglycaemia

Glucagon: It is a polypeptide (a single chain 29 amino acid peptide). It is synthesized and secreted by the alpha cells of the pancreatic islets. Blood concentration of glucagon is higher in diabetics than in non-diabetics. Its important actions are:
- It causes glycogenolysis in the liver by activating phosphorylase and glucose is released into the blood. One milligram of glucagon normally increases blood sugar by 50–80 mg% with gradual decline in 90 minutes or so.
- It inhibits glycogen synthesis.
- It induces lipolysis and ketogenesis.
- It stimulates release of insulin.

Uses: It may be used:
- As an alternative to glucose in hypoglycaemia, especially in insulin shock therapy. It is given subcutaneously or intramuscularly in a dose of 0.5 to 2.0 mg.
- In cardiogenic shock
- In spasm of sphincter of Oddi
- In diverticulitis
- Prior to radiographic examination of gut
  However, the use of glucagon in all these conditions is very limited.

Somatostatin: It is a growth hormone-release inhibiting factor. It inhibits secretion of:
- Growth hormone
- Insulin
- Glucagon

So it can be used:
- To reduce fasting hyperglycaemia in insulin deficient juvenile diabetics.
- To block the hormone release in endocrine-secreting tumours such as insulinomas, glucagonomas, vasoactive intestinal peptidomas, and carcinoid tumours. However, the important limiting factor in its use is its short biological half-life (3–6 minutes. So its longer acting analog,

octreoide (sandostin) is used to treat the above tumours and also checks excess secretion of growth hormone. Octreoide is also used to treat bleeding oesophageal varices, peptic ulcer, and postprandial orthostatic hypotension because it decreases blood flow to gastrointestinal tract.

Diazoxide: It is an antihypertensive and a potent hyperglycemic agent. Its hyperglycemic action is due to its ability to interact with an ATP-sensitive K^+ channel and keeps the channel open for a long period. This is an action opposite to sulphonylureas. It is used to treat various forms of hypoglycaemia in doses of 3 to 8 mg/kg per day.

Points for Dental Students

1. Overall, diabetic patients respond to most dental treatments similarly to the way non-diabetic patients respond. However, glycemic control appears to play an important role in response to periodontal therapy.
2. So the dental practitioner must establish the level of glycemic control early in the treatment process.
3. Endogenous production of epinepherine and cortisol is increased during stressful situations. These hormones elevate blood glucose levels and interfere with glycemic control. Adequate pain control and stress reduction are therefore important in treating diabetic patients.
4. Profound anaesthesia reduces pain and minimizes endogenous epinepherine release. Dental local anaesthetic with small amount of epinepherine (1: 100,000 concentration) have no significant effect on blood glucose.
5. For extremely anxious patients, conscious sedation should be given.
6. Antibiotics are indicated in the presence of acute infection.

7. In cases of extensive dental therapy, diet adjustment is necessary in consultation with patient's physician. Similarly adjustment of the dose of insulin or oral agents may be needed in this situation in consultation with patient's physician. Physicians often recommend reduction in the dose of insulin that immediately precedes lengthy or extensive dental procedures.
8. It is generally best to plan dental treatment to be carried out either before or after periods of peak insulin activity to minimize the risk of stress induced hypoglycaemia.
9. Hypoglycaemia is the most common diabetic emergency in dental clinic. It is a potentially life-threatening complication that must be managed accordingly. Confusion, sweating, tremors, agitation, anxiety, dizziness, tingling or numbness and tachycardia are the signs and symptoms. Severe hypoglycaemia may result in seizures or loss of consciousness. It should be treated immediately as under:
   - Administer approximately 15 gm of oral carbohydrate in a form that will be absorbed rapidly. A source of sugar (e.g. a candy or chocolate) should be readily available for such patients.
   - If oral route is not available administer 25 to 50 ml of 50% dextrose solution i.v. or 1 mg of glucagon i.v.
   - If i.v. route is not available, administer glucagon (1 mg) s.c. or i.m.
   - Usually patient recovers in 10 to 15 minutes. The patient should be observed for 30 to 60 minutes after recovery and then discharged.
10. A dentist must have the knowledge of common oral complications of diabetes such as paraesthesia, burning pain, xerostomia, delayed healing of oral lesions,

susceptibility to infection, increased incidence of gingivitis, dental caries, periapical abscess, candidiasis and periodontal disease. This will help him to manage his cases judiciously.

TO REMEMBER

1. Insulin and oral hypoglycaemic agents reduce blood sugar levels. Insulin is used to treat type-I diabetes (juvenile onset) as well as type-II diabetic patients where dieting has failed. Oral hypoglycaemics are used in type-II (maturity onset) diabetes.
2. Glucagons, adrenaline, glucocorticoids and thyroxin increase blood sugar levels.
3. Sulphonylureas are effective only in patients who have residual insulin in their pancreatic beta cells because they act by stimulating them.
4. Biguanides are used in type-II diabetes mellitus. They act by inhibiting glucose absorption from gut and hepatic gluconeogenesis; accelerates peripheral uptake of glucose provided insulin is present.

5. Glucagon is synthesized and released by the alpha cells of the pancreatic islet. It may be used as an alternative to glucose in hypoglycaemia, especially in insulin shock.
6. Somatostatin is growth hormone release inhibiting factor and also inhibits secretion of both insulin and glucagon. So it can be used to reduce fasting hyperglycaemia in insulin deficient juvenile diabetics as well as to block the hormone release in endocrine-secreting tumours. However, it has a short biological half-life, so its longer acting analog, octreotide is preferred for the treatment of all these conditions.
7. Diazoxide has potent hyperglycaemic action, so it is also used in the treatment of hypoglycaemia.
8. Newer antidiabetic agents are aldose reductase inhibitors (e.g. tolrestat), thiazolidindione derivatives (e.g. rosiglitazone, pioglitazone, and troglitazone), α-glucosidase inhibitors (e.g. acarbose, miglitol) and insulin secretagogues (e.g. nateglinide, repaglinide).

Chapter 44

Gonadal Hormones

Androgens are steroid hormones. Testosterone is the major natural androgen. It is mainly secreted by the interstitial cells of testes. It is also secreted in smaller amounts by ovary and adrenal cortex. Important physiological functions of testosterone are:

1. It is responsible for the development of male genital organs and secondary sex characteristics such as growth of facial, pubic and body hair.
2. Androgens lower vocal pitch through laryngeal enlargement and thickening of vocal cord.
3. Androgens are responsible for the growth of long bone during puberty and closure of their epiphyses.
4. Testosterone possesses anabolic effects as under:
   - It causes enhancement of protein synthesis and decrease in protein breakdown within the body. It is indicated by reduced excretion of nitrogen in urine.
   - It leads to sodium and water retention.
   - It increases bone density and skeletal muscle mass.
   - It induces increase in haem synthesis.
5. Testosterone is required for spermatogenesis. FSH controls spermatogenesis while LH stimulates androgen secretion. Testosterone and its metabolite, 5-alpha-dihydrotestosterone, induce feedback inhibition of gonadotropin releasing hormone in hypothalamus and of gonadotropins in anterior pituitary.
6. Metabolic effects of androgen are:
   - Increased synthesis of clotting factors, triglyceride lipase, α_1-antitrypsin and hepatoglobulin in liver
   - Decreased HDL levels
   - Accelerated erythropoiesis by increasing erythropoietin production and haemoglobulin synthesis

Mechanism of Action

Testosterone is converted to 5-α-dihydrotestosterone (DHT) in skin, prostate, seminal vesicles and epididymis. So DHT is the dominant androgen in these tissues. Testosterone and DHT bind to the intracellular androgen receptor and initiate a series of events which lead to spermatogenesis, sexual differentiation, and sexual maturation at puberty, external virilization and godadotrophin regulation. They also initiate formation of tissue specific proteins after forming an androgen receptor complex.

Preparations, Doses and Pharmacokinetics

- **Testosterone:** If given orally, it undergoes extensive hepatic first pass metabolism. Testosterone enanthate is a long acting preparation that is given intramuscularly in dose of 250 mg every 2–3 weeks.

Testosterone implants (100–600 mg) are done for longer duration (7–8 months) of action.

- **Methyltestosterone:** It is more resistant to hepatic metabolism. It is given sublingually in doses of 30–50 mg daily.
- Fluoxymesterone, mesterelone and stanolone can be administered orally because they are resistant to hepatic metabolism. Dose of fluoxymesterone is 2.5 to 10 mg daily.

Clinical Uses

1. **Hypogonadism:** It is useful in primary (testicular with elevated levels of LH and FSH) or secondary (abnormalities of the hypothalamic-pituitary axis with low levels of LH and FSH) hypogonadism. Testosterone is given for 2–3 years or until adequate sexual maturation takes place.
2. **Cryptorchism** (failure of testicular descent into the scrotum) and delayed puberty: Human chorionic gonadotropin treatment for 6 weeks or testosterone administration helps in testicular descent.
3. Androgens also enhance libido, sexual performance, and stimulate spermatogenesis. However, the use of androgens in impotency has to be based on proper assessment of endocrine deficiency as a cause of impotency.
4. Androgens are used with varying success in premenopausal breast carcinoma in females.
5. Androgens have also been used to treat refractory anaemias because natural androgens stimulate erythrocyte production. However, recombinant erythropoietin has largely replaced the androgen for this purpose. Earlier androgens were used to treat selected cases of osteoporosis along with oestrogens because they reduce Ca^{++} ion excretion sharply. However, at present bisphosphonates are employed for this purpose.

Side effects: They cause fluid retention, increase in weight and jaundice. Virilization and menstrual irregularities occur in women. Acne and growth disturbances are seen in children. Excessive administration in males may suppress spermatogenesis and cause azoospermia.

Antiandrogens: Oestrogens and progestins have antiandrogenic activity; oestrogens induce this effect by inhibiting gonadotropin release while progestins produce this effect by competing with testosterone for target organ androgenic receptors.

ANDROGEN RECEPTOR ANTAGONISTS

- **Danazol:** It is an ethisterone derivative. It has weak androgenic, progestational, antioestrogenic and anabolic actions. It inhibits ovulation, spermatogenesis and testosterone secretion by inhibiting synthesis and release of gonadotropin. It is used:
  1. Mainly in the treatment of endometriosis
  2. In the long-term management of hereditary angioneurotic oedema
  3. For mammary dysplasia and gynecomastia where other measures have failed

  It is used in a dose of 200–800 mg per day in divided doses.
- **Cyproterone acetate:** It is a progesterone derivative. It has weak progestational activity. It acts as a partial agonist on androgen receptors and competes with 5-alpha dihydrotestosterone for these receptors. It inhibits spermatogenesis and produces reversible infertility by suppressing synthesis and release of gonadotropins. It is used in the treatment of:
  1. Hypersexuality in males
  2. Severe hirsutism in women

  In the former condition, it is given in doses of 50 mg twice a day and in later condition in a dose of 2 mg per day along with an oestrogen.

- **Flutamide:** It is a potent antiandrogen. It is used in the treatment of prostate carcinoma. Mild gynecomastia and mild reversible hepatotoxicity may frequently occur as side effects.
- **Spironolactone:** Its important features are:
  - A competitive inhibitor of aldosterone
  - Competes with dihydrotestosterone for the androgen receptors in target tissues
  - Lowers plasma levels of testosterone and androstedion by reducing 17α-hydroxylase activity. It is used to treat hirsuitism in women in doses of 50 mg per day.
- **5-alfa reductase inhibitors:** They inhibit conversion of testosterone into dihydrotestosterone. The drugs are :
  - *Finasteride:* It is selective for 5-α-reductase type-2 isoenzyme which predominates in male urogenital tract. It decreases prostate size and increases urinary flow rate in 50% patients. Maximum symptomatic relief occurs at 6 months. With continued therapy benefit is maintained for two years or more.

It is effective orally. It is metabolized in liver and metabolites are excreted in urine and faeces.

It is well tolerated. Side effects are decreased libido, impotence and decreased volume of ejaculation; skin rashes and swelling of lips.

Dose: 5 mg once daily.

Its other uses are:
- Male pattern baldness
- Acne
- Prostate cancer
  - Dutersteride: It is a 4-azosteroid. It is a selective and potent inhibitor of type 1 and 2 isoforms of 5-α reductase. It is more potent than finasteroide in reducing serum dihydrotestosterone.

On oral administration, it is well absorbed. It is widely distributed in the body and is highly bound to plasma proteins (> 99.5%). It is metabolized in liver and its metabolites are mainly excreted in faeces.

It is contraindicated in children, adolescent and severe hepatic impairment. Blood concentration of dutersteroid are increased in presence of ritonavirus, ketoconazole, verapamil, diltiazime and ciprofloxacin.

It is indicated for the treatment of symptomatic benign prostate hypertrophy in men to:
- Improve symptoms
- Reduce the risk of acute urinary retention
- Reduce the risk of related surgery

Dose: 0.5 mg orally daily; can be given with or without food.

ANABOLIC STEROIDS

These steroids have marked anabolic and weak androgenic activity. These drugs are mostly used for their protein anabolic effect characterized by increased protein synthesis and skeletal muscle development. However, they are not commonly used as tonics or body builders because of their side effects such as cholestatic jaundice (on prolonged use), increased risk of coronary heart disease and instances of sudden death in young athletes. Other side effects are testicular atrophy, sterility, gynecomastia in men and inhibition of ovulation, hirsutism, deepening of voice, alopecia and acne in women.

Preparation and Doses

- **Methandienone (dianabol):** Dose 5–10 mg oral; 25 mg/ml. i.m.
- **Nandrolone (durabolin):** Dose: 25–50 mg/ week i.m.
- **Nandrolone decanoate:** Dose: 25–50 mg/3 weeks i.m.
- **Ethyloestrenol (orabolin):** Dose: 2–4 mg/ day orally.
- **Oxymetholone:** Dose: 5–15 mg/day orally.
- **Stanozolol:** Dose: 5 mg/day orally.

Uses

They are used:

1. For the treatment of osteoporosis in elderly males.
2. In catabolic states such as acute illness, severe trauma and major surgery.
3. In renal insufficiency to reduce nitrogen load on the kidneys.
4. In hypoplastic anaemias.
5. In breast cancer.
6. To decrease itching of chronic biliary obstruction.
7. To stimulate growth in children.
8. To correct weakness and muscle wasting in AIDS patients with low testosterone levels.
9. To prevent attacks of hereditary angio-neurotic oedema due to their ability to increase synthesis of compliment C-1 esterase inhibitor. One course should not exceed more than 2 to 3 weeks and protein rich diet must be given along with them for full desired effect.

OESTROGENS

The major oestrogens are oestradiol, oestrone, and oestriol. They are produced by Graafian follicle, placenta, and to small extent by testes and adrenal cortex. The primary source of oestradiol is ovaries. In the liver, oestradiol is biotransformed into oestrone and oestriol. Since they are subjected to extensive first pass hepatic metabolism, they are not effective by oral route. However, synthetic oestrogens as well as non-steroidal compounds with oestrogenic activity exhibit less first-pass metabolism and are available by oral route. Binding with specific intracellular receptors, oestrogens induce DNA-directed messenger RNA synthesis which in turn determines specific protein synthesis. These receptors are present in female reproductive organs and breasts, as well as in the hypothalamus and pituitary. Progestins decrease the number of these receptors, whereas prolactin increases their number in mammary glands but not in the uterus. Oestrogens can induce the synthesis of progesterone receptors in the female reproductive organs, hypothalamus and anterior pituitary.

Actions

1. Oestrogens play an important role in the development and maturation of female reproductive organs, breast and secondary female sex characters.
2. They are required for the proliferative phase of the endometrium and for maintenance of pregnancy and concomitant growth of breast.
3. They are responsible for the rapid growth of the long bones during puberty and also influence psychological and emotional behaviour.
4. In the non-pregnant premenopausal woman, the rate of oestrogen synthesis in the corpus luteum is modulated by both follicle stimulating hormone (FSH) and luteinizing hormone (LH). LH stimulates formation of androgens by the theca cells while FSH facilitates the conversion of androgen to oestrogens in the granulosa cells.
5. During pregnancy, oestrogen is mainly formed in the corpus luteum for the first 9–10 weeks and thereafter by placenta.

All clinically used oestrogens are well absorbed from gut. In plasma, they are bound with globulin and albumin. They are metabolized in liver and are excreted in urine as glucuronide and sulphate conjugates.

Clinical Uses

1. Oestrogens are used to treat woman who have abnormally low oestrogen such as in primary ovarian failure and female hypogonadism.

2. Vasomotor instability, headache and emotional liability are seen in a few per cent of women during and after menopause. If these symptoms are severe, oestrogen therapy may be used and the dose should be individually adjusted. Overdose may cause troublesome toxic effects.

3. Oestrogen-progestogen combination is useful in the treatment of pelvic endometriosis, dysmenorrhea and habitual abortion.

4. High doses of oestrogens have been employed in the treatment of primary and metastasis forms of the carcinoma of prostate.

5. They have also been used in the treatment of female hirsutism, acne in females, senile vaginitis, epistaxis, atrophic rhinitis and male hypersexuality.

6. For oral contraception, they may be employed in combination with progesterone or given alone.

Adverse effects: These include feminization in males; sodium retention, oedema, aggravation of hypertension and congestive cardiac failure, increase in migraine, nausea, vomiting, diarrhoea; cholestasis and gallbladder disease, thromboembolism; endometrial carcinoma on long-term use during menopause.

They are contraindicated in premenopausal breast cancer and in patients with history of thromboembolism. They should be cautiously used in presence of hypertension, hepatic dysfunction, diabetes mellitus, migraine and uterine fibroid because all of them may be aggravated by them.

Preparations and doses: Parenteral oestrogen preparations are now rarely used. Commonly used preparations with therapeutically equivalent doses in clinical practice are :

- Ethinyl estradiol 5–10 µg (oral)
- Conjugated oestrogen 0.625 mg (oral)
- Micronized estradiol 1 mg (oral)
- Estradiol valerate 2 mg (oral)
- Estradiol (transdermal) 50 µg

These are average doses for women in their sixties for bone and cardioprotection. Larger doses may be needed for younger women while smaller doses for older women.

Antioestrogens

Although several effects of oestrogen are antagonized by androgens and progestin, drugs which have selective effect on oestrogen receptors as competitive antagonists are:

1. **Clomiphen citrate:** It is structurally related to stilbestrol. It acts as a partial antagonist by blocking oestrogen receptors in hypothalamus and anterior pituitary. Thus it reduces the feedback effect of oestrogens on the secretion and release of gonadotropins. It is employed in anovulatory sterility, in the dose of 50 mg/day for 5–7 days starting from day 5 of the menstrual cycle. It has also been used in premenopausal breast cancer. Multiple pregnancy and polycystic disease of ovary may occur.

2. **Cyclofenil** has actions similar to those of clomiphen.

3. **Selective oestrogen receptor modulators**

They are called selective oestrogen receptor modulators because they have differential oestrogen agonistic and antagonistic activities. They are:

- **Tamoxifen** is a competitive partial agonist and inhibitor of estradiol at the oestrogen receptor. It is mainly used for treatment of oestrogen dependent breast cancer in doses of 20–40 mg/day. Vaginal bleeding and menopausal syndrome like symptoms may occur as side effects.

- **Raloxifene** is recommended for prevention of osteoporosis in a dose of 60 mg per day. Common adverse effects are hot flushes and leg cramps. Rarely may it cause deep venous thrombosis and pulmonary embolism.

PROGESTINS (PROGESTOGENS)

The major natural progestogen is progesterone. It is secreted by the ovarian corpus luteum and placenta in females, by testes in males, and adrenal cortex in both the sexes. Progestins convert the uterine endometrium from the proliferative to the secretory phase. During pregnancy, progesterone is essential for its maintenance. Progesterone itself is seldom used in clinical practice because of extensive first pass metabolism. Synthetic progesterones or progestins can be administered orally but they are usually less selective because they may have some oestrogenic or androgenic activity.

Progesterone first combines with specific receptor proteins in target cells and then induces synthesis of specific proteins via messenger RNA.

Actions

1. Acting on oestrogen primed endometrium, progesterone prepare it for implantation and growth of the fertilized ovum.
2. Progesterone changes the oestrogen induced watery cervical secretion to a viscid secretion which attenuates sperm penetration.
3. Together with oestrogens, progesterone induces glandular development of mammary gland during pregnancy.
4. If conception occurs, progesterone inhibits further ovulation by feedback inhibition of LH secretion, decreases uterine contractions and reduces uterine sensitivity to oxytocin.
5. Progesterone produces slight increase in body temperature of about 0.5°C and has some degree of anabolic activity due to androgenic activity.
6. Progesterone stimulates lipoprotein lipase activity and leads to fat deposition.

7. There occurs sodium and water retention by progesterone due to its ability to indirectly stimulate aldosterone release by adrenal cortex.
8. Progesterone and related steroids have depressant and hypnotic effect on the brain.

Preparations and Pharmacokinetics

Progestins are of two types:
1. **Progesterone and progesterone derivatives:**
   - Hydroxy progesterone
   - Medroxy progesterone
   - Allyloestrenol
   - Dydrogesterone
   - Megestrol
   - Chlormadinone
2. **Nortestosterone derivatives:**
   - Norethisterone
   - Ethynodiol (prodrug, converted into norethisterone)
   - Norethynodrel
   - Ethinylestrenol
   - Norgestrel
   - Gestronol
   - Norgestimate.

Synthetic progestins are well absorbed from gut and are excreted in urine as glucuronide and sulphate conjugates.

Clinical uses: They have been employed:
- As oral contraceptives either alone or in combination with oestrogens
- To treat habitual or threatened abortion
- In functional uterine bleeding
- In menstrual disorders
- In endometrial carcinoma
- In endometriosis

There may be sodium retention, oedema, hypertension, thrombophlebitis, mental depression, and adverse effect on blood lipids on prolonged use.

Antiprogestins

- Mifepristone is progesterone receptor as well as glucocorticoid receptor antagonist. It is mainly used to terminate early pregnancy. It can also be used as a contraceptive when given once a month during the mid luteal phase. Important side effects are nausea, vomiting, abdominal pain and severe uterine bleeding.

Treatment of Menstrual Disorders

1. Amenorrhoea is treated with cyclical replacement therapy of oestrogens and progesterones.
2. Postponement of menstruation is achieved by giving norethisterone (5 mg thrice daily) starting 3 days prior to expected date of onset and continued through desired period. Withdrawal bleeding ensues 2–3 days after stoppage.
3. Dysfunctional uterine bleeding is controlled by giving norethisterone (5 mg/day) for 7 to 10 days. Norethisterone can also be used prophylactically in doses of 10 mg/day from day 19 to 26 of the menstrual cycle for 2 to 3 cycles. Danazol and non-steroidal anti-inflammatory drugs have also been used.
4. Dysmenorrhoea is treated by inhibiting ovulation (norethisterone or the conventional oral pill) or by non-steroidal anti-inflammatory drugs.
5. Premenstrual tension is treated with combined oral pill, non-steroidal anti-inflammatory drugs, thiazide diuretics and bromocriptine.

> **Types of oral contraceptives**
> - Combination of oestrogen with progestin
> - Sequential regimen
> - Phased regimen preparations
> - Progestin pill (minipill)
> - Oestrogen pill (postcoital or morning after pill.)

ORAL CONTRACEPTIVES

Types of oral contraceptives:

1. **Combination of oestrogen with progestin (oral pills):** This combination therapy is very convenient, relatively less expensive and highly effective. The combination is taken for 21 consecutive days, starting on day-5 of menstruation, followed by 7 days gap during which menstrual bleeding takes place. Various preparations that are available in the market are given in Table 44.1.
2. **Sequential regimen:** In this, oestrogen alone is given for 15–16 days followed by 5 days of oestrogen progesterone combination. At present these preparations have been withdrawn following reports of increased incidence of endometrial carcinoma.
3. **Phased regimen preparations:** These are biphasic or triphasic preparations where the oestrogen and progesterone content of the pill is varied at different time periods to mimic hormonal changes during the normal menstrual cycle. They are regarded as more physiological than the conventional fixed dose combination preparations with lesser incidence of break through

Table 44.1: Some oral contraceptive preparations containing oestrogen-progestogen

Oestrogen	Progestogen	Trade name
Ethinylestradiol (0.05 mg)	Norgestrol (0.5 mg)	Ovral
Ethinylestradiol (0.5 mg)	Ethynodial (1 mg)	Ovulen-50
Ethinylestradiol (0.05 mg)	Lynestrenol (1 mg)	Noracyclin
Mestranol (0.1 mg)	Ethynodiol (1 mg)	Ovulen
Ethinylestradiol (0.05 mg)	Norethisterone (1 mg)	Orlest

bleeding. They are recommended for women above the age of 35 years.

4. **Progestin pill (minipill):** Norethindrone is generally used daily in small doses. Medroxy progesterone is long acting synthetic progestogen which is given intramuscularly once (150 mg) in every 6 weeks for three doses. This will provide long-term contraception. However, contraceptive effect was less reliable and there was increased incidence of breakthrough bleeding.

5. **Postcoital or morning after pill:** High dose estrogen and/or high dose progestin are quite effective in emergency contraception when given immediately after unprotected coitus (rape or condom rupture).

   Following three regimens are available:

   a. Two tablets of the progestin levonor-gestrel (0.75 mg each) are used. The first tablet must be taken as soon as possible (within 48 hours of the coitus) and the second tablet is taken later on but within 72 hours of the coitus. This is more effective (98.75%) and better tolerated than high dose estrogen + progestin combination.

   b. Ethinyl estradiol (50 µg each tablet) + Levonorgestrel (250 µg each tablet) combination is used. Two such tablets are to be taken within 72 hours of the unprotected coitus and then next two tablets after 12 hours. However, success rate is low (90–91 %) and incidence of severe nausea and vomiting is more.

   c. Mifepristone (600 mg) single dose taken within 72 hours of unprotected intercourse is an effective method to prevent pregnancy with lesser side effects. It interferes with implantation of fertilized ovum.

   Mechanism of action:

   - The oestrogen-progestin combination pill prevents ovulation by inhibiting gonadotropin secretion. The main site of their action is hypothalamus. The oestro-

gens induce feedback inhibition of FSH secretion and progestins inhibit the secretion of LH.

- Oestrogen and progesterone inhibit implantation of fertilized ovum on endometrium.
- Progestins induce thick viscid cervical secretion which is less conducive for passage of the sperms.
- Prevention of normal fertilization may occur due to hypermotility of fallopian tube and uterus. This may be the mode of action of postcoital pill.

Side effects: Several adverse reactions to combined type oral contraceptives have been reported. These are:

- Bleeding irregularities
- Amenorrhea
- Nausea, vomiting and gastrointestinal symptoms
- Oedema
- Weight gain
- Mental depression
- Changes in libido
- Thrombophlebitis and pulmonary embolism
- These drugs may alter liver function and may interfere with the metabolism of other drugs.
- There is also risk of developing hypertension in women who are on oral contraceptives.
- Premenstrual migrainous headaches may be aggravated. High incidence of cancer has also been reported.

Oral contraceptives are contraindicated in thromboembolic disease, breast cancer, hepatic dysfunction, cerebral vascular disease, myocardial infarction, coronary artery disease and abnormal uterine bleeding.

Some drugs may induce contraceptive failure either by increasing the metabolism of oral contraceptives by causing enzyme induction (rifampicin, phenytoin, barbiturates, ethanol and carbamazepine) or by suppression of gut microflora (broad-spectrum antibiotics) and hence interfering with enterohepatic cycling of oestrogens.

Oral contraceptives reduce clinical efficacy of antihypertensive and antidiabetic agents as well as antidepressant drug therapy.

6. **Centchroman (ormeloxifene):** It is a nonsteroidal antagonist or selective estrogen receptor modulator. Its brand name is "SAHELI". Each tablet contains 30 mg of centchroman. It is taken twice in a week for first three months and then once a week subsequently to be continued as long as contraception is desired. The first tablet should be taken on the first day of menstrual cycle (e.g. Sunday). Then the second tablet should be taken on 4th day of the cycle (i.e. Wednesday). Subsequent tablets should be taken every Sunday and Wednesday for first three months, followed by once a week on the same day every week, i.e. Sunday or Wednesday. Contraceptive effect of centchroman is readily reversible within 6 months and subsequent pregnancy is normal.

Centachroman is a potent competitive antagonist at peripheral estrogen receptors and suppress proliferative stage of endometrium. It also accelerates ovum transport without affecting ovulation. Summarily, it desynchronizes the event of ovum transport with endometrial phases of development.

It is devoid of all the side effects of steroidal oral contraceptives. It does not exhibit androgenic, antiandrogenic or progestational properties; likewise it does not affect the secretions of pituitary, thyroid or adrenal hormones in its oral contraceptive doses. Important contraindications are:

- Jaundice or hepatic dysfunction
- Polycystic ovarian disease
- Cervical hyperplasia
- Tuberculosis
- Renal disease
- Hypersensitivity with centachroman

TO REMEMBER

1. Natural sex hormones are not available by oral route. Although they are readily absorbed from gut, they are rapidly metabolized in the liver.

2. Androgens are used in premenopausal carcinoma; oestrogens are used in primary and metastatic forms of prostate carcinoma; and progesterones are used in endometrial carcinoma.

3. Cyproterone is a progesterone derivative which suppresses gonadotropin synthesis and release, leading to suppressed spermatogenesis and testosterone synthesis. It is effective in treating precocious puberty, acne, masculinization in females.

4. Danazol is an ethisterone derivative which also inhibits gonadotropin synthesis and release. It is the first choice drug in endometriosis.

5. Clomiphene, cyclofenil and tamoxifen are selective competitive antagonists of oestrogen on oestrogen receptors. They increase gonadotropin activity and are used in anovulatory sterility. Tamoxifen is mainly used to treat oestrogen dependent breast cancer.

6. Mifepristone is a progesterone antagonist which is used in termination of early pregnancy as well as a contraceptive when given once a month during the mid luteal phase.

7. Contraceptive failure may be induced either by increasing the metabolism of oral contraceptives by causing enzyme induction by rifampicin, phenytoin, barbiturates, ethanol and carbamazepine or by suppression of gut microflora by broad-spectrum antibiotics and hence interfering with enterohepatic cycling of oestrogen.

Section 12

Chemotherapy

Chapter 45

General Considerations

Definitions

1. **Chemotherapy:** Paul Ehrlich was the person who coined the term chemotherapy. It denotes systemic treatment of specific infective conditions by chemical substances which injure the invading organisms without causing injury to host. These chemical substances are called chemotherapeutic or antimicrobial agents.

2. **Antibiotics:** These are chemical substances. They are produced by microorganism such as fungi, bacteria and actinomycetes. They suppress the growth of other microorganisms and may eventually destroy them. Although antibiotics are mainly produced by microorganisms, many are now obtained semisynthetically and some, e.g. chloramphenicol, can be completely synthesized. So it will be more appropriate to use the term antimicrobial agent (AMA) for both synthetic as well as naturally obtained drugs that attenuate microorganisms.

3. **Bacteriostatic agents:** These antibiotics/antimicrobials do not kill the organisms. They reversibly inhibit the growth and multiplication of susceptible microorganisms. Antifungal agents are known as fungistatic. Examples of bacteriostatic drugs are macrolide group of antibiotics, oxazolidine, chloramphenicol, tetracyclines, sulphonamides, trimethoprim, clindamycin, nitrofurantine and ethambutol.

4. **Bactericidal agents:** These antimicrobials irreversibly damage and kill the susceptible microorganisms. They act best against multiplying organisms. Fungicidal is the term used for antifungal agents. Examples of bactericidal drugs include beta-lactam antibiotics, cotrimoxazole, aminoglycosides, fluoroquinolones, vancomycine, polymyxin, bacitracin, isoniazid, pyrazinamide, and rifampicin.

Mechanism of Action of Antimicrobials

1. Inhibition of bacterial cell wall synthesis leading to loss of viability and cell lysis, e.g. penicillins, cephalosporins, monobactams, carbapenams and glycopeptide group of antibiotics (vancomycin, teicoplanin and daptomycin).

2. Interfering with cell membrane function leading to leakage of intracellular compounds, e.g. polymyxin B, amphotericin B and colistin.

3. Interfering with DNA-RNA synthesis. The nucleic acid synthesis can be inhibited by five different mechanisms as under:
   - By inhibiting the synthesis of folate (e.g. sulfonamides and trimethoprim), purine and pyrimidine.
   - By altering the base pairing properties of the template, e.g. acriflavin antiseptic. These agents intercalate (get inserted) in the DNA and inhibit its synthesis.
   - By inhibiting either DNA or RNA polymerase, e.g. rifampicin acts by

inhibiting the bacterial RNA polymerase and foscarnet acts by inhibiting the viral RNA polymerase.

- By inhibiting DNA gyrase enzyme (topoisomerase II in gram-negative bacteria and topoisomerase IV in gram-positive bacteria). Example is fluoroquinolones. In therapeutic doses, fluoroquinolones only inhibit bacterial topoisomerase and not mammalian topoisomerase.
- By directly damaging DNA and its functioning, e.g. metronidazole, an antiprotozoal drug, that acts partly by this mechanism.

4. Inhibition of protein synthesis or structure in a reversible manner, e.g. erythromycin, tetracyclines and chloramphenicol.
5. Interfering with initiation complex and causing misreading of mRNA, e.g. amino glycoside antibiotics.

Antimicrobial agents (penicillin, aminoglycosides, rifampicin and polymyxin B) that induce alteration in chemical structure of the cell wall, membrane or interference with nucleic acid (DNA or RNA) lead to lysis and cidal (lethal) effect on the microbes. They are called bactericidal drugs. On the other hand, inhibitors of protein synthesis (erythromycin, tetracycline, and chloramphenicol), structure or metabolism (sulphonamides and trimethoprim) prevent growth and replication. They are called bacteriostatic agents.

Superinfection and Pseudomembranous Colitis (PMS)

The natural indigenous bacterial flora is present in gastrointestinal tract and oral cavity. It provides resistance to colonization and limits the growth of other pathogenic flora. Antibiotic therapy markedly inhibits natural bacterial flora. Due to this, there occurs invasion of opportunistic organisms such as Proteus, resistant staphylococci and Pseudomonas, etc. This is called superinfection. It is manifested as antibiotic induced diarrhoea and colitis. Superinfection due to *Clostridium difficile* or Candida (a fungus) is more serious and leads to pseudomembranous colitis (PMS). It is characterized by bloody diarrhoea, abdominal distension with pain, dehydration and leukocytosis. This occurs with amoxicillin, third generation cephalosporins and clindamycin. It is treated with metronidazole (500 mg orally, three times a day for 10 days) or with vancomycin (125 mg orally four times a day for 10 days). Other drugs have also been tried such as vancomycin + rifampicin, teicoplanin, bacitracin and re-establishment of colonial flora by lactobacilli and *Saccharomyces boulardii* (probiotics).

Bacterial Resistance to Antimicrobial Drugs

A state of insensitivity or decreased sensitivity of microorganisms to drug is called bacterial resistance. It occurs after repeated use of the drug.

Genetic methods of antibiotic resistance:

Mutation: It may occur in originally sensitive microorganisms which undergo a genetic change. Mutation is the common cause of resistance to antimicrobial agents. It is a stable and heritable genetic change. It occurs spontaneously and randomly among microorganisms. Few mutant cells in any sensitive population are selectively preserved because they require higher concentration of AMA for inhibition. They get a chance to proliferate when sensitive cells are removed by AMA. It may be a single step mutation resulting in a high degree of resistance as seen in case of streptomycin, and rifampin. In other cases, it may be a multiple step mutation in which resistant mutants may emerge by a slow stepwise process, e.g. in case of penicillin.

Plasmids: These are actually vectors that serve as a carrier of DNA molecule. Most bacteria contain such extrasomal genetic elements which can replicate independently and freely in cytoplasm. 'R'-plasmids carry genes resistant to antibiotics (r-genes). These r-genes can get readily transferred from one 'R'-plasmids to another plasmid or to chromosome. This can occur as under:

Transfer of 'r'-genes from one bacterium to another: This can occur in one of the following ways:

• **Conjugation:** This is the main method of transfer of 'r'-gene from one bacterium to another by conjugating plasmids (extrachromosomal genetic elements), which can cause the bacterium to make a connecting tube between bacteria, through which the plasmid itself (and other plasmids) can pass.
• **Transduction:** It is the transmission of an 'r' gene-carrying plasmid into a bacterium by a bacterial virus (phage).
• **Transformation:** In this case, a resistant bacterium may release the resistance carrying DNA into the medium which may be imbibed by another sensitive organism. Due to this later becomes unresponsive to drug.

Transfer of 'r'-genes between plasmids within the bacterium:

• **By transposons:** Transposons are DNA segments of genetic material with insertion sequences at the end of gene. They cannot self-replicate. However, they can self transfer between plasmids or from plasmid to chromosomes. In this case, the donor plasmid, containing a transposon, co-intigrates with the acceptor (or target) plasmid. During this process, the transposon can replicate. The plasmids then separate and each contains the r-gene carrying the transposons. Some strains of staphylococci and enterococci can acquire resistance by transposons and cause

virtually untreatable noscomial (those acquired in hospital) infections.
• **By integrons:** "Intigron" is a larger mobile DNA unit. It can be located on a transposon. It is packed with multiple gene cassettes which are encoded with several bacterial functions including resistance and virulence.

Biochemical mechanisms may be responsible for drug resistance as under:

1. The antibiotics can be inactivated by enzymes synthesized by a large number of organisms. Classical examples are:
   • Beta-lactam antibiotics are inactivated by beta lactamases which are produced by staphylococci and enteric gram-negative rods.
   • Aminoglycosides are inactivated by several enzymes which are produced by both gram-positive and gram-negative organisms.
   • Chloramphenicol is inactivated by chloramphenicol acetyltransferase, produced by resistant strains of gram-positive and gram-negative organisms.
2. Both gram-positive and gram-negative bacteria may develop resistance to tetracycline, aminoglycosides, betalactamases, chloramphenicol and polymyxins due to biochemical alteration of their envelope. Due to this, accumulation of drug in the bacteria is decreased.
3. Organism may show resistance to penicillin, erythromycin, aminoglycosides, rifampin, etc. due to mutation of their drug binding sites.
4. Staphylococci and many other bacteria may show resistance to sulphonamides and trimethoprim by developing alternative metabolic pathways.

Cross-resistance is seen in microorganisms resistant to a certain antimicrobial agent. They will also show resistance to other chemically related drugs having the same mechanism of antimicrobial action, e.g. cross-resistance amongst different sulphonamides, tetracyclines, beta-lactam antibiotics, aminoglycosides, etc.

Combination of Antimicrobial Drugs

The simultaneous use of two or more antimicrobial agents is some times justified. Combination should be judiciously chosen keeping in mind their effect on the microorganisms as well as the host. Attempt should be made to use only bactericidal drugs. However, indiscriminate use of such combinations is to be avoided because of the following disadvantages:

- Increased toxicity
- Possibility of superinfection
- Antagonism of antibacterial action on concomitant use of bacteriostatic and bactericidal drugs
- Development of resistance against both drugs
- Erroneous dosage (excessive amounts or suboptimal dose)

Combinations of antimicrobial agents may be indicated in:

- Treatment of mixed bacterial infections as in the case of abdominal, pulmonary or urinogenital tract infections.
- To severe infections of unknown etiology as in septic shock with urinary tract infection.
- To prevent the development of resistant microorganisms as in case of treatment of tuberculosis where combination of three antimicrobial agents is used.
- To enhance antibacterial activity (synergistic combinations) as:
  - In the treatment of enterococcal endocarditis (penicillin and streptomycin)
  - In therapy of pseudomonas infection (carbenicillin plus gentamicin)

- Combination of sulphonamides with trimethoprim against infections caused by microorganisms that are resistant to sulphonamides alone
- Amphotericin B and rifampin in antifungal infection
- Amoxycillin and clavulanic acid to enhance antibacterial spectrum

Selection of an Antimicrobial Drug

An ideal chemotherapeutic agent should be selectively toxic to the organism without producing any harmful effect to the host. So the physician should select a proper antimicrobial agent based on clinical judgment, microbiological factors and the pharmacological features of the drug. It is really very unfortunate that these precautions are not always taken care of while prescribing antimicrobial agents. Hence serious side effects and bacterial resistance may appear due to irrational prescribing. Whenever clinician is not certain about the infecting organism, he should take the help of bacteriological diagnosis based on cultures of blood, urine and other body fluids.

Points for Dental Students

Antimicrobial agents are frequently prescribed in clinical practice. So a dental student must learn the general principles of chemotherapy thoroughly for their rational use. This will help him while prescribing these drugs in dental practice. A dentist must take care of the following points while prescribing antimicrobial agents in dental practice:

1. Indiscriminate use of antimicrobial agents should be avoided.
2. These drugs should be given in proper doses for a full duration.
3. Concomitant use of antimicrobial agents or fixed dose combinations should be used on strict rational basis as discussed above.

4. Some antimicrobial agents suppress normal non-pathogenic bacterial flora of gut, oral cavity and respiratory tract. Hence inorder to avoid superinfection with opportunistic pathogenic organisms proper measures must be taken as discussed above.

5. Failure of drug therapy on prolonged use may be due to development of bacterial resistance to the drug. This may require dose adjustment or change of drug.

6. Antimicrobial agents are also used for prophylaxis. Specific indications for chemoprophylaxis in dental practice have been discussed in Chapter 75.

TO REMEMBER

1. Chemotherapy denotes systemic treatment of specific infective conditions by chemical substances, which are called chemotherapeutic agents.

2. Antibiotics are chemical substances which are produced by microorganisms and suppress the growth of other microorganisms and may eventually destroy them.

3. Bacteriostatic antimicrobials reversibly inhibit the growth and multiplication of susceptible organisms.

4. Bactericidal antimicrobials irreversibly damage and kill the microorganisms.

5. An antimicrobial agent may act by: (i) inhibition of cell wall synthesis; (ii) interfering with cell wall function; (iii) interfering with DNA-RNA synthesis; (iv) inhibition of protein synthesis or structure; (v) causing misreading of mRNA; and (vi) inhibiting the bacterial metabolism.

6. Bacterial resistance means insensitivity or decreased sensitivity of micro-organisms to drugs. A sensitive microorganism may become resistant by undergoing a genetic change. Further, in some cases biochemical mechanisms may be responsible for drug resistance.

7. When an antibiotic removes natural antibiosis of non-pathogenic organisms against pathogenic ones in the intestine, respiratory and genitourinary tracts, superinfection may occur.

8. The simultaneous use of two or more antimicrobial agents is some times justified. However, indiscriminate use of such combinations is to be avoided.

9. An ideal chemotherapeutic agent should be selectively toxic to the organism without producing any harmful effect to the host.

Chapter 46

Sulphonamides and Trimethoprim

SULPHONAMIDES

Sulphonamides were the first chemotherapeutic agents. They were introduced in 1935 and were employed systematically for the prevention and cure of bacterial infection in man. But, with the development of hosts of safe and effective antibiotics and emergence of sulphonamide resistant strains, their importance as chemotherapeutic agents has decreased.

Sulphonamides are derivatives of p-aminobenzoic acid (PABA). They are prepared either substituting the amido- or the p-amino group. Sulphonamides are bacteriostatic agents. They competitively inhibit bacterial dihydrofolate synthetase enzyme and block the utilization of PABA. Due to this, they prevent the synthesis of folic acid which is essential to bacterial growth. Human beings do not synthesize folic acid. They obtain it through their diet. Hence sulphonamides selectively inhibit microbial growth. Sulphonamides are effective against gram-negative and gram-positive microorganisms. Their antibacterial activity can be reversed by the presence of pus, tissue fluids and drugs that contain PABA. Bacterial resistance to sulphonamides has emerged due to widespread indiscriminate use, especially in cocci and some gram-negative bacilli. Resistance may be due to mutation of dihydrofolate synthetase, over production of PABA or loss of bacterial plasma membrane.

Pharmacokinetics

Most of the sulphonamides are readily absorbed from the gastrointestinal tract with the exception of sulphasalazine and pthalylsulphathiazole which are designed for their local actions in bowel. Sulphonamides are widely distributed throughout all tissues of the body. They can cross placental barrier and reach the fetal circulation. Sulphadiazine and sulfisoxazole are effective in meningeal infections because they can reach in adequate concentrations in cerebrospinal fluid. All sulphonamides are bound to plasma proteins, particularly to albumin by varying degrees. They are metabolized in liver and excreted in the urine in free (active) and acetylated (inactive) forms.

Adverse Reactions

Headache, fever, skin rashes, gastrointestinal upsets, stomatitis, eosinophilia, etc. are common side effects. Rarely allergic reactions such as agranulocytosis, thrombocytopenia and vasculitis have been reported. Stevens-Johnson syndrome is a manifestation of long acting sulphonamides which are now not used. Less soluble sulphonamides induce urinary tract disturbances due to crystalluria. Drug interactions may occur due to plasma protein binding property of sulphonamides. In presence of deficiency of glucose-6-phosphate dehydrogenase, sulphonamides may lead to haemolytic anaemia.

Preparations and Doses

I. **Rapidly absorbed and rapidly eliminated sulphonamides:** Sulphadiazine, sulfisoxazole, sulphamethoxazole. All of them are used in doses of 2–4 gm followed by 1 gm 6 hourly orally.

II. **Well absorbed but poorly excreted sulphonamides:** Sulphamethoxy pyridazine, sulphamoxole, sulphaphenazole. They are given in doses of 1 gm (initially) followed by 0.5 gm daily orally. Sulphamethoxine is given in single dose of 2 gm every 7th day.

III. **Poorly absorbed sulphonamides:** Phthyalylsulphathiazole, and succinylsulphathiazole are used for intestinal disinfection in doses of 10–20 gm daily in divided doses. Sulphasalazine is another sulphonamide which is employed in intestinal disorders in doses of 2–8 gm per day (ulcerative colitis and regional enteritis).

IV. **Sulphonamides for topical use:**
   a. *Sulphacetamide:* Its sodium salt is extensively used in the management of ophthalmic infections. Ophthalmic solutions of 10, 20 and 30% concentrations and ointment (10%) are used. Usual dose is 1–2 drops three to four times a day.
   b. *Silver sulphadiazine:* It is used topically in concentration of 1% to reduce the microbial infections of wounds from burns.
   c. *Mefenide:* It is used in concentrations of 2–5% cream locally for reducing the infection of burn wound.

TRIMETHOPRIM

It is a pyrimidine derivative. It inhibits the enzyme dihydrofolate reductase which catalyses the conversion of dihydrofolic acid to tetrahydrofolic acid, essential for bacterial growth. It is bacteriostatic and effective against most common bacterial pathogens. Resistance to trimethoprim develops due to mutation of bacterial dihydrofolate reductase. It is commonly used in combination with selected sulphonamides. Its pharmacokinetics is similar to that of sulphonamides. However, it is highly concentrated in prostatic and vaginal fluids due to its relatively acidic nature. Nausea, vomiting and skin rashes are common adverse reactions. Rarely megaloblastic anaemia occurs which can be prevented by folinic acid.

Cotrimoxazole

It is a combination of trimethoprim (80 mg) and sulphamethoxazole (400 mg). Both the drugs are well absorbed from gastrointestinal tract. About 75% of trimethoprim and 65% of sulphamethoxazole are bound to plasma proteins. Up to 60% of trimethoprim and 25–50% of sulphamethoxazole are excreted in the urine in 24 hours.

There are many advantages of this combination such as:
- The combination has bactericidal effect due to sequential block of bacterial tetrahydrofolate synthesis.
- Antimicrobial spectrum is wider (active against salmonella)
- Toxicity is less because of reduced doses in the combination.
- Chances of drug resistance are reduced due to dual mode of action.

Therapeutic Uses of Sulphonamides and Trimethoprim

These drugs are effective against gram-positive and gram-negative bacteria, Chlamydia and Nocardia. Individual uses of sulphonamides and trimethoprim are very limited. For systemic therapy, the most widely used drug is cotrimoxazole. Sometimes a combination of sulphadiazine (410 mg) and trimethoprim (90 mg) is used. Trimethoprim can be used alone for genitourinary infections (UTI, prostatitis, or vaginitis).

1. **Topical/local:** Sulphonamides alone are used but their topical applications may lead to allergic sensitization, especially of the skin.
    i. Sulphacetamide solution (30%) or ointment (10%) is used to treat conjunctivitis and trachoma.
    ii. Silver sulphadiazine and marfanil are employed topically to protect burned skin surface from infecting bacterial flora.
    iii. Sulphasalazine (salicylazosulphapyridine) is widely used to treat ulcerative colitis and other inflammatory bowel disorders. Sulphasalazine splits into 5-aminosalicylate (anti-inflammatory) and sulphapyridine (antibacterial) by colonic bacterial flora.

2. **Systemic:**
    i. Most commonly used preparation is cotrimoxazole which is employed in doses of 2 normal tablets/12 hours or 1 double strength (DS) tablet/12 hour. *Important indications are:*
    - Urinary tract infections, cystitis, and pyelonephritis, if uncomplicated and previously untreated, are effectively treated by cotrimoxazole.
    - Respiratory tract infections such as bronchitis and pneumonia. It is drug of choice in Nocardia infection. It is also used in whooping cough.
    - Intestinal infections such as shigella dysentery and cholera. It is an alternative drug for the treatment of enteric fever.
    - Meningitis, caused by meningococci or Haemophilus.
    - Other bacterial infections such as beta-haemolytic streptococcal infection, methicillin resistant staphylococcal infection, brucellosis, granuloma inguinale, otitis media, gonorrhoea, prostatitis and bacterial vaginitis.
    ii. Pyrimethamine + a sulphonamide (sulphadoxine, or sulphadiazine or sulfisoxazole) are in use for resistant malaria of falciparum origin.
    iii. Although dermatitis herpetiformis is not an infective disorder, it responds to sulphapyridine.

Points for Dental Students

Sulphonamides should not be prescribed in patients receiving primaquine antimalarial drug to avoid haemolytic effect. At present cotrimoxazole is not used in the treatment of orofacial infections.

TO REMEMBER

1. Sulphonamides are derivatives of para-aminobenzoic acid (PABA). They are bacteriostatic and selectively inhibit microbial growth of gram-positive and gram-negative organisms.
2. Trimethoprim is a pyrimidine derivative and a bacteriostatic drug.
3. Individual uses of trimethoprim and sulphonamides are very limited. They are often used in combination. One such commonly used combination is cotrimoxazole. In combination, they exert a bactericidal effect due to sequential block. Sulphonamides competitively inhibit dihydrofolate synthetase enzyme and block the utilization of PABA in micro-organism and thus prevent synthesis of folic acid. Trimethoprim inhibits the enzyme dihydrofolate reductase which catalyses the conversion of dihydrofolic acid to tetrahydrofolic acid, essential for bacterial growth.

4. Cotrimoxazole is used in urinary, respiratory and gastrointestinal infections, meningitis, and other bacterial infections.
5. Pyrimethamine plus sulphonamide are used in resistant malaria of falciparum infection.
6. Sulphasalazine is widely used to treat ulcerative colitis and other inflammatory bowel disorders.
7. Sulphacetamide solution is used topically to treat conjunctivitis including trachoma.
8. Silver sulphadiazine and marfanil are used topically to protect burned skin surface from infecting bacterial flora.
9. In general the importance of sulphonamides as chemotherapeutic agents has decreased due to development of hosts of safe and effective antibiotics and emergence of sulphonamide resistant strains.

Chapter 47

Beta-Lactam Antibiotics

PENICILLINS

Although penicillin was discovered by Alexander Fleming from Penicillium mould in 1928, it was first used as antibacterial therapy by Chain and Florey in 1941. The basic nucleus of all penicillins is 6-aminopenicillanic acid. Pencillins have:

- A thiazolidine ring
- A beta-lactam ring and
- A side chain.

The penicillins are bactericidal. They act by inhibiting bacterial cell wall peptidoglycan synthesis by inhibiting the transpeptidation reaction which is catalyzed by penicillin binding proteins (PBPs). These proteins are transmembrane surface enzymes present in bacteria. Peptidoglycan is composed of parallel "glycan" (polysaccharide) chain which is cross-linked by "peptide chains" by a pentoglycin bridge. The process of cross-bridging is called as the transpeptidation reaction. The penicillins are classified as:

I. Narrow Spectrum Penicillins

a. β-Lactamase sensitive natural penicillins
  i. *Acid stable:*
    - Penicillin-V (phenoxymethyl penicillin; oral)
  ii. *Acid labile:*
    - Penicillin-G (benzyl penicillin; i.m., i.v.)

- Procaine penicillin-G (i.m., depot inj.)
- Benzathine penicillin-G (i.m., depot inj.)

b. β-Lactamase resistant (anti-staphylococcal penicillins)
  i. *Acid stable* (oral, i.m.)
    - Cloxacillin
    - Dicloxacillin
    - Flucloxacillin
  ii. *Acid labile* (i.m., i.v.)
    - Methicillin
    - Naficillin

II. Extended Spectrum Penicillins

All are sensitive to β-lactamase degradation.
  i. *Acid stable*—aminopenicillins (oral/ parenteral)
    - Ampicillin
    - Bacampicillin
    - Talpicillin
    - Amoxycillin
  ii. *Acid labile*—antipseudomonal penicillins (parenteral)
    - Carbenicillin
    - Ticarcillin
    - Piperacillin
    - Mezlocillin
    - Azlocillin

III. Reverse Spectrum Penicillins

(Mainly active against gram-negative bacilli such as *E. coli, Enterobacter, Klebsiella, Salmonella*

and *Shigella*; *Pseudomonas*, indole-positive *Proteus*, *Serratia* and enterococci are resistant). These are acid stable penicillins.
- Mecillinam (amdinocillin)
- Pivmecillinam (Prodrug; oral)

Pharmacokinetics

With the exception of penicillin V and acid resistant penicillins such as ampicillin, cloxacillin, amoxycillin, etc. most penicillin congeners are poorly absorbed from gastrointestinal tract. Since food delays absorption of oral penicillins, these should be given half to one hour before or 1–2 hour after meal. So other penicillins are given parenterally. Penicillins are widely distributed in the body. However, they do not cross the blood–brain barrier being lipid insoluble. In the presence of inflammation, the permeability into CSF is increased. Penicillins cross the placental barrier. Penicillins are not metabolized in the body. They are rapidly excreted in urine. About 90% of renal excretion is by active tubular excretion. Probenecid prolongs the duration of action of penicillins by competitively inhibiting its tubular secretion. Nafcillin can be given in renal failure because 80% is excreted in bile.

Adverse Drug Reactions

- The most important side effects of the penicillins are hypersensitivity reactions (seen in 5–8% patients). These are due to: (a) major antigenic determinant—penicilloic acid or (b) minor determinants—benzyl penicillin itself or sodium benzyl penicillioate +host proteins (become antigenic). These can be classified as:
  i. Immediate (most common; occur within 20 minutes of parenteral administration; mediated by IgE antibodies against the minor determinants): Urticaria, pruritus, wheezing, sneezing, and rhinitis which

may pass over to anaphylaxis in 0.5% cases.
  ii. Accelerated (within 72 hours; mediated by IgE antibodies against major antigenic determinants): Rash, fever, and urticaria; rarely usually non-fatal angioneurotic oedema)
  iii. Late (after 72 hours; mediated by IgE and IgM antibodies against the major antigenic determinants): Morbidiform urticaria or erythematous eruption, local inflammatory reactions, lymphadenopathy, splenomegaly, serum sickness and Coomb positive haemolytic anaemia.

There is cross-allergy amongst all penicillins. In case the use of penicillin is essential, intradermal skin test (Penicilloyl polylysine+ penicillin) must be carried out to test for penicillin sensitivity. In cases of severe anaphylactic shock, adrenaline is the therapy of choice.
- Broad-spectrum penicillins may lead to superinfections with Pseudomonas, staphylococci, Proteus or *Candida albicans*.
- Ampicillin may give rise to diarrhoea and macular rashes (not allergic in nature).
- Methicillin and nafcillin cause nephritis.
- Carbenicillin may give rise to hypokalaemic alkalosis and bleeding.
- When penicillin is injected in a syphilitic patient (particularly secondary syphilis) it may produce Jarisch-Herxheimer reaction (shivering, fever, myalgia, exacerbation of lesions, even vascular collapse), due to sudden release of spirochetal lytic products. Aspirin and sedation will relieve symptoms.

Therapeutic Uses

1. **Coccal infections:** Streptococcal infections, gonorrhea, pneumonia, pneumococcal meningitis, non-beta-lactamase producing staphylococcal infections and bacterial endocarditis.

2. **Gram-positive rods:** Tetnus, anthrax, gas gangrene.
3. **Spirochaetes:** Yaws, syphilis, leptospirosis.
4. **Actinomycetes:** Actinomycosis.
5. **Cloxacillin** is used to treat betalactamase producing staphylococcal infections.
6. Penicillin G benzathine is a long acting penicillin. It is employed to treat or for prophylaxis of streptococcal pharyngitis in doses of 1.2 million units per week intramuscularly.
7. Amoxycillin and ampicillin are broad spectrum penicillins. Out of the two, amoxicillin is preferred because it is better absorbed orally and is less liable to cause diarrhoea. In addition to the above mentioned indications, they are also used for urinary tract infection (coliforms), Shigella dysentry, salmonella and Haemophilus infections.
8. Carbenicillin or ticarcillin is employed to treat Pseudomonas infection.
9. Amoxycillin and penicillin V are used to treat odontogenic infections such as dental alveolar abscess, acute necrotizing ulcerative gingivitis, Vincent angina, etc.
10. Penicillins are some times combined with other drugs either to improve pharmacokinetics of penicillin or increase drug sensitivity, e.g.
    a. To improve pharmacokinetics: Ampicillin + probenecid.
    b. To increase drug sensitivity:
       • Pencillin + gentamicin for bacterial endocarditis.
       • Carbenicillin+gentamicin for Pseudomonas infection
    c. To extend antibacterial spectrum to betalactamase producing bacteria:
       • Amoxycillin + clavulanic acid.
       • Ampicilliin + sulbactam
       • Ampicillin + cloxacillin
       • Amoxycillin + cloxacillin.

11. Prophylactic uses:
    • Rheumatic fever: Benzathine penicillin 1.2 MU i.m. every 4 weeks till 18 years of age or 5 years after attacks whichever is more.
    • Gonorrhoea or syphilis: Procaine penicillin or benzathine penicillin 2.4 MU i.m. (single dose) before or within 12 hours of contact.
    • To prevent bacterial endocarditis in patients with valvular heart disease that is likely to occur during dental extraction, endoscopies, catheterization and other surgical procedures.
    • Agranulocytosis: Penicillin may be used alone or in combination with an aminoglycoside antibiotic.
    • Surgical infections: Procaine penicillin 1 MU with an aminoglycoside i.m. 1 hour before and 8 to 12 hours after surgery.

Doses of Penicillins

• Penicillin G: 300–600 mg (0.5–1 million units)/6 h i.m.
• Procaine penicillin: 360 mg (0.6 million units)/12 to 24 h i.m.
• Penicillin V: 130–250 mg/6 h oral
• Ampicillin: 250–500 mg/6 h oral
• Amoxycillin: 250–500 mg/8 h oral
• Cloxacillin: 250–500 mg/6 h oral
• Carbenicillin: 1–2 gm/6 h i.m.
• Becampicillin: 400–800 mg/day oral
• Dicloxacillin: 250 mg/6 h oral.
• Oxacillin: 500–1000 mg/6h oral
• Azlocillin: 4 g i.v.

CEPHALOSPORINS

Cephalosporium acremonium mould produces cephalosporins. The basic nucleus of cephalosporins is 7-aminocephalosporanic acid. Antibacterial activity of cephalosporin is similar to broad-spectrum penicillins. Like penicillin, they also act by inhibiting the bacterial cell wall peptidoglycan synthesis. They resist attack by betalactamases. They are inactivated by cephalosporinase enzyme.

Some cephalosporins (e.g. cephalexin, cefadroxil, cephradine, cefaclor, cefuroxime, cefixime) are absorbed orally. Most others have to be given intravenously. Intramuscular injections are painful and avoided. These drugs are excreted in the urine except cefuperazone and ceftriazone which are excreted through bile. Probenecid blocks the renal excretion of cephalosporins.

The antibacterial activity of different cephalosporins is widely variable. Depending on this, they are classified as under:

1. First generation (cephalexin, cefadroxil, cefazolin, cephaloridine, cephradine, cephalothin, cephapirin): These cephalosporins are active against gram-positive cocci, some gram-negative bacteria (*E. coli*, *Klebsiella*, *Proteus*), some anaerobes (cocci).

2. Second generation cephalosporins (cefuroxime, cefaclor, cephamandole, cefotetan, cefonicid, ceforamide, cefoxitin) are active against organisms affected by 'first generation drugs but less potent against gram-positive bacteria. Some of them (cefuroxime, cefaclor) are active against *H. influenzae* and some others (cefoxitin, cefotetan) against *B. fragilis* and *N. gonorrhoeae*. These can be used against betalactamase producing organisms and anaerobes.

3. Third generation cephalosporins (ceftriazone, cefotaxime, cefuperazone, cefuroxime, cefixime, ceftizoxime, ceftazidime, moxalactam, latamoxef) provide extended coverage against gram-negative organisms and most of these reach the central nervous system. These are also active against *Pseudomonas*, *Haemophilus* and *Nisseria*. Ceftizoxime act against *B. fragilis*.

Therapeutic Uses

1. First generation cephalosporins are used in urinary tract infection, bronchitis, and minor infections.

2. Second generation cephalosporins can be used against beta-lactamase producing organisms and anaerobes.

3. Third generation cephalosporins are used to treat meningitis caused by pneumococci and *H. influenzae*, resistant urinary tract infection and penicillin resistant gonococci.

4. Fourth generation cephlosporins (cefpirome) is used in the treatment of serious and resistant hospital acquired infections such as septicemia, lower respiratory tract infection, etc.

5. These antibiotics have proved useful in preventing infection at the time of biliary surgery, orthopedic surgery on fracture and particularly in heart surgery. The older agents, i.e. cephalothin and cepharin are not useful as prophylactic agents.

6. Cephalexin is used in odontogenic infection.

Doses: The doses vary with the severity of the disease. The commonly used doses are:
a. For oral agents 0.25–0.5 gm 6 hourly;
b. For parenteral agents 0.5–1 gm i.v. 6 hourly; can also be given intramuscularly.
c. For betalactamase resistant agents: 0.5 to 1.0 gm i.v. 6–8 hourly.

Adverse Effects

- The primary side effect of cephalosporins is hypersensitivity.
- Prolonged use of cephalosporins may produce blood dyscrasias (neutropenia, thrombocytopenia) and nephritis.
- Second and third generation cephalosporins may cause superinfection with resistant staphylococci, enterococci and candida on prolonged use.

- Disulfiram-like reactions may sometimes be seen on ingestion of alcohol.

CARBAPENEMS

Imipenem: It is a beta-lactam antibiotic. It is not inactivated by betalactamase enzyme. It is given intravenously because its oral bioavailability is erratic and poor. It is widely distributed in body tissues and fluids. It is inactivated by dihydropeptidase of renal tubules. So it is given in combination with cilastatin, an inhibitor of dihydropeptidase. This combination is used to treat infections caused by gram-positive and gram-negative aerobes and anaerobes. Common adverse reactions are gastrointestinal tract upsets, allergic reactions, confusion and convulsions.

Meropenem: It is not inactivated by dihydropeptidase. So it is not given in combination with cilastatin. Another clinical advantage is the lower likelihood of convulsions which are associated with imipenam.

Carbacephems: Loracarbef (Lorabid) belongs to carbacephem class. Its chemical structure is similar to that of cefaclor and its antibacterial spectrum resembles those of the second generation cephalosporins. It is given orally. It is excreted in urine.

Monobactams: Aztreonam, carumonam and tigemonam are monobactams. They are resistant to betalactamases. Out of these, aztreonam is used clinically intravenously. It is active against gram-negative rods including *Haemophilus*, *Nesseria* and *Pseudomonas*. It is not effective against gram-positive bacteria and anaerobes. Adverse drug reactions are allergy, gastrointestinal upsets, hepatitis and blood dyscrasias.

Betalactamase inhibitors: Clavulanic acid, sulbactam and tazobactam are betalactamase inhibitors. They do not have any antimicrobial activity. They protect penicillins from degradation by binding covalently to betalactamases. So they are employed in combination with penicillins (ampicillin, amoxycillin, or ticarcillin) for treating betalactamase producing organisms, such as *H. influenzae*). The combination in use is:

- Amoxycillin + clavulanic acid
- Ampicillin + sulbactam
- Ticarcillin + clavulanic acid
- Piperacillin + tazobactam

These drugs do not inhibit betalactamases produced by *Pseudomonas aeruginosa* and Enterobactor species. Further, methicillin resistant staphylococci are not susceptible to these drugs.

Points for Dental Students

Commonly used β-lactam antibiotics in dental practice are:

1. Amoxicillin is used to treat orofacial infections.
2. Amoxicillin + clavulanic acid or erythromycin or roxithromycin or clindamycin is used for orofacial infection caused by β-lactamase producing bacteria.
3. Amoxicillin + metronidazole or amoxicillin + clavulanic acid + metronidazole is used to treat periodontal infections (polymicrobial in nature).
4. Cefuroxime (II generation), cefpodoxime and cefixime (III generation) with or without metronidazole have good activity against orofacial pathogens while limited activity against oral anaerobes.
5. A combination of one of the above cephalosporins + clavulanic acid with or without metronidazole is used for severe polymicrobial infection.
6. Meropenem (i.v.) has very wide-spectrum and not hydrolysed by most β-lactamases. It is used for acute aerobic + anaerobic orofacial infections.

TO REMEMBER

1. The penicillins are bactericidal drugs and act by inhibiting bacterial cell wall synthesis.

2. The most important side effects of penicillin are hypersensitivity reactions that extend from rashes to occasional anaphylactic shock which can be fatal. So in cases where use of penicillin is essential, intradermal skin test must be carried out to test for 'penicillin sensitivity.

3. Carbenicillin or ticarcillin is employed to treat *Pseudomonas* infection.

4. Antibacterial activity of cephalosporins is similar to broad-spectrum penicillins. They also act by inhibiting the bacterial cell wall synthesis. The primary side effect of cephalosporins is hypersensitivity.

5. Disulfiram like reaction may occur with cephalosporins on ingestion of alcohol.

6. Imipenem is a beta-lactam antibiotic which is not inactivated by betalactamase enzyme. It is given i.v. because its oral bioavailability is erratic and poor.

7. Monobactams are resistant to beta-lactamase and are given i.v. Commonly used drug is aztreonam.

8. Clavulanic acid, sulbactam and tazobactam are betalactamase inhibitors. They do not have any antimicrobial activity but are used to protect penicillins from degradation from betalactamases.

Chapter 48

Aminoglycoside Antibiotics

Aminoglycoside antibiotics contain amino-sugars in glycosidic linkage. Aminoglycosides which end up with suffix 'mycin' are obtained by various streptomyces while those which end up with suffix 'micin' are obtained by other sources such as natural, synthetic or semisynthetic. Drugs included in this group are streptomycin, paramomycin, kanamycin, neomycin, tobramycin, amikacin, gentamicin, netilmicin and sisomicin. Gentamicin and sisomicin are produced by the mould *Micromonospora purpurea*. Netilmicin is a synthetic drug.

Important Features of these Antibiotics

- All these drugs share many chemical, antimicrobial, pharmacological and toxic characteristics.
- All these antibiotics are bactericidal.
- They are active against gram-positive and gram-negative organisms.
- Mycobacterium tuberculosis infection responds to streptomycin and kanamycin, while amikacin, gentamicin and tobramycin are active against *Streptococcus faecalis* and *Pseudomonas aeruginosa* also.
- Aminoglycoside antibiotics act directly on the bacterial ribosomes where they inhibit protein synthesis by interfering with translation of genetic code. For this purpose initially, the aminoglycosides enter the bacteria by passive diffusion. When given along with β-lactam antibiotics, there occurs synergistic action because β-lactam antibiotics weaken the bacterial cell wall by inhibiting its synthesis and further facilitate the passive diffusion of aminoglycosides. Subsequently, energy and oxygen dependent active transport is needed for the transport of aminoglycosides across the cytoplasmic membrane to reach the ribosomes. So aminoglycosides are inactive against anaerobic bacteria due to lack of oxygen.
- Aminoglycosides are water soluble and more active at alkaline pH probably due to improved transport of the antimicrobial agents inside the bacterial cell.
- Human ribosomes are unaffected.
- Development of resistance against amino-glycosides is very common in gram-negative bacteria and mycobacteria.
- Aminoglycosides show post-antibiotic effect for several hours even when their serum concentration falls below their MIC. This is due to disruption in 30S ribosomal function and resumption of bacterial ribosomal function requires time for the synthesis of new ribosomes. So it is suggested that these drugs can be given in a single daily dose despite their short half-life (1–3 hours). A single daily dose results in a higher peak tissue concentration than if the total daily dose is divided and given at 8 or 12 hourly intervals.

- Absorption of aminoglycosides from gastrointestinal tract is poor. However, they are rapidly absorbed from intramuscular and subcutaneous sites of injection.
- They reach to all body fluids but do not cross the blood–brain barrier. So they do not reach the CSF or eye.
- Neomycin is not used systemically. It is applied topically.
- Aminoglycosides are not metabolized. They are mainly excreted by kidney.
- The most important adverse effects are:
  - *Ototoxicity (cochlear damage:* tinnitus, hearing disturbances, complete deafness; *vestibular damage:* vertigo, nystagmus, balancing problem and ataxia): Streptomycin, gentamicin, and tobramycin mainly affect vestibular function whereas cochlear function is mainly affected by kanamycin, amikacin and neomycin. They should be given carefully to pregnant mothers because they cross the placenta and can cause fetal eight nerve damage.
  - *Nephrotoxicity:* These drugs may lead to tubular necrosis. Nephrotoxicity is enhanced by simultaneous use of loop diuretics or cephalosporins with aminoglycosides.
  - Aminoglycoside antibiotics possess neuromuscular blocking property. So rarely they may lead to skeletal muscular weakness and respiratory weakness. These drugs, therefore, should not be used in patient with myasthenia gravis or along with neuromuscular blocking agents.

Therapeutic Uses

Systemic: With the availability of broad-spectrum penicillins, cephalosporins and fluoroquinolones, therapeutic uses of aminoglycosides are very much limited.

> **Gentamicin combinations**
>
> Gentamicin + Metronidazole: For pelvic sepsis
> Gentamicin + Penicillin: For septicaemic sepsis
> Gentamicin + Ampicillin: For coliform infection
> Gentamicin + Penicillin: For bacterial endocarditis
> Gentamicin + Carbenicillin: For pseudomonas infection

Streptomycin and kanamycin are still kept reserved for resistant tubercular infections. Gentamicin is used in some selected systemic infections. Tobramycin is an alternative. Important indications of gentamicin are:

- For severe infections (septicaemia or abdominal or pelvic sepsis) gentamicin + penicillin are used. In pelvic infections, gentamicin may be combined with metronidazole (active against *B. fragilis*).
- To treat acute coliform infections of urinary tract or other places, gentamicin is used along with ampicillin or cephalosporin.
- For treatment of bacterial endocarditis, caused by *Streptococcus viridans* or *Streptococcus faecalis*, gentamycin is used along with penicillin.
- To treat *Pseudomonas* infection, gentamycin is used in combination with carbenicillin or ticarcillin. However, tobramycin is preferred to gentamicin.
- Gentamicin may also be used to treat plague, brucellosis and tularaemia.

In gentamicin or tobramycin resistant cases, amikacin or nitilmicin may be used.

Doses of gentamicin or tobramycin: 40–80 mg/ 8 hr i.m. or i.v.

Topical: Neomycin, framycetin or even gentamicin is used as ointment or solution for infection of mucous membranes (eyes or ear) or skin (burns or wounds). Neomycin is also used orally to sterilize bowel before abdominal surgery and also in hepatic failure. In the later condition, sterilization of bowel minimizes production of bacterial toxins and resultant hepatic coma.

Aminoglycosides have no use in the management of orofacial infections in dental practice.

TO REMEMBER

1. Aminoglycosides contain amino sugars in glycoside linkage. Drugs included in this group are streptomycin, kanamycin, gentamicin, paromomycin, amikacin and neomycin.
2. They are effective against gram-positive and gram-negative organisms. *Mycobacterium tuberculosis* infection responds to streptomycin and kanamycin, while amikacin, gentamicin and tobramycin are active against *Streptococcus faecalis* and *Pseudomonas aeruginosa* also.
3. They act directly on bacterial ribosomes where they inhibit protein synthesis and interfere with translation of genetic code.

4. Development of resistance against aminoglycosides is very common in gram-negative bacteria and *Mycobacterium*.
5. The most important adverse effects are ototoxicity, and nephrotoxicity.
6. With the availability of broad-spectrum penicillins, cephalosporins and fluoroquinolones, therapeutic uses of aminoglycosides are very much limited.
7. Streptomycin and kanamycin are still kept reserved for resistant tubercular infections.
8. Gentamicin (alternative—tobramycin) is used in some severe systemic infections such as septicaemia, sepsis, bacterial endocarditis, *Pseudomonas* infection, etc.
9. Neomycin, framycetin or even gentamicin are used as ointment or solution for infection of mucous membranes (eyes or ear) or skin (burns or wounds).

Chapter 49

Tetracyclines and Chloramphenicol

TETRACYCLINES

The tetracyclines are broad-spectrum antibiotics. They have different chemical structures and are produced by different species of *Streptomyces*. They are effective against gram-positive and gram-negative bacteria including anaerobes, Spirochaetes, Mycoplasma, Chlamydia and Rickettsia. Two serious limitations of these drugs are:

• Bacteriostatic activity
• Significant adverse drug reactions

All tetracyclines are similar in mechanism of action, antimicrobial activity, pharmacology, therapeutic uses, cross-resistance and adverse drug reactions. However, they may differ in pharmacokinetics.

Tetracyclines enter the microorganisms by passive diffusion through the hydrophilic channels in case of gram-negative bacteria and an energy dependent tetracycline active transport system in case of gram-positive bacteria. However, doxycycline and minocycline diffuse through the bacteria by porin channels as well as by passive diffusion being more lipid soluble. Subsequently tetracyclines are transported by a protein carrier system across the inner cytoplasmic membrane from periplasmic space. Then they bind reversibly to 30S subunit of the bacterial ribosome. Due to this, all tetracyclines act by inhibiting bacterial protein synthesis by blocking the attachment of aminoacyl tRNA to the "A" site (acceptor site on the 50S subunit

of ribosome). As a result of this, the peptide chain fails to grow. Since the binding to ribosomes is reversible, they are bacteriostatic. Bacterial resistance may develop which is primarily plasmid-mediated and is an inducible trait. It may be due to:

• Decreased accumulation of tetracycline because the permeability barrier of the cell envelope does not allow tetracyclines to concentrate intracellularly.
• Presence of ribosome protection proteins which decrease access of tetracycline to the ribosome.
• Inactivation of tetracyclines by enzyme.

The commonly available tetracyclines are classified on the basis of their duration of action as under:

a. **Shorter duration of action (6–10 hrs):**
   • Tetracycline
   • Chlortetracycline
   • Oxytetracycline
b. **Intermediate duration of action (12–13 hrs):**
   • Demeclocycline
   • Methacycline
c. **Longer duration of action (18–20 hrs):**
   • Doxycycline
   • Minocycline

All the tetracyclines are substituted derivatives of a polycyclic structure (four 6-membered rings).

Most of the tetracyclines are partially absorbed from the gastrointestinal tract. However, in case of minocycline and doxycycline, absorption is complete. Since they form insoluble chelates with calcium, magnesium, and other metal ions, they should not be administered with milk (calcium), magnesium hydroxide, and aluminium hydroxide or iron preparations. Tetracyclines tend to alter the intestinal bacterial flora due to partial absorption and thus lead to superinfection. Food delays absorption. Tetracyclines are widely distributed in tissues and body fluid. They cross the placental barrier but not the blood–brain barrier. With the exception of chlortetracycline, all other tetracyclines do not undergo metabolism. Tetracyclines differ widely in the amount excreted in urine. These are also secreted in bile and a significant amount is excreted via the faeces.

Therapeutic Uses

1. Tetracyclines are used in the treatment of infections caused by:
   - Chlamydia(trachoma, psittacosis, lymphogranuloma venereum)
   - Mycoplasma pneumoniae (pneumonia)
   - Rickettsia (typhus fever, Q fever)
   - Spirochaetes (relapsing fever, lyme disease)
   - Gram-negative infections (brucellosis, tularaemia, plague and cholera).
2. Tetracyclines have been employed for intestinal amoebiasis, actinomycosis and *P. falciparum* malaria.
3. Minocycline is used to treat meningococcal carrier state for 5 days. However, rifampicin is preferred.
4. Demeclocycline has a special use to treat chronic hyponatraemia due to syndrome of inappropriate antidiuretic hormone secretion.
5. Post-radiation osteonecrosis may occur as complication of treatment of oral squamous cell cancer. Topical tetracycline rinses may reduce the potential local irritation from the microbial flora.
6. Tetracycline has been used topically for treatment of recurrent aphthous stomatitis and periodontitis.
7. Usually tetracyclines are not recommended in acute orofacial infections due to their bacteriostatic action. However, doxycycline can be used to treat localized juvenile periodontitis (LJP) due to actinomyces.

At present their use has decreased due to development of resistant strains of bacteria and the availability of newer antimicrobial agents. They have no place as prophylaxis to prevent individuals with viral illness from developing a bacterial infection. These are not to be used for pharyngitis and for staphylococcal infections.

Adverse Drug Reactions

- On oral administration, tetracyclines may cause nausea, vomiting, diarrhoea, epigastric burning, and hepatotoxicity.
- Superinfection with Candida, Proteus and Pseudomonas may occur.
- With the exception of doxycycline, tetracyclines should not be used in the presence of renal dysfunction because they may cause renal necrosis.
- Photosensitization often occurs with demeclocycline.
- Minocycline may produce vestibular disturbances such as dizziness, vertigo, nausea and vomiting.
- Tetracyclines readily chelate calcium and get deposited in newly formed bone and teeth. So they should not be prescribed to pregnant women and to children less than 6 years of age.

Doses (Oral)

- Tetracycline, chlortetracycline and oxytetracycline: 250–500 mg/6 hr.
- Doxycycline: 200 mg on first day, then 100 mg/day

- Minocycline: 100 mg /12 hr.
- Demeclocycline and methacycline: 300 mg/ 12 hr.

CHLORAMPHENICOL

Chloramphenicol is a broad-spectrum antibiotic. Originally, it was derived from streptomyces venezuelae but now it is produced entirely by synthetic process.

Chloramphenicol is a bacteriostatic drug to most organisms but is bactericidal to *H. influenzae*. It acts by inhibiting bacterial protein synthesis. It inhibits peptide bond formation by preventing binding of aminoacyl t-RNA to 50S ribosomal subunits. The drug can also inhibit protein synthesis in mammalian mitochondrial cells by binding to 70S ribosomes. Bacterial resistance to chloramphenicol develops slowly. It may be due to:

- Decreased permeability to the drug as a result of permeability barrier of the envelope of the cell.
- Protection of ribosome by ribosome protection proteins. This leads to decreased affinity of chloramphenicol to the binding site.
- Inactivation of the drug by chloramphenicol acetyltransferase enzyme produced by resistant organisms.

Chloramphenicol is effective against Rickettsia, Chlamydia, Mycoplasmae, large number of gram-positive and gram-negative organisms, *Salmonella typhi* (however, more susceptible to chloramphenicol).

On oral administration, it is completely absorbed. Peak plasma concentration occurs at 2 hours and the plasma half-life is 2–4 hours. It is widely distributed in the body fluids and tissues including brain and CSF. It is metabolized in liver either by conjugation with glucuronic acid or by reduction to inactive aryl amines. Free and metabolites of chloramphenicol are excreted in urine.

Therapeutic Uses

Because of its adverse drug reactions, chloramphenicol is no longer the drug of choice for any disease. However, it is an alternative drug for several diseases such as:
- Enteric (typhoid) fever
- *H. influenzae* meningitis
- Severe rickettsial infection
- Infections by anaerobic organisms (sepsis)
- Pneumonia or laryngotracheitis caused by Haemophilus.
- It can be used topically for eye and ear infections as drops and ointment.

Dose: Chloramphenicol—500 mg/6 hr oral. Chloramphenicol is not indicated in orofacial infections.

Adverse Drug Reactions

- Chloramphenicol may cause skin rash, drug fever, angioneurotic oedema, dermatitis and haemorrhage.
- Dose related bone marrow depression is a serious adverse reaction. Due to this there may occur anaemia, leukopenia, thrombocytopenia, agranulocytosis and aplastic anaemia. So it is advisable to do regular blood smear examinations during the therapy.
- Non-dose related or idiosyncratic aplastic anaemia may occur very rarely due to genetic cause. It is a serious adverse effect which is irreversible and even fatal. Usually it occurs after repeated courses of the drug. However, sometimes it may occur after ocular administration or after a single dose.
- Chloramphenicol should not be used in neonates and infants because it produces *Gray baby syndrome* which is characterized by anorexia, vomiting, lethargy, abdominal distension, irregular respiration, hypothermia, peripheral vascular collapse, gray cyanosis, shock-like condition and death. It occurs because liver enzymes are not fully developed in neonates and infants.

Drug Interactions

- Chloramphenicol inhibits liver microsomal enzymes. So it prolongs half-life of phenytoin, tolbutamide, chlorpropamide, and possibly warfarin.
- Simultaneous use of tetracycline or chloramphenicol with a bactericidal agent (penicillin or aminoglycoside) may reduce the bactericidal action of the later.
- Chloramphenicol should not be prescribed to a patient receiving primaquine anti-malarial drug to avoid haemolysis.

TO REMEMBER

1. Tetracyclines and chloramphenicol are broad-spectrum antibiotics, i.e. they are effective against gram-positive and gram-negative bacteria including anaerobes, Spirochaetes, Mycoplasma, Chlamydia and Rickettsia.
2. Two serious limitations of these drugs are:
    - Bacteriostatic property
    - Significant adverse drug reactions.
3. Tetracyclines and chloramphenicol act by inhibiting bacterial protein synthesis at 30S ribosomes and 50S ribosomes, respectively.
4. The use of tetracyclines has decreased due to development of resistant strains of bacteria and the availability of newer antimicrobial agents. They should not be used to prevent bacterial infection during viral illness as well as for pharyngitis and staphylococcal infection.
5. Tetracyclines may lead to super infection with Candida, Proteus and Pseudomonas.
6. With the exception of doxycycline, tetracyclines should not be used in the presence of renal dysfunction because they may cause renal necrosis.
7. Tetracyclines should not be given to pregnant women and to children under 6 years of age because they readily chelate with calcium and get deposited in bones and teeth.
8. Chloramphenicol is no longer the drug of choice for any disease because of its serious adverse reactions such as bone marrow depression. However, it is an alternative drug for several diseases such as enteric fever, *H. influenzae* meningitis, anaerobic sepsis, etc.
9. It should not be used in neonates and infants because it produces Gray baby syndrome.

Chapter 50

4-Quinolones and Fluoroquinolones

Nalidixic acid is a 4-quinolone derivative. It was introduced in 1963. The other members of the group are oxolinic acid and cinoxacin. Since systemic antibacterial levels of 4-quinolone derivatives are not achieved, they are only useful as urinary antiseptic. Later on fluorinated derivatives of 4-quinolones have been introduced. They are called fluoroquinolones. The important features of fluoroquinolones are:

- Wide antibacterial spectrum
- High bacterial sensitivity
- Desirable pharmacokinetics
- Low toxicity

Classification: Based on their introduction:

Group I
- Ciprofloxacin
- Norfloxacin
- Pefloxacin
- Ofloxacin

Group II
- Lomefloxacin
- Levofloxacin

Group III
- Sparfloxacin
- Gatifloxacin

Group IV
- Moxifloxacin

Mechanism of Action

Fluoroquinolones enter the bacterial cell by passive diffusion through porin channels. Intracellularly, in gram-negative bacteria, they block DNA synthesis by inhibiting DNA gyrase enzyme. They also inhibit topoisomerase IV, mainly in gram-positive bacteria and thus interfere with DNA function. They are bactericidal. Resistant organisms emerge rapidly during therapy with 4-quinolones (nalidixic acid). In case of fluoroquinolones, development of resistance is slow. It occurs either due to change in permeability of the bacterial envelope or a change in target enzyme. No cross-resistance exists between these drugs and non-quinolone drugs. So they are very useful in the treatment of multidrug resistant infections.

On oral administration, all the quinolones are well absorbed. Fluoroquinolones are widely distributed in most of the tissues and body fluids. They also cross the placental barrier. 80% of 4-quinolones is metabolized in liver and 20% is excreted in urine in free form. About 20% of fluoroquinolones is metabolized and 80% of these drugs are excreted as such in urine. Some amount of the drug is eliminated in bile also.

Antibacterial Spectrum

Group I

These are mainly effective against aerobic gram-negative bacilli (*E. coli*, *Klebsiella*, *Proteus*, *Pseudomonas*, *Schigella*, *H. influenzae*, *Salmonella typhi*) and gram-negative cocci (*N. gonorrhoeae*). These are less effective on gram-

341

positive cocci and have no effect on MRSA and anaerobes.

Group II

In addition to group I antibacterial spectrum these are also effective against gram-positive cocci (*Streptococcus pneumoniae*), *Chlamydia*, and *Mycoplasma*.

Group III

In addition to group I antibacterial spectrum, these are also effective against gram-positive cocci (*Streptococcus, Staphylococcus*), *Entrococcus*, anaerobes, *Mycobacterium avium* complex in AIDS, sexually transmitted disease in males e.g. gonoccocal urethritis.

Group IV

In addition to group III antibacterial spectrum, it is also used in community acquired pneumonia.

Therapeutic Uses

1. 4-quinolones (nalidixic acid) are used in urinary tract infection caused by coliform organisms.
2. Important uses of fluoroquinolones:
   i. Therapeutic uses common to all fluoroquinolones:
      • Multi-antibiotic resistant infections
      • Salmonella infections (enteric fever including carrier state)
      • Dysentery due to Shigella infection
      • Pseudomonas infections (urinary tract infection and others)
      • N-gonorrhoea (a single dose is sufficient)
      • Septicaemia (severe infection)
   ii. Special therapeutic features to individual drug:
      a. *Norfloxacin:* It is not good for systemic infection due to poor availability. It has limited uses only such as urinary tract infection due to coliform organisms, diarrhoea, prostatitis and gonorrhoea.
   b. *Ciprofloxacin:* It is drug of first choice for typhoid fever. It also cures carrier state. So there are less chances of relapse. It is also used as drops or ointment in eye infections. It is also used in odontogenic infection.
   c. *Ofloxacin:* It is very useful in uretheritis, cervicitis, and odontogenic infection.
   d. *Pefloxacin:* It is accumulated in CSF. So it is useful in meningitis and N. meningitides.
   e. *Lomefloxacin:* It has similar uses as that of ciprofloxacin.
   f. *Levofloxacin:* It is also effective in gram-positive cocci (*Streptococcus pneumoniae*), *Chlamydia* and *Mycoplasma*.
   g. *Sparfloxacin and gatifloxacin:* These are also used in infections caused by gram-positive cocci (*Streptococcus, Staphylococcus, Enterococcus*), anaerobes, *Mycobacterium avium* complex in AIDS, sexually transmitted disease in males, e.g. gonococcal urethritis. Gatifloxacin is used in odontogenic infections.
   h. *Moxifloxacin:* It is also used in community acquired pneumonia.

Adverse Drug Reactions and Contraindications

Toxicity profile is same with 4-quinolones and fluoroquinolones. However, incidence of adverse reactions is low with fluoroquinolones. These drugs may cause rash, pruritus, photosensitivity, headache, drowsiness, confusion, convulsions and gastrointestinal upsets. Ciprofloxacin may be hepatotoxic. Superinfection may also occur.

Absorption of fluoroquinolones is inhibited by antacids (Al^{++} and Mg^{++} salts), Zn^+ and iron while probenecid inhibits renal clearance of these drugs. With the exception of ofloxacin, fluoroquinolones increase half-life of theophylline and warfarin by inhibiting hepatic metabolizing enzymes.

Fluoroquinolones are contraindicated:

- In children, during pregnancy and lactating mothers because these drugs may cause arthropathy in infants and children.
- In patients of epilepsy and cerebral arteriosclerosis because they may precipitate convulsions.

  Doses of these drugs should be reduced in presence of renal dysfunction.

Special Features of Fluoroquinolones and Doses

1. **Ciprofloxacin:** Widely used. Dose: 250–750 mg/12 hours orally. Single dose (250 mg) treatment for gonorrhoea.
2. **Norfloxacin:** Absorption is partial. Dose: 400 mg/12 hours oral. Single dose (800 mg) is curative for gonorrhoea.
3. **Pefloxacin:** Its clearance from body is inhibited by cimetidine. Dose: 400 mg/12 hours oral.
4. **Ofloxacin:** Its absorption is complete. It does not inhibit hepatic metabolizing enzymes. Dose: 200–400 mg/day oral.
5. **Levofloxacin:** It is levoisomer of ofloxacin having improved antibacterial spectrum. Its t½ is 10 hrs. Dose: 500 mg/day oral.
6. **Sparfloxacin:** It is difluorinated quinolone. Its t½ is about 20 hrs. Dose: 200–400 mg orally in one or two divided doses.
7. **Lomefloxacin:** It is also difluorinated quinolone. Its t½ is 10 hrs. Dose: 400 mg once daily orally.
8. **Gatifloxacin** has enhanced activity as sparfloxacin. Its t½ is 8–12 hrs. Dose: 400 mg on first day followed by 200 mg once daily for 7 to 10 days.
9. **Moxifloxacin:** Its t½ is 12 hrs. Dose: 400 mg once daily for 7 to 10 days.

Points for Dental Students

1. With the exception of ofloxacin, fluoroquinolones increase half-life of theophylline and warfarin by inhibiting hepatic metabolizing enzymes. A dentist must keep this point in mind while prescribing drug from this group to a patient who is receiving either theophylline or warfarin.
2. Ciprofloxacin + tinidazole or ofloxacin + ornidazole are used for refractory periodontitis associated with Enterobacteriacea.

TO REMEMBER

1. Nalidixic acid and 4-quinolones are only useful as urinary antiseptics because systemic antibacterial levels are not achieved.
2. However, fluorinated derivatives of 4-quinolones are bactericidal and have wide antibacterial spectrum, high bacterial sensitivity, desirable pharmacokinetics, low toxicity and slow emergence of bacterial resistance.
3. Fluoroquinolones are very useful in the treatment of multi-drug resistant infections.
4. Fluoroquinolones are contraindicated in children, during pregnancy, and in lactating mothers because these drugs may produce arthropathy in infants and children.
5. Ciprofloxacin is widely used while norfloxacin is used for urinary tract infection and gonorrhoea due to its partial absorption.
6. Acrosoxacin and enoxacin are used in single dose in gonorrhoea.
7. Levofloxacin is indicated in community acquired pneumonia and exacerbations of chronic bronchitis.
8. Cimetidine inhibits the clearance of perfloxacin from the body while ofloxacin does not inhibit the hepatic metabolizing enzymes.

Chapter 51

Erythromycins and other Antimicrobial Drugs with Special Indications

ERYTHROMYCINS

Erythromycins are macrolide antibiotics, consisting of lactone ring to which sugars are attached. The antibacterial spectrum is similar to that of penicillin. They are effective against gram-positive organisms (streptococci, pneumococci, staphylococci, corynebacteria and anthrax) and gram-negative organisms (*Neisseria*, *Helibactor*, *Legionella*, *Mycoplasma*, *Chlamydia*, *Spirochaetes*). They act by inhibiting bacterial protein synthesis at 50S ribosome subunits and interfere with 'translocation'. They may have bactericidal or bacteriostatic activity depending on the microorganism and concentration of the drug used. Bacterial resistance to erythromycins is common especially amongst staphylococci. It occurs due to chromosomal mutation of the binding site on 50S subunit of bacterial ribosome or plasmid mediated (becomes less permeable to erythromycin or produce an erythromycin esterase).

They are readily absorbed on oral administration. Erythromycin base is broken down by gastric acidity. So acid stable preparations such as stearate, succinate, and estolate esters of erythromycin and enteric coated tablets are used. Erythromycin is primarily excreted in the bile and thus appears in the faeces.

Newer macrolide derivatives have been synthesized. They have better pharmaco-

> **Limitations of erythromycin**
> - Narrow spectrum
> - Gastric intolerance
> - Acid labile
> - Low oral bioavailability
> - Poor tissue penetration
> - Shorter half-life

kinetics and lower incidence of adverse drug reactions. However, antibacterial spectrum is same.

Preparations, Doses and Special Features

- Erythromycin—acid labile, short half-life.
  Dose: 250 mg/6 hours oral.

Newer Macrolides

[Better pharmacokinetics; less adverse drug reactions]

- Roxithromycin—acid stable, better absorption, longer half-life, plasma protein binding 95%.
  Dose: 150 mg/12 hours oral.
- Azithromycin—longer half-life, given once a day, plasma protein binding is lowest, relatively wider antibacterial spectrum.
- Clarithromycin—long half-life, metabolites also active, relatively wider antibacterial spectrum.
- Dirithromycin—acid stable, longer acting, given once daily.

- Troleandomycin and oleandomycin—pharmacokinetic features similar to erythromycin; 80% excreted in faeces via the bile and 20% unchanged through urine.
- Spiramycin—incompletely absorbed from gut but is given orally as well as i.v.; metabolized in liver; 90% excreted in bile and only 10% in urine; plasma half-life 8 hrs.
- Telithromycin—the enhanced activity of this drug is most likely due to:
  - Tighter binding of ketolides to ribosome
  - Additional ribosome binding sites
  - Slow dissociation from the ribosome
  - Rapid drug accumulation

Therapeutic Uses

Erythromycins and newer macrolides are drugs of choice for:
- Diphtheria
- Plague
- Mycoplasma
- Pneumonia
- Chlamydia
- Trachoma
- Genital infections
- Odontogenic infections

Clarithromycin is also used:
- As a component of triple drug regimen to eradicate *H. pylori* infection
- As first line drug in the combination regimen for *Mycobacterium avium* complex (MAC) infection in AIDS patients
- As second line drug for other atypical mycobacterial diseases as well as leprosy

Azithromycin is also used in combination for prophylaxis and treatment of MAC infections in AIDS patients.

Non-chemotherapeutic uses:
- Erythromycin may be useful in rheumatoid arthritis, cystic fibrosis, chronic sinusitis and asthma due to its anti-inflammatory effects by decreasing proinflammatory cytokines release from phagocytes.
- Erythromycin may be used to improve gastric emptying in cases of diabetic gastroparesis, being a motiline receptor agonist. Motiline is a regulatory peptide of gastrointestinal tract that stimulates contraction of the stomach in phases leading to enhanced gastric empting.

Uses of macrolides in dental practice:
- Erythromycin or roxithromycin or clarithromycin is used in β-lactam antibiotic allergic patients with acute orofacial infections.
- Clarithromycin is also useful for endocarditis prophylaxis.
- Azithromycin is effective against oral spirochetes and gram-negative anaerobes found in orofacial infection. It also has lesser chances of drug interactions.
- Clarithromycin is most effective against gram-positive anaerobes (e.g. *Actinomyces*).

Adverse Effects

- Erythromycins estolate may cause allergic reactions (fever, eosinophilia, skin eruptions); less common with other salts of erythromycin or with other macrolides.
- Epigastria distress due to stimulation of gastric smooth muscle motiline receptors; less with azithromycin and clarithromycin.
- Obstructive jaundice/cholestatic hepatitis is common with erythromycin estolate than with other macrolides; less with clarithromycin and rare with azithromycin.
- Reversible ototoxicity (hearing loss) with erythromycin in a dose exceeding 4 gm/day. It may be seen with other macrolides in patients with AIDS.
- Intravenous administration of erythromycin may cause thrombophlebitis.

These drugs increase half-life of warfarin, theophylline, digoxin, carbamazepine and cyclosporine by inhibiting cytochrome P-450.

OTHER ANTIMICROBIAL DRUGS WITH SPECIAL INDICATIONS

Treatment of Anaerobic Infections

i. **Lincomycin and clindamycin:** Lincomycin is an antibiotic. It is obtained from streptomyces lincolnensis. Clindamycin is chlorinated derivative of lincomycin and is more potent. So clindamycin is used clinically.

Clindamycin is readily absorbed from gastrointestinal tract. It is widely distributed in the body except CSF. It is excreted in urine and bile with some enterohepatic circulation. Its metabolites are also active. It acts by inhibiting protein synthesis due to its attachment with 50 S subunit of bacterial ribosomes. It is effective against gram-positive cocci and anaerobes. It is used in the treatment of severe anaerobic infection caused by Bacteroides and other anaerobes. It is combined with an aminoglycoside to treat mixed infection. In dentistry, it is used to treat odontogenic infections resistant to β-lactam antibiotics. Its dose is 150–300 mg/6 hour oral.

Common adverse reactions are gastrointestinal upsets and rashes. Some times it causes neutropenia and hepatic dysfunction. The most severe reaction is clindamycin associated pseudomembranous enterocolitis due to *Clostridium difficile* superinfection which is potentially fatal complication. It should be promptly treated with oral vancomycin or metronidazole.

ii. **Metronidazole:** It is a synthetic antiprotozoal drug. By reduction of its nitro group, it is converted into active form which prevents nucleic acid formation combining with DNA. It is used for the treatment of anaerobic infection (caused by Bacteroids and Clostridia) and mixed infections in combination with cephalosporins. In dentistry, its combination with β-lactam antibiotics is frequently used to treat chronic refractory periodontitis as well as serious acute orofacial infections. Dose is 50 mg/8 hour oral. Tinidazole is another antiprotozoal drug which is used for same purpose as metronidazole.

Treatment of Penicillin Resistant Infection

i. **Spectinomycin:** Chemically, it is related to aminoglycosides. It is a bacteriostatic antibiotic. It is effective against grampositive and gram-negative organisms. It attaches to 30 S subunit of ribosomes and inhibits bacterial protein synthesis. It is only used as an alternative treatment for penicillin-resistant gonorrhoea. Since it is not absorbed orally, it is administered i.m. Allergy, nephrotoxicity, dizziness and insomnia may occur as adverse effects.

ii. **Vancomycin:** It is glycopeptide. It is produced by streptomyces orientalis. Oral administration is restricted to treat antibiotic associated entrocolitis because it is not absorbed from gut. It is given intravenously for systemic effects and is widely distributed in the body. However passage to CSF is irregular. It is excreted in urine. It is effective in gram-positive and gram-negative cocci and *C. difficile*. It acts by inhibiting bacterial cell wall synthesis. It is used parenterally to treat resistant staphylococcal sepsis or endocarditis and orally to treat antibiotic associated pseudomembranous entrocolitis. Dose is 125 mg/6 hour. To avoid diffuse flushing infusion should be given over a period of 1 hour. Phlebitis, mild ototoxicity and nephrotoxicity may occur.

iii. **Fusidic acid (sodium fusidate):** It is steroid antibiotic which is active against gram-positive bacteria. On oral administration, it is readily absorbed and widely distributed. It is metabolized. It acts by inhibiting protein synthesis and is mainly employed to treat penicillin-resistant staphylococcal infections, especially osteomyelitis because it is concentrated in bones. It is available as ointment for skin infections. Gastrointestinal upsets, skin rashes and jaundice may occur as adverse effects. It is given in doses of 50 mg/8 hours.

iv. **Teicoplanin:** It has structural resemblance with vancomycin. It is effective against gram-positive bacteria. It is given once a day because it has prolonged half-life (50 hours). It is given systemically for endo-carditis and peritonitis.

Treatment of Urinary Tract Infection (UTI)

Urinary tract infections are caused by coliforms (*E.coli, Proteus, Klebsiella, Enterobactor*), *Pseudomonas aeruginosa*, enterococci and *Staph. Saprophyticus* commonly. They are quite common and sometimes difficult to treat because of rapid emergence of resistant strains and recurrence of UTI in women, enlarged prostate, structural abnormality of urinary tract, and due to ineffective treatment. A drug will be effective when excreted in urine in active form. Low doses of suitable antimicrobials may be effective in lower urinary tract infection while full dose of a drug is required for upper urinary tract infection.

Systemic antimicrobial can be used for upper or lower urinary tract infection while

---

Prophylaxis for urinary tract infection

This may be required during:
- Catheterization or instrumentation
- Use of indwelling catheters
- Presence of uncorrectable abnormalities of urinary tract
- Inoperable enlarged prostate
- Urinary stasis due to chronic obstruction

---

urinary antiseptics are useful for lower urinary tract infection. Following antimicrobials are effective in the treatment of urinary tract infection. They have already been discussed in detail.

- Cotrimoxazole
- Ampicillin
- Amoxycillin
- Carbenicillin
- Third generation cephalosporins
- Gentamicin
- Nalidixic acid
- Norfloxacin
- Trimethoprim
- Sulphonamides

All of them are effective against coliform while carbenicillin, cephlosporins, gentamicin and norfloxacin are also effective against Pseudomonas infection. In addition to the above nitrofurantoin, mendelamine, 4-quinolones and acidifying agents are also used to treat urinary tract infection.

i. **Nitrofurantoin:** It is a synthetic nitrofuran derivative. On oral administration, it is readily absorbed, metabolized and excreted in urine. It is only useful as urinary antiseptic because of its rapid excretion. It is used to treat lower UTI caused by coliforms. For acute UTI, it is given in doses of 100 mg four times a day while for chronic UTI as well as a prophylactic in recurrent UTI, it is administered in doses of 100 mg per day. It should be administered with meals. The action of nalidixic acid is antagonized by nitrofurantoin. It may cause gastric upsets, haemolytic anaemia in glucose-6-phosphate dehydrogenase deficiency and rarely neuropathies and allergic reactions. It is contraindicated in renal insufficiency.

ii. **Methenamine mandelate (mandelamine):** It is a salt of mandelic acid and methenamine. It is employed only as a urinary antiseptic for lower UTI. It is effective due to formaldehyde, released in acidic urine. On oral administration, it is readily absorbed and excreted in urine. For desired effect, urine must be made acidic by giving ascorbic acid (4–12 gm/day). It is effective against most of the urinary organisms except proteus because this organism makes the urine alkaline. Sulphonamides should not be given along with it because they form an insoluble compound with formaldehyde. Gastritis and cystitis may occur as side effects. It should not be used in the presence of renal and hepatic failure. It is kept reserved to treat chronic and recurrent UTI not responding to other drugs.

iii. **4-quinolones (already discussed):** They are used to treat UTI caused by *E. coli* and some of other coliforms. Nalidixic acid, oxolinic acid and cinoacin are 4-quinolones which are employed to treat lower UTI as urinary antiseptics.

iv. **Acidifying agents** are required to keep the urine acidic while using nitrofurantoin or mandelamine. They also keep down bacteriuria which may be useful in chronic or recurrent UTI. For this purpose, ascorbic acid and ammonium chloride are used.

Linezolid

It is an oxazolidinones. It is effective against gram-positive pathogens only because they lack specific efflux pumps. It is not effective against gram-negative bacteria because it efflux out the antibiotic. It acts by binding to the 50S subunit and thus it inhibits the formation of tertiary initiation complex and prevents translation. On the other hand, a number of old antibiotics control bacterial growth through the inhibition of prokaryotic RNA transcription and protein translation. Due to different mechanism of action linezolid is free from cross-resistance.

It is recommended in the treatment of:
- Vancomycin resistant Enterococcus infections
- Pneumonia caused by gram-positive bacteria
- Skin and soft tissue infection caused by gram-positive bacteria
  Dose: 60 mg i.v. or oral every 12 hours.

Common adverse effects are nausea, vomiting, diarrhoea, headache, oral candidiasis and pain at the infection site. Rarely it causes enzyme induction, atrial fibrillation, renal failure, thrombocytopenia.

TO REMEMBER

1. Erythromycins are macrolide antibiotics and have similar antibacterial spectrum as that of penicillin.
2. They act by inhibiting bacterial protein synthesis at 50 S ribosomal level.
3. Erythromycin is acid labile and has short half-life; roxithromycin, azithromycin, clarithromycin have longer half-life.
4. Erythromycins are primarily used as an alternative to penicillin and to treat respiratory tract infections.
5. Clindamycin is chlorinated derivative of lincomycin. It acts by inhibiting bacterial protein synthesis at 50S ribosomes. It is used in the treatment of severe anaerobic infection caused by Bacteroids and other anaerobes either alone or in combination with an aminoglycoside. It may cause pseudo-membranous entrocolitis which is potentially a fatal complication. Metronidazole is another drug which is used in anaerobic infections.
6. Spectinomycin (aminoglycoside) is only used as an alternative treatment for penicillin resistant gonorrhoea.
7. Vancomycin (glycopeptide) is used parenterally to treat resistant staphylococcal sepsis and endocarditis and

orally to antibiotic associated pseudo-membranous enterocolitis.

8. Fusidic acid (steroid antibiotic) is mainly employed to treat penicillin resistant staphylococcal infections specially osteomyelitis because it is concentrated in bones.

9. Cotrimoxazole, ampicillin, amoxicillin, carbenicillin, third generation cephalo-sporins, gentamicin, nalidixic acid and norfloxacillin are effective against coliforms of urinary tract infection while carbenicillin, third generation cephlo-sporins, gentamicin and norfloxacin are effective against Pseudomonas infection of urinary tract.

10. Nitrofurantoin and mandelamine are used to treat lower urinary tract infection caused by coliforms.

11. Linezolide is a oxazolidinones. It is effective against gram-positive pathogens only because they lack specific efflux pumps. It acts by inhibiting the formation of tertiary inhibition complex by binding to the 50S subunit and prevents translation.

Chapter 52

Antifungal Drugs

Recently there is steady increase in local and systemic fungal infections. In fact most of them are opportunistic infections due to two reasons:

- Immunosuppression due to AIDS or intensive use of corticosteroids or during cancer chemotherapy
- Indiscriminate use of 'broad' or 'extended' spectrum antibiotics which eliminate or decrease non-pathogenic bacterial population that normally compete with fungi.

Many fungal infections occur in poorly vascularized or avascular skin, in nails, and hair. The systemic fungal infections include localized or disseminated blastomycosis, cryptococcosis, candidiasis and other invasive infections.

Systemic Antifungal Drugs

1. **Amphotericin B:** It is obtained from streptomyces nodosus. It is amphoteric polyene macrolide antibiotic. It is insoluble in water and unstable at 37°C. It inhibits fungi through an interaction with fungal membrane sterols. It is ineffective in bacteria because bacterial membrane does not contain these sterols.

   Amphotericin B is used orally only for gastrointestinal infections because it is poorly absorbed from gastrointestinal tract. For systemic infections, it is given by i.v. infusion of a colloidal suspension. It is highly protein bound and is slowly excreted in urine. On parenteral administration, it may cause fever, anorexia, nausea, vomiting, hypokalaemia, nephrotoxicity and inflammation at the site of injection. For external use, it is available as 3% cream, lotion and ointment. For systemic infection, it is given by slow i.v. infusion over 4–6 hours in a dose of 0.3–0.7 mg/kg body weight. It is given intrathecally in meningitis caused by cocidioides.

   Amphotericin B is used to treat systemic fungal infections caused by Cryptococcus, Histoplasma, Candida and Blastomyces. The therapy is usually for 6–10 weeks and may be extended to 3–4 months, if needed.

2. **Flucytocine:** It is a synthetic antifungal drug. It is a narrow spectrum antifungal drug. Since resistance develops rapidly, it is usually used in combination with amphotericin B for the treatment of systemic candidiasis and cryptococcus. Fungal cells convert it into 5-fluorouracil which acts as an antimetabolite and inhibits thymidylate synthetase and DNA synthesis. It is well absorbed from the gut. Side effects are uncommon but mild bone marrow depression can occur. So weekly blood counts should be done. It is given orally in a dose of 150–200 mg/kg daily in divided doses.

3. **Azoles:** They are synthetic antifungal agents. They have a broad-spectrum activity. All the three azoles, ketoconazole, fluconazole, and intraconazole are readily absorbed from gut. So they are employed for systemic fungal infection. All azoles act by blocking synthesis of ergosterol of fungal cell membrane because they interact with the enzymes essential for the conversion of lanosterol to ergosterol. So the membrane is altered due to its fluidity and the action of membrane associated enzymes is disturbed. So finally there occurs inhibition of replication. They are effective in cryptococcosis, paracoccidioimycosis, histoplasmosis, blastomycosis, aspergillosis, sporotrichosis and also candidiasis. They are also effective against dermatophytosis. Orally used azoles may give rise to gastric upsets. Important features of each azole are as under:

- *Ketoconazole:* It is metabolized in liver by microsomal enzymes and excreted in bile and urine. It may cause lethal hydrogen peroxide accumulation in fungal cells. Since ketoconazole inhibits steroidogenesis it is also useful in prostatic cancer and hyperadrenal corticism. It may cause hepatic impairment and gynaecomastia. It is given orally in doses of 200 mg once or twice daily. It is contraindicated in pregnancy, lactation or children below 2 years.

- *Fluconazole:* It can be administered orally or i.v. It is drug of choice for most types of fungal meningitis because it passes to CSF in effective concentrations. Its oral doses are:
  a. For oropharyngeal candidiasis—50 to 100 mg daily
  b. For oesophageal candidiasis—100 to 200 mg
  c. For cryptococcal meningitis in AIDS patients—200 mg daily

- *Itraconazole:* It has close resemblance to ketoconazle. It is used orally. It has fewer side effects than ketoconazole. It is preferred over ketoconazole for the treatment of non-meningeal histoplasmosis.

- *Miconazole:* Although miconazole can be used for systemic infections (by i.v. infusion) and gastrointestinal fungal infections (orally), it is no more used for them with the advent of newer agents. At present it is mainly used topically.

Antifungal Drugs for Superficial Infections

Superficial fungal infections are dermatophytosis (skin, scalp and nails) and candiasis (mouth, vagina, mucocutaneous, intestinal and skin).

- **Griseofulvin:** It is an antibiotic which is produced by *Penicillium griseofulvum*. It is selectively concentrated in newly formed keratin precursor cells of the skin, hair follicles and nailbeds which become resistant to fungal infections. It is drug of choice for widespread or intractable dermatophyte infections. It is readily absorbed on oral administration but is inactive when applied locally. Treatment should be continued for several weeks to months in doses of 0.5–1 gram daily in divided doses. It is a relatively safe drug. Rarely may it give rise to gastrointestinal upsets, CNS symptoms, heptotoxicity, leucopenia, photosensitivity, allergy, etc.

- **Nystatin:** It is polyene macrolide antibiotic. It is not absorbed from gut, skin or mucous membranes. It is too toxic for parenteral use. So it is only used for superficial candidiasis of skin, mouth, vagina and intestinal canal as ointment, suppositories and oral tablets. It acts in the same way as amphotericin.

- **Azoles:** Topical azoles used for superficial candidiasis and dermatophytosis are clotrimazole, econazole, troconazole, sulconazole and miconazole. These are available as dermatologic cream, spray, powder, lotion or suppositories.

• Other topical antifungal drugs:
  – Candidicin and natamycin are alternative topical antifungal drugs used for superficial candidiasis as ointments and suppositories.
  – Undecylenic acid, naftifine and tolnafate are used for dermatophytosis. Tolnafate is especially useful for athlete's foot (dermatophytosis).
  – Haloprogin and ciclopirox ointments are used for candidiasis and dermatophytosis.

Points for Dental Students

1. Ketoconazole or itraconazole is used for 6–12 weeks to treat oral manifestation of histoplasmosis.
2. Amphotericin B (i.v.) is used for 10 weeks in severe cases of oral manifestations of histoplasmosis.
3. Amphotericin B is used systemically for three months in oral manifestation (ulceration of palate) of mucomycosis.
4. Ketoconazole (200 mg once daily) or fluconazole (100 mg once daily) or itraconazole (100–200 mg once daily) is used for 2 weeks to treat acute and chronic oral candidiasis.
5. Nystatin rinse (3–4 times daily) is useful in oral candidiasis.
6. Topical antifungal drugs are used in oropharynx candidiasis, e.g. nystatin lozenges (200,000 units) 4 to 6 times a day; miconazole solution (2%); clotrimazole (1%) lotion.
7. Oral fluconazole (100–200 mg/day) or oral itraconazole (200 mg/day) is also effective in oral candidiasis resistant to polyenes (nystatin, amphotericin-B) and imidazoles (ketoconazole, miconazole or clotrimazole) group of antifungal drugs.

8. For denture stomatitis nystatin ointment (100,000 units/gm) can be applied topically every 6 hours to the tissue surface of the denture.
9. Topical antifungal + topical corticosteroid (e.g. clobetasol and triamcinolone) preparation is also used to treat oral candidiasis with lichen planus.
10. Chlorhexidine oral rinses may also be used as supportive therapy for treating oral candidiasis.
11. Ketoconazole, itraconazole and fluconazole require acid medium for their absorption from gut. Hence they should not be administered along with antacids, H_2 receptor antagonists or proton pump inhibitors which increase pH. If antifungal drugs have to be given along with these drugs they should not be administered together. Proper time interval should be observed between the administrations of these drugs.
12. Enzyme inducers such as barbiturates, rifampin, phenytoin, etc. increase the metabolism of ketoconazole, fluconazole and itraconazole. So for desired therapeutic effect of these antifungal drugs, their doses have to be adjusted on concomitant administration of any one of these drugs.

TO REMEMBER

1. There are two reasons for steady increase in local as well as systemic fungal infections viz. (i) immunosuppression due to AIDS or intensive use of corticoids, or during cancer therapy and (ii) indiscriminate use of broad or extended spectrum antibiotics.
2. Amphotericin is used orally for gastrointestinal infection and parenterally (by slow infusion) for other

systemic infections caused by Cryptococcus, Histoplasma, Candida and Blastomyces.

3. Flucytosine is a narrow spectrum antifungal drug which is usually used in combination with amphotericin-B for the treatment of candidiasis and cryptococcus. Since it can cause bone marrow depression, weekly blood count should be done.

4. Azoles are synthetic broad-spectrum antifungal agents. They are available by oral route for systemic fungal infections.

5. Since fluconazole passes to CSF in effective concentrations, it is used to treat meningitis.

6. Ketoconazole is also used to treat prostate cancer and hyperadrenal corticism as it inhibits steroidogenesis.

7. For superficial fungal infections such as dermatophytosis (skin, scalp, and nails) and candidiasis (mouth, vagina, mucocutaneous intestinal and skin), griseofulvin, nystatin, azoles (clotrimazole, econazole, triconazole, sulconazole and miconazole) are commonly used.

8. Other topical antifungal drugs are candidicin, natamycin, undecylenic acid, naftifine, tolnafate, haloprogin and ciclopirox.

9. Tolnafate is especially useful for athlete's foot (dermatophytosis).

Chapter 53

Antiviral Drugs and
Pharmacology of AIDS

All viruses are composed of a nucleic acid core, either DNA or RNA plus nucleoproteins. They are enclosed by a protein coat, the capcid. They do not have intracellular materials for basic cellular metabolism and division. So they are dependent on the host cells for survival and replication. They are obligate intracellular parasites. The different targets of drug interventions are the several steps of the process of viral replication such as:

- Adsorption
- Penetration
- Uncoating
- Synthesis of viral nucleic acid and proteins
- Assembly
- Release

Viral infections are common but unfortunately there are no specific chemotherapeutic agents available for the treatment of viral infections. Most of the drugs available are chemoprophylactic agents. Commonly used drugs are as under:

1. **Those causing inhibition of viral adsorption to cells and cellular penetration:**
   - *Gamma globulins:* They are pooled gamma globulins (immunoglobulins). They can combine with the antigenic protein coating of the free viral particle, if administered before infection. Thus they prevent their adsorption to and penetration into susceptible cells and imparts passive immunization to the host for 2 to 3 weeks. They may attenuate or prevent measles, viral hepatitis B, rabies, poliomyelitis, vaccinia and varicella-zoster if used before the onset of signs and symptoms.
   - *Amantadine:* It is a synthetic tricyclic primary amine. Rimantadine is another related drug. They are used orally for the chemoprophylaxis of influenza A. Amantadine releases dopamine from dopaminergic nerve endings. So it is also used in some cases of parkinsonism. Important side effects are gastrointestinal upsets, insomnia, nervousness and dizziness. It is contraindicated in epilepsy and gastric ulcer. It should be used with utmost care in cardiovascular, hepatic, renal and psychiatric disorders. Adult dose is 200 mg daily for 10 days. Rimantadine is similar to amantadine and may have fewer adverse effects.

2. **Those causing inhibition of viral nucleic acid synthesis:**
   - *Acyclovir (acycloguanosine):* It is a synthetic purine nucleoside derivative. It is highly specific for herpes simplex and varicella-zoster viruses. It is available for oral administration, as an ointment (0.5%) and for i.v. use. In genital herpes, it is given in a dose of 200 mg orally for 10 days. For i.v. use it should be given slowly (5 mg/kg every 8 hours) by infusion. In dentistry, it is

used to treat hairy leukoplakia, oral ulcerative or bullous disease, herpetic gingivostomatitis and recurrent intraoral herpes simplex. Adverse effects include nausea, headache and rarely encephalopathy.

- *Ganciclovir:* It is a guanine derivative. It is chemically related to acyclovir and also has same mechanism of action. It is more active against cytomegalovirus (CMV) than acyclovir. It is specifically used for cytomegalovirus infections (retinitis, pneumonia and gastrointestinal lesions). It is given i.v. It is more toxic than acyclovir and causes gastrointestinal upsets and bone marrow depression.

- *Vidarabine (adenine arabinoside):* It is least toxic and most effective of the purine analogues. It acts principally by relatively selectively inhibiting viral DNA polymerase. It is, thus, effective against DNA viruses. It is indicated in immunosuppressed patients for the treatment of serious infections caused by herpes simplex and varicella-zoster viruses, e.g. herpes keratitis, encephalitis, neonatal disseminated herpes simplex, herpes zoster. It is applied either topically (3% ophthalmic ointment) as in the eye infections or administered i.v. as a slow infusion (10 mg/kg) for 5 days. It may cause gastrointestinal upsets, neurological effects like tremors, ataxia, hallucinations, confusion and coma in some patients.

- *Idoxuridine and bromovinyldeoxyuridine:* They are analogues of thymidine. Idoxuridine is phosphorylated by cellular kinase and the activated triphosphate derivative acts on viral as well as host DNA. So it is only used topically to treat herpes simplex lesions of the skin, eye and external genitalia. On the other hand, bromovinyldeoxyuridine is a very potent antiviral drug and has the advantage of acting on viral DNA only. Local application of idoxuridine may be associated with irritation, itching, oedema, and photophobia. It is available as 0.1% ophthalmic solution and as a 0.5% ophthalmic ointment. One drop of the solution is instilled hourly during the day and every 2 hourly at night for two weeks.

- *Trifluorouridine (trifluridine):* It is a pyrimidine analogue. Its actions are similar to idoxuridine but less toxic. So it is preferred to idoxuridine in herpetic keratitis.

- *Cytarabine(cytosine arabinoside):* It is similar to idoxuridine in actions. It is more potent but more toxic than idoxuridine. So it is only used in idoxuridine resistant cases of herpetic keratitis.

- *Ribavirin:* It is a synthetic nucleoside which has structural resemblance with guanosine. It is effective against both RNA and DNA viruses because it interferes with the synthesis of early viral mRNA and also causes inhibition of DNA polymerase. It is indicated to treat influenza (A) and (B), herpes simplex, and respiratory syncytical virus (RNA myxovirus). It is drug of choice for Lassa fever and is potential drug for HIV infection.

- *Forcarnet (phosphonoformate):* It is a pyrophosphate analogue. It acts by binding with pyrophosphate binding site on viral DNA polymerase. It is effective against herpes viruses, hepatitis B virus and retroviruses. It is also useful in AIDS. Its use is limited because it causes nephrotoxicity.

3. **Those causing inhibition of viral protein synthesis:**
   - *Interferons:* They are small glycoproteins. They are produced within the body in response to viral infection. There are at least three types of interferons:
     - Alpha (type-I from human leucocytes)
     - Beta (type-I from human fibroblasts)
     - Gamma (type-II from T lymphocytes)

   They act by inhibiting translation of the viral mRNA into proteins. Endogenous interferons are primarily responsible for making most viral infections 'self-limiting'. Stimulation of production of 'endogenous' interferon has been unsatisfactory. 'Exogenous' human interferon is being produced in pooled leucocytes, cultured fibroblasts, lymphoblast cultures and now in large amounts by recombinant DNA technology in bacterial cultures. They are used as adjunct in the treatment of viral diseases including AIDS. They may cause gastrointestinal symptoms, cardiovascular disturbances, anaemia, myalgia, headache, etc. as side effects.

1. **Methisazone:** It is a thiosemicarbazone derivative. It acts by inhibiting synthesis of viral structural proteins. It is an active prophylactic agent for smallpox. However, it has no therapeutic value, once smallpox has developed. It is given in doses of 100 to 200 mg/kg daily in divided doses orally. It is also useful in the treatment of vaccinia.

2. **Immunomodulators:** Interferons also act as immunostimulants. They also modify cell regulatory mechanisms and inhibit neoplastic growth.

3. **Inosine:** It increases macrophage activity and stimulate beta and T lymphocyte differentiation. It also potentiates action of interferon. It has been used for mucocutaneous herpes simplex and genital warts.

Pharmacology of AIDS

AIDS (acquired immunodeficiency syndrome) is the end stage of chronic viral infection. It is caused by HIV (human immunodeficiency virus) which is an RNA retrovirus. The virus enters several types of cells, e.g. lymphocytes, macrophages, Langerhans cells and neurons within central nervous system.

The illness is due to destruction of the helper T lymphocytes by the replicating virus particles and impairment of functioning of the surviving helper T cells. HIV is most commonly transmitted by:

- Sexual intercourse, either heterosexual or homosexual
- By contaminated syringes and needles
- By blood transfusions and blood products
- From the infected mother to the fetus during pregnancy as well during childbirth.

Acute HIV infection is followed by months or years of chronic infection with no symptoms and only a few signs. There occurs gradual but remorseless destruction of the immune system due to lymphotropic and neutrotropic properties of the virus. As the disease progresses, there occurs recurrent common infections. In the final stage, the patient suffers from opportunistic infections (candidiasis, tuberculosis, *Pneumocystitis carinii* pneumonia, cryptococcal meningitis and toxoplasmosis of the central nervous system) and unusual tumours (Kaposi's tumour). HIV infection is not self-limiting infection and the end result is invariably death. The important measures to fight HIV infections are:

- Preventive measures against sex, blood transfusion and drug abuse
- Antiviral drugs
- Immunomodulator drugs

Salient Features of Drugs

1. **Zidovudine (ZVD):** It is a thymidine analogue. After phosphorylation in the body, zidovudine triphosphate is formed which selectively inhibits viral transcriptase (RNA dependent DNA polymerase) in preference to cellular DNA polymerase. Resistance to ZVD occurs by point mutations which reverse transcriptase enzyme. It is given orally every 4–6 hours. It is readily absorbed and gets distributed throughout the body including CSF. It is partly metabolized by glucuronidation in liver and excreted in urine. It acts as DNA chain terminator by integrating into developing virus DNA chain. Continuous treatment with the drug can extend survival time in patients of AIDS who have advanced AIDS-related complexes. However, on stoppage of therapy there is a reversal of all signs and symptoms. ZVD has no effect on Kaposi's tumour. It may cause bone marrow depression (neutropenia, anaemia), neurotoxicity (peripheral neuropathy, seizures and asthenia), myalgia and myositis as adverse effects. It is contraindicated in neutropenia and anaemia. It should be used carefully in patients of hepatic and renal impairment. It is given in doses of 500 mg/day in 2–4 divided doses.

2. **Didanosine, zalcitabine and stavudine:** They are nucleoside analogues. They also go intracellular conversion to the active triphosphate derivatives which inhibit viral reverse trnscriptase. Thus they terminate proviral DNA of HIV. They are second line therapy in cases of ZVD failure or toxicity. They cause myelosuppression, neurotoxicity and pancreatitis.

3. **Foscarnet:** It is used in combination with ZVD in AIDS-related complexes.

4. **Interferon-alpha:** It has shown synergism with ZVD and foscarnet in AIDS.

5. **Monoclonal antibodies:** A technique for production of monoclonal antibodies (antigp 41 and antigp 120) is being developed.

6. **Vaccine:** Anti-idiotype vaccine is at an advance stage. It would act by binding to HIV and thus can neutralize it.

7. To increase efficacy and reduce toxicity, ZVD has been used in combination with acyclovir, foscarnet, didanosine or interferon-alpha.

TO REMEMBER

1. All viruses are composed of a nucleic acid core, either DNA or RNA plus nucleoproteins. They are enclosed by a protein coat, capsid.

2. Viral infections are common but unfortunately no specific chemotherapeutic agents are available for their treatment. Most of the available drugs are chemoprophylactic agents.

3. Gamma globulins, amantadine and rimantadine act by inhibiting viral adsorption to cells and cellular penetration.

4. If used before the onset of signs and symptoms, gamma-globulins may attenuate or prevent measles, viral hepatitis, rabies, poliomyelitis, vaccinia and varicella-zoster.

5. Amantadine is used orally for the chemoprophylaxis of influenza-A.

6. Acyclovir, ganciclovir, vidarabine, idoxuridine, bromovinyldeoxyuridine, trifluorouridine, cytorabine, ribavirin and foscarnet act by causing inhibition of viral nucleic acid synthesis.

7. Interferons and methisazone act by causing inhibition of viral protein synthesis. Interferons are used as adjunct in the treatment of viral diseases including AIDS. Methisazone is effective prophylactic agent for smallpox.

8. Interferons also act as immuno-stimulants and inosine increases macrophage activity and stimulates beta and T lymphocyte differentiation.

9. AIDS (acquired immunodeficiency syndrome) is caused by HIV (human immunodeficiency virus). It is treated with zidovudine (first line therapy) or didanosin (second line therapy). These drugs act as DNA chain terminator.

10. To increase efficacy and reduce toxicity, zidovudine has been used in combination with acyclovir, foscarnet, didanosine interferon-alpha.

Chapter 54

Chemotherapy of Malaria

Four species of the protozoa *Plasmodium (P. vivax, P. falciparum, P. malariae* and *P.ovale)* cause malaria. Two commonest forms of malaria are benign tertian (BT) and malignant tertian (MT). The former is caused by *P. vivax* and latter by *P. falciparum*. In both the types the infected individual develops fever, with rigors every third day and are called "Tertian". Infections due to *P. ovale* and *P. malariae* are not common in man.

A large number of sporozoites are present in the salivary glands of the infected female anopheles mosquitoes. An individual is infected by malarial parasites through the bite of a female anopheles mosquito. Sporozoites thus inoculated into the bloodstream disappear rapidly from the circulation and invade the parenchymatous cells of the liver and the reticuloendothelial cells. They multiply there to form tissue schizonts (primary exo-erythrocytic form or pre-erythrocytic stage). After this stage (incubation period 5–7 days in case of *P. falciparum* and 8 days to several months in case of *P. vivax*), merozoites are released into the bloodstream. They then invade erythrocytes and undergo further developments and multiplication giving rise to erythrocytic schizonts (a sexual erythrocytic stage) known as trophozoites.

Eventually infected blood cells rupture and release merozoites along with metabolic and toxic substances which cause fever with chills and rigor followed by feeling of heat and sweating. The merozoites released in blood may invade fresh erythrocytes to undergo erythrocytic schizogony repeatedly; some of them are differentiated into male (microgametocyte) and female (macrogametocyte) sexual forms which when taken by another female mosquito develops into zygotes to form oocyst which ultimately gives rise to sporozoites. In case of *P. vivax* infection, some of them enter new liver cells and continue exo-erythrocytic stage. They are termed hypnozoites which are responsible for relapses.

Classification of antimalarial drugs according to their chemical structure:

1. 4-aminoquinolines
   - Chloroquine
   - Amodiaquine
   - Hydroxychloroquine
2. 8-aminoquinolines
   - Primaquine
3. Diaminopyrimidines
   - Pyrimethamine
   - Trimethoprim
4. Biguanides
   - Proguanil
   - Chlorproguanil
   - Cycloguanil
5. 4-quinoline methanol
   - Mefloquine
   - Halofantrine
6. Cinchona alkaloids
   - Quinine

7. Sulphonamides and sulphones
   - Sulphadoxine
   - Sulphalene
   - Sulphamethoxazole
   - Dapsone
8. Acridine
   - Mepacrine
9. Miscellaneous
   - Artemisinin (quinghaosu)
   - Yinghaosu
   - Doxycycline
   - Norfloxacin

Eradication of malaria may be done by the use of drugs in the following way:

Causal prophylaxis is achieved by drugs (beta aminoquinolines, diaminopyrimidines, and biguanides) which act at exo-erythrocytic stage. They destroy the sporozoites within the infected hepatic cells and prevent the invasion of erythrocytes. There is no drug (true causal prophylactic) available, which can kill the sporozoites before they can infect the cells of reticuloendothelial system.

Suppressives are drugs (4-aminoquinolines, quinine, mefloquine, sulphonamides, sulphones, quinghaosu, biguanides, and diaminopyrimidines) which act at erythrocytic stage and prevent the rupture of the infected cells.

Gametocidal drugs (primaquine) destroy the sexual forms of malarial parasites and eradicate both the vivax and falciparum gametocytes.

Clinical cure is achieved by schizontoicides which interrupt erythrocytic schizogony of the malarial parasite and terminate the clinical attack.

Radical cure is achieved by drugs which act on both erythrocytic and exerythrocytic parasites. Primaquine may be used with chloroquine for better results. Prolonged use of suppressive therapy (1 month) can achieve radical cure in case of falciparum malaria.

Antimalarial Drugs

Chloroquine

It is a 4-aminoquinoline derivative. On oral administration, it is completely and rapidly absorbed from gut. It is concentrated in the liver, spleen, kidney, lungs, red blood cells, leucocytes and other tissue proteins. Plasma half-life is 3–7 days. It is slowly excreted by kidney.

Malarial parasites thrive on haemoglobin. Chloroquine acts by degrading haemoglobin and prevent the parasites to be able to utilize it. It also blocks the synthesis of amino acids essential to parasites. Chloroquine is used to suppress and clinically cure malaria caused by all four species of malarial parasites. It is also effective against gametocytes of *P. vivax*, *P. ovale* and *P. malariae*, but not of *P. falciparum*. It also has antiamoebic, antigiardial and anti-inflammatory actions. In high doses, it depresses myocardium and has a relaxant effect on smooth muscle.

Therapeutic Uses

- Chloroquine is a drug of choice for the treatment of acute attack of malaria and is also used for its suppressive prophylaxis.
- Extra-intestinal amoebiasis
- Giardiasis
- Collagen disorders: rheumatoid arthritis and discoid lupus erythmatosus
- Lepra reactions
- Photogenic reactions
- Infectious mononucleosis

Chloroquine may cause mild headache, nausea, vomiting, anorexia, abdominal pain, pruritus, deafness, skin rash, psychosis, hypotension, photoallergy and myopathy as side effects. Blurring of vision, diplopia and temporary loss of accommodation are rare and reversible. If used in high doses for a along period as in case of collagen diseases chloroquine may cause lenticular opacity, sub-capsular posterior cataract retinopathy. These effects are irreversible. It is contraindicated in patients of psoriasis and porphyria.

Dose: Acute attacks of malaria: 600 mg (base) is given initially followed after 6 hours by 300 mg, then 150 mg twice daily for next two days. If required it can be given i.m. or by slow i.v. injection in a dose of 200–300 mg (base).

Hydroxychloroquine and amodiaquine have similar pharmacokinetic, pharmacological and adverse effects as that of chloroquine.

Primaquine

It is 8-aminoquinoline derivative. On oral administration, it is readily absorbed and is highly concentrated in liver and lungs. It is metabolized in liver and excreted in urine within 24 hours. Its plasma half-life is 3–6 hours. It acts on malarial parasites through its intermediates (quinoline-quinone derivatives) which are oxidants. It is also effective against persistent tissue phase of *P. vivax* and *P. ovale* and primary exoerythrocytic stage of *P. falciparum*. Being a toxic drug, it is only used as a radical curative against *P. vivax* malaria after the patient has left the endemic area. Gastrointestinal upsets are the common side effects. Important toxic hazard is intravascular haemolysis in individuals with deficiency of glucse-6-phosphate dehydrogenase enzyme. Primaquine is contraindicated in pregnancy, in patients suffering from rheumatoid arthritis and DLE and also in patients receiving haemolytic drugs such as analgesics, sulphonamides, chloramphenicol, nitrofurans and methotrexate.

Dose: 15 mg/day for 15 days.

Pyrimethamine

Being most potent dihydrofolate reductase enzyme inhibitor, it prevents the synthesis of tetrahydrofolate in malarial parasite. It is effective causal prophylactic for *P. falciparum* and *P. vivax*. It also acts as radical curative for *P. vivax*. It is an effective blood schizonticidal and gametocidal only to *P. falciparum*. Its action is enhanced when used in combination with sulphonamide due to sequential blockade of folic acid synthesis. On oral administration, it is readily absorbed and gets concentrated in kidney, liver, lungs and spleen. It is slowly eliminated. Although drug is well tolerated, rarely it may cause megaloblastic anaemia and thrombocytopenia.

Therapeutic Uses

1. For chemoprophylaxis of malaria in doses of 25 mg per week.
2. To treat acute attack of malaria caused by chloroquine resistant strains in combination with sulphonamide or quinine.
3. To treat toxoplasmosis, it is given along with trisulphapyrimidine for 3–4 weeks.

Chloroguanide (Proguanil)

It is another dihydrofolate reductase enzyme inhibitor. It is a prodrug. It cyclises and gets converted into triazine, cycloguanil. It is now rarely used because of two important limitations, i.e.

- Rapid development of resistance
- Slow action

Trimethoprim: It has similar action as that of pyrimethamine but weaker in nature. It may be used in combination with a sulphonamide, e.g. cotrimoxazole.

Sulphonamide and Sulphones

They are not effective anti-malarial drugs. When combined with pyrimethamine they produce supra-additive synergistic combination due to sequential block. The combination is employed for prophylaxis and treatment of chloroquine-resistant malaria. The combination should not be used in late pregnancy because of the risk of provoking kernicterus.

Mefloquine

It is a synthetic 4-quinoline methanol derivative. It is a strong schizonticidal drug. On oral administration, it is well absorbed and is extensively bound to plasma proteins. It undergoes enterohepatic circulation and has a long half-life of 17 days. It is recommended to use for the treatment of multidrug resistant *P. falciparum*. A single dose of 1 to 1.5 gm is quite effective. It may induce nausea, abdominal discomfort, diarrhea, vertigo and hypotension. Rarely may it cause acute psychosis and transient encephalopathy with convulsions.

Halofantrine

It is a phenanthrine methanol derivative. It is employed to treat multidrug resistant *P. falciparum* and *P. vivax* malaria. It has no advantage over mefloquine.

Qinghaosu

It is a sesquiterpene lactone. It is obtained from Chinese herbal medicine,' Artemisia annua'. Its derivatives artemisinin and related compound artesunate (oral and i.v. preparation) and artemether (i.m. preparation) have undergone clinical trials. They are effective blood schizonticides. They are specially useful in cerebral malaria due to *P. falciparum*. They act by damaging cellular membrane of the parasite.

Yinghaosu

It is also derived from Chinese herb. It is similar in properties to those of quinghaosu.

Antibiotics

* **Doxycycline (100 mg):** It is employed along with chloroquine, quinine or antifolate drugs to treat multidrug resistant malaria.

It may be used alone for prophylaxis during stay in endemic areas.
* **Norfloxacin:** It is effective against chloroquine resistant *P. falciparum* infection.

Quinine

It is an alkaloid which is obtained from cinchona bark. With the invent of safer drugs, it is only used to treat chloroquine resistant strains of *P. falciparum*. On oral administration, it is completely absorbed and peak plasma level occurs in 1–3 hours. Seventy per cent is bound to plasma proteins. It is metabolized in the liver and then completely excreted by the kidney within 24 hours. Plasma half-life is 10 hours. Quinine is rapidly acting schizonticidal drug and is gametocidal for *P. vivax* and *P. malarae*. It is a protoplasmic poison. It may act by inhibiting protein synthesis in the malarial parasites. It has mild analgesic, antipyretic and quinidine like depressant action on the heart. It has local irritant action and curare like relaxant action on skeletal muscles. It stimulates uterine muscle during third trimester of pregnancy.

Therapeutic Uses

* Used to treat severe (cerebral malaria) and complicated *P. falciparum* malaria resistant to chloroquine by rate controlled i.v. infusion.
* Used to relieve skeletal muscle spasm in myotonia congenita, a hereditary myopathy.
* Also effective in nocturnal muscle cramps.
* Used as a sclerosing agent in varicose veins.

It may cause nausea, vomiting, abdominal pain, pruritus, angioneurotic oedema and asthmatic attacks. It may cause cinchonism which is characterized by headache, ringing of ears, blurring of vision, disturbance of coloured vision, photophobia, amblyopia. It is contraindicated in myasthenia gravis and during pregnancy.

Chemoprophylaxis

It should be started 1–2 weeks before going to endemic area, continued throughout the period of stay and for a further period of 6 weeks after return from that area. Drugs used are:

- Chloroquine 300 mg (base) once a week (drug of choice) or pyrimethamine 25 mg per week.
- In chloroquine resistant *P. falciparum* areas, pyrimethamine (25 mg) plus sulphadoxine (500 mg) or sulphamethoxypyridazine (500 mg) or dapsone (100 mg) once a week.

Treatment of Cerebral Malaria

i. **Specific treatment:**
- Quinine dihydrochloride is the drug of choice. 600 mg salt of the drug is diluted with 200–500 ml of 5% glucose solution and infused i.v. over 2–3 hours. This may be repeated after 8 hours with a maximum dose of 2 gm of the salt in 24 hours.
- Alternatively in case of chloroquine sensitive parasites chloroquine, 200 mg (base) in adults, is diluted in 5% dextrose and infused over 8 hours, followed by 15 mg/kg which is infused over 24 hours.
  Parenteral chloroquine should be avoided in children because it may lead to convulsions and death.

ii. **Supportive measures:**
- Shock and deep coma:
  - Adequate glucose fluid and electrolyte replacement should be given.
  - Dexamethasone acetate is given in doses of 8 mg i.v. followed by 4 mg 8 hourly. After 24 hours, it is tapered off.
  - Dopamine is given by i.v. infusion with constant monitoring of blood pressure.
- Convulsions:
  - Diazepam is given in doses of 10 mg i.v.
- Hyperpyrexia:
  - Ice sponging
  - Paracetamol 0.5 mg i.m. 8 hourly or by slow i.v. infusion with monitoring of blood pressure, with utmost care.

TO REMEMBER

1. Chloroquine is the drug of choice for the treatment of acute attack of malaria except in chloroquine resistant cases.
2. Mefloquine is used to treat multidrug resistant *P. falciparum* infection. It should not be used as a prophylactic because of the danger of development of mefloquine resistant malarial parasite.
3. Another drug which is used to treat multi drug resistant *P. falciparum* and *P. vivax* malaria is halofantrine. It has no advantage over mefloquine.
4. Quinine is the drug of choice for the treatment of severe (cerebral) and complicated (*P. falciparum* malaria resistant to chloroquine) malaria. It should not be given by i.v. bolus injection. It is always given by rate controlled i.v. infusion.
5. Chloroquine (300 mg base once a week) or pyrimethamine (25 mg per week) is used for the chemoprophylaxis of malaria.
6. In chloroquine resistant *P. falciparum* areas. pyrimethamine (25 mg) plus sulphadoxin (500 mg) or sulphamethoxypyridazine (500 mg) or dapsone (100 mg) combination is used once a week for prophylaxis of malaria.
7. Primaquine is used as a radical curative against *P. vivax* malaria after the patient has left the endemic area.
8. The most significant toxic danger with primaquine is intravascular haemolysis in individuals with deficiency of glucose 6-phosphate dehydrogenase enzyme.

Chapter 55

Chemotherapy of Amoebiasis

Amoebiasis is an infectious disease. Both intestinal and extraintestinal form of amoebiasis are caused by *Entamoeba histolytica*. It mainly infects colon. Liver, lungs and brain may also be involved once the disease advances. Acute amoebic dysentery is characterized by blood and mucous in stools, abdominal pain and a persistent desire to pass stool. In chronic cases, anorexia, abdominal pain, and intermittent diarrhea or constipation are the main symptoms. Many amoebic carriers remain symptom less but they do pass cystic form of the protozoa in faeces.

Classification of Drugs

1. **Drugs used in intestinal amoebiasis:**
   - *Nitroimidazoles:*
     - Metronidazole
     - Tinidazole
     - Omidazole
     - Secnidazole
   - *Halogenated hydroxyquinolines:*
     - Di-iodohydroxyquinoline
     - Iodochlorohydroxyquinoline
     - Hydroxyquinoline
   - *Emetine*
   - *Dihydroemetine*
   - *Diloxanide furoate*
   - *Antibiotics:*
     - Parmomycin
     - Tetracyclines
     - Erythromycin

2. **Drugs used in extraintestinal amoebiasis:**
   - Nitroimidazoles
   - Chloroquine
   - Emetine

Nitroimidazoles

- **Metronidazole (flagyl):** It is a safest drug of choice for acute intestinal and extra-intestinal amoebiasis. On oral administration, it is rapidly absorbed. Protein binding is 20% and it is metabolized in the liver. Plasma half-life is 7½ hours. It is excreted in urine. It is readily taken up by sensitive protozoa and anaerobic bacteria. In these organisms, its nitro group is chemically reduced by ferridoxin into products which are lethal to these organisms by reacting with various macromolecules inside the cells. Since metronidazole interacts with free radicals, it has a radio-sensitizing effect on tumour cells.

Anorexia, diarrhoea, epigastric distress and metallic unpleasant taste are the common side effects. The tongue may become fury and glossitis and stomatitis may occur. It may also cause dizziness, lassitude and neurotoxicity. It has disulfiram-like effect with alcohol.

Therapeutic Uses

1. It is effective and drug of choice in all forms of amoebiasis. It is given in doses of

750 mg three times a day for 5–7 days. In children, the dose is 35–50 mg/kg per day in divided doses.

2. Giardiasis
3. Trichomoniasis
4. Balantidiasis
5. Trichomonal vaginitis
6. Anaerobic infections (surgical and gynecological sepsis)
7. Pseudomembranous enterocolitis due to *Cl. difficile*
8. In conditions due to both anaerobic and aerobic infections such as acute ulcerative gingivitis, cancrum oris, decubitus ulcer, phagedenic leg ulcers
9. Trench mouth
10. *Helicobacter pylori* gastritis/peptic ulcer
11. Guinea worm infestations
12. Vincent's angina and acute necrotizing ulcerative gingivitis.

For anaerobic infections, the recommended dose is 15 mg/kg initially i.v. which is followed 6 hours later with a maintenance dose of 7.5 mg/kg i.v. every 6 hours for 7–10 days. For other infections, it is used in doses of 250 mg orally three times a day for 5–7 days.

- **Tinidazole, omidazole and secnidazole:** They are structurally related to metronidazole and have similar therapeutic range. They have longer half-life (tinidazole—13 hours; secnidazole—21 hours) and lower incidence of side effects. Tinidazole is given 600–800 mg orally three times a day for 5–10 days in amoebic dysentery. Secnidazole is given in a single once only dose of 2 gram.
  Omidazole is given in a dose of 500 mg twice daily for 5–10 days.

Emetine hydrochloride and emetine bismuth iodide: Since emetine has a narrow margin of safety and produces severe cardiovascular and gastrointestinal side effects, its use has large been replaced by metronidazole. Emetine hydrochloride is given by deep or subcutaneous or intramuscular injection in doses of 30–60 mg daily for 10 days to treat acute amoebic dysentery. Emetine bismuth iodide is given orally in a dose of 60–120 mg daily for 12 days.

Dehydroemetine: It is equally effective but less toxic due to its more rapid excretion and lower concentration in cardiac tissue. It is given in a dose of 1.0 mg/kg i.m. daily for 5–10 days.

Chloroquine: Since chloroquine is highly concentrated in liver and lungs, it is effective in hepatic and pleuropulmonary amoebiasis. The recommended dose is 1 gm daily for 2 days followed by 500 mg daily for 2–3 weeks. Better results are seen in combination with emetine and metronidazole.

Halogenated hydroxyquinolines: This group includes di-iodohydroxyquinoline (iodoquinol), iodochlorohydroxyquinoline (vioform), hydroxyquinoline, and chlorohydroxyquinoline. They are used as alternative drugs for the treatment of asymptomatic or mild to moderate amoebiasis. Their absorption in the gut is variable and most of the drug is excreted in the faeces. The dose of halogenated quinolines varies from 600–750 mg daily in divided doses for 10–20 days.

Commonest side effects are nausea, vomiting, skin rash, fever, peripheral neuropathy and enlarged thyroid. Optic neuritis, optic atrophy and subacute myelooptic neuropathy (SMON) have been reported with iodoquinol in Japan after long-term use. It is also effective against giardiasis and *E. coli* infection.

Diloxanide furoate: It is drug of choice for treating asymptomatic and mild intestinal amoebiasis. On oral administration, it is rapidly absorbed, undergoes glucuronide conjugation and excreted in urine. Flatulence, nausea, vomiting, dryness of mouth, urticaria, diarrhoea and tingling sensations may occur as side effects. It is not recommended during pregnancy and children below 2 years of age.

Antibiotics

- Paromomycin is an aminoglycoside. It has direct amoebicidal property as well as acts indirectly by inhibition of normal intestinal flora essential for the multiplication of the amoeba. It is not absorbed from gut. It is given in doses of 25–35 mg/kg in divided doses at meal time for 7 days. It may cause diarrhoea, candidiasis, renal damage and ototoxicity.
- Tetracyclines and erythromycin act indirectly by inhibiting the intestinal normal flora. They are used as adjunct to main drugs. Tetracyclines should not be used during pregnancy and in children under 8 years of age.

TO REMEMBER

1. Metronidazole is the drug of choice for acute intestinal amoebiasis (dysentery), amoebic hepatitis and liver abscess and other extraintestinal amoebiasis.

2. Tinidazole, omidazole and secnidazole are other drugs structurally related to metronidazole and are used for the same purpose. These drugs may have better patient compliance due to better oral absorption, longer half-life, lesser dose and lower incidence of side effects.

3. Other important uses of metronidazole are giardiasis and anaerobic infection.

4. Most troublesome side effects of metronidazole are metallic taste and gastrointestinal disturbances.

5. Metronidazole has disulfiram-like effects, so alcohol should not be consumed during its use.

6. Chloroquine is effective in hepatic and pleuropulmonary amoebiasis.

7. Diloxanide furoate is the drug of choice for treating asymptomatic and mild intestinal amoebiasis.

8. Halogenated hydroxyquinolines may be used as alternative drugs for treatment of asymptomatic or mild intestinal amoebiasis.

Chapter 56

Chemotherapy of Tuberculosis

Tuberculosis is a chronic systemic disease. It is caused by *Mycobacterium tuberculosis*. It commonly involves the respiratory system but it can affect other organs as well. Although a large number of drugs are available for its treatment, there are certain problems also, viz.

- If single drug is employed, drug resistant strains emerge rapidly. So 2, 3 or 4 drugs are used in combination.
- Since organisms may lie dormant intra-cellularly for long period, drugs which cross cell membranes are used.
- Drug toxicity and patient compliance are also problems.
- To treat tubercular meningitis, appropriate combination of drugs is selected because all the drugs do not cross blood-brain barrier.
- It is problematic to treat high-risk groups, contacts, HIV infected, etc.

However, with the advent of chemotherapy, tuberculosis once almost certainly fatal is now a curable disease.

Primary Drugs (Main Line Drugs)

1. **Streptomycin (SM):** It is an amino-glycoside. It has already been discussed in detail. The major problems to treat tuberculosis by streptomycin are:
   - Parenteral administration
   - Non-penetration into cells (macro-phages) and CSF; so not effective on intracellular bacilli.

- Toxicity
- Not active in acid medium
- Development of bacterial resistance

So at present it is kept reserved in the main line drugs.

2. **Rifampicin (rifampin; RMP):** It is a highly effective semisynthetic derivative of one of the rifamycins produced by sterpto-myces mediterranei. It is bactericidal against sensitive organisms. It acts by inhibiting DNA dependent RNA synthesis in bacteria. It can also kill intracellular organisms by entering into phagocytic cells. Thus it is effective on intracellular and extracellular bacilli. It has tuber-culocidal effect in acid medium. If given singly, bacterial resistance develops either due to bacterial permeability barrier or to a mutation of DNA dependent RNA polymerase.

Rifampicin is rapidly absorbed from gut and widely distributed in tissues and fluids including cerebrospinal fluid. It is eliminated in bile and undergoes entrohepatic circulation. It is mainly excreted in faeces and only a little amount is excreted in urine. Nausea, vomiting and diarrhea are common side effects. It may impart a harmless orange colour to urine, sweat, tears and sputum. It may produce flu-like syndrome including chills, fever, dizziness and bone pain. Rarely jaundice and thrombocytopenia may occur. It is contraindicated in hepatic dysfunction. It induces microsomal enzymes. So it reduces the activity of several drugs, e.g. oral contraceptives, oral antidiabetics, warfarin, phenytoin, etc.

It is effective against gram-positive and gram-negative cocci, gram-negative bacilli, *M. tuberculosis*, *M. leprae*, *Chlamydia* and poxviruses. Its important uses are:

- *Tuberculosis:* It is always used in combination with other antimyco-bacterial agents in a dose of 600 mg/24 hours orally.
- *Leprosy:* It is used in combination with dapsone.
- *Other uses:*
  - Meningococcal carriers: 600 mg twice a day for two days.
  - *H. influenzae* prophylaxis: 20 mg/kg/24 hours for 4 days.
  - Brucellosis: used in combination with doxycycline.
  - Systemic fungal infections: used to enhance the effect of amphotericin B.

3. **Isoniazid (INH—isonicotinic acid hydrazide):** It has structural resemblance with pyridoxine and nicotinic acid. It is bactericidal against actively growing tubercular bacilli. It acts by interfering with the synthesis of mycobacterial cell wall due to its ability to inhibit synthesis of mycolic acid. It is effective in both acid and alkali media. It is effective on intracellular and extracellular bacilli. It also inhibits atypical mycobacterium. On oral administration, it is readily absorbed from gut and is well distributed in body fluids and tissues. It is metabolized in liver by acetylation. The activity of acetyl transferase enzyme is genetically determined. So the blood levels of isoniazid depend on the rate of acetylation. In 'slow acetylators', neurotoxicity is more while in 'rapid acetylators' hepatotoxicity is more. It is excreted in urine partly in free form and partly in the form of metabolites.

It may cause neurotoxicity, hepatotoxicity and allergic reactions. Peripheral neuritis may be prevented with pyridoxine (20–50 mg daily). It should be employed with care in presence of liver and kidney disease, epilepsy, alcoholism and to breastfeeding mothers.

Dose: 300 mg/24 hours; in children 10 mg/kg/24 hours; for chemoprophylaxis it is given alone in dose of 300 mg/24 hours for one year.

4. **Ethambutol (ETB):** It is a synthetic tuberculostatic drug. If used alone, bacterial resistance emerges rapidly. On oral administration, about 75–80% of the dug is absorbed and widely distributed in tissues and fluids including CSF. Partly it is metabolized. It is excreted in urine. It is employed in the treatment of tuberculosis in combination with other antitubercular drugs. Recommended adult dose is 15 mg/kg, given once a day.

It may cause optic neuritis and retinal damage. It may increase blood urate concentration due to reduced uric acid excretion. Other adverse effects are gastrointestinal disturbances, giddiness, mental disturbances and rarely allergic reactions. It should be avoided in very young children and elderly patients.

5. **Pyrazinamide (PZA):** It is a synthetic derivative of nicotinic acid. It is a bactericidal drug. It is particularly useful in tubercular meningitis because of good meningeal penetration. On oral administration, it is well absorbed and widely distributed in tissues including macrophages and CSF. It is excreted in urine. If used alone bacterial resistance emerges rapidly. Hepatotoxicity, arthralgia, nausea and vomiting may

appear as side effects. It is given in doses of 20–30 mg/kg daily.

Alternative Second Line Reserve Drugs

They are relatively more toxic and less effective drugs. They are only employed when:
- Organisms have developed resistance against the main line drugs
- Patient fails to respond to primary drugs

1. **Ethionamide:** It is structurally similar to isoniazid. It is administered orally up to 1 gram daily in divided doses. It may cause gastric irritation, hepatitis, neurological symptoms and postural hypotension.
2. **Morphazinamide:** It is chemically related to pyrazinamide. It is given in a dose of 2–3 gm per day along with isoniazid or PAS.
3. **Antibiotics:**
   - *Kanamycin, amikacin, viomycin and capreomycin:* First two are aminoglycosides while last two are peptides. All of them have similar pharmacokinetics and adverse effects. Since not absorbed on oral administration, they are given i.m. They are excreted in urine. They do not cross blood–brain barrier. All of them cause ototoxicity and nephrotoxicity. Cross-resistance exist amongst each other but not against main line drugs except streptomycin. They are given i.m. in a dose of 1 gm daily except viomycin which is given in a dose of 2 gm twice weekly.
   The importance of amikacin has increased with multidrug resistance cases because most of the drug resistant strains are susceptible to amikacin. Cross-resistance is not seen between streptomycin and amikacin. However, it must be used with other antitubercular drugs.
   - *Cycloserine:* It is a structural analogue of D-alanine. It acts by inhibiting bacterial cell wall synthesis by competing with D-alanine. It is given in a dose of 250 mg

twice a day. It may produce vertigo, tremors, convulsions and acute psychosis. It is contraindicated in epilepsy, depression and anxiety. Pyridoxin (150 mg/day) is administered to prevent occurrence of peripheral neuropathy and central nervous system side effects.
- *Fluoroquinolones:* Ciprofloxacin and levofloxacin are specially effective. These drugs are used in combination with other drugs such as pyrazinamide in multidrug resistant tuberculosis. Ciprofloxacin is given in a dose of 750 mg twice daily while levofloxacin is used in a dose of 500 mg once a day.
- *Rifabutin (ansamycin):* It is a derivative of rifampicin and its activity is also similar to rifampicin. Cross-resistance exists between the two drugs. It is used to treat atypical mycobacterial infection. It is a preferred drug where HIV-infection co-exists. It is administered in a dose of 300 mg per day.
- Rifapentine is also rifampicin analogue. It is identical to rifampicin in all respects. It is used in a 3 to 4 drug combination regimen in doses of 600 mg/day thrice a week.

4. **Para-aminosalicylic acid (PAS):** It is a synthetic drug. Its sodium salt is readily absorbed on oral administration and widely distributed in body fluids. It has two main disadvantages, i.e. weak bacteriostatic activity and a very high dose (8–12 gm/24 hours). After the discovery of rifampicin and many other antitubercular drugs, it is now obsolete. Important side effects are gastrointestinal upsets, kidney and liver damage and myxoedema.

Status of Antitubercular Drugs

A. **As per recommendations of WHO, tubercular patients are treated as under:**
   - New (untreated) smear positive and smear negative (seriously ill) pulmonary

tuberculosis and seriously ill extrapulmonary tuberculosis cases are treated for 6 months as under:

- Intensive phase (2 months): INH + RMP + PZA + ETB followed by,
- Continuous phase (4 months): INH + RMP

• New (untreated) smear negative (not seriously ill) pulmonary tuberculosis and less severe cases of extrapulmonary tuberculosis are treated for 6 months as under:

- Intensive phase (2 months): INH + RMP + PZA followed by,
- Continuous phase (4 months): INH + RMP

• Smear positive retreatment group due to: (a) treatment failure; (b) relapse default are treated for eight months as under:

- Intensive phase (2 + 1 months):
• 2 months: INH + RMP + PZA + ETB + SM
• 1 month: INH + RMP + PZA + ETB
- Intensive phase (5 months): INH + RMP + ETB

B. **Multi-drug resistant case is one where there is resistance to:**

(a) INH (b) RMP (c) INH + RMP (d) More number of drugs, if sensitivity of tubercular bacilli is known, treat as under:

• For INH resistance: RMP + PZA + ETB for 12 months.
• For RMP resistance: INH + PZA + ETB for 12 months.
• For both INH + RMP resistance: PZA + ETB + SM or ethyonamide + ciprofloxacin or ofloxacin or levofloxacin for 12 to 18 months.

C. **Chemoprophylaxis is indicated to:**
• House hold members
• Close contacts of potentially infected patients
• Neonate of tubercular mother

Any of the following regimens may be followed:
• INH 300 mg/day (5 mg/kg/day for children) for 6 to 12 months.
• INH (5 mg/day) + RMP(10 mg/kg/day) for 6 months

D. Latent tuberculosis infected patient is one whose skin test is positive but no evidence of disease. For this, regimens are:
• INH 300 mg/ day (5 mg/kg/ day for children) for 9 months or
• RMP 600 mg/ day (10 mg/kg/day for children) for 9 months

E. Treatment should not be withheld due to pregnancy because INH, RMP, PZA and even ETB are safe in pregnancy. However, ETB should be added during last trimester of pregnancy not earlier.

F. **Indications for corticoids are:**
• In AIDS patients with serious illness.
• In meningeal or renal tuberculosis or pleural effusion to minimize inflammation and exudation.

They should not be used in routine cases of tuberculosis. These drugs should be withdrawn gradually.

Points for Dental Students

1. Rifampin causes enzyme induction. So a dentist must remember about following drug interactions on concomitant use of other drugs:
• Reduces the activity of oral antidiabetics
• Responsible for oral contraceptive failure
• Decreases the effect of oral anticoagulants such as warfarin
• Diminishes the effect of phenytoin

2. Corticosteroids should not be used in routine cases of tuberculosis to avoid spread of infection. However, these are used for short period in meningeal or renal tuberculosis or tubercular pleural effusion to minimize inflammation and exudation rapidly.

TO REMEMBER

1. Tuberculosis is a chronic systemic disease, caused by *Mycobacterium tuberculosis*.
2. To avoid emergence of drug-resistant strains rapidly, multidrug therapy is indicated in tuberculosis.
3. Drugs, which cross cell membrane, are used because tubercular bacilli may lie dormant intracellularly for long periods. Similarly to treat tubercular meningitis, those drugs are selected which cross blood–brain barrier.
4. Streptomycin is kept reserved among the main line drugs for tuberculosis due to its parenteral administration, slow penetration into cells and CSF, toxicity and emergence of bacterial resistance.
5. All drug regimens have two components; a short intensive therapy (2 months) of 3 or 4 drugs and a longer maintenance (4 months) of 2 drugs. If the response of treatment is not satisfactory, the duration of therapy should be extended to 9 months (3 + 6 months).
6. In short course chemotherapy regimen, commonly used drugs are isoniazid, rifampicin, and pyrazinamide (2 months) plus isoniazid and rifampicin (4 months).
7. In high resistance cases, chemotherapy consists of isoniazid, rifampicin, ethambutol and pyrazinamide (2 months) plus isoniazid and rifampicin (4 months).
8. For chemoprophylaxis, isoniazid (300 mg/day/oral) alone is given for 1 year.
9. To prevent neurotoxicity 10 mg of pyridoxine for every 100 mg of isoniazid may be given.

Chapter 57

Chemotherapy of Leprosy

Leprosy is caused by *Mycobacterium leprae*. There are two major types, viz.

1. Lepromatous leprosy (multibacillary type) with extensive involvement. Lapromine reaction is negative.
2. Tuberculoid leprosy (paucibacillary type) with single or few skin lesions and neurological involvement. Lepromine reaction is positive.

Dimorphic (borderline) and indeterminate are other types of leprosy. It is a chronic disease and its treatment is very long (even it has to be given life long). In India, leprosy was being treated with chaulmoogra oil/hydnocarpus oil for centuries. But for the last 50 years, these oils are no more used because of the advent of antilepra chemotherapy. The main antileprotic drugs are dapsone, rifampicin and clofazimine.

- **Dapsone:** It is diamino diphenyl sulphone (DDS). It acts by inhibiting folate synthesis by competing with PABA. To avoid development of bacterial resistance, it is used in combination with rifampicin. It is slowly but completely absorbed from gut and widely distributed in the body. It is acetylated as well as undergoes glucuronide and sulphate conjugation in liver. It is excreted in urine as conjugated metabolites. It undergoes enterohepatic circulation also. Common side effects are anorexia, nausea, vomiting. Intravascular haemolysis occurs in patients with glucose-6-phosphate dehydrogenase deficiency. It may induce peripheral neuropathy, hepatitis, allergic skin reactions and psychosis. In lepromatous leprosy, it may precipitate erythema nodosum leprosum which may be suppressed by corticosteroids or by clofazimine. Its other use is to treat chloroquin resistant malaria in combination with pyrimethamine.

- **Rifampicin:** It is also effective against *M. leprae*. It rapidly makes leprosy patients non-contagious. However, it should not be used alone because some bacilli persist even after prolonged treatment and become resistant to the drug. So it is given as combination therapy to prevent drug resistance and to shorten duration of treatment of leprosy. It has already been discussed in detail.

- **Clofazimine:** It is phenazine derivative. It has leprostatic and anti-inflammatory properties. It probably produces its effect by interfering with template function of DNA. Its absorption from gut is variable. It is stored in reticuloendothelial tissues and skin. It is released from these sites very slowly and excreted in urine and bile. It is used in patients who are resistant to sulphones. Since it has anti-inflammatory property, it is useful in preventing the development of erythema nodosum leprosum. It is also used in combination therapy to treat atypical mycobacterial infection caused by *M. avium-intracellulare* specially in patients of AIDS. It is given in a dose of 100–300 mg daily by oral route. Treatment may continue for one year. It may cause gastrointestinal upsets and red-brown to nearly black discolouration of skin. Clofazimine should be avoided during early pregnancy and in patients with liver and kidney damage.

- **Other antilepra drugs:** These are used only as alternative drugs in multiple drug therapy regimens. These drugs are:
  - *Ofloxacin:* It is a fluoroquinolone. It is highly active against *M. leprae*. It is used as a component of multidrug regimen in case rifampicin cannot be used or to shorten the duration of therapy. It is given in doses of 400 mg per day orally.
  - *Minocycline:* It is a tetracycline. Being highly lipophilic, it is active against *M. leprae*. It is used as an alternative in multidrug therapy regimens. It is given in doses of 100 mg per day orally.
  - *Clarithromycin:* It is a macrolide antibiotic which has significant activity against *M. leprae*. It is used as an alternative in multidrug therapy regimens. It is given orally in doses of 500 mg per day.
  - *Ethionamide:* It has significant antileprotic activity. However, it should be used only when absolutely necessary because it causes hepatotoxicity in 10% patients.

TO REMEMBER

1. Leprosy is caused by *Mycobacterium leprae*. Two major types of leprosy are lepromatous (multibacillary type) and tuberculoid (paucibacillary type) leprosy.
2. The guiding principles of chemotherapy of leprosy are:
   - Prevention of development of resistance
   - Making the patient non-infective as quickly as possible
   - Shortening the duration of therapy
3. Paucibacillary (tuberculoid) leprosy is treated with dapsone (100 mg/day) + rifampicin (600 mg/month) for 6 months.
4. Multibacillary (lepromatous) leprosy requires treatment for two years. Drug therapy consists of dapsone (50–100 mg/day) + rifampicin (600 mg/month) + clofazimine (50 mg/day and 300 mg/month).
5. Other antilepra drugs are only considered for use when patients do not tolerate standard antileprotic drugs.

Chapter 58

Chemotherapy of other Protozoal Infections

1. Giardiasis

Flagellate protozoan *G. lamblia* is responsible for causing giardiasis. Mostly it lives as a commensal in the intestine. However, sometimes it causes diarrhoea and requires treatment. Effective drugs are:

- **Metronidazole:** It is the drug of first choice. Dose: 400 mg three times a day for seven days.
- **Tinidazole:** Dose: 2 gm as single dose.
- **Secnidazole:** Dose: 2 gm as single dose.
- **Furazolidone (furoxone):** It is a 5-nitrofuran derivative. It is highly effective against gram-negative bacteria including Salmonella and Shigella and some protozoa such as Giardia and Trichomonas. It is partly absorbed on oral administration and partly excreted in urine. It imparts orange colour to the urine. It is given in a dose of 100 mg four times a day for 5–7 days to treat bacterial enteritis, giardiasis, food poisoning, bacillary dysentery and diarrhoea. It is employed as an alternative drug to treat typhoid fever in a dose of 200 mg 4 times a day for 2 weeks. It is used in combination with infuroxine for topical treatment (as a powder or suppository) of vaginal trichomoniasis and candidiasis. It causes nausea, vomiting, diarrhoea, skin rash and disulfiram like effect as side effects.
- Being toxic, mepacrine is no more used in giardiasis and malaria.

2. Trichomoniasis

Vulvovaginitis is caused by *Trichomonas vaginalis*. Effective drugs are:

- **Metronidazole (drug of choice):** Dose: 400 mg twice daily for 7 days.
- **Tinidazole:** Dose: 0.3 gm once daily for 7 days or 2 gm as a single dose.
- Intravaginal drugs are metronidazole, hamycin, clotrimazole and iodoquinol.

3. Trypanosomiasis

Following drugs are used to treat trypano-somiasis:

- **Suramin sodium:** It is benzidine derivative. It is drug of choice for early stages of African trypnosomiasis. Initially give a small dose (200 mg) i.v. slowly as a test dose. It is followed by 1 gm i.v. slowly every week for 5 weeks.
- **Arsenicals:** They affect the cellular structure and functions by combining with sulph-hydral groups in proteins.
- **Melarsoprol** is an organic trivalent arsenical. It is drug of choice to treat late stage of trypnosomiasis. It may cause reactive encephalopathy and serious haemolytic anaemia (in patients deficient in G-6Ph-dehydrogenase enzyme).
- **Tryparsamide** is a pentavalent arsenical which is also used in the late stages of trypanosomiasis. Side effects are hepatitis,

gastrointestinal upsets, skin rashes, hemeralopia, transient emblyopia and total blindness.

- **Nifurtimox:** It is a nitrofuran derivative which is used to treat acute as well as chronic forms of American trypanosomiasis. On oral administration, it is readily absorbed from gut and is rapidly metabolized.

4. Leishmaniasis

The vector in the life cycle of the protozoan is a phlebomatoxs sandfly. Visceral leishmaniasis (kala-azar) is caused by *L. donovani*. Cutaneous leishmaniasis or oriental sore is induced by *L. tropica* and mucocutaneous leishmaniasis is caused by *L. braziliensis*. Following drugs are used in the treatment of leishmaniasis:

- **Sodium stibogluconate** is pentavalent antimonial and is the drug of choice. It is given in doses of 20 mg/kg body weight daily i.v or i.m. for 20 days. Nausea, vomiting, metallic taste, headache, bradycardia, arthralgia, respiratory arrest and shock may occur as side effects. It is contraindicated in patients of tuberculosis and renal and hepatic failure.
- **Pentamidine isothionate** is an aromatic diamidine. It is used to treat antimony resistant kala-azar with tuberculosis. It is also useful in trypnosomiasis, African sleeping sickness and *Pneumocytosis carinii* pneumonia in AIDS patients. It is given in doses of 4 mg/kg body weight slowly i.v. or i.m. on alternate days for 12–15 days and repeated after 3 weeks, if necessary. It is a very toxic drug. It may cause hypotension, tachycardia, headache, breathlessness, diarrhoea, abdominal pain, fainting attacks, trigeminal neuropathy, haematological disturbances, hypocalcaemia, hypoglycaemia, pancreatitis, impaired hepatic and renal functions and local reactions at the site of injection.

- **Amphotericin-B:** It is employed in cases of kala-azar not responding to antimonials and pentamidine. It is given in doses of 5–10 mg, gradually increased by 5–10 mg each day, till a dose of 0.5 mg/kg body weight is reached. Then give it on alternate days till a total of 1–3 gm is achieved.
- **Ketoconazole:** It is used to treat drug resistant kala-azar and dermal leishmaniasis in dose of 200 mg thrice daily for 4 weeks.
- **Allopurinol:** It is used as an adjunct to standard anti-leishmaniasis drugs.

TO REMEMBER

1. Giardiasis is caused by *G. lamblia*. Metronidazole is the drug of choice. Tinidazole, secnidazole and furazolidone are the other drugs. Mepacrine is no more used due to its toxicity.
2. Vulvovaginitis is caused by *T. vaginalis* and responds to metronidazole and tinidazole.
3. Suramin, arsenicals, and nifurtimox are used to treat trypanosomiasis.
4. Sodium stibogluconate is the drug of choice to treat visceral leishmaniasis (kala-azar). Second alternative is pentamidine isothionate. If patient is not responding to these drugs amphotericin-B or ketoconazole are used.

Chapter 59

Anthelmintics

Cestodes (flatworms or tapeworms), nematodes, and trematodes (flukes) parasitize man. In man, helminths (worms) infection is generally limited to the intestinal lumen but in certain situations they can migrate to other tissues. A group of compounds used to eradicate parasitic worms from the human body are called anthelmintic drugs. Anthelmintic drugs that kill the worms are known as vermicide while those that expel the worms are called vermifuge. The commonly used drugs are being described individually.

Treatment of Infections caused by Cestodes

Taenia saginata, T. solium and *Diphyllobothrium latum* are the common cestodes (tapeworms) that infest man. Their life cycles are complex. No symptoms are seen in majority of the patients. However, some patients may suffer from abdominal discomfort, indigestion, anorexia, and vitamin B deficiency.

Drug of choice for tapeworm infestations is nicolosamide.

Nicolosamide: It acts by affecting the scolex (head) and proximal (tail) segments of the worm through which the worm attaches to tissue. It produces its effect by inhibiting oxidative phosphorylation in mitochondria and interfering anaerobic generation of ATP by tapeworm. Due to this, the worm is detached from the intestinal wall and ultimately expelled from the body. It is administered in a dose of 2 gm orally. To prevent visceral cysticercosis, a purgative may be administered. There is no systemic toxicity. The drug can be given safely during pregnancy.

Treatment of Infestation caused by Nematodes

Nematodes are also called roundworms (*Ascaris lumbricoides*—intestinal nematode, filarial and guineaworms blood, lymphatic and other tissues), hookworms (*Ancylostoma duodenale*), and pinworms (*Enterobius vemiculosis*).

A group of newly developed drugs (mebendazole, albendazole, pyrantal pamoate, levamisole, tetramisole and thiabendazole) are broad-spectrum anthelmintics. These drugs are well tolerated and very effective. They do not need preparation of the patients prior to their administration. Further, purgative is not required to be given during post-drug period.

1. Mebendazole

- It is a broad-spectrum anthelmintic.
- It is highly effective in roundworm, hookworm (both species), Enterobius and Trichuris infestations. It is also the first drug of choice in the treatment of echinococcosis.
- It acts by reversibly impairing glucose uptake because it inhibits microtubule in nematodes. Due to this, parasites are immobilized and die slowly.

- On oral administration, it is poorly absorbed from gut and 90% of the drug is excreted in the faeces and 10% is eliminated in the urine unchanged or as metabolites.
  - Although drug is remarkably safe, it may cause mild nausea, vomiting, diarrhoea and abdominal discomfort.
  - It is given in doses of 100 mg twice daily for 3 days. It may be repeated 2–3 weeks later, if needed.
  - It is contraindicated during pregnancy and in children below 2 years of age due to teratogenic and embryotoxic properties.

2. Albendazole

- It is a congener of mebendazole. Its spectrum of activity and mechanism of action are similar to mebendazole with the advantage of single dose administration.
- On oral administration, it is rapidly absorbed from the gut; metabolized mainly to its sulphoxide, excreted in urine.
- It is given in a single dose (400 mg) for roundworm, hookworm, enterobius and trichuris; 400 mg for 3 days in strongloides and tapeworms and 400 mg twice daily for 4 weeks in hydatid disease.
- It is an alternative drug to praziquantel in neurocysticercosis (15 mg/kg/24 hr for one month).
- It should be given carefully in patients with liver or renal disease.
- It is contraindicated in pregnancy.
- Epigastric distress, diarrhoea, headache, nausea, dizziness and insomnia are mild side effects.

3. Pyrantel Pamoate

- It is highly effective against roundworm, hookworm and pinworm infestations.
- Pyrantel and its analogues act by causing neuromuscular block and cause spastic paralysis of the worms. Finally these worms are expelled from the gut.

- On oral administration, it is poorly absorbed from the gut and mainly excreted in faeces.
- It may cause headache and gastrointestinal discomfort.
- Its recommended dose is 11 mg/kg body weight.
- It should be used carefully in hepatitis and contraindicated in pregnancy.
- Fasting and purgative are not required with the use of this drug.

4. Tetramisole (Racemic Isomer) and Levamisole (l-Isomer)

- These drugs are used in a single dose of 150 mg to treat ascariasis. In case of hookworm infestation, they are given in two doses of 150 mg at 12 hours interval.
- They cause tonic paralysis by stimulating the ganglia in worms. This helps in expulsion of live worms.
- Levamisole has also been used in rheumatoid arthritis due to its immuno-stimulant property.
- They are well tolerated. However, there may be giddiness and drowsiness rarely. Skin rash, agranulocytosis and proteinuria may occur on prolonged use.

5. Piperazine

- It is available as hexahydrate, citrate and phosphate salts.
- Due to large dose and narrow spectrum, it is a drug of second choice to treat roundworm and pinworm infestations. A single dose of 4 gm of piperazine hydrate is effective in roundworm infestation while in pinworm infestation a 7 days course (2 gm daily) is required for complete eradication.
- It acts by causing flaccid paralysis of the roundworms by blocking neuromuscular transmission because it prevents action of acetylcholine and causes hyperpolarization. Due to this, the worms are then expelled alive; to facilitate expulsion of the worms often a purgative is given after drug.

- It may cause gastrointestinal symptoms, paresthesia, and muscular incoordination.
- It can be given safely in pregnancy but contraindicated in epilepsy and renal insufficiency.

6. Thiabendazole

- It is effective against roundworm, hookworm, pinworm, threadworm and whipworm infestations.
- It acts by interfering with the carbohydrate metabolism in the worms and there occurs loss of intracellular microtubules of the worm.
- It also has analgesic, antipyretic, and anti-inflammatory properties which gives total comforting effect to the patient.
- It is the drug of choice for the treatment of threadworm (*Strongyloides stercoralis*) infestation and when *Trichinella spiralis* larvae migrated to skin and skeletal muscle.
- It is given orally in dose of 25 mg/kg twice daily for two days.
- Nausea, vomiting, diarrhoea, vertigo, hallucinations may occur as side effects. Rarely may it cause Stevens-Johnson syndrome.

7. Bephenium (Alcopar)

- It is effective against roundworm and hookworm infestations.
- It is administered in a single dose of 2.5 gm orally.
- Its use has declined as better and less toxic drugs are available.

8. Diethylcarbamazine (Hetrazan)

- This is highly selective drug against microfilaria and adultworms.
- It is piperazine derivative.
- It has muscle paralyzing effect on the worm. Due to which, worm is dislodged from its site.
- On oral administration, it is rapidly absorbed, metabolized and excreted in urine.

- It is given in a dose of 2 mg/kg three times a day for 14–21 days. The drug should be taken after meals.
- Headache, nausea and vomiting appear as side effects.

9. Ivermectin

- It is the drug of choice in strongyloidiasis. It is also useful in the treatment of other forms of filariasis and cutaneous larva migrants.
- It is given in a single dose of 200 µg/kg and produces 60–100% cure.
- Fatigue, dizziness, nausea, vomiting, and abdominal pain may occur as side effects.
- It is contraindicated in pregnancy.
- Since ivermectin enhances GABA activity, it potentiates the action of benzodiazepines, barbiturates, and related drugs.

Treatment of Infestations caused by Trematodes

Trematodes are non-segmented flattened, helminths. Schistosomiasis is the commonest infestation. It is caused by schistosomes (blood flukes) group of trematodes. Following drugs are useful:

1. Praziquantel:
   - A wide spectrum of cestodes and trematode infestations respond to this drug.
   - It is the first drug which is useful in the treatment of neurocysticercosis.
   - On oral administration it is rapidly absorbed, crosses blood–brain barrier, rapidly metabolized in liver and excreted mostly in urine.
   - Abdominal discomfort, headache, dizziness appear as side effects.
   - Its important uses are:
     – It is first drug of choice for schistosomiasis clonorchiasis, opisthorchiasis and paragonimiasis. It is given in a dose of 20 mg three times a day for 1–3 days.

– It is the only drug of proven efficacy in the treatment of neurocysticercosis and subcutaneous cysticercosis. It is given orally in a dose of 50 mg/kg daily in three divided doses for 15 days. To decrease cerebral and meningeal inflammation due to release of toxic substances from the killed cysticerci, corticosteroids are given.

– It is used in a single dose to treat *H. nana* (25 mg/kg), taeniasis (10 mg/kg) and diphylobothriasis (25 mg/kg).

2. **Bithinol:** It is given orally in a dose of 40–50 mg/kg every other day for up to 15 doses.

3. **Oxaminiquine:** To treat schistosomiasis, it is administered in a dose of 12–15 mg/kg orally.

4. **Niridazole:** To treat schistosomiasis, it is given orally in a dose of 25 mg/kg daily in divided doses for 7 days. It may cause headache, gastrointestinal disturbances, insomnia and psychiatric disturbances.

5. **Antimony potassium tartrate:** To treat all the three species of schistosomiasis infestation, it is given intravenously in a dose of 8 ml of a 0.5% solution; gradually dose is increased every day up to 360 ml of the solution. It is contraindicated in cardiac, hepatic and renal insufficiency.

TO REMEMBER

1. Anthelmintics are a group of compounds which are used to eradicate parasitic worms from the human body.

2. Niclosamide is the drug of choice for tapeworm infestations. To prevent visceral cysticercosis, a purgative may also be administered along with niclosamide.

3. Mebendazole and albendazole are broad-spectrum anthelmintics and are used to treat roundworm, hookworm, Enterobium and Trichuris infestations.

4. Diethylcarbamazine is highly selective drug against microfilaria and adult-worms.

5. Ivermectin is the drug of choice in strogyloidiasis and is also useful in the treatment of other forms of filariasis as well as cutaneous larva migrants.

6. Praziquantel is the first drug of choice to treat a wide spectrum of cestodes and trematodes infestations. Further, it is the only drug of proven efficacy in the treatment of neurocysticercosis and subcutaneous cysticercosis.

7. Bithinol, oxaminquine, niridazole, and antimoney potassium tartrate are alternative drugs for the treatment of schistosomiasis infestation.

Chapter 60

Chemotherapy of Malignancy

It differs from the treatment of bacterial and parasitic infection in many respects such as:

- The malignant cell is a variant of the normal human cell. So its biochemical characteristics are same as that of normal cell. It means all agents who are deleterious to cancer cells are injurious to many normal human cells also. They do not have selective action against malignant cells as is seen in bacterial and parasitic infection.

- Moreover defense mechanisms of the body play an important role in disposing of the bacteria and parasite. So in microbial infections, a chemotherapeutic agent reduces the total number of micro-organisms and checks their multiplication and the body defense mechanism may take care of the remaining pathogenic organisms. Such body defense mechanism does not exist for cancer cells.

- So a single cancer cell, if remaining, may multiply and cause a relapse or recurrence of the disease. It is, therefore, important to use antineoplastic drugs in doses which reach the limit of tolerance. However, under these circumstances, there occurs attenuation of body defense mechanisms as to permit the development of a secondary bacterial invasion.

At present, picture is not so gloomy. Chemotherapy along with surgery and/or radiotherapy has enhanced chances of survival of cancer patients. Proper chemotherapy at least lead to long-term remissions in acute leukaemia in children, Hodgkin's disease, choreocarcinoma, Wilms' tumour, neuroblastoma, and rhabdomyosarcoma.

Classification of Cytotoxic Drugs

1. **Alkylating agents:** Cyclophosphamide, ifosfamide, mechlorethamine, chlorambucil, busulphan, melphalan, carmustine, lomustine, semustine, decarbonizes, thiotepa, temozolomide, streptozocin, estramustine, cisplatin, carboplatin

2. **Antimetabolites:** Methotrexate, 6-thioguanine, 6-mercaptopurine, cytarabine, 5-fluorouracil, fludarabine, pentostatin, cladribine, 5-fluorouracil, cytarabine, ftorafur.

3. **Natural substances:**
   - Alkaloids: Vincristine, vinblastine, L-asparaginase.
   - Epipodophyllotoxins: Etoposide, teniposide
   - Taxanes: Paclitaxel, docetaxel
   - Camptothecins: Topotecan, irinotecan
   - Enzyme: Asparaginase

4. **Antibiotics:** Mitomycin, mithramycin, doxorubicin, daunorubicin, bleomycin, actinomycin-D, pilcamycin, epirubicin, idarubicin, mitoxantrone

5. **Hormones and hormone antagonists:** Glucocorticoids, oestrogen, androgens and their analogues (fluvestrant, nilutamide, bicaluamide), progestins, tomoxifen,

flutamide, cyproterone acetate, gonado-tropin releasing hormone (agonists: goserelin, buserelin, leuprolide and antagonists: cetrorelix, ganirelix, abarelix), somatostatin analogues (e.g. octreotide, lanreotide).

6. **Miscellaneous:** Hydroxyurea, amsarrine, mitoxantrone, mitotane, radioactive isotopes (P^{32}, I^{131}, AU^{198}).

General Comments

Basically anticancer drugs are of two types:

i. Those which act only against dividing cells and not against resting cells. They are called cell cycle specific (CCS) drugs.

ii. Those which act against multiplying as well as resting cells. They are known as cell cycle non-specific (CCNS) drugs.

So the anticancer drug is selected on the basis of knowledge whether the growth fraction (dividing) of the malignancy concerned is large or small. In general, it is small in case of solid tumours. Since antineoplastic agents have non-specific action they have deleterious effect on rapidly dividing normal cells. However, these effects are usually reversible and recovery takes place during the time interval between two courses. Following are adverse reactions which are common to most of the anticancer drugs and are due to their effect on rapidly proliferating normal tissues.

• Bone marrow depression: granulo-cytopenia, thrombocytopenia, aplastic anaemia, and agranulocytosis.

• Lymphocytopenia and immunosup-pression occur due to suppression of reticuloendothelial system.

• Gastrointestinal tract upsets such as stomatitis, diarrhoea, vomiting, ulcer, haemorrhages.

• Fetus: abortion, teratogenicity, fetal death.

• Skin: alopecia, dermatitis.

• Hyperuricaemia as a result of massive cell destruction. This may lead to gout and urate stones in the urinary tract.

• Gonades: sterility and impotence.

• Secondary cancer may develop after several years due to depression of cell mediated and humoral blocking factors against neoplasia.

Alkylating Agents

The alkylating agents are so called because they possess highly reactive alkyl groups through which they can get linked with large molecules such as DNA, i.e. they can "alkylate" the macromolecules. Since they induce changes similar to radiation they are also known as radiomimetics.

They undergo intramolecular cyclization in neutral or alkaline solution and give rise to highly reactive ethyleneimmonium cation which is soluble in fat. The cation alkylate covalently with groupings like amino, sulphydryl, hydroxy or phosphate of the cellular constituents. Hence there occurs inhibition of DNA replication, breaking of DNA strand, miscoding of the gene and production of defective proteins.

Therapeutic Uses

1. **Mechlorethamine** is used to treat Hodgkin's disease, lymphoma and lung cancer. It is given in a dose of 0.4 mg/kg i.v. in any one course; it may be given at one time or in half the quantity on two successive days.

2. **Chlorambucil:** It is a very slowly acting alkylating agent. It is commonly used to treat chronic lymphatic leukaemia, Hodgkin's disease, carcinoma ovary, non-Hodgkin's lymphoma. It is given in a dose of 5–10 mg daily for 3–6 weeks. Maintenance dose is 2–4 mg daily.

3. **Cyclophosphamide:** It is inactive as such. It is transformed into active metabolites

(aldophosphamide, phosphoramide mustard) in the liver which exert anti-tumour action. It is a prominent immuno-suppressant also. It is very commonly used to treat wide range of haematological malignancies, non-Hodgkin's lymphomas, and solid tumours. It is given in a dose of 50–100 mg daily orally. It is also available as injectable (100–500 mg per vial).

4. **Ifosfamide:** It is a congener of cyclophos-phamide. It is longer acting and causes less alopecia and is less emetogenic than cyclophosphamide.

5. **Melphalan:** It is employed in the treatment of multiple myeloma at intervals of 4–6 weeks in a dose of 10 mg daily.

6. **Busulphan:** It is alkyl sulphonate. It is used in the treatment of chronic myeloid leukaemia and polycythemia vera. Initially the dose is 4–12 mg/day, and the maintenance dose varies from 1–4 mg/day.

7. **Thiotepa:** It is mainly used by intracavitary instillation in the manage-ment of effusions; also used to treat bladder tumours and ovarian carcinoma. It is available as injectable (15 mg per vial).

8. **Nitrosoureas** (carmustine, lumustine, and semustine): These are highly lipid soluble alkylating agents which cross blood–brain barrier. They are used to treat brain tumours and myeloma. Doses: Carmustine 50–200 mg/m^2 surface area by i.v. infusion; lumustine 100–300 mg/m^2 body surface area by single oral dose; semustine 100–200 mg/m^2 body surface area by single oral dose. Second course is repeated after 6 weeks.

9. **Cisplatin:** It is a metal complex. It is employed to treat testicular teratoma, carcinoma of ovary, lung, cervix, bladder, head and neck. It is hydrolysed intra-cellularly to produce a highly reactive moiety which causes cross-linking of DNA. It reacts with-SH groups in proteins and has radiomimetic property also. It is given in a dose of 50 mg/sq meter body surface at 3 weekly interval. It is diluted in 5% dextrose or normal saline and slowly infused.

10. **Carboplatin:** It is less reactive second generation platinum compound. It is better tolerated and has low toxicity. It is used in ovarian carcinoma, squamous carcinoma of head and neck, small cell lung cancer and seminoma. It is given in doses of 400 mg/m^2 by i.v. infusion over 15 to 60 minutes. Second course is repeated after 4 weeks.

11. **Oxaliplatin:** It is a new class of platinum agent. It consists of a platinum atom complexed with oxalate and diamino-cyclohexane. It is effective in testicular, ovarian, bladder, lung, prostate, colorectal, head and neck cancer.

12. **Decarbazine:** Unlike other alkylating agents, it has primary action on RNA and protein synthesis (others mainly affect DNA). It is used in malignant melanoma in doses of 3.5 mg/kg/day i.v. for 10 days. Second course is repeated after 4 weeks.

13. **Temozolomide:** It is employed in brain tumour and melanoma.

14. **Streptozocin:** It is used in islet cell carcinoma of pancreas.

Adverse effects of alkylating agents are same as described earlier.

Antimetabolites

They are structural analogues of chemical substances that take part in normal cellular activities. They inhibit synthesis of nucleic acid either competing with the natural substances for specific enzymes or become incorporated into the RNA or DNA.

1. **Methotrexate:** It is a folic acid analogue. It prevents the formation of tetrahydrofolate by competing with folic acid for the

enzyme dihydrofolate reductase. Thus it causes cell death by preventing the synthesis of purine, thymidylate and DNA. On oral administration, it is readily absorbed; 50% is bound with plasma protein and excreted in urine. Its toxicity is increased by sulphonamides, salicylates and tetracycline which displace it from plasma proteins and inhibit its tubular excretion. It is used to treat acute lymphoblastic leukaemia, early breast cancer, choriocarcinoma, bladder, head and neck cancers. It is also employed in psoriasis and mycosis fungoides. It is given in a dose of 10–25 mg weekly orally. It is also available for injection. Adverse effects are same as described earlier. They can be reduced if folinic acid is administered within 24 hours of the administration of the drug.

2. **Purine analogues:** They are 6-mercapto-purine, 6-thioguanine, fludarabine, pentostatin, and cladribine.

   Mercaptopurine and *thiogunine* are structural analogues of hypoxanthine. They act by suppressing DNA synthesis. On oral administration, they are readily absorbed, metabolized by xanthine oxidase in the liver and excreted as metabolites. Their toxicity is increased by allopurinol which inhibits xanthine oxidase enzyme. 6-mercaptopurine is used to treat acute lymphatic leukaemia and in chronic myeloid leukaemia refractory to busulfan. It is given orally in a dose of 2.5 mg/kg daily. 6-thioguanine is employed to treat myeloid leukaemia. In addition to those adverse effects described earlier, hyperuricaemia may occur.

   Fludarabine is purine analogue of antiviral drug vidarabin. It is converted intracellularly to its active metabolite (-a triphosphate derivative) by deoxycytidine kinase. This metabolite interferes with DNA synthesis by inhibiting various enzymes such as DNA polymerase-α and ribonucleotide reductase leading to apoptosis. It is used in chronic lympho-cytic leukaemia. Myelosuppression, mild nausea, alopecia, and stomatitis may occur as side effects.

   Pentostatin: This purine analogue is isolated from Streptomyces antibiotics. It interferes with utilization and DNA synthesis by inhibiting adenosine deaminase enzyme. This enzyme also converts adenosine to inosine and this inhibition leads to an inhibition of methylation and other reactions. It is used in hairy leukaemia. Adverse reactions are myelosuppression, nephrotoxicity, skin reaction and nausea.

   Cladribine: It is a synthetic purine analogue. It is phosphorylated by deoxycytidine kinase to active metabolite which exhibits its cytotoxic action by fraudulent incorporation into DNA. It is used also in hairy cell leukaemia. Myelosuppression may occur as side effect.

3. **Pyrimidine antagonists: 5-fluorouracil:** It is a fluorine substituted analogue of uracil. In the body, it is converted to its active ribonucleotide that blocks the formation of thymidylic acid, a crucial precursor of DNA, by inhibiting the enzyme thymi-dylate synthetase. It is used to treat solid tumours (breast cancer, adenocarcinoma of cervix, bladder and prostate). It is given orally or by infusion. By oral route, it is given in a divided doses of 1 gm per day on alternate day.

Cytarabine: It is an analogue of cytidine. It is phosphorylated in the body to corres-ponding nucleotide which blocks the generation of cytidilic acid and inhibits DNA polymerase. It is employed for the treatment of acute myeloid leukaemia in combination with 6 thioguanine or daunorubicin. It is given intravenously in a dose of 3–6 mg/kg per day in two divided doses daily for 5–10 days.

Ftorafur: It is a 5-fluorouracil congener. It is used in the treatment of breast and gastrointestinal cancers in doses of 0.8–1.2 gm/day orally.

Natural Substances

Natural substances, used in the treatment of malignancy, are complex chemical structures such as alkaloids, resins, glycosides, antibiotics, enzymes, etc. They are derived from a wide variety of plants and lower organisms (*Streptomyces* species).

1. **Alkaloids:** They act on various phases of the cell cycle and block mitosis. They interfere with microtubular function by binding to tubulin. Due to this, they stabilize cell microtubules and prevent their depolymerization. Thus they disrupt cell growth and cell function.

   Vinca rosea alkaloids are vincristine and vinblastine. Vinorelbine is semisynthetic derivative of vinblastine. They act by causing mitotic arrest at M phase.
   - Vincristine is the major drug in the management of leukaemias and lymphomas. It is also employed to treat a variety of solid tumours. It is given intravenously and maximum recommended dose is 2 mg. Adverse effects are neurotoxicity, inappropriate ADH secretion, tissue necrosis, alopecia, colicky abdominal pain.
   - Vinblastine is often used as a substitute for vincristine in the treatment of lymphomas. Advanced teratoma is also treated by vinblastin. Its usual dose is 0.1–0.2 mg/kg per week intravenously. Adverse effects are myelosuppression, tissue necrosis, GIT upsets, dermatitis, alopecia and inappropriate ADH secretion.

   - Vinorelbine has similar uses as that of vinblastine. In addition, it is also effective in non-small cell lung carcinoma. Adverse effects are same as that of vinblastine except lesser neurotoxicity.

2. **Epipodophyllotoxins:** Etoposide and teniposide are semisynthetic derivatives of podophyllotoxin, which is a plant glycoside. They act by arresting cells in the G_2 phase. They also cause DNA breaks by stimulating DNA topoisomerase II. They are used in testicular tumours, lung cancer, Hodgkin's, other lymphomas, and carcinoma bladder. Teniposide is also used in acute lymphoblastic leukaemia in children. Their main toxicity includes alopecia, leucopenia, and gastrointestinal disturbances. Teniposide may also cause neuropathy.

3. **Texanes:** Paclitaxel and docetaxels are complex diterpin texanes. They are obtained from bark of the western yew tree. By enhancing polymerization of tubulin, they stabilize microtubules and prevent their depolymerization. Due to this, they block interphase and mitotic functions by inhibiting normal dynamic reorganization of the microtubule network. They are used in:
   - Metastatic ovarian and breast carcinoma
   - Head and neck cancer
   - Small cell lung cancer
   - Oesophageal adenocarcinoma
   - Hormonal refractory prostate cancer

   Dose of paclitaxel is 175 mg/m² by i.v. infusion over 3 hours or 24 hours, repeated every 3 weeks.

   Their main toxicity includes reversible myelosuppression, neuropathy, chest pain, arthralgia, myalgia, mucositis and oedema.

4. **Camptothecins:** Topotecan and irinotecan are semisynthetic derivatives of campto-

thecins, isolated from an ornamental Chinese tree. They inhibit topoisomerase I and lead to an irreversible double strand DNA break. They cause mitotic arrest of cells in S-phase of cell cycle. They are used in:

- Ovarian cancer
- Colon and lung cancers
- Small cell lung cancer

Myelosuppression, flu-like symptoms, nausea and vomiting may occur as side effects.

5. **Enzyme:** Asparaginase is an enzyme. It is obtained from *E. coli*. It hydrolyses the amino acid L-asparagine to aspartic acid and ammonia. Asparagine is not an essential amino acid for normal cells which can synthesize it. Certain types of neoplastic cells cannot synthesize asparazine being deficient in L-asparaginase synthetase enzyme. So they cease to grow and multiply if deprived of this amino acid. It is used to treat acute lymphoblastic leukaemia.

In addition to usual adverse effects of cytotoxic drugs, it may give rise to allergic reactions, hepatotoxicity, pancreatitis, and mental depression.

Antibiotics

They are obtained from *Streptomyces* species. They act by:

- Blocking the synthesis of new DNA
- Blocking DNA dependent RNA synthesis
- Breaking DNA strands

Following antibiotics are used in the treatment of cancer:

1. **Mitomycin C:** It is employed to treat resistant cases of gastrointestinal tumours, breast, head, neck and lung carcinoma. It is available as injectable (2 mg/vial). Adverse effects include myelosuppression, stomatitis, pulmonary toxicity, tissue necrosis, alopecia and rarely hepato-toxicity.

2. **Actinomycin D:** It is used in childhood solid tumours, soft tissue sarcoma and testicular teratoma. It is given in doses of 15 µg/kg per day intravenously for 5 days. It may be repeated after 4 weeks, if necessary.

3. **Bleomycin:** It is used in head and neck, larynx, cervix, vulvovagina, skin and penis cancers. It does not cause bone marrow depression. However, it may cause nausea, vomiting, alopecia, skin rash, fever and pulmonary toxicity. It is given in doses of 15 mg/m^2 twice weekly to a total dose of 200 mg/m^2.

4. **Doxorubicin:** It is employed to treat carcinoma of breast, bronchi, urinary bladder, and thyroid gland. It is given in a total dose of 550 mg/sq meter body surface area intravenously. Its unique adverse effects are cardiotoxicity and radiation recall reaction.

5. **Mitoxantrone:** It is an analogue of doxorubicin with lower cardiotoxicity. It is used in acute non-haemolytic leukaemia, chronic myelogenous leukemia, non-Hodgkin lymphoma, and cancer breast.

6. **Mithramycin:** Its use is restricted to embryonic testicular tumour, disseminated cancer with bony metastasis and hypercalcaemia. It is given in doses of 25 µg/kg by slow i.v. infusion daily or on alternate days (total 8–10 doses).

7. **Daunorubicin and idarubicin:** They are employed to treat acute myelocytic leukemia. Adverse effects are myelosuppression, alopecia, cardiotoxicity, stomatitis, tissue necrosis.

8. **Pilcamycin:** It is used in metastatic testicular carcinoma, and hypercalcaemia of malignancy. Myelosuppression, hypocalcaemia, nausea, vomiting, hepatotoxicity, nephrotoxicity, skin rash, and stomatitis may occur as adverse effects.

9. **Epirubicin:** It is used in breast cancer. Myelosuppression, GIT distress, skin rash, cardiotoxicity, and stomatitis may occur as adverse effects.

10. **Mitoxantrone:** It is used in breast cancer, ovarian cancer, non-lymphocytic leukaemia, and secondary progressive multiple sclerosis. Adverse effects are similar to epirubicin plus rarely hepatotoxicity.

Hormones and Hormone Antagonists

- Hormones are not cytotoxic agents.
- They only affect the environment or cancer cells—favourably or adversely.
- They are employed as adjunct to cytotoxic chemotherapy and/or surgery.
- They have only palliative value.

  1. **Glucocorticoids:** Prednisone and prednisolone are used in the treatment of acute lymphoblastic leukaemia and non-Hodgkin's lymphoma. They quickly lower the white cell count due to their lympholytic effect. They also control toxemia and improve the patient's general condition due to the non-specific "antistress" effect. In chronic lymphocytic leukaemia, they are used to control autoimmune hemolytic anemia and thrombocytopenia. The average dose of prednisolone is 40–100 mg per day.

  2. **Androgens:** Androgens may be used to treat inoperable premenopausal carcinoma breast which is oestrogen dependent. They act by inhibiting endogenous oestrogen production from ovaries by suppressing the release of FSH from anterior pituitary. They also have a direct inhibitory effect on the tumour cells. Drug of choice is testosterone propionate which is given in a dose of 50–100 mg intramuscularly three times a week. Fluoxymesterone may be given orally in a dose of 5 mg four times a day. There may be hoarseness of voice, hirsutism, masculinisation and clitorial hypertrophy.

  3. **Oestrogens:** They are used to treat carcinoma of prostate and post-menopausal breast cancer. They act by inhibiting the endogenous production of androgen by suppressing the release of interstitial cell stimulating hormone from anterior pituitary. They also depress the growth of the neoplasm directly. Most commonly used oestrogen is stilbestrol. Its initial dose is 5 mg three times a day. The dose is reduced to 1 mg thrice a day on substantial improvement. Feminization, impotence and gynecomastia often occur as side effects.

  4. **Progestins:** They are used to treat carcinoma of the endometrium. Derivatives of 17 hydroxyprogesterone are the agents of choice because they are devoid of either androgenic or oestrogenic activity.

  5. **Estrogen receptor antagonists:**

     - *Tamoxifen* and *toremifene* are non-steroidal antioestrogen. They act by binding to and decreasing the availability of oestrogen receptors. They also suppress serum levels of insulin-like growth factors and up regulate local production of transforming growth factor-β. These are used to treat oestrogen dependent breast cancer, male breast carcinoma postoperatively and endometrial cancer. Transient flare of tumour activity initially, oedema, hot flushes, deep vein thrombosis and endometrial hyperplasia occur as side effects. Tamoxifen is given in doses of 10–20 mg/day orally.

     - *Fluvestrant* is a steroidal selective estrogen receptor down regulator and is termed as "pure antiestrogen". It is used for estrogen receptor metastatic breast cancer that has progressed despite tamoxifen therapy. Oedema and hot flushes occur as side effects.

6. **Androgen receptor antagonists:** *Flutamide, nilutamide* and *bicalutamide* are non-steroidal compounds. They act by inhibiting binding of testosterone to nuclear androgen receptors. They are effective in the management of prostatic cancer. Flutamide is given in oral doses of 250 mg three times a day. The other two drugs are given once daily. The adverse effects are nausea, vomiting, loss of libido, sexual impotence, hot flushes, mild gynaecomastia and transient elevation of liver enzymes.

7. **Somatostatin analogues** such as octreotide and lanreotide are occasionally used in the management of: (a) metastatic carcinoid tumours by inhibiting secretions of various autacoids (e.g. serotonin) and (b) islet cell carcinoma by inhibiting peptide hormones (e.g. gastrin, VIP, insulin).

8. **Gonadotropin-releasing hormone (GN-RH) agonists** (goserelin, buserelin and leuprolide) have been used in certain hormone dependent cancers, e.g. cancer of prostate and breast. These agonists act by inhibiting gonadotrophin (FSH/LH) release and suppress gonadal functions due to down regulation and desensitization of GN-RH receptors. Hot flashes, osteoporosis, oedema, headache, nausea, loss of libido and allergic manifestations may appear as side effects.

9. **Gonadotropin-releasing antagonists** (cetrorelix, ganirelix, abarelix) act as competitive antagonist at pituitary GN-RH receptors. These are used in prostatic carcinoma. Pain and swelling at the injection site may appear as side effects.

Miscellaneous Drugs

1. **Hydroxyurea:** It is used to treat chronic myelogenous leukaemia and melanoma. It acts by inhibiting ribonucleotide reductase enzyme which is essential for DNA synthesis.

2. **Mitotane:** It is employed to treat inoperable adrenal cancer. It acts by destroying normal and neoplastic adrenocortical cells. It may cause gastrointestinal disturbances, dermatitis and mental depression.

3. **Amsarrine:** It is used to treat myelogenous leukaemia, resistant to other drugs, advanced ovarian cancer and lymphomas. It acts by binding to DNA and causing chromosome breakage.

4. **Mitoxantrone:** It is employed to treat acute myelogenous leukaemia refractory to other drugs, non-Hodgkin's lymphomas and breast cancer. It acts by inhibiting both DNA and RNA synthesis.

5. **Radioactive isotopes:**

   i. P^{32} *(phosphotope):* It is used to treat polycythemia vera, chronic lymphocytic and granulocytic leukaemia in a dose of 3–5 millicuries intravenously. The physical half-life is 14 days and it emits beta radiation.

   ii. I^{131} *(iodotope):* It is employed in hyperthyroidism and thyroid cancer in a dose of 4–10 millicuries for thyrotoxicosis and 50–100 millicuries for thyroid cancers. The physical half-life is 8 days. It emits beta and gamma rays.

   iii. Au^{198} *(aureotope):* It is used to treat pleural and peritoneal effusions. 35–100 millicuries are injected intrapleurally or intraperitoneally. The physical half-life is 3 days. It emits beta and gamma radiations.

6. **Newer drugs:**
   i. *Imatinib:* It is tyrosine kinase inhibitor. It has specific activity against BCR-ABL tyrosine kinase which is responsible for uncontrollable proliferation of and reduced apoptosis of malignant white blood cells. Thus it stops cell proliferation and can induce apoptosis of tumour cells. Imatinib acts as a competitive inhibitor of ATP. So it blocks the binding of ATP and inhibits kinase activity.

   On oral administration, it is well absorbed. It is mostly metabolized in liver. About 68% of the dose is excreted in faeces as metabolite and 5% is excreted unchanged in urine. It has been found useful in the treatment of:
   - Chronic myeloid leukemia (400 mg per day)
   - Chronic accelerated phase of chronic myeloid leukemia as well as in blast crisis chronic myeloid leukemia (400–600 mg per day)
   - Ph+ acute lymphoblastic leukemia
   - Patients with metastatic gastrointestinal stromal tumours (400–600 mg per day) because it also inhibits the receptor tyrosine kinase for c-kit

   Side effects are nausea, vomiting, haemorrhage, severe fluid retention (controlled by diuretics), neutropenia, thrombocytopenia, and hepatotoxicity. Regular blood counts are therefore needed. It is contraindicated in hypersensitivity, pregnancy and lactation. It should be given cautiously in hepatic impairment, geriatric patients and children.

   ii. *Capecitabine:* It is a new anticancer therapy for oral administration. It is a fluoro pyrimidine, which is converted into 5-fluorouracil (5-FU) once inside the tumour. The drug takes the advantage of the higher thymidine phosphorylase activity in malignant tissue. It acts by inhibiting cell division because it inhibits the formation of thymidylate which is essential for the synthesis of DNA. It also interferes with RNA processing and protein synthesis. On oral administration, it is rapidly and completely absorbed unchanged from gastrointestinal tract. It is metabolized in liver and tumour tissue. It is eliminated mainly through kidney. It is used in colorectal carcinoma, breast cancer, pancreatic cancer. Capecitabine is administered orally in doses of 1250 mg/m^2 (range- 313–1250 mg/m^2) twice a day for 14 days starting on day-1 (total dose per cycle 3500 mg/m^2), followed by a 1 week rest period given as 3 week cycle. Side effects are diarrhoea, nausea, vomiting, stomatitis, abdominal pain, upset stomach, constipation, loss of appetite and dehydration.

   iii. *Hexamethyl-melamine* (altretamine) is used to treat ovarian cancer. It acts by selectively inhibiting the incorporation of thymidine and uridine into DNA and RNA inhibiting their synthesis. Adverse effects are gastrointestinal toxicity, neurotoxicity and myelosuppression.

   iv. *Arsenic trioxide* and *tretinoin* are retinoids. These are used in acute promyelocytic leukaemia by upgrading the genes involved in apoptosis.

   v. *Bexarotenep (retinoids)* and *denileukin diftitox* (immunotoxin) are used in cutaneous T cell lymphoma.

   vi. *Thalidomide* has been used in multiple myeloma and melanoma. It acts by inhibiting angiogenesis, tumour necrosis factor-α production, stimulating T cell proliferation and increasing interferon as well as IL-2 release and erlotinib.

vii. *Gefitinib* is used in metastatic non-small cell lung cancer and other solid tumours. These drugs act by inhibiting epidermal growth factor receptor linked tyrosine kinase pathway by inhibiting to tyrosine kinase-ATP binding site.

viii. *Bortezomibis* is used to treat refractory and relapsed multiple myeloma. It acts by inhibiting proteosome (large multiprotein complex in plasma and nucleus) and prevents degradation of intracellular proteins leading to activation of signaling cascades, cell cycle asset and apoptosis.

ix. *Monoclonal antibodies (MAbs):* Malignant cells often have unique antigens which are exposed on their surface. These are called tumour associated antigens. Monoclonal antibodies are single species of antibody that recognize and react with a specific antigen only. The cytotoxic effect of MAbs may be attributed to their antibody dependent cellular toxicity (ADCC) or due to complement-dependent cytotoxicity (CDC) and also because of direct induction of apoptosis.

   a. *Naked monoclonal antibodies* do not carry any immunotoxin or radiopharmaceutical warheads to be used as missile. Clinically used naked MAbs are:

   - *Rituximab* is used in B cell lymphoma, chronic lymphocytic leukaemia. Side effects are hypersensitivity reactions and neutropenia.
   - *Alemtuzumab* is used in B cell chronic lymphoid leukaemia and T cell lymphoma. Immunosuppression and hypersensitivity reactions may occur as side effects.
   - *Trastuzumab* is used in breast cancer. Hypersensitivity reaction, gastrointestinal toxicity and cardiomyopathy may occur as adverse effects.
   - *Cetuximab* is useful in colorectal cancer, non-small cell lung carcinoma, breast and pancreatic carcinoma. Infusion related toxicity and skin rash are the adverse reactions.
   - *Bevacizumab* is used in metastatic colorectal cancer with 5-Fu, renal cell carcinoma and breast cancer (along with chemotherapy). Adverse effects are hypertension, mild neutropenia, congestive heart failure, pulmonary haemorrhage and proteinuria.

   b. *Gemtuzumab ozogamicin* (conjugate of MAb against CD33 antigen+ calicheamicin antibiotic) is used to treat acute myeloid leukaemia. Toxicity includes infusion related, myelosuppression and helps to toxicity.

   c. *Radioisotope-based MAbs* are ibritumomab-Y^{90} (yttrium90–radionucleotide conjugated to ibritumomab) and testitumomab-I^{131} (iodine radionucleotide conjugated to tostitumomab). These have additional advantage of providing targeted delivery of radioactive particles to nearby tumour clusters in which blood circulation fails to deliver MAbs. Since Y^{90} emits β-radiation only, it is easier and safer to use even in outpatient settings. It also has better radiation penetration in lymphomas of large diameter. These are used in follicular low grade non-Hodgkin's lymphoma. Adverse effects are neutropenia, infusion related toxicity, hypothyroidism (with I^{131}).

x. *Protectants:* They have been developed to treat or reduce adverse effects which are produced during chemotherapy or radiotherapy of cancers. These are as under:

- *Colony stimulating factors (CSF):* Filgrastim (human recombinant granulocyte CSF) and sargramostim (human recombinant granulocyte and macrophages CSF) are used to prevent chemotherapy-induced neutropenia, to increase neutrophil counts and to prevent infection by enhancing neutrophil functions and accelerating bone marrow repopulation. Side effects are fever, myalgia, pericardial effusion and bone pain.

- *Amifostine* is a thiophosphate cytoprotectant. It is administered before cisplatin to reduce incidence of nephrotoxicity and before radiation therapy for head and neck cancer to reduce xerostomia. It is metabolized by membrane bound alkaline phosphatase into an active free thiol which is rapidly accumulated in normal tissues by facilitated diffusion as compared to neoplastic tissues. So it protects normal tissue by covalently binding to cisplatin, taxanes and anthracycline group of anticancer drugs. Hypotension, nausea and vomiting may occur as side effects.

- *Mesna:* Acrolein is a nephrotoxic metabolite of cyclophosphamide and ifosfamide, causing haemorrhagic cystitis. Mesna prevents haemorrhagic cystitis by conjugating with acrolein in urine. Nausea and vomiting may occur as side effects.

- *Dexrazoxane* is coadministered with doxorubicin in patients of breast cancer to reduce the incidence of cardiomyopathy. It acts by helping natural defence mechanisms such as action of superoxide dismutase against free radicals by chelating the iron which catalyses the production of free radicals anthracycline group of antibiotics. Myelosuppression may occur as side effect.

- *Oprelvekin* (recombinant human IL-11) and thrombopoietin (high molecular weight glycoprotein) are thrombopoietic growth factors. These are used to prevent chemotherapy-induced thrombocytopenia. Oprelvekin acts by stimulating megakaryocytes and their precursors in the bone marrow while thrombopoietin acts being primary regulator of platelet production. Both decrease the need for platelet transfusions in cancer patients receiving highly myelosuppressive chemotherapy such as carboplatin or cyclophosphamide. Adverse effects include peripheral edema, palpitation, fatigue, dyspnoea, myalgia, arthralgia and immunogenicity.

- *Levamisole* is combined with 5-FU to improve survival of patients of colorectal cancer due to its ability to enhance T cell functions and cellular immunity. Flu-like symptoms, nausea and vomiting are side effects.

Points for Dental Students

1. Oral squamous cell cancer (SCC) is the outcome of a multistage process from normal to dysplastic lesions and ultimately to SCC.

2. A premalignant or precancerous lesion is defined by the WHO as a morphologically altered tissue in which cancer is more likely to occur and includes oral leukoplakia, oral erythroplakia and

possibly oral lichen planus. Leukoplakia is a white patch of oral mucosa that cannot be characterized clinically or pathologically as anyother diagnosed disease.

3. Main line of treatment of SCC is surgery and/or radiation.

4. Chemotherapy has been considered for treatment of individuals with advanced tumour or recurrent disease in whom surgery or radiation unlikely to result in cure.

5. Chemotherapy is used as induction therapy prior to local therapies, as simultaneous chemoradiotherapy and as adjunct chemotherapy after local treatment. The objective of adding chemotherapy is to promote initial tumour reduction and to provide early treatment of micrometastases.

6. The principal agents that have been studied alone or in combination are methotrexate, bleomycin, taxol and its derivatives, cisplatin and platinum derivatives and 5-fluorouracil.

7. Nasopharyngeal carcinoma is treated by chemotherapy and immunotherapy, in combination with radiation therapy.

8. Complications of cancer treatment include:

   a. **Mucositis:** Ulcerative mucositis is a painful condition that is a dose and rate limiting toxicity of cancer therapy. Its management includes use of:
      * *Diluting agents:* Saline, bicarbonate rinses, frequent water rinses, dilute hydrogen peroxide rinses.
      * *Coating agents:* Kaolin-pectin, aluminium chloride, aluminium hydroxide, magnesium hydroxide, hydroxypropyl cellulose, sucralfate
      * *Lip lubricants:* Water-based lubricants, lanolin.
      * *Topical agents:* Dicyclomine hydrochloride, xylocaine hydrochloride, benzocaine hydrochloride, diphenhydramine hydrochloride.
      * *Analgesic agents:* Benzydamine hydrochloride.
      * Pain due to oropharyngeal mucositis frequently requires the use of opioid analgesics.

   b. **Xerostomia (hyposalivation):** Salivary secretion can be stimulated by:
      * Pilocarpine that acts on muscarinic cholinergic receptors of salivary gland acinar cells.
      * Bethanechol may be used as sialagogue. It does not cause gastrointestinal upsets.

   c. Oropharynx candidiasis is treated with topical antifungals because it does not lead to systemic infection unless the patient is immunocompromised.

   d. Caries associated with hyposalivation typically affect the gingival third and incised cusp tips of the teeth. In such cases, give treatment of dental caries.

   e. Soft tissue necrosis may involve any oral site, including the cheeks and tongue.

   f. Post-radiation osteonecrosis (PRON) may be chronic or progressive. It is treated as under:
      * Avoid mucosal irritants.
      * Discontinue the use of dental appliances if they contact the area of the lesion.
      * Topical antibiotic (tetracycline) or antiseptic (chlorhexidine) rinses may reduce the potential local irritation from the microbial flora.
      * Hyperbaric O_2 therapy to increase oxygenation of tissues.
      * Provide appropriate analgesia.

   g. Other complications are speech and mastication problems, mandibular dysfunction and dentofacial abnormalities.

9. Oral pain in cancer patients may be due to:
   • Tumor
   • Cancer therapy
   • Radiotherapy
   • Chemotherapy

It may be unrelated to cancer or cancer therapy. Oral pain can be treated by analgesics. When required, it should be provided on a regular basis. In general, non-narcotic analgesics should be provided to all patients even if potent opioids are required because this may allow a lower dose of narcotic medication. Adjunct medication such as tricyclic anti-depressants may enhance the analgesic effects of other agents, possess analgesic potential themselves and promote sleep which is often disrupted by pain. Adjunct medications directed at the aetiology of the pain should be used whenever possible. For example, for neuralgia-like pain, anticonvulsant medication should be included.

Possible side effects, such as constipation due to opioids, should be anticipated and treated.

TO REMEMBER

1. Two important differences between chemotherapy of malignancy and chemotherapy of bacterial and parasitic infections are:
   a. Chemotherapeutic agents for the malignancy are non-selective
   b. Body defense mechanisms do not play any role to dispose of a malignant cell.
2. Bone marrow depression, lympho-cytopenia, immunosuppression, gastro-intestinal upsets, alopecia, hyperuri-caemia, sterility and impotence are common adverse effects of anticancer drugs due to their effect on rapidly proliferating normal tissue.
3. Mechlorethamine is commonly used to treat Hodgkin's disease.
4. Cyclophosphamide is commonly emplo-yed in lymphomas and carcinoma of ovary and breast.
5. Chlorambucil is the drug of choice to treat chronic lymphatic leukaemia.
6. Busulphan is drug of choice to treat chronic myeloid leukaemia.
7. Melphalan is indicated in multiple myeloma.
8. Nitrosoureas (carmustine, lomustine, semustine) are very useful in brain tumours.
9. Decarbazine is useful in malignant melanoma.
10. Cisplatin is used to treat testicular teratoma, carcinoma of ovary and bladder.
11. Vinblastin is useful in Hodgkin's disease while vincristine is used in acute lymphoblastic leukaemia, choriocar-cinoma, Hodgkin's and non-Hodgkin's lymphomas.
12. Dactinomycin is useful in Wilms' tumour, and choriocarcinoma.
13. Doxarubicin and daunorubicin are used to treat acute myeloid leukaemia. The former is also employed in lymphomas, sarcomas and cancer of lung and thyroid.
14. Asparaginase is useful in acute leukemia of children.
15. Hydrocortisone is used in acute leukaemia and prednisolone is employed to treat Hodgkin's disease and lymphomas.
16. Flutamide is used to treat prostate cancer.
17. Testosterone is employed to treat premenopausal breast cancer.
18. Cancer prostate is also treated with leuprolide and diethylstilbestrol.
19. Progestins are employed to treat endometrial metastatic cancer.
20. Tamoxifen is used to treat postmeno-pausal breast cancer.

Antiseptics

Treatment of Dentoalveolar Abscess, Gingivitis and

Ulceration and Inflammation

Therapeutic Considerations in the Use of Drugs

Toothbrushing Techniques

Section 13

Dental Pharmacology and Therapeutics

Chapter 61

Antiseptics

Antiseptics and disinfectants are anti-infective agents. They are used to reduce the bacterial population. They are usually used topically on the skin or mucous membrane or inanimate objects. Antiseptic agent is applied on a living tissue to inhibit the bacterial growth. On the other hand, disinfectant is used to inhibit or kill bacteria in inanimate objects. Disinfectants inhibit the growth of bacteria when used in dilute solution.

Sepsis means the presence of bacteria while asepsis implies an entire freedom from bacteria. Sterilization is the process of freeing an article, surface, or a medium from bacteria, by removing or killing all micro-organisms, both in vegetative and sporing states. It can be achieved by boiling in water or by cold sterilization (dettol, methylated spirit).

Antiseptics act as protoplasmic poisons, i.e. they destroy the protoplasm of cells. Some antiseptics (e.g. carbolic acid) will poison both the bacterial as well as host cells indiscriminately. However, cetrimide, furan compounds and the antibiotics such as soframycin, etc. are recently introduced newer antiseptics. They have a selective action, i.e. they will have a greater effect on the protoplasm of the bacteria than on the protoplasm of the host cells. No doubt an ideal antiseptic will be one that inhibits the action of bacteria without affecting the tissue cells at all.

A number of factors may modify the activity of antiseptic such as:
- Temperature and pH (antiseptics are more effective in warm or hot environment)
- The number and virulence of the bacteria present
- The presence of blood, pus, tissue debris, saliva, etc. (dilute the antiseptic and makes penetration difficult)
- Period of contact of antiseptic with microorganisms
- Size of innoculum and nature of microbe involved
- Concentration of the antiseptic solution

Properties of an ideal antiseptic agent should be:
- Chemically stable and cheap
- Wide range of activity against bacteria, fungi, viruses, protozoa
- Rapid in action and exert sustained protection
- Non-staining with agreeable colour and odour
- Non-irritating to tissues and should not delay healing
- High solvent action for grease, i.e. a low surface tension so that it can penetrate deeply
- Non-absorbable, produce minimum systemic toxicity
- No loss of potency in presence of organic material such as blood, pus, exudates and excreta

- Non-sensitizing (no allergy)
- Active in very dilute solution at ordinary temperature
- No deterioration of potency on keeping
- Compatible with soaps and other detergents

Classification

Physical Agents

- Heat such as superheated steam
- Irradiation such as ultraviolet rays, sun light
- Surface active agents such as soaps and detergents
- Substances exerting osmotic pressure, e.g. concentrated solution of sugar and salt

Chemical Agents

1. **Inorganic:**
   - Oxidizing agents and inorganic halogen compounds such as hydrogen peroxide, potassium permanganate
   - Acids and alkalis such as strong mineral acids, boric acid and caustic alkalies
   - Metallic salts such as silver nitrate, colloidal silver salt, silver sulphadiazine, nitromersol, thimersol, mercurochrome, zinc sulphate, calamine.
2. **Organic:**
   - Alcohols such as ethanol, isopropanol
   - Aldehydes such as formaldehyde, guitar aldehyde
   - Phenols and simple aromatic compounds such as phenol, cresol, chlorxylenol, hexachlorphene, chlorhexidine
   - Halogens such as iodine, povidone iodine, chlorine, chlorophores
   - Dyestuff such as acriflavine, proflavine, gentian violet, brilliant green
   - Nitrofurans such as nitrofurantoin, nitrofurazone, furazolidine, nifuroxane
   - Miscellaneous such as balsams, volatile oils

Redeal Walker's test (RW test): This test is performed to determine the activity of an antiseptic by comparing it with the potency of phenol. A coefficient is determined as follows:

$$\text{KW coefficient} = \frac{\begin{array}{l}\text{Maximum dilution of the}\\ \text{unknown substance which kills}\\ \text{24 hr old culture of bacillus}\\ \text{Typhosus at 37°C in 71/2}\\ \text{minutes}\end{array}}{\begin{array}{l}\text{Maximum dilution of phenol}\\ \text{which kills a similar culture}\\ \text{under identical conditions}\end{array}}$$

Higher the coefficient greater is the antiseptic property.

Chick Martin's test: It is more useful because it employs admixture with organic matter at room temperature. Many antiseptics are inactivated in the presence of organic matter.

Uses of Local Anti-infective

1. As disinfectants of surgical instruments:
   - Formaldehyde is used for delicate electrical instruments.
   - Lysol is employed for sharp instruments such as knife, needles, etc.
   - Oxycyanide of mercury (0.5%) is also used for sharp instruments.
2. As antiseptic wash and dressing:
   - Cetrimide (1%)
   - Gentian violet (2 to 5%)
   - Methylene blue (1 to 3%)
   - Mercurochrome (1 to 2%)
   - Acriflavin (0.1%)
   - Thiomersol (0.1%)
   - Triple dye (brilliant green 1% + gentian violet 1% + acriflavine 0.1%)
   - Weak iodine solution
3. As cleansing agent for wound:
   - Hydrogen peroxide (10–20%)
   - Potassium permanganate (0.5%)
   - Chloramine (0.5 to 1%)
4. As preservative:
   - Phenol or cresol (0.5%) for serum, vaccine, etc.

- Sodium metabisulphite (0.05 to 0.1%)
- Chlorbutol (0.3%)

5. As parasiticides:
   i. Fungicides
      - Antifungal antibiotics
      - Salicylic acid (2%)
      - Chrysorbin (5%)
      - Dithranol (1%)
      - Undecenoic acid (5%)
   ii. Scabicides
      - Benzyl benzoate emulsion (25%)
      - Sulphur ointment (10%)
      - Gammaxane lotion (1%)
   iii. Pediculocides: (Lice infection)
      - Gamma benzene hexachloride (0.2%)
      - Dicophane (2 to 4%)
      - Benzyl benzoate (25%)
      - Xylol (20 to 25%)

6. As insecticides:
   - Pyrethrum
   - Dicophane (DDT) 5 to 10% powder
   - Gammexane
   - Dibutyl phthalate
   - Dimethyl phthalate

Individual Agents

Only those antiseptics will be discussed which are of importance in dental practice.

1. **Hydrogen peroxide (H_2O_2):** It is a colourless and odourless liquid. It produces thick froth in mouth. Since sulfuric acid is added as a preservative, it is slightly acidic in nature. In order to prevent its ready dissociation in light, water and oxygen, it should be kept in dark bottles, away from sun light and in a cool place. It is available as 3% aqueous solution.

Pharmacological actions:
- *Antiseptic:* In the body tissues, hydrogen peroxide is dissociated into water and oxygen. The newly liberated oxygen is called as nascent oxygen. It is more active than atmospheric oxygen. It causes considerable effervescene (frothing action). It is used to clean suppurating wounds and inflamed mucous membranes because the froth loosens adherent deposits. It is a powerful antiseptic for anaerobic bacteria.
- *Bleaching agent:* Hydrogen peroxide changes pigments into colourless material by chemical reaction.
- Hydrogen peroxide acts as *deodorant* by oxidising the odorous gasses which arise from the breakdown of protein.
- *Haemostatic:* Strong solution of hydrogen peroxide (25–30%) acts as local haemostatic (styptic). It has very weak haemostatic properties if 3% solution is used.

Uses: It is used in dental practice as under:
- As antiseptic to treat general acute gingivitis and acute ulcerative stomatitis. For this purpose, it is applied either locally (3% undiluted solution) or as mouthwash (one part of 3% hydrogen peroxide to four parts of water).
- To remove superficial stains on teeth in combination with pumice and glycerine.
- To control gingival seepage during cavity preparation (3% solution of hydrogen peroxide is employed as haemostatic).

Contraindications: It is contraindicated in the following situations in dental practice:
- To avoid infection into deeper tissues due to liberation of oxygen; not used in deep cavities or wounds, e.g. sockets.
- To avoid breakdown, it is not employed on fresh granulating tissue.
- As mouthwash following tooth extraction because hydrogen peroxide breaks down blood clot.
- Avoid frequent use of hydrogen peroxide because it may cause decalcification of enamel due to presence of sulfuric acid.

398 Principles of Pharmacology for Dental Students

2. **Potassium permanganate (Condy's crystals):** It exists as dark purple crystals with a metallic luster and is a strong oxidising agent which is readily soluble in water. It has *antiseptic* and *deodorant* actions which are produced by the liberation of nascent oxygen and by metallic action of manganese. Its chief disadvantage is staining properties.

Uses: It may be used:

- As a mouthwash for stomatitis and Vincent's infection due to its antiseptic and deodorant properties. For this purpose, a few crystals of potassium permanganate are dissolved in a glass of warm water to make a rose-coloured liquid or a solution of potassium permanganate or it can be obtained commercially as Condy's fluid. However, at present it is seldom used as a mouthwash and has been replaced by dettolin and peroxide mouthwashes.
- As antiseptic, fungicidal and disinfectant due to its ability to oxidize organic matter
- For gargles in concentration of 1:5000
- For uretheral and vaginal irrigation in concentration of 1:5000
- As wet dressings in the treatment of ivy poisoning and for weeping skin lesions
- For stomach wash in poisoning with drugs like alkaloids (such as morphine, atropine, cocaine) and chloral hydrate in concentration of 1:5000
- As a first aid treatment locally in form of solid crystals in case of snake bite to destroy the venom
- As disinfectant to wash tumblers, vegetables and fruits in concentration of 1:5000

3. **Formaldehyde (formalin):** It is available as an aqueous solution which contains 10% formaldehyde gas. It is a clear colourless liquid with pungent taste. It may turn yellow on standing and deteriorates with age. So fresh solution should be obtained frequently.

Pharmacological actions:

- Being a protoplasmic poison, it acts as an *antiseptic*.
- Formaldehyde precipitates metallic silver from ammoniacal silver nitrate and acts as *reducing agent*.
- Because of its caustic action, it should not be employed as a desensitizing agent for dentine because it may kill the pulp.
- In concentrated solution, it is a very powerful *disinfectant*.
- Its vapours are intensely irritating to the mucous membranes of the nose and eyes. It is also not used as a component of mouth-wash due to its irritant action to mucous membranes.

A 10% solution of formaldehyde may be used to reduce ammoniacal silver nitrate solution (Howe's solution) with care so that excess formalin may not irritate the pulp.

Commonly used Antiseptics in Dental Practice

These can be grouped on the basis of their mechanism of action. The possible use(s) is also mentioned.

I. **Which act by precipitating bacterial proteins:**
   - *Phenols:* It is used as 2% aqueous solution or 4% solution in glycerine on skin but not on damaged skin.
   - *Lysol:* It is available as soap in combination with 2% cresol; used as hand wash in operation theatre.
   - *Dettol:* It is a 5% chlorinated phenol which is used as hand wash.
   - *Hexachlorophene:* It is used as 3% powder in soaps and talcum powders.
   - *Alcohols:* 70–80% ethyl alcohol or 50–60% isopropyl alcohol is used for cleaning skin before injections.
   - *Zinc calamine lotion (ZnO + Fe$_2$O$_3$):* It is used on sun burns.

II. Which act by "complexing" with sulfhydryl (SH) groups of bacterial enzymes:

- *Mercurochrome:* It is used as 2% solution on the skin.

III. Which act by "oxidizing" the sulfhydryl (SH) groups of bacterial enzymes:

- *Povidon iodine (Betadine):* It is an iodophore, i.e. it releases I_2 slowly. It is used as 5% lotion to clean wound and as 1% lotion in mouthwash.
- *Tincture iodine:* It is a combination of KI+ I_2 in aqueous ethyl alcohol. It is also an iodophore, i.e. it releases iodine. It is used on cuts and wounds.
- *Sodium hypochlorite ($NaHClO_3$):* It is a chlorophore, i.e. it releases Cl_2. A 4% solution is used in root canal treatment. It is also used to bleach silver pigments on teeth.
- H_2O_2: It liberates oxygen. It is used in mouthwash.
- $KMNO_4$ *(potassium permanganate):* It is used as 0.1% lotion in mouthwash.

IV. Which alter property of bacterial cell wall:

- *Cetrimide:* It is used as 1–3% solution to clean surgical instruments. It is a multipurpose antiseptic.
- *Chlorhexidine:* It is used as hand wash; applied on preoperative skin; and in mouthwash.
- Savlon is a combination of cetrimide and chlorhexidine.
- Benzylkonium chloride is used in eye-drops, eardrops and in mouthwash.

V. Miscellaneous:

- *Acriflavin:* It is used as 0.1% cream in burn dressing.
- *Nitrofurazone (furacin):* It is used as 0.2% ointment in burn dressing.
- *Gentian violet:* It is rarely used as antiseptic for gram-positive organisms or fungi.

TO REMEMBER

1. Antiseptics (inhibit the bacterial growth) and disinfectants (inhibit or kill bacteria) are anti-infective agents, which are used to reduce the bacterial population.
2. Sepsis means the presence of bacteria while asepsis implies an entire freedom from bacteria.
3. Sterilization is the process of freeing an article surface, or a medium from bacteria by removing or killing microorganisms, both in vegetative and sporing states.
4. Antiseptics act as protoplasmic poisons, i.e. They destroy the protoplasm of the cell. Recently introduced antiseptics (e.g. sofframycin) have a selective action, i.e. they will have greater effect on the protoplasm of bacteria than on the protoplasm of the host cells.
5. Redeal Walker's test and Chick Martin's test are used to determine the activity of an antiseptic.
6. Antiseptics are used: (a) as disinfectants of surgical instruments, (b) as antiseptic wash and dressings, (c) as cleansing agent for wound, (d) as preservative, (e) as parasiticides, and (f) as insecticides.
7. In dental practice, antiseptics of importance are hydrogen peroxide, potassium permanganate and formaldehyde (formalin), sodium hypochlorite, and chlorhexidine.
8. Hydrogen peroxide (3% solution) is used: (a) as antiseptic to treat general acute gingivitis and acute ulcerative stomatitis, (b) to remove superficial stains on teeth, and (c) to control gingival seepage during cavity preparation.
9. Potassium permanganate may be used as mouthwash for stomatitis and Vincent's infection.
10. A 10% solution of formalin is used as antiseptic and reducing agent.

Chapter 62

Dental Caries

Dental caries is a degenerative condition. It is characterized by decay of the hard and soft tissues of the teeth.

Aetiology

- Infection and decaying food are two main aetiological factors.
- Xerostomia is also responsible for development of dental caries.
- Carbohydrates particularly act as decaying food due to bad hygienic habits. Acids are produced in the mouth due to fermentation of carbohydrates. These acids then react with the insoluble calcium salts of the teeth and convert them into soluble salts. Solution and fracture can easily remove these soluble salts of calcium.
- *Streptococcus mutants*, principally, along with other bacteria colonize the organic buffering film on the tooth surface to produce plaque. If not removed by brushing or the natural cleaning action of saliva and oral soft tissues, proteolytic enzymes are produced by these bacteria. These enzymes digest the organic enamel matrix. Thus they further enhance the action of acids. Fissures and pits on the occlusion surfaces are the most frequent sites of decay. Surfaces adjacent to tooth restorations and exposed roots are also vulnerable.
- In other words, the proteolytic enzymes digest the organic matter of the dentine and organic acids of the mouth destroy the inorganic matter.
- Over time, dental caries extend to the underlying dentin, leading to cavitation of the enamel and finally penetration to the tooth pulp, producing acute pulpitis. At this early stage, the tooth becomes sensitive to percussion and hot or cold. At this time, the pain is immediately relieved as soon as irritating stimulus is removed.
- Irreversible pulpitis occurs, if infection spreads throughout the pulp and leads to pulp necrosis. At this late stage, the patient suffers with severe, sharp or throbbing visceral pain which may be worse when patient lies down. Pain may be constant once pulp necrosis is complete. Finally, with the advancing decay, infection may reach in the body through lymph and blood circulation.

It is always better to adopt prophylactic measures to prevent dental carries. The best way is to educate the public regarding dental hygiene. It is still better if school children are educated because this will go a long way to eradicate this disease. Important points for maintenance of oral dental hygiene are:

- Teeth should be properly cleaned after each meal.
- Brushing of the teeth every morning and before retiring is equally necessary.
- Proper instructions should be given for the use of tooth brush.

– Carbohydrates (soluble) should be avoided by the patient especially if one is suffering from dental caries.

Treatment

- Dental caries is treated using various chemical agents.
- Urea is one of the oldest chemical which has been used for this purpose.
- To reduce the incidence of dental caries, ammonium ions are applied to the oral cavity. They decrease the number of acid producing pathogen, reduce the acidity of the mouth and dissolve the dental plaques. Some of the dentifrices contain ammonia or ammoniated substances which liberate ammonia in the mouth such as dibasic ammonium phosphate, and urea carbamide. Urease is present in some dentifrices. Urea is broken down to ammonia by urease.
- **Fluorides:** It has been observed that the incidence of caries is high if water supply is deficient in fluorides. So incidence of caries can be reduced by adding fluorides to the water supply (one part of fluoride to million parts of water). Although exact mode of action of fluorides in dental caries is not fully understood, it is suggested that fluorides may act in two ways:
  - By preventing acid decalcification of the tooth structure. This is achieved by fluorides by inhibiting bacterial enzymes which produce lactic acid.
  - By increasing tooth resistance to acid decalcification. Hydroxy apatite of enamel, dentine or bone is changed to fluorapatite by sodium fluoride applied either internally or externally. Thus the fluorapatite is more resistant to lactic acid attack than the hydroxyl apatite.

For prophylaxis, one part of fluoride to one million part of water is considered sufficient. It is used in the form of sodium fluoride.

By this method, incidence of caries is reduced over 50%. During development of teeth structure fluoride is carried to the teeth through the bloodstream and is laid down as acid resistant fluorapatite in the actual structure of teeth. When water fluoridation is not possible, fluoride supplements can be provided for prevention of caries. For this purpose, chewable tablets of sodium fluoride (0.55 mg or 1mg) or sodium fluoride drops (0.55 mg/drops) or sodium fluoride lozenges (2.2 mg) are used. For prophylaxis, 1 tablet or 1 ml of drops or 1 lozenges is taken every day during the period of tooth development by nursing mothers and afterwards by children up to the completion of calcification of third molars.

For prophylaxis of caries, self-applied topical fluoride tooth paste and gels or fluoride mouth rinses may also be used.

For therapeutic purpose, 2% sodium fluoride solution/gel or 8% stannous fluoride solution/gel or acidulated phosphate fluoride (containing 1.23% fluoride) solution/gel/foam is used by the dentist. Among them, most popular form of fluoride therapy by the dentist is the application of acidulated phosphate fluoride. It is applied topically to the teeth after thorough cleaning. This leads to the absorption of fluorine on the enamel surface as calcium fluoride. The procedure is repeated every 6 months. This will lead to 40% reduction in the incidence of dental caries.

Above mentioned agents are saliva miscible aqueous formulations. For therapeutic purpose, non-aqueous solutions in the form of fluoride varnishes (2% sodium fluoride lacquer in alcoholic solution of natural resins or difluorosilane agent containing 0.7% fluoride) can also be applied.

Sodium fluoride is a poisonous substance. So it should be used carefully. Acute poisoning with fluoride may cause nausea, vomiting and burning abdominal pain. These patients are treated by giving a full glass of milk. If necessary give artificial respiration.

When fluorine is ingested for a long period it may cause chronic fluoride poisoning. This is seen when drinking water contains more than one part per million. It affects enamel and dentine of developing teeth.

- **Chlorophyll:** It is present in many tooth pastes and tooth powders with the belief of as a protective against dental carries. It is a green colouring matter of plants.

- **Antibiotics** may be present in dentifrices. They are being used to reduce the bacterial count of the mouth and thereby reducing the incidence of dental caries. For this purpose, penicillin, bacitracin, aureomycin, chloramphenical and streptomycin have been used.

- **Hexachlorophene:** It has not been found useful to reduce oral bacterial population or incidence of dental caries. Since it has been found very toxic, it is advised not to use it for any toilet and cosmetic purpose.

- **Silver nitrate:** Before using it clean debris and decaying material. It is applied on the deciduous teeth.

TO REMEMBER

1. Dental caries is a degenerative condition which is characterised by decay of the hard and soft tissues of the teeth. It is mainly caused by infection and decaying food.

2. To prevent dental caries, it is always better to educate the public regarding dental hygiene.

3. To reduce the incidence of dental carries, ammonium ions are applied to the oral cavity. They decrease the number of acid producing pathogens, reduce the acidity of the mouth and dissolve dental plaques.

4. Incidence of caries can be reduced by adding fluorides in water supply (one part of fluoride to million part of water). Fluorides may act: (a) by preventing acids decalcification of the tooth structure and (b) by increasing the resistance to acid decalcification.

5. For therapeutic purposes, 2% sodium fluoride solution is used topically to the teeth after thorough cleaning.

6. Other agents used to treat dental caries are chlorophyll, antibiotics and silver nitrate.

Chapter 63

Dental Abrasives

Dental abrasives are fine powder preparations.
- They help the scouring action of toothbrush mechanically.
- Some of them are utilized in the manufacture of toothpastes and tooth powder.
- Their help is also taken for cleaning, polishing and fittings the teeth.

To avoid scratching of enamel, they should not contain gritty particles. They should be in a form of fine powder that passes through a 60 mesh powder sieve.

Commonly used dental abrasives are:
- Calcium carbonate (precipitated chalk)
- Creata (prepared chalk)
- Heavy and light magnesium carbonate
- Kaolin
- Calcium phosphate and dibasic calcium phosphate
- Heavy and light magnesium oxide
- Milk of magnesia
- Stanic oxide
- Charcoal
- Ferric oxide
- Powder pumice

Among all these agents, dibasic calcium phosphate has the least scratching or abrasive action. Calcium carbonate and chalk scratch surfaces of the hardness of cementum and dentine. The pastes made of with calcium phosphate, magnesium carbonate and oxide have a greater scratching power but most of these scratch surfaces of the hardness of enamel.

Following are the characteristics and pharmaco-therapeutics of the most commonly used dental abrasives:

1. **Pumice:** It is of volcanic origin. It is a light porous stone. It consists of complex silicates of aluminium, potassium and sodium chiefly. It exists as very light, hard, rough porous grayish masses or a gritty, grayish powder of several grades of fitness. It is odourless, tasteless and stable in air. It is insoluble in water and is not attacked by acids or alkali hydroxide solutions. It is available as pumice with glycerine which is used to polish, fill and clean teeth. Being a powerful abrasive, it should not be employed for every day use.

2. **Precipitated calcium carbonate:** It is white, odourless, tasteless, high quality finely ground microcrystalline chalk, which is prepared by double decomposition of calcium chloride and sodium carbonate in aqueous solution. Various grades of fineness, weight and colour of precipitated calcium carbonate will depend on the process of manufacture. Commercial form of calcium carbonate is available as heavy and light forms. Its dose is 1–5 gm that is repeated in accordance with the need of the patient. It absorbs insignificant amount of moisture at 25°C

at relative humidity up to 90%. It is practically insoluble in water and alcohol. It is dissolved with effervescence in dilute acetic, hydrochloric or nitric acids. It is a mild abrasive. It is employed to give the final polish to silver amalgam fillings. To have maximum effect, it is used either dry or mixed with little alcohol. Its other important use is in the manufacture of toothpaste and tooth powders.

TO REMEMBER

1. Dental abrasives are fine powder preparations which pass through a 60 mesh powder sieve.

2. Dental abrasives are used: (a) to help the scouring action of toothbrush mechanically and (b) for cleaning, polishing and filling the teeth.

3. Most commonly used dental abrasives are pumice and precipitated calcium carbonate.

4. Pumice consists of silicates of aluminium, potassium and sodium chiefly. To polish, fill and clean teeth, the pumice with glycerine is employed.

5. Precipitated calcium carbonate is a mild abrasive which is employed to give the final polish to silver amalgam fillings. It is also used to prepare toothpastes and tooth powders.

Chapter 64

Dentifrices

Dentifrices are therapeutic mechanical aids which are available as either tooth powder or tooth paste. These may be prepared in the form of bulk powder, generally containing a soap or detergent, mild abrasive and anti-carcinogenic agent.

Properties of Ideal Good Oral Preparations

It should be:
- Non-caustic to the mucous membrane
- Non-decalcifying and non-overabrasive to the teeth
- Non-poisonous to the body as a whole

It must not:
- Inhibit the secretion and alter the reaction of saliva
- Destroy the ferments of saliva

It should have:
- Pleasant taste, odour and consistency
- Sufficient cleansing action

Since all these properties are not found in a single oral preparation, many ingredients are used together to prepare tooth powder or tooth paste. These various ingredients are:

1. **Abrasive agents:** Already discussed in previous chapter.
2. **Detergents:** These are cleaning agents. They can be classified on the basis of their mechanism of action:
   i. *Sodium bicarbonate:* It acts by dissolving the proteins. It is a mild alkali.

ii. *Hydrogen peroxide:* It acts by liberating oxygen.
iii. *Hard soaps:* They act by lowering the surface tension. They are prepared by heating any vegetable oil or their fatty acids with sodium hydroxide. They are grayish white or yellowish white in colour. They are available as odourless solid or powder. They are partially soluble in water. They are completely soluble in alcohol. They are incompatible with strong acid and heavy metal salts.

They are commonly used detergents in tooth powders and tooth pastes. The proportion of hard soap in most tooth powders and tooth pastes varies from 5 to 25%. Hard soap has multipurpose actions:

- It is an excellent cleansing agent. To achieve this goal, it acts by dissolving fatty substances, mucous plaques, and lowering surface tension.
- It causes loosening of debris adhering to teeth.
- It also acts as lubricant when scrubbed over the teeth and gums.

Sodium fitinakats, sapomollis, spoani-males, alkylsulphite, etc. are the hard soaps, used for preparing tooth powder and pastes.

iv. Since saponins (e.g. senega, quillcia, etc.) lower the surface tension, they can also be used as cleansing agents.

3. Perborates are substances which liberate oxygen and act as deodorant. They act by detaching the debris and exfoliating epithelium.
4. **Antiseptics:** In dentifrices, the value of antiseptic is limited because it can be used in very little amount due to safety reasons. Commonly used antiseptics are:
   - Volatile oils (thymol, menthol, eugenol, cinnamon—up to 1%)
   - Benzoic, potassium chlorus, salol, acid boric, magnesium and calcium peroxide (2–5%)
   - Myrrh (15%)
5. **Sweetening agents:** Saccharine is commonly used sweetening agent. The other sweetening agents are sucrose and lactose. Out of the two, sucrose causes less fermentation.

   Saccharine sodium is a synthetic sweetening agent. It is white effervescent crystal or a white odourless or faintly aromatic crystalline powder with intensely sweet taste. It is soluble 1 in 1.5 of water and 1 in 50 of alcohol. It is insoluble in chloroform and ether. Solutions are sterilized by autoclaving and are stored in tight container to prevent fermentation. It is used as a synthetic sweetening agent. It is more palatable and free from after taste of saccharine. It has no food value. So it can be used in place of glucose or sucrose by diabetic and obese patients. Its daily intake should not exceed 1 gm. It has carcinogenic effect and may cause cancer of bladder.
6. **Colouring agents:** To make the preparation attractive and acceptable, the colouring agents are used. Commonly used colouring agents are:
   - Liquor azorubri, liquor rubri, liquor caramini or tincture cocci (1 to 3%) are used to impart red colour.
   - Methylene blue (0.001%) is used to impart blue colour.
   - Magenta (0.05%) is used to give red colour to acid mouth washes.

Following is the formula for a popular tooth powder (1000 gm):

Precipitated calcium carbonate	935 gm
Hard soap	50 gm
Soluble saccharine	2 gm
Cinnamon oil	2 ml
Peppermint oil	4 ml
Methyl salicylate	8 gm

Following is commonly used formula for a popular tooth paste (100 gm):

Dicalcium phosphate	54 gm
Sodium lauryl sulphate	2.5 gm
Carboxy methyl cellulose	0.9 gm
Methyl paraben	0.1 gm
Saccharine sodium	0.1 gm
Propylene glycol	18.0 gm (17.4 ml)
Glycerine	1.0 gm (0.8 ml)
Peppermint oil	0.3 gm (0.3 ml)
Liquid paraffin	1.0 gm (0.85 ml)
Purified water	13.5 ml

This is the basic formula for preparing tooth paste. No doubt various mechanical agents are added to some proprietary brands of tooth paste with the claim of reducing the incidence of dental caries. So far these claims are futile. However, addition of a fluoride compound to tooth paste (stannous fluoride) has recently been reported as reducing the incidence of dental caries.

TO REMEMBER

1. Dentifrices are therapeutic mechanical aids which are available as either tooth powder or tooth pastes.
2. To achieve all the properties of an ideal good tooth powder or tooth paste, many ingredients are used together to prepare them.
3. Important ingredients of tooth powder or tooth pastes are: (a) abrasive agents, (b) detergents (e.g. sodium bicarbonate, hydrogen peroxide, hard soaps, saponins, etc.), (c) antiseptics, (d) sweetening agents, and (e) colouring agents.

Chapter 65

Root Canal Filling Materials

It is most important that root canal filling materials should be rendered aseptic before using them for the root canal. They should be insoluble, non-irritant and able to seal the apex of the root, the dentinal foramina and tubules. In fact, they are employed to act as firm barrier against moisture and bacteria. Commonly used root canal filling materials are:

- Gutta-percha points
- Chlorapercha (10% gutta-percha in chloroform)
- Eucopercha (10% gutta-percha in eucalyptol)
- Silver amalgam
- Silver points

Usually two or more than two root canal filling materials are combined and used for filling purpose.

Earlier pastes were used for this purpose. For example, oxpera paste containing equal parts of formaldehyde, creosote and alcohol mixed with a powder composed of alum, thymol, zinc oxide, each 25 parts. Triformal, asto, and euphenco are the other combinations.

TO REMEMBER

1. Root canal filling material should be aspetic, insoluble, non-irritant and able to seal the apex of the root, the dentine foramina and tubules.

2. They act as firm barrier against moisture, and bacteria.

3. Commonly used root canal filling materials are gutta-percha points, chlorapercha, eucopercha, silver amalgam and silver points. Usually two or more than two are combined and used for filling purpose.

Chapter 66

Obtundents and Desensitizing Agents

OBTUNDENTS

In order to make the excavation painless, the dentine sensitivity is either diminished or eliminated by some agents. These agents are called obtundents. Some important facts about obtundents are:

- A good obtundent should not stain the dentine and should be free from any irritation or pain.
- Further to remove dentine sensitivity, it should penetrate the dentine sufficiently.
- However, if irritant obtundent is applied for a long period, it may cause formation of secondary dentine and the pulp may shrink.
- At present, the use of obtundents has declined due to the availability of local anaesthetics. Xylocaine is now widely used for painless excavation. It can be used either by hypodermic injection or surface application.

Classification

Obtundents can be classified as under according to their mechanism of action:

1. Those which act by paralysing the sensory nerve endings such as:
   - Phenol
   - Camphor
   - Menthol
   - Thymol
   - Creosote
   - Olive oil
   - Benzyl alcohol

2. Those which act by precipitating proteins such as:
   - Silver nitrate
   - Zinc chloride
3. Those which act by destroying the nervous tissue, e.g. absolute alcohol.

Important Features of Individual Obtundents

1. **Ethyl alcohol:**
   - Its 70% solution is used.
   - It penetrates rapidly but not deeply.
   - It is painless and non-toxic to the pulp.
   - It does not cause staining.
   - It acts by precipitating the proteins in the dentinal tubules.
   - Allow the alcohol to evaporate and carry out the painless excavation.
2. **Benzyl alcohol:**
   - Due to its local anaesthetic action, it is useful as obtundent.
   - It can be either used alone or in mixture with chloroform and ethyl alcohol in proportion of 5:3:2, respectively.
3. **Phenol:**
   - It has protoplasmic poisonous nature which is responsible for its obtundent action.
   - On application, it causes irritation followed by numbness.
   - Although it acts rapidly it does not penetrate deeply.
   - It dose not stain the healthy dentine but the infected dentine is darkened.

- It may be used alone or in combination with chloroform and olive oil in proportion of 2:4:10, respectively.
- Its penetrability is increased by combining with equal parts of potassium hydroxide and glycerine. The mixture will make a paste.

4. **Creosote:**
   - Its properties and actions are similar to phenol.
   - The advantage is that its penetrability is relatively more.

5. **Camphor, thymol and menthol:**
   - All of them are volatile oils.
   - They are used as mixture by combining in a proportion of 1:2:1. This mixture has a rapid action and is especially useful for dry dentine.
   - Some times phenol may be used in place of menthol.
   - The mixture acts initially stimulating and then paralysing the sensory nerve endings.

6. **Clove oil:**
   - Like volatile oils, it acts by paralysing the sensory nerve endings after a brief initial stimulation.
   - Eugenol is an active constituent of clove oil and has similar action.
   - The penetrability of clove oil is increased on prolonged contact.
   - It is non-irritating.
   - It stains the dentine yellow.
   - It is often mixed with several other obtundents.

7. **Zinc chloride:**
   - It is an astringent, which is used in a concentrated form.
   - Initially, it causes sharp pain for a brief period which is followed by rapid desensitization.
   - It acts primarily by precipitating dentinal proteins and liberating acid.
   - It does not penetrate deeply and the teeth are not stained.

- It is useful for shallow cervical cavities in front teeth.

8. **Paraform (paraformaldehyde):**
   - It is a prodrug which acts by slow liberation of formaldehyde.
   - Formaldehyde combines with and precipitates proteins.
   - Its onset of action is slow.
   - It does not cause pain.
   - Its main drawback is that formaldehyde may penetrate the pulp and cause inflammation.
   - It is combined with zinc oxide and clove oil or phenol to make a paste.
   - It may be incorporated into cement for temporary filling.

9. **Silver nitrate:**
   - It is similar in action as that of zinc chloride.
   - However, it is less painful.
   - Its drawbacks are poor penetrability and staining the dentine black.
   - It is available as crystal or solution.
   - Its contact with gums should be avoided.

DESENSITIZING AGENTS

A sensitive dentine is recognized by pain. Pain is produced by various stimuli such as touch, cold, sour or sweet food. It is due to exposure of dentine which occurs either by removal of enamel or denudation of root surfaces.

Dentine tubule contains fluid. There occurs rapid movement of fluid within the tubule by a blast of air or hot and cold stimuli. This leads to deformation of the odontoblastic process and adjacent nerve fibers cause pain.

Desensitizing agents, used to treat sensitive dentine, are:

1. **Strontium chloride:** It is added to toothpaste in 10% concentration. Strontium ions have a strong affinity for calcified tissue. They also accelerate the rate of calcification. When toothpaste is applied on teeth, the strontium ions obliterate dental tubules and relieve pain.

2. **Stannous fluoride:** It is available in the form of gel which is applied on teeth. It acts:
   - By inactivating enzymes within the odontoblastic process.
   - By inducing mineralization within the dentine tubules and creates a calcified barrier on the surface of the dentine.
3. **Sodium fluoride** is available as paste or gel. It is rubbed into previously dried sensitive area and left on for about 3 minutes, before rinsing. It may increase secondary dentine formation. Thus it reduces sensitivity by blocking dentine tubules.
4. **Formaldehyde toothpaste** contains 1.3–1.4 % formaline. When used, it reduces the sensitivity by precipitating proteins in the dental tubules. Disadvantage is that it has an unpleasant taste.
5. **Tresiolan:** It is a mixture of two silloxane esters. It is applied to the sensitive surface of dentine after drying by means of pledget of cotton wool. There it polymerizes and forms an organosiloxane resinuous skin in presence of moisture. In turn this material plugs the orifices of the dental tubules, forming a mechanical barrier against exogenous stimuli.

TO REMEMBER

1. Obtundents are agents which are used to either diminish or eliminate the dentine sensitivity in order to make the excavation painless.
2. They may act: (i) by paralysing the sensory nerve endings, e.g. phenol, camphor, menthol, thymol, creosote, olive oil, benzyl alcohol, etc.; (ii) by precipitating proteins, e.g. silver nitrate, zinc chloride; and (iii) by destroying the nervous tissue, e.g. absolute alcohol.
3. At present, the use of obtundents has declined due to the availability of local anaesthetics (e.g. xylocaine) for painless excavation.
4. A sensitive dentine is recognized by pain which is produced by touch, cold, sweet or sour food. It occurs due to removal of enamel or denudation of root surface.
5. Sensitive dentine is treated by desensitizing agents such as sodium fluoride gel or paste, stannous fluoride gel, tresiolan, strontium chloride and formaldehyde toothpaste.

Chapter 67

Mummifying Agents

Astringents and antiseptics are employed to harden and dry tissues of the pulp and root canal in order to maintain the tissues in an aseptic condition so that the tissues are resistant to infection. These are called as mummifying agents when used for this purpose. They are particularly used when it is not possible to remove the pulp and contents of the root canal completely. Since a single drug may be insufficient to accomplish the desired goal, these are generally employed in the form of a paste.

Mummifying Agents—Used Clinically

1. **Paraform:** It is employed in following combinations:
     i. Paraform + zinc oxide + glycerine or
    ii. Paraform + creosote + zinc oxide + zinc sulphate.
   It acts by slow liberation of formaldehyde.
2. **Iodoform:**
   - It has both antiseptic and local anodyne properties.
   - It acts by slow liberation of iodine.
   - It is used as mummifying agent in the form of a paste.
   - The paste consists of iodoform, tannic acid, phenol, eugenol, cinnamon oil and glycerine.
3. **Liquid formaldehyde:**
   - It is not used alone because it is irritant and penetrates dentine and apical formation.

- Being volatile, it is used as paste with zinc oxide, glycerine and a local anaesthetic.
- It hardens the tissue without causing its shrinkage.
- It is diluted with four parts of water before use.
4. **Tannic acid:**
   - It is an astringent.
   - It is prepared from tannin which is usually obtained from nutgalls. The nutgalls are the excrescences produced on the young twigs of *Quercus infectoria olivier* and allied species of *Quereus linne* (*Fam. fagaceae*).
   - Tannin is yellowish white to light brown amorphous powder, glistening scales or spongy masses.
   - It gradually darkens on exposure to air and light.
   - One gram is soluble in 0.35 ml of water or 1 ml of glycerine.
   - It is very soluble in alcohol and practically insoluble in chloroform and ether.
   - It hardens the tissues and precipitates proteins.
   - In this way, it avoids bacterial action.
   - It causes shrinkage of tissues.
   - On absorption, it may cause liver damage.

Creosote and ammonia-silver nitrate are other agents which may be used alone or in combination with other mummifying agents.

TO REMEMBER

1. When astringents and antiseptics are used to harden and dry tissues of the pulp and root canal in order to maintain the tissues in an aseptic condition, they are called mummifying agents.
2. To accomplish the desired goal, more than one drug will be employed in the form of a paste.
3. Clinically used important mummifying agents are paraform, iodoform, liquid formaldehyde, tannic acid, cresol, and ammonia-silver nitrate.
4. Mummifying agents are particularly used when it is not possible to remove the pulp and contents of root canal completely.

Chapter 68

Bleaching Agents and Disclosing Agents

BLEACHING AGENTS

To remove pigmentation of the teeth, bleaching agents are employed. Some of them are as under:

1. A saturated solution of sodium thiosulphate (hyposulphate) is a reducing agent. It is used to remove superficial stains with silver, iodine or permanganate.

2. Perhydrol (30% hydrogen peroxide in water), pyrozone (25% hydrogen peroxide in ether), sodium peroxide (50% aqueous solution) are oxidizing agents. Among them, sodium peroxide has the advantage of forming sodium hydroxide on loosing oxygen. Due to this, a preliminary use of fat solvent is not necessary when sodium peroxide is employed to remove pigmentation of the teeth.

3. Chlorinated lime is a chloride compound. It acts by evolution of chlorine. A drop of acetic acid is added to hasten the evolution of chlorine. Clinically, it is packed into the cavity as a dry powder. Though liquor sodium chlorinate is available but less effective than powder.

4. To bleach the dentine from a carbon or mercury arc lamp ultraviolet rays have been used.

Removal of Special Stains of the Teeth

- Weak ammonia or sodium thiosulphate solution is used to remove iodine stains.

- Silver stains on the teeth are either grey or black. A hypochlorite or iodine solution is used to remove them. After application of the solution, the teeth are washed with a saturated solution of sodium thiosulphate.

- Hypocholorites are used to remove iron stains of teeth. If residual stains are still present, they can be removed by oxalic acid.

- Chlorinated lime and acetic acid are used to remove aniline dyes easily.

DISCLOSING AGENTS

In order to make the dental plaque visible (supragingival), certain dyes are used. These are called disclosing agents. For this purpose, solution of these dyes is used by various ways such as:

- Paint the teeth with cotton swab, dipped in the solution of dye or

- Rinse the mouth with dye or

- Dissolve tablet consisting of dye in saliva by chewing

  After using dye rinse the mouth with water.

Various disclosing agents are:

- **Erythromycin:** It stains the plaque red. Disadvantage is that it may also stain soft tissues.

- **Fluoroscine dye:** It stains the plaque yellowish which can be seen by using ultraviolet light. Advantage is that it does not stain the soft tissues.

- **Two-tone dyes:** It is a solution which is composed of a combination of drugs. Advantage is that old plaques are blue while new plaques are stained red.

TO REMEMBER

1. Bleaching agents are used to remove pigmentation of the teeth.
2. Reducing agent (hyposulphate), oxidizing agents (perhydrol, pyrozone, sodium per oxide), chlorinated lime (evolution of chlorine) and ultraviolet rays have been used to bleach the dentine.
3. Iodine stains on teeth are removed by weak ammonia, or sodium thiosulphate solution.
4. A hypochlorite or iodine solution is used to remove silver stains on the teeth.
5. Iron stains on teeth are removed by hypochlorites.
6. To remove stains of dyes, chlorinated lime and acetic acid are used.
7. Disclosing agents are used to make the dental plaque visible (supragingival). This is achieved by using certain dyes such as erythromycin (stains the plaque red), fluoroscine dye (stains the plaque yellow), two-tone dyes (stains-old plaque blue and new plaque red).

Chapter 69

Mouthwashes

To rinse the mouth, a mouthwash is used. It is generally used in conjunction with a tooth brush. Approximately 15 to 30 ml of mouthwash is used for single mouthful of rinse. Usually one-half to one minute should be spent for single mouthful of rinse. A mouthwash can be used for either therapeutic or cosmetic purposes. Therapeutic rinses or washes can be formulated to reduce plaques, gingivitis, dental caries and stomatitis. Cosmetic mouthwashes may be formulated to reduce bad breath through the use of antimicrobial and/or flavouring agents.

Recent information indicates that mouthwashes are being used as a dosage form for a number of specific problems in the oral cavity, for example:

- Mouthwashes containing a combination of antihistamine, hydrocortisone, nystatin and tetracyclines have been prepared from commercially available suspensions, powders, syrups or solutions for the treatment of stomatitis and painful side effect of cancer therapy.
- Other drugs, added to mouthwashes, are:
  - Allopurinol for the treatment of stomatitis
  - Pilocarpine for xerostomia
  - Tranexamic acid for the prevention of bleeding after oral surgery
  - Amphotericin B for the treatment of oral candidiasis

  - Chlorhexidine gluconate for plaque control
  - Hexatidine as an antibacterial and antifungal agent

Since medicines are added in mouthwashes, they should only be used under the direction of a dentist. Some mouthwashes are employed to relieve soreness by hardening sensitive mucous membranes. To achieve this, astringent mouthwashes may be used alone or in combination with antiseptic. They are required for the treatment of:

- Sensitive gingival oral burns
- Soreness under dentures, etc.

Mouthwashes generally contain five groups of excipients as suggested by Tricca.

i. **Alcohols:**
   - It is often present in the range of 10–20%.
   - It functions as solubilizing agent for some flavouring agents as well as a preservative.
   - It enhances flavour and provides certain sharpness to the taste. It aids in masking unpleasant taste of active ingredients.

ii. **Humectants (such as glycerine and sorbitol):**
   - They may form 5–20% of the mouthwash.
   - These agents increase the viscosity of the preparation and provide a certain body or mouthful to the product.
   - They also enhance the sweetness of the product.

- Along with the ethanol, they improve the preservative qualities of the product.

iii. **Surfactants:**
- They are usually of non-specific class.
- They are employed because they help in the solubilization of flavours and in the removal of debris by providing foaming action.
- The concentration range is 0.1–0.5%.
- An occasionally used anionic surfactant is sodium lauryl sulfate.
- Cationic surfactants such as acetylpyridinium chloride are used for their antimicrobial properties but these tend to impart a bitter taste.

iv. **Flavours:**
- To overcome disagreeable taste, they are used along with alcohol and humectants.
- The principle flavouring agents are peppermint oil, spearmint oil, cinnamon oil, wintergreen oil, methanol and methyl salicylate.
- Other flavouring agents may be used singly or in combination.

v. **Colouring agents:** They are also used in these products.

Following mouthwashes may be prescribed for daily use for prevention of infections, halifosis, post-surgical impactation:

1. Sodium chloride   1 teaspoonful
   Milk of magnesia   1 teaspoonful
   Lime water   1 teaspoonful
   Warm water   1 glassful
   To this colouring, flavouring and sweetening agents may be added.

2. **Detergent mouthwash:**
   Boric acid   90 ml
   Sodium perborate   90 ml
   This is used as a mouthwash after meals. For this purpose, one tea spoonful is added in half glassful of warm water.

3. **Obtundent mouthwash:**
   Saccharine sodium   6 gm
   Peppermint water   250 ml

To use it as a mouthwash after meals, it is diluted with equal parts of warm water.

4. Dilute H_2O_2 (0.6%) mouthwash is used to clean oral debris due to its frothing effect.

Therapeutic mouthwashes:

1. **Antiseptic and astringent mouthwash:**
   i. Zinc chloride   5 gm
       Resorcinol   10 ml
       Peppermint water   250 ml
   ii. Pot. chlorate   8 ml
       Zinc sulphate   4 ml
       Aqua camphor   120 ml
   iii. 1% povidone I_2 mouthwash
   iv. 0.25% chlorhexidine mouthwash

2. **Anticaries mouthwashes:**
   i.   Fluorinated mouthwash consisting of flavouring agent + alcohol + sodium fluoride (0.5%) + sodium monophosphate (0.07%).
   ii. Antiseptic anti-caries mouthwash consisting of sodium fluoride + chlorhexidine
   iii. Antiplaque anti-caries mouthwash consisting of sodium fluoride + triclosan
   iv. Anti-caries antiplaque antiseptic mouthwash consisting of triclosan + chlorhexidine + sodium monofluorophosphate
   v.   Mouthwash for prevention of caries and sensitizing tooth consisting of sodium fluoride + potassium nitrate

3. **Antiplaque mouthwash:**
   i. 0.03% triclosan mouthwash with flavouring agent and alcohol
   ii. 0.25% chlorhexidine mouthwash with flavouring agent + alcohol

4. **Mouthwashes for gingivitis:**
   i. 0.1–0.2% chlorhexidine mouthwash
   ii. 1% povidone I_2 mouthwash

5. **Multipurpose mouthwashes:**
   i. Sodium fluoride + chlorhexidine mouthwash—anticariogenic and antiseptic

ii. Triclosan + sodium fluoride mouthwash—antiplaque and antiseptic

iii. Chlorhexidine + sodium fluoride mouthwash—antiseptic and anticariogenic

iv. Chlorhexidine +sodium fluoride + triclosan mouthwashantiseptic, anticariogenic and antiplaque

TO REMEMBER

1. A mouthwash is used to rinse the mouth.
2. Therapeutic mouthwashes are prepared to reduce plaques, gingivitis, dental caries and stomatitis.
3. Cosmetic mouthwashes are formulated to reduce bad breath.
4. Recently mouthwashes are being used as a dosage form for a number of specific problems in the oral cavity. For this purpose, certain medicines are added to these mouthwashes.
5. Mouthwashes generally contain five groups of excipients: (i) alcohols, (ii) humectants, (iii) surfactants, (iv) flavours and (v) colouring agents.
6. Alcohol is used as solubilizing agent for some flavouring agents as well as a preservative.
7. Surfactants are non-specific substances which are used to help in the solubilization of flavours and in the removal of debris by providing foaming action.
8. Flavours are used to overcome disagreeable taste.
9. Colouring agents are used to give a pleasing colour to mouthwash.

Chapter 70

Dental Protectives and Dressings

Dental protectives and dressings are used:
- As protective linings for cavities in order to prevent staining or chemical irritation of the dentine
- As varnishes over synthetic fillings to protect them from secretions until setting is complete
- To help in pulp healing.

In the dental operative procedures, following dental protectives and dressings are employed:

1. **Zinc oxide:** It is a tasteless, odourless, white powder which is insoluble in water. It is important to keep the bottle of zinc oxide well stoppered because it gradually absorbs carbon dioxide from air. It is a weak antiseptic and is used as basis for ointments and cements.

   Uses:
   - In combination with carbolised resin, it is used as a sedative dressing in cavities for the treatment of bleeding sockets following extraction and also for the treatment of dry sockets.
   - It acts as basis of different zinc cements, e.g. oxyphosphate of zinc cement.
   - In combination with eugenol, it is used as an obtundent dressing. Such dressing is required in sensitive teeth and unfinished cavity preparation. For a copper amalgam filling in a deciduous tooth, zinc oxide and eugenol may be cut down to a lining after setting. After

setting, they may be cut down to prelining in a permanent tooth.
   - Zinc oxide and eugenol combination is available as zonalin. It is employed in deep deciduous cavities to have a lining with sedative qualities and to complete the filling at the same time.

2. **Resin:** It is a fine crystalline powder which is obtained as residue left after distilling oil of turpentine. It is available as carbolised resin and cavity varnish.

   i. *Carbolic resin* consists of chloroform (three parts), carbolic acid (four parts) and resin (four parts). It is used as an obtundent dressing. Carbolic acid is responsible for its obtundent properties and also causes some degree of anaesthesia in nerve endings. It is used in combination with zinc oxide as:
   - An obtundent dressings in cavities
   - A haemostatic to plug bleeding sockets
   - A soothing and antiseptic dressing in the treatment of dry socket.

   ii. *Cavity varnish:* It is prepared by dissolving resin in a volatile solvent (ether, chloroform or acetone). It is applied to silicate filling to protect the gel formation from moisture during the primary setting period. In this procedure, resin is left as a covering for the filling due to evaporation of volatile solvent.

418

3. **Calcium hydroxide:** It exists as odourless, tasteless white powder. For dental use, only sterile powder is employed. So its sterility must be maintained. It is available as bland pulp capping material. For capping pulp material, calcium hydroxide is used in the form of a paste with sterile water. It has advantages over other pulp capping materials because:

   - It is alkaline in reaction and
   - Also stimulates odontoblastic activity

   Capping with calcium hydroxide leads to complete pulp healing in suitable cases. With its use as capping, no sign of inflammation is seen in pulp tissue and dentine bridge is formed beneath the calcium hydroxide which closes the exposure completely.

4. **Glycerine:** It is a clear, colourless, odourless and sweet liquid. It is obtained by decomposition of vegetable or animal fats. It is of a thick syrupy consistency and oily to the touch.

   Uses:

   - Used as a solvent for drugs, e.g. borax (one part) and glycerine (6½ parts) which is applied to the oral tissues for the treatment of thrush. Since glycerine is readily absorbed into the tissues, it carries the dissolved borax with it.
   - Used as a vehicle:
     - With pumice for polishing teeth and filling
     - To manufacture toothpastes.
   - Applied to carbolic acid burns in the mouth following the application of alcohol to remove the caustic effect of carbolic acid.
   - Applied to cracked or dry lips before carrying out dental operations.

5. **Petroleum (vaseline):** It exists as a white or yellow viscous substance which readily liquefies a few degrees above body temperature.

   Uses:

   - Applied to cracked or dry lips during dental surgery to avoid pain to the patient.
   - Used on discs or strips to protect silicate and cement fillings while polishing them.
   - After the cavity has been filled with the silicate cement, a celluloid matrix strip covered with vaseline is placed in position.
   - For applying to a matrix band before inserting a cement filling.
   - To prevent rusting, vaseline is applied on instruments kept in storage.
   - Put vaseline on instruments before placing a carbolised resin dressing.
   - Apply vaseline around the puncture hole before placing rubber dam over the tooth to prevent its tearing.

6. **Gutta-percha:** It is a coagulated milky juice. It is obtained from certain types of rubber trees. Purified gutta-percha is a white, tasteless, odourless inert mass. It hardens on cooling and softens on heating. It is dissolved in oil of eucalyptus and chloroform. It is used:

   - As a cavity dressings for completed or lined cavities, both deciduous and permanent.
   - To maintain space between approximating teeth.

TO REMEMBER

1. Dental protectives and dressings are used:
   - As protective linings for cavities
   - As varnishes over synthetic filling
   - To help in pulp healing.
2. Zinc oxide is a weak antiseptic and is used as basis for ointment and cements.

3. Resin is available as carbolic resin and cavity varnish. Former is used as an obtundent dressing and later is employed to protect the gel formation from moisture during the primary setting period.

4. Calcium hydroxide is available as bland pulp-capping material, which leads to complete pulp healing in suitable cases.

5. Glycerine is used:
   - As a solvent for drugs
   - As vehicle with pumice for polishing teeth and filling
   - To remove the caustic effect of carbolic acid
   - To apply to cracked or dry lips

6. Petrolatum (vaseline) is used:
   - For application on dry and cracked lips
   - To protect silicate and cement fillings
   - For applying to matrix band before inserting a cement filling
   - To prevent rusting of surgical instruments.

7. Gutta-percha is used:
   - As a cavity dressing
   - To maintain space between approximating teeth.

Chapter 71

Demulcents and Protectives

A demulcent is used to protect and lubricate mucous membrane. It is a drug of a viscid nature. Following drugs are used to produce this effect.

1. **Acacia (gum acacia):**
   - It acts as a mucilage.
   - When applied on mucous membrane, it coats its surface with a gummy layer to protect them from irritation.
   - To treat catarrhal infections of the mouth it is used as a demulcent in antiseptic pastilles.
   - It is also used as suspending agent in mixtures and emulsifying agent for preparing emulsions.

2. **Glycerine:** It is clear, colourless, non-volatile, hygroscopic liquid syrup. It is also odourless and has sweet taste. It is miscible with water, alcohol, propylene glycol. It is soluble in acetone and insoluble in methyl chloride, ether and fixed and volatile oil. So it is helpful in reducing oedema. Being hygroscopic, it absorbs moisture. If used as such, initially it causes irritation to skin and mucous membrane. It is, therefore, generally used hydrated with two parts of rose-water. It is available as:
   - Glycerine of borax
   - Glycerine of starch
   - Glycerine tannic acid
   - Glycerine alum.

It is employed:
- As an emollient and protective to the skin
- As a protective demulcent and mild antiseptic for mucous membrane
- Because of astringent action, glycerine tannic acid and glycerine alum are painted on oral ulcers
- As a mild laxative and demulcent
- As a sweetening agent in mixture
- As an ingredient in some tinctures and paste
- For decreasing intraocular tension in glaucoma
- As per rectum enema to promote peristalsis and evacuation of bowels
- In toilet creams and jelly due to its water retaining and emollient property
- As anti-inflammatory in boils, carbuncles and other inflammatory conditions
- As a solvent or vehicle for eardrops because it softens the ear wax
- In jelly to be used as lubricant in endoscopic instruments

3. **Tragacanth (gum tragacanth):** It is a dried gummy exudation from the stems and branches of *Acacia arabica*. It contains Ca^{++}, K^+ and Mg^{++} salts of Arabic acid. It is used:
   - To emulsify fats in emulsion.
   - As suspending agent to suspend resins and insoluble powders in water.
   - As a demulcent on mucous abrasions arising from friction.

- As a valuable fixative for the denture when first worn. For this purpose, either powdered tragacanth or the compound powder is dusted upon the moistened palatal surface of an upper denture. On application, it forms a gelatinous mass which is squeezed towards the edges of the denture under pressure. Due to this, it minimizes air leakage and increases adhesions by suction.

TO REMEMBER

1. A demulcent is used to protect and lubricate mucous membranes.
2. Acacia protects mucous membrane from irritation by coating its surface with a gummy layer. So it is used to treat catarrhal infections of the mouth.
3. Glycerine is used hydrated with two parts of rose water in order to avoid irritation to skin and mucous membranes. It is used as an emollient and protective to skin and as a protective demulcent and mild antiseptic to mucous membrane.
4. Tragacanth is applied on mucous abrasions arising from friction. It forms a valuable fixative for the denture when first worn. It minimizes air leakage and increases adhesions by suction forming a gelatinous mass.

Chapter 72

Astringents

Astringents are used to diminish the excretion or exudation of superficial cells. They act by precipitating proteins in superficial cells, which are thus hardened. The insoluble layer of precipitated proteins has following actions:

- Resists bacterial attack
- Forms a sedative protective coating over the underlying tissue against irritants
- Delays absorption from the surface

They are also used:

- As mummifying agents
- As haemostatics. For haemostatic action, they are applied on bleeding surfaces. They promote clotting by precipitating blood proteins.

There are two types of astringents: vegetable and metallic.

Vegetable Astringents

1. **Tannic acid:** It acts as an active astringent by precipitating proteins and gelatin as tennates owing to its acid radical. It hardens the superficial cells and forms pellicle on them. Due to this, it checks exudation of serum. Although it is slightly antiseptic, its albuminous precipitate resists bacterial growth. Its other actions are:
- Reduces mucous secretion
- Prevents absorption of toxins
- Acts as a protective coating
- Decreases inflammatory reaction
- Retards exuberant granulation

It is available as 3 to 5% lotion which is used as:

- Astringent mouth wash
- Astringent dentifrices
- Mummifying agent
- Obtundent
- Haemostatic

At present, its use has declined on account of hepatic toxicity on absorption.

2. **Catechu:** It has similar actions as that of tannic acid. It is used as an astringent mouthwash.

Metallic Astringents

1. **Alum:**
- It is available as 1–2% solution.
- It has astringent, antiseptic and haemostatic properties.
- It may be used as an astringent mouth wash to harden the gums or for inflamed and ulcerated gums.
- Powder alum is applied on cotton wool to the gum as a haemostatic.

2. **Copper sulphate:**
- It is available as astringent mouth wash in strength of ½ to 2%.
- It is also used to treat indolent ulcers of gums or to syringe pyorrhoeal pockets.

3. **Zinc chloride:** It is available as 5–10% solution. It is a caustic astringent. It is useful for:

- Ulcerative gingivitis
- Apthous ulcers
- Pyorrhoeal pockets

4. **Zinc sulphate:** It is available in strength of 0.5–1%. It is used:
   - As astringent paint for mastoiditis
   - As mouthwash for stomatitis
   - As lotion for chronic alveolar abscess

   The advantage of zinc salts is that they do not stain the teeth.

5. **Ferric chloride solution:** Since it stains teeth, it is rarely used as oral astringent. However, it is employed as haemostatic.

6. Lead acetate is also used as astringent.

7. Silver nitrate is a weak astringent.

8. Mercuric chloride is a weak astringent.

TO REMEMBER

1. Astringents are used to diminish the excretion or exudation of superficial cells by precipitating proteins. They are also used as mummifying agents and haemostatics.
2. Tannic acid, in the form of 3–5% lotion, is used as astringent mouthwash, astringent dentifrices, mummifying agent, obtundent and haemostatic.
3. Catechu is used as astringent mouthwash.
4. Metallic astringents are alum, copper sulphate, zinc chloride, zinc sulphate, ferric chloride, lead acetate, silver nitrate and mercuric chloride.
5. The advantage of zinc salts is that they do not stain the teeth.

Chapter 73

Caustics

Caustics are protoplasmic poisons. They cause local necrosis or/and death of the tissues. Liquification of tissues may sometimes be produced by them. Following are some of the important caustics:

1. **Strong acids:**
   - They cause dehydration of cells and precipitation of cellular proteins which is followed by dissolution as soluble acid albumin.
   - Alkalies are neutralized by them.
   - They are very toxic.
   - So they must be used with great care. At present, they are seldomly used. However, sometimes they may be employed to devitalise pulp and to enlarge the root canals.

   Important strong acids are:
   i. *Sulphuric acid (strong):* It has similar actions and uses as that of other strong acids.
   ii. *Trichloroacetic acid:* It has rapid caustic and antiseptic action. Since it is less painful, it is more suitable than mineral acids for mucous membranes. Its important uses are:
      - To cauterize granulation tissue, small polyp or gum growths and to treat aphthous ulcers. For this purpose, 50% of the trichloroacetic acid is used.
      - While 5 to 20% of trichloroacetic acid is employed for pyorrhoeal pockets,

Vincent's infection and to prevent wetting of cervical cavities.
      - In order to remove tobacco stains, a very dilute solution of the acid is used.
   iii. *Lactic acid:* Since it has very low general toxicity, it is very useful for the treatment of:
      - Gingivitis
      - Leukoplakia
      - Pyorrhoeal pockets
      - Aphthous ulcers
   iv. *Chromic acid:* It has caustic, antiseptic and oxidizing properties. Although irritative, it can be used after diluting it with equal parts of water.
      - For treating acute ulcerative gingivitis, 10 to 20% of chromic acid is used.
      - To treat Vincent's infection, cancrum oris, and papilloma of the mouth, 2 to 3% of the acid is employed.

2. **Strong alkalis:** Strong alkalis such as sodium hydroxide, sodium carbonate, potassium carbonate form soluble alkali albumins with proteins. They also make soaps with fats. They are used occasionally:
   - To liquefy pulp polypus.
   - They are put on the epithelial lining of the pyorrhoeal pockets as watery solution. Although not painful they can penetrate deeply. The wound is gelatinised and heals slowly.

3. **Soluble metallic caustics:** They cause precipitation of surface proteins. They are metallic on toxicity. They do not penetrate deeply. However, they are painful. Important metallic caustics are:
   i. *Silver nitrate:* Acting on the surface of the cells, they precipitate silver albuminate and silver chloride. A 10% solution is used to treat:
      - Polyp
      - Aphthous ulcer
      - Exuberant granulation
      - Dental ulcer

      They are desensitizer of cementum of exposed roots. It is relatively a safe caustic and is not very painful. If proper care is not observed, it may cause recession of gums.
   ii. *Zinc chloride:* It acts on the surface of the cells and causes precipitation of zinc albuminate and zinc chloride. Its uses are same as that of sliver nitrate. For clinical use, 5 to 10% solution is used. It is less painful and does not stain the teeth or gums.
   iii. *Copper sulphate:* It also acts on the surface of the cell and causes precipitation of copper albuminate. It is painful. It is used:
      - To treat exuberant granulations
      - As antiseptic for pyorrhoeal pockets.

4. **Specific protoplasmic poisons:**
   i. *Arsenic acid:* It acts as protoplasmic poison. It causes necrosis of tissues (coagulation necrosis). It is too toxic and very painful, so it is not used.
   ii. *Carbolic acid:* It acts as antiseptic, obtundent, caustic and styptic. It is used as carbolic resin which consists of 4 parts of carbolic acid (9%) + 4 parts of resin + 3 parts of chloroform. It should be used with great care because it can cause internal and external white burns. It is used:
      - For removal of pieces of hypertrophied gum tissues such as gum polypus
      - To control gingival seepage during cavity preparation

TO REMEMBER

1. Caustics are protoplasmic poisons which cause local necrosis and/or death of the tissues.
2. Strong acids sometimes may be used to devitalize pulp and to enlarge the root canal.
3. Trichloroacetic acid is less painful than mineral acids for mucous membranes. So it is often used in dental practice as caustic and antiseptic.
4. Lactic acid is useful in gingivitis, leukoplakia, pyorrhoeal pockets and aphthous ulcer.
5. Chromic acid has caustic, antiseptic and oxidizing properties. It is used to treat gingivitis, Vincent's infection, cancrum oris and papilloma of the mouth.
6. Strong alkalis are occasionally used to liquefy pulp polypus.
7. Soluble metallic caustics precipitate surface proteins.
8. Silver nitrate is relatively a safe caustic and is not very painful.
9. Zinc chloride is less painful caustic and does not stain the teeth or gums.
10. Copper sulphate is painful. It is used in exuberant granulations and as antiseptic for pyorrhoeal pockets.

Chapter 74

Treatment of Dentoalveolar Abscess, Gingivitis and Xerostomia

DENTOALVEOLAR ABSCESS

It is a periodontal infection in a sac like alveolar around the tooth. The organisms most often encountered are:

- Streptococcus viridans
- Streptococcus (anaerobic species)
- Staphylococcus aureus
- Actinomycetes (Nocardia asteroids)
- Gram-positive and gram-negative bacilli including anaerobes
- Fusiform bacteria
- Spirochaetes

Treatment

Most cases of dentoalveolar abscess are resolved in early stages by administering combination of ofloxacin (200 mg twice daily) + ornidazole (500 mg twice daily). If patient does not respond the line of treatment will be:

- Incise and drain the abscess
- Use 0.1–0.2% chlorhexidine mouth wash or 1% povidine iodine mouth wash as adjunctive treatment after incision and drainage
- Suitable antibiotic regimen is carried out for 7 days orally unless mentioned otherwise. Selection of antibiotic depends on following particular situation.
  - a. For patients who are not allergic to penicillin:
    - Early symptoms within 3 days: Penicillin V (adult: 500 mg 6 hrly;

children: 25–50 mg/kg in 6 hrly divided doses.
  - No improvement within 36 to 48 hours—augmentin (amoxicillin 500 mg + clauvulinic acid 125 mg) adult: 1 capsule 8 hrly; children: 20–40 mg/kg 8 hrly in divided doses or alternatively administer penicillin V (doses as above) + metronidazole (Adult: 400 mg 8 hrly; children 35–50 mg/kg 8 hrly in divided doses).
  - b. For patients who are allergic to penicillin or do not respond to penicillin:
    - Early or late symptoms:
    - Administer one of the following antibiotics.
      - i. Clindamycin (adult: 150–450 mg 6 hrly; children: 8–20 mg/kg in 6 hrly divided doses or
      - ii. Clarithromycin (adult: 500 mg 12 hrly; children: 15 mg/kg 12 hrly in divided doses or
      - iii. Azithromycin (adult: 500 mg once daily orally for 3 days; children: 10 mg/kg once daily for 3 days).
    - Alternatively administer doxycycline (100 mg twice daily on first day followed by 100 mg once daily for 6 days) + metronidazole (doses as above).
  - c. In severe cases where infection has spread into facial planes, meropenam

can be used to avoid impending septicemia (Adult: 1 gm 8 hrly by slow i.v. injection; children: 10–20 mg/kg 8 hrly by slow i.v. injection).

GINGIVITIS

Gingiva is the covering tissue of periodontium (fibrous ligament which anchors the tooth into skeleton). It allows the penetration of teeth into an intact mucosa. Inflammation of gingiva is called gingivitis which occurs due to accumulation of microorganisms on the tooth surface along the gingival margin. Frequent appearance of gingivitis can lead to other form of more destructive periodontal disease. Hence, prevention and cure of gingivitis is important.

Treatment

- The most common method is to remove mechanically the microorganisms found in dental plaque via tooth brush and floss.
- Pharmacological agents are used to prevent or reduce plaque in order to effectively prevent or eliminate gingival inflammation. Plaque primarily consists of micro-organisms in an organized matrix of organic and inorganic components. The organic matrix of plaque consists of polysaccharide, protein and lipid components and inorganic matrix is composed of primarily of calcium and phosphorus ions. The microorganisms associated with gingivitis are gram-positive rods and cocci as well as spiral organisms and spirochetes. Hence, it is important to remove plaques.

Antiplaque Agents

1. Chlorhexidine is a bisbiguanide. Its digluconate salt is highly water soluble. It binds strongly to hydroxyapatite (the mineral component of tooth enamel), the organic pellicle on the tooth surface, salivary proteins and bacteria. Low concentration of chlorhexidine is bacteriostatic due to its binding to the negatively charged bacterial cell wall (e.g. lipopolysaccharides). Due to this, it interferes with membrane transport system. Higher concentration has bactericidal effect due to its ability to cause intracellular protein precipitation and cell death.

It is available as 0.1 to 0.2% mouth wash. It is used to facilitate the patient's effort to fight new plaque formation and to resolve gingivitis. After one mouth rinse with 10 ml of 0.2% aqueous solution, the anti-bacterial effect lasts for about 5 hours. Important adverse effects are:
   - Development of yellow to brownish extrinsic stain on the teeth and soft tissue of some patients.
   - Desquamation of soft tissue lesions on prolonged application.
   - Impaired taste sensation.

2. Hydrogen peroxide and sodium perborate are oxygen releasing agents. These have been used to treat periodontal disease-acute ulcerative gingivitis caused by anaerobic agents.

3. Antimicrobial agents:
   - Triclosan is a broad-spectrum non-ionic bisphenol antimicrobial compound. It is effective against a broad range of oral gram-positive and gram-negative bacteria. It acts by binding to cell membrane targets and inhibit enzymes associated with phosphotransferase and protein force systems. Triclosan (0.3%) plus polyvinyl methyl ether maleic acid copolymer (PVM/MA-2%) is available in tooth paste. The substantivity (the period of contact of a drug with a particular state in the oral cavity) of triclosan is increased to 12 hours in the oral cavity

due to its combination with copolymer. The use of this tooth paste leads to:

a. 15 to 20% plaque reduction

b. 25 to 35% reduction in calculus formation

c. 50% reduction in gingivitis. This effect appears to be by a mechanism independent of its plaque activity.

- Metronidazole or tinidazole (given systematically) inhibits plaque accumulation and the development of gingivitis.

- Tetracyclines (as a mouth wash or by direct irrigation or given systemically) reduce bacterial colonization of teeth and periodontal pockets.

4. **Essential oils:** A mixture of essential oils (such as listerine) consisting of thymol 0.06%, eucalyptol 0.09%, methyl salicylate 0.06% and menthol 0.04% in an alcohol based vehicle (26.9%) provides the plaque inhibiting properties of rinsing agents. Essential oils may act: (a) by inhibiting bacterial enzymes, (b) by reducing the amount of endotoxin; the alcohol is probably responsible for denaturing the bacterial cell walls. Adverse reactions include bitter taste, burning sensation in the oral cavity, aggravation of oral lesions and desiccation of mucous membranes on regular use.

5. **Dentifrices** containing stannous fluoride have been shown to inhibit plaque formation because stannous ion may interfere with bacterial membrane function, bacterial adhesions and glucose uptake.

6. **Enzymes:** Mucinases (extracts from dried pancreas containing trypsin, chymotrypsin, amylase, lipase and nuclease) and dextranase breakdown the plaque matrix, consisting of proteins and carbohydrates and disperse microorganisms. These are incorporated in tooth pastes and chewing gum. However, plaque control by enzymes is poor.

Acute Ulcerative Gingivitis (Trench Mouth)

It is commonly seen in teenagers and young adults. The patient complains of moderate gingival pain, spontaneous bleeding, halitosis (bad breath), bad taste with increased salivation due to necrosis and ulceration of gingiva. It is caused by *Selenomonas, Fusobacteria, Treponema, Prevotella, Bacteroides, Eikenella, Veillonella, Actinomyces* and *Streptococci.*

Acute Necrotising Ulcerative Periodontitis

It is usually a condition of patients having severe immunosuppression with low CD4 counts. It is characterized by deep seated bone pain, spontaneous gingival bleeding, halitosis and tooth mobility.

Line of treatment of acute necrotising ulcerative gingivitis and acute necrotising ulcerative periodontitis is same. It consists of:

- Remove necrotic soft and hard tissue.
- Use one of the following treatment for 7–10 days with a follow-up for scaling and debridement:

  a. Tetracycline (250–500 mg every 6 hr, orally)

  b. Tetracycline + metronidazole (400 mg every 6–8 hrs, orally)

  c. Oral penicillin V potassium (500 mg)

- A systemic fungal drug, fluconazole (150 mg once daily) may be prescribed as an adjunct due to high risk of fungal infection.

- Chlorhexidine (0.12%) gluconate mouth wash may be used as maintenance therapy.

XEROSTOMIA

Xerostomia means dry mouth. The causes of xerostomia are:

- Damage to or disease of the salivary glands.
- Drugs with antimuscarinic effects such as atropine and its substitutes, tricyclic antidepressants, antipsychotics, clonidine, etc.
- Irradiation of the head and neck.

Treatment

Xerostomia can be treated as under:

- Take frequent sips of cold drinks.
- Sucking of pieces of ice or sugar free fruit drops.
- Use artificial saliva. It consists of electrolytes which correspond to the composition of natural saliva approximately.
- Xerostomia due to irradiation is best treated by pilocarpine tablet (5 mg) which is administered three times a day with or after meals.
- Cevimeline hydrochloride is another parasympathomimetic agonist. It has been recently approved for the treatment of xerostomia.
- The use of topical fluorides as preventive therapy in a patient with salivary gland hypofunction is absolutely critical to control dental caries.

TO REMEMBER

1. Alveolar abscess is a periodontal infection, caused by streptococci, staphylococci, Actinomycetes, fusiform bacteria, Spirochaetes, gram-positive and gram-negative bacilli.

2. Alveolar abscess is treated by using suitable antibiotic drug(s) or drug combinations.

3. After drainage of pus, local application of antiseptic to the periodontal pocket may be of value also.

4. Gingiva is the covering tissue of periodontium (fibrous ligament) which anchors the tooth into skeleton.

5. Inflammation of gingiva is called gingivitis which occurs due to accumulation of microorganisms on the tooth surface along the gingival margin.

6. Gingivitis is treated as under:
   - Mechanically remove the microorganisms found in dental plaque
   - Use pharmacological agents to prevent or reduce plaque in order to effectively prevent or eliminate gingival inflammation

7. Antiplaque agents, used, are:
   - Chlorhexidine
   - Hydrogen peroxide and sodium perborate
   - Anti-microbial agents such as tetracycline, metronidazole, tinidazole and triclosan
   - Essential oils and enzymes
   - Stannous ion in tooth paste

8. Xerostomia (dry mouth) is caused by damage to or disease of salivary glands, drugs with antimuscarinic effects, and irradiation of the head and neck.

9. Xerostomia is treated by frequent sips of cold drinks, sucking of pieces of ice or sugar free fruit drops and use of artificial saliva. Pilocarpine is used to treat xerostomia due to irradiation.

Chapter 75

Chemoprophylaxis in Dental Practice, Drugs for Oral Ulceration and Inflammation

CHEMOPROPHYLAXIS IN DENTAL PRACTICE

Transient bacteraemia is provoked by dental practice and seemingly innocent activities such as brushing the teeth or chewing toffee. In such cases, the risk of infection is low but the consequences of infection would be disastrous. So such cases may be protected by antimicrobials used prophylactically.

Chemoprophylaxis may be Required

1. **To prevent development of endocarditis in presence of following cardiac conditions:**
   - Prosthetic heart valves
   - Previous bacterial endocarditis
   - Complex cyanotic congenital heart disease (tetralogy of Fallot)
   - Congenital cardiac malformation
   - Rheumatic valvular heart disease
   - Mitral valve prolapse with valvular regurgitation or thickened leaflets

2. **In following dental oral procedures:**
   - Extraction of tooth
   - Periodental surgeries, subgingival placement of antibiotic fibers and rod planning
   - Implant placement
   - Tooth reimplantation
   - Placement of orthodontic bands (not brackets)

- Endodontic instrument beyond apex/surgery
- Intraligamentary injection
- Any procedure where bleeding is anticipated

Chemoprophylaxis is Not Recommended:

1. **Endocarditis prophylaxis is not recommended in presence of following cardiac conditions:**
   - Isolated atrial septal defect
   - Ventricular septal defect and PDA
   - Previous coronary artery bypass graft surgery performed more than 6 weeks prior to dental procedure
   - Mitral valve prolapse without valvular regurgitation
   - Physiologic, functional heart murmurs
   - Cardiac pacemakers and implanted defibrillators

2. **Chemoprophylaxis is not required in following dental procedures:**
   - Operative and prosthodontic procedures with/without retraction cord
   - Non-intraligamentary local anaesthesia injection
   - Intracanal endodontic procedure (post and core build up)
   - Placement of remoprostho and ortho appliances

- Impression taking
- Exfoliation of milk teeth
- Oral radiography
- Fluoride treatment
- Postoperative suture removal

For chemoprophylaxis, drugs are given as a short course in high dose at the time of the procedure to coincide with the bacteraemia. The purpose is to avoid emergence of resistant organisms.

Chemoprophylaxis during Dental Procedures

1. **Those carried out under local or no anaesthesia:**
   - *Amoxicillin:* 3 gm orally 1 hour before the procedure. It is given to adults: (a) who are not allergic to penicillins and (b) who have not taken penicillin more than once in the previous month (including those with a prosthetic valve). However, it is not given to those patients who have endocarditis in the past.
   - *Clindamycin:* 600 mg orally one hour before the procedure. It is given to patients: (a) who are allergic to penicillins or (b) who have taken penicillin more than once in the previous month.
2. **Those carried out under general anaesthesia:** Amoxicillin is used in patients: (a) who are not allergic to penicillins and (b) who have not taken penicillin more than once in the previous month. The procedure followed will be:
   - *Amoxicillin:* 1 gm i.m. or i.v. at induction of anaesthesia and 0.5 gm orally 6 hours later.
   Or
   - *Amoxicillin:* 3 gm orally together with 1 gm of probenecid by mouth 4 hours before the procedure. Probenecid delays the renal excretion of amoxicillin and thus maintains a high blood concentration.

Or
- *Amoxicillin:* 3 gm may be followed by another 3 gm dose as soon as possible after the procedure.
3. **Chemoprophylaxis in Special Risk Patients:** Special risk patients are those who are with prosthetic valves or with previous endocarditis. They should be treated.
   - *Amoxicillin:* 1 gm i.m. or i.v. and gentamicin 120 mg at induction; followed by amoxicillin 0.5 gm orally 6 hour later.
   Patients who are allergic to penicillin or have received penicillin more than once in the previous month should receive:
   - *Vancomycin:* 1 gm i.v. over 100 minutes; then gentamicin 120 mg i.v. at induction or 15 minutes before the procedure.
   Or
   - *Teicoplanin:* 400 mg i.v. plus gentamicin 120 mg i.v. at induction or 15 minutes before the procedure.
   Or
   - *Clindamycin:* 300 mg over at least 10 minutes at induction or 15 minutes before the procedure; then it is followed by clindamycin 150 mg i.v. or by mouth 6 hours later.

DRUGS FOR ORAL ULCERATION AND INFLAMMATION

Causes for oral mucosal ulceration are:
- Trauma (physical or chemical)
- Recurrent aphthae (small white spots on the mucous membrane of mouth) due to thrush, sprue or Vincent's infection
- Infection
- Carcinoma
- Nutritional deficiencies
- Gastrointestinal diseases
- Haemopoietic disorders
- Drug therapy

Treatment

Establish diagnosis and treat the cause. Local treatment is given to protect the untreated area, relieve pain and reduce inflammation as under:

A. **General:**
- To relieve pain in traumatic ulceration use a saline or compound thymol glycerine mouth wash
- To protect and promote the healing of recurrent aphthae, use chlorhexidine or povidine-iodine mouth wash
- Apply carmellose gelatin paste to provide mechanical protection
- Hydrocortisone lozenges or triamcinolone dental paste is useful in recurrent aphthae, discoid lupus erythematosus, erosive lichen planus, etc.
- Use lignocaine (5% ointment) or lozenges or benzydamine mouth wash or spray or choline salicylate gel to relieve severe pain of oral ulceration due to major aphthae

B. **Specific:**
  i. *Vincent's angina:* It is an acute ulceromembranous stomatitis or acute ulcerative gingivitis and stomatitis (caused by *Borrelia vincentii*, an anaerobic spirochaete and fusiform gram-negative rods which are normal pathogens of oral cavity. It is treated as under:
  - Improve nutrition
  - Hydrogen peroxide mouth wash helps in washing away the membrane.
  - Inject penicillin G (10 lakh i.m. 6 hourly) for 6–7 days.
  - Since they are anaerobic microorganisms, inject metronidazole in doses of 400 mg three times a day for 7–10 days.

  ii. *Erythema multiforme (EM) minor and major (Stevens-Johnson syndrome):* It is primarily present on the oral mucosa and skin of the hands and feet. It is characterized by intraoral ruptured bullae surrounded by an inflammatory area; lips may show haemorrhagic crusts; the "iris" or "target" lesion on the skin is pathogenic; patient may have severe signs of toxicity. Onset is very rapid. Usually idiopathic, but may be triggered such as drug reaction (e.g. NSAIDs, sulphonamides, anticonvulsants, trimethoprim-sulphonamide combinations, allopurinol and penicillin, etc.). The condition may last 3–6 weeks. If not treated the mortality in case of EM major is 5–15 %. Treatment of oral lesions consists of:
  - In mild cases, topical anaesthetic mouth washes are sufficient.
  - For moderate to severe cases of oral EM, a short course of corticosteroids is given, if not contraindicated.
  - In severe cases of recurrent EM, treat with dapsone, azathioprine, levamisole, or thalidomide.
  - If EM has been triggered by progesterone, treat with tamoxifen.

  iii. *Stomatitis:*
  a. **Allergic stomatitis:** The treatment consists of:
  - In mild cases, removal of allergen suffices.
  - In severe symptomatic cases, the use of topical corticosteroid is helpful to speed healing of painful lesions.
  b. **Recurrent aphthous stomatitis:** It is treated as under:
  - In mild cases with 2 or 3 small lesions:
    - Use protective emollient such as orabase.

– Relieve pain with use of topical local anaesthetic agent or topical diclofenac.
- In severe cases:
  – Use a high potency topical steroid preparation such as fluocinomide, betamethasone or clobetasol.
  – When major aphthae or severe cases of minor aphthae is not responding to topical therapy, give systemic drugs such as colchicine, pentoxifylline, dapsone, short bursts of systemic steroids and thalidomide.

iv. *Recurrent aphthous ulcers:* These are usually present on non-keratinized oral mucosa (buccal and labial mucosa, floor of mouth, soft palate, lateral and ventral tongue). These are characterized by single or clusters of painful ulcers with surrounding erythematous border. These are idiopathic oral ulcers. They may develop either due to hypersensitivity to the oral bacterial flora or transient depression of immune system by trauma, anxiety or stress. These are of two types:

Minor recurrent aphthous ulcers:
- **Size:** Smaller than 10 mm in diameter
- **Site:** Tongue or lips
- **Appearance:** Yellowish-grey with erythematous halo of inflammation tissue surrounding the ulcer
- **Duration:** 7–14 days; heal up without scaring
- **Treatment:**
  a. Use local anaesthetic mouth rinses, e.g. 2–4% viscous xylocaine solution or 5–10 % benzocaine suspension (swished and spitted)
  b. Apply locally 5% amlexanox paste, a locally acting anti-inflammatory drug or swish and spit out

maltodextrin oral gel as a protective adherent barrier
  c. Replacement therapy with folic acid and vitamin B_{12}

Major recurrent aphthous ulcers:
- **Size:** Larger than 10 mm in diameter
- **Site:** Any area of the oral mucosa
- **Appearance:** Shallow or deep and round with indurated margin; usually single ulcer except in immunosuppressed cases (many)
- **Duration:** More than 21 days; heal leaving scar formation
- **Treatment:**
  a. Topical application of corticoids (clobetasol or flucocinolone gel or dexamethasone elixir mouth rinse (10 mg/100 ml)
  b. For AIDS-associated major ulcers or for steroid resistant ulcers, use 100–200 mg of thalidomide alternatively
  c. Concurrently use antibiotics and antifungal drugs to prevent bacterial or fungal infection
  d. Supplement B_{12} and folic acid

v. *Oral lichen planus:* It is immunologically mediated mucocutaneous disease. It is characterized by white striae in mouth. Occasionally oral mucosal ulcers and erosive gingivitis may develop. Treatment consists of:
- Topical medication with 0.05% fluocinonide and 0.05% clobetasol is very useful.
- Systemic steroids are rarely indicated for brief treatment of severe exacerbations or for short periods of recalcitrant cases that fail to respond to topical steroids. Prednisone is used in doses of 40–80 mg daily for 10 days without tapering.

Number of drugs such as antimicrobials (dapsone, tetracycline, ketoconazole, etc.), antihypertensive drugs (ACE inhibitors, labetalol, hydrochlorthiazide, etc.), anxiolytic (lorazepam), NSAIDs (ibuprofen, naproxen, etc.), uricosuric agent (allopurinol), and sulfonylureas may precipitate lichenoid reactions which may resolve promptly when the offending drug is eliminated.

vi. *Mucous membrane pemphigoid:* It typically produces marked gingival erythema and ulceration. Other areas of oral cavity may also be affected. There occurs painful, grayish-white collapsed vesicle or bullae of full thickness epithelium with peripheral erythematous zone. The gingival lesions desquamate and leave ulcerated area. It has protracted course with remissions and exacerbations. Glucocorticoids may temporarily reduce symptoms but do not control the disease.

vii. *Pemphigus vulgaris:* It is mostly seen in older adults. Usually (> 70%) the condition presents with oral lesions, which are fragile, ruptured bullae and ulcerated oral areas. With repeated development of bullae, toxicity may lead to cachexia, infection and death within 2 years. It is often controllable with oral glucocorticoids.

TO REMEMBER

1. Chemoprophylaxis during dental procedure is important to control transient bacteraemia. It may lead to infection which would be disastrous, e.g. infection of prosthetic joints or prosthetic heart valves.

2. Drugs used for chemoprophylaxis are amoxicillin, clindamycin, vancomycin or teicoplanin. Drugs are given as a short course in high doses at the time of procedure to coincide with the bacteraemia to avoid emergence of resistant organisms.

3. Oral ulceration and inflammation may be produced by physical or chemical trauma, recurrent aphthae, infection, carcinoma, nutritional deficiencies, gastrointestinal tract and haemopoietic disorders and due to drug therapy.

4. Treat the cause of oral ulceration and inflammation. Local treatment is given to protect the untreated area, relieve pain and reduce inflammation by various mouthwashes (saline or compound thymol glycerine mouthwash; chlorhexidine or povidine-iodine mouthwash; benzydamine mouthwash), pastes (carmellose gelatin paste; triamcinolone dental paste), lozenges (hydrocortisone; lignocaine) and choline salicylate gel.

Chapter 76

General Dental Considerations in the Use of Drugs

1. **Teach to the patients:**
   - Importance of good oral hygiene to prevent soft tissue inflammation and minimize gingival overgrowth
   - Caution to prevent injury while using oral hygiene aids
2. Assess salivary flow as a factor in caries, periodontal diseases and candidiasis.
3. Monitor vital signs on every appointment due to cardiovascular and respiratory side effects of drugs.
4. When chronic dry mouth occurs, advise patient:
   - Avoid mouth rinses with high alcohol content due to drying effects
   - To use daily home fluoride products for anticaries effect
   - To use sugarless gum, frequent sips of water or salivary substitutes
5. Use lower doses to geriatric patients because they are more susceptible to drug effects.
6. Patients on chronic drug therapy may rarely present with symptoms of blood dyscrasias, which can include infection, bleeding and poor healing.
7. Instruct patient to report to physician, if significant xerostomia side effects occur such as:
   - Increase caries
   - Sore tongue
   - Problems to eating or swallowing
   - Difficulty wearing prosthesis

   In such cases, it is important to consider a change in medication.
8. If an epileptic patient is on valproate sodium therapy, evaluate for clotting ability during gingival instrumentation because inhibition of platelet aggregation may occur.
9. If dental surgery is anticipated, avoid use of non-steroidal anti-inflammatory drugs such as aspirin, ibuprofen, etc. before operative procedure due to risk of bleeding.
10. When fluoroquinolone anti-infective agents are used, following precautions should be taken:
    - Do not use ingestible sodium bicarbonate products such as the air polishing system (prophy jet) unless 2 hours have passed since flouroquinolones.
    - Examine for oral manifestations of opportunistic infections.
    - Avoid dental light in patient's eyes; offer dark glasses for patient's comfort.

Chapter 77

Therapeutic Agents Commonly Prescribed in Dental Practice

There are quite limited numbers of drugs which are prescribed for dental and oral diseases.

Drug	Indications
1. Antibacterial agents	
• Amoxicillin	Endocarditis, odontogenic infections
• Amoxicillin+ Clavulanic acid	Orofacial infections caused by β-lactamase producing bacteria
• Amoxicillin + Metronidazole	Periodontal infections (Polymicrobial in nature)
• Amoxicillin + Clavulanic acid + Metronidazole	Periodontal infections (Polymicrobial in nature)
• Penicillin V	Endocarditis, odontogenic infections
• Erythromycin	Endocarditis, odontogenic infections
• Roxithromycin	Endocarditis, odontogenic infections
• Clarithromycin	Endocarditis, odontogenic infections due to gram-positive anaerobes
• Azithromycin	Orofacial infections caused by spirochetes and gram-negative anaerobes
• Clindamycin	Gram-negative anaerobic bacilli; odontogenic infections
• Cephalexin	Odontogenic infections
• Cefuroxime	Odontogenic infections
• Cefpodoxime	Odontogenic infections
• Cefixime	Odontogenic infections
• Meropenem	Acute aerobic + anaerobic orofacial infections

Drug	Indications
• Doxycycline	Topical for recurrent aphthous stomatitis, juvenile periodontitis (LJP) due to *Actinomyces* and *Actinobacillus*
• Vancomycin	Endocarditis, odontogenic infections; rescue from clindamycin colitis
• Metronidazole	Chronic, refractory periodontitis (antiprotozoal drug)
• Ciprofloxacin+ Tinidazole	Refractory periodontitis associated with Entrobacteriacea
• Ofloxacin+ Ornidazole	Refractory periodontitis associated with Entrobacteriacea
2. Antifungal agents	
• Nystatin	Oral candidiasis
• Clotrimazole	Oral candidiasis
• Ketoconazole	Oral candidiasis
• Fluconazole	Oral candidiasis
• Miconazole	Oral candidiasis
• Itraconazole	Oral candidiasis
3. Antiviral agents	
• Acyclovir	Herpes simplex, varicella zoster, hairy leukoplakia Oral ulcerative or bullous disease
4. Analgesics	
• Aspirin	Mild pain
• Acetaminophen	Mild pain
• Ibuprofen	Mild pain
• Codeine	Moderate pain
• Hydrocodone	Moderate pain

Drug	Indications
• Oxycodone	Moderate pain
• Meperidine	Moderate pain
• Hydromorphone Hydrochloride	Severe pain
• Carbamazepine	Trigeminal neuralgia

5. **Anti-inflammatory agents: Steroids and sulpha drugs**

Drug	Indications
• Triamcilone	Oral ulcerative or bullous disease
• Fluocinonide	Oral ulcerative or bullous disease (topical)
• Clobetasol	Oral ulcerative or bullous disease (topical)
• Dexamethasone	Oral suspension topical rinse for ulcerative or bullous diseases
• Prednisone	Oral ulcerative or bullous disease (systemic use)
• Methylpred-nisolone	Oral ulcerative or bullous disease (systemic)
• Dapsone	Mucous membrane pemphigoid
• Azathioprine	Severe oral ulcerative or bullous disease

6. **Anxiolytic agents**

Drug	Indications
• Benzodiazepines	Preoperative sedation in anxious patients, muscle relaxation in craniofacial and cervical myalgia

7. **Muscle relaxants**

Drug	Indications
• Baclofen	Muscle relaxation for craniofacial and cervical myalgia
• Chlorzoxazone	Muscle relaxation for craniofacial and cervical myalgia
• Cyclobenzamine	Muscle relaxation for craniofacial and cervical myalgia

8. **Antidepressants**

Drug	Indications
• Tricyclics and tetracyclic	Burning mouth syndrome, atypical facial pain and odontalgia
• Fluoxetine	Burning mouth syndrome, atypical facial pain and odontalgias

9. **Sedative-hypnotics**

Drug	Indications
• Chloral-hydrate	Preoperative paedriatic sedation
• Barbiturates	Intermediate acting for preoperative sedation in adults

10. **Antihistamines**

Drug	Indications
• Diphenhydramine	To reverse type I allergic reactions, e.g. penicillin reaction, stomatitis
• Promethazine	To reverse type I allergic reactions, e.g. penicillin reaction, stomatitis

11. **Antineoplastic agents**

Drug	Indications
• Fluorouracil cream	Actinic cheilitis, actinic keratosis

12. **Sialogogues**
   • Pilocarpine hydrochloride

13. **Mouth rinse preparations**

Drug	Indications
• Antihistamines (promethazine and diphenhydramine syrup or elixir, 50/50 kaopectate)	Palliative mouth rinse for oral ulcers and erosions
• Anaesthetic: 2% lidocaine viscous	Sore mouth, oral ulcerations and erosions
• Chlorhexidine gluconate	Periodontal disease, gingivitis, candidiasis, aphthous ulcers
• Tetracycline oral suspension	Recurrent aphthous stomatitis

14. **Emergency drugs:** These are kept in every dental clinic. These drugs are:
   a. Adrenaline
   b. Atropine
   c. Aminophylline injection
   d. Dopamine
   e. Dexamethasone
   f. Fortvin (pentazocine i.m. injection)
   g. Fluids (ringers; normal saline)
   h. Glucose
   i. Hydrocortisone
   j. Nifedipine
   k. Nitroglycerine
   l. Propranol
   m. Prednisolone

Chapter 78

Toothbrushing Techniques

There are several techniques for tooth-brushing. They are as under:

- Scrub technique
- Roll's technique
- Fone's technique
- Bass method (sulcus cleaning technique)
- Vibratory techniques
  1. Modified Stillman's method
  2. Charter's method
- Smith physiological technique
- Miscellaneous technique
  1. Leonard's technique
  2. Powdered motor driven tooth brushing Technique
- Combination technique

Scrub technique: It is probably the most popular method of brushing. In this technique, the brush is held firmly and the ends of bristles are rubbed vigorously over all surfaces of teeth and gum in a manner somewhat similar to that used to scrub a wooden floor. It is not recommended for occlusal surfaces of the teeth. Further this technique should not be preferred because it does not adequately clean the teeth.

Roll's technique: In this technique, the bristles of toothbrush are placed as high in the vestibule as possible in the buccal region with the side of the bristles touching gum tissue. Now exert as much pressure as possible with side of bristles that can be tolerated and simultaneously the brush is moved towards occlusal surface so that it approaches plane of occlusion. Then brush is removed slowly so that ends of brush touch enamel of the teeth. This technique cleans the tooth adequately and gives amorphous management to gingival tissue.

Fone's technique: In this technique, brush is held in occlusion to teeth. To brush, the bristles are pressed rather vigorously against teeth and gums. Then these are revolved in circular manner with large diameter as far as possible. It is particularly effective in case of children of younger age because they cannot use complex techniques. The technique is contraindicated in post-surgery and periodontal diseases.

Bass method (sulcus cleaning method): In this method, the bristles of the brush are placed at the gingival margin. Establish an apical angle of 45° to the long axis of the teeth. Exert gentle vibratory pressure in the long axis of bristles and force the end of the bristles into the facial gingival sulci as well as interdental spaces. This should produce perceptible blenching of gingiva. Activate the brush with short back and forth motion without dislodging the tips of the bristles. Complete twenty such strokes in the same portion. This process is commonly used to all tooth surfaces. The advantages of this technique are:

- It is easy to learn because of easy and short motion of elbow movements.

- It concentrates on the cervical and interdental portion of teeth where microbial plaque is detrimental to gingiva.
- This technique can be recommended to individuals with or without periodontal ailments.

Vibratory Techniques

1. **Modified stillman's method:** In this method, the bristles of the brush are placed partly on the cervical portion of teeth and partly on gingiva. Adjacent to gingiva point the brush is held in apical direction at the oblique angle to the long axis of teeth. Pressure is applied laterally against gingival margin to produce perceptible blenching to give short back and forth strokes, more towards crown along the attached gingiva. Sides of bristles are used and their penetration into gingival margin is avoided. This technique is recommended for cleaning the areas for progressive gingival recession as well as for gingival message in cases of root exposure in order to prevent abrasive tissue.

2. **Charter's method:** In this method, brush is placed on the tooth with the bristles pointed towards the crown with a 45° angle to the long axis of the teeth. Then brush is activated in short circular or back and forth strokes. It is especially recommended for gingival message and for cleaning interproximal areas of healing gingival wound especially following gingivectomy or flap surgery.

Smith's physiological technique: In this technique, gingival surfaces are brushed from crown towards the root in gentle sweeping movement.

Miscellaneous techniques: These are used for occasional patients who cannot carry out complete instructions for gingival message.

In motor driven tooth brushing technique, electric tooth brushes are used. Brushing is done by reciprocal back and forth or both types of motion (circular elliptical motions). This technique is recommended for individuals lacking manual dexterity, e.g. small children, handicapped or hospitalized patients who need to have their teeth cleaned by someone and patients with orthodontic appliances.

Combination techniques: In this method, all the patients start with scrub technique. This is then followed by:

i. Fone's method for young children who have no periodontal problem
ii. Roll's technique for young adults
iii. Stillman and Roll techniques for periodontic patients

Note: The teeth should be brushed properly after meals twice a day. They should be brushed properly, carefully and thoroughly.

TO REMEMBER

There are several techniques for toothbrushing. The salient features of each are given bellow:

1. In scrub technique, the brush is held firmly and the ends of bristles are rubbed vigorously over all surfaces of teeth and gum in a manner somewhat similar to that used to scrub a wooden floor.
2. Roll's technique cleans the tooth adequately and gives amorphous management to gingival tissue.
3. Fone's technique is particularly effective in children of younger age because they cannot use complex techniques.
4. Bass method is commonly used to clean all tooth surfaces. It is easy to learn and helps to remove the microbial plaque which is detrimental to gingival. This technique is recommended to individuals with or without periodontal ailments.

5. Modified Stillman's method is recommended for cleaning the areas for progressive gingival recession as well as for gingival massage in cases of root exposure to prevent abrasive tissue.
6. Charter's method is recommended for gingival massage and for cleaning interproximal areas of healing gingival wound.
7. Motor driven tooth brushing is recommended for individuals lacking manual dexterity, e.g. small children, handicapped or hospitalized patients.

Section 14

Miscellaneous Topics

Section 14

Miscellaneous Topics

- Vitamins

- Antioxidants in Health

- Treatment of Heavy Metal Poisoning

Chapter 79

Vitamins

Vitamins are organic compounds which do not produce energy. These are essential for normal human metabolism. So these must be supplied in small quantities in diet. Vitamin deficiencies occur due to:

- Inadequate intake
- Increased tissue needs
- Increased excretion
- Malabsorption
- Certain genetic abnormalities
- Drug-vitamin interaction

Vitamins as drugs are used in the prevention and treatment of deficiency diseases. These are divided into two groups:

i. **Fat soluble (A, D, E, K) vitamins:** Important features are:
   - Stored in the body for prolonged periods
   - Liable to cause cumulative toxicity, if administered in large amounts regularly
   - Some interact with specific cellular receptors which are analogous to hormones

ii. **Water soluble (B-complex, C) vitamins:** Important features are:
   - Meagerly stored in the body
   - Little chance of toxicity because excess is excreted
   - Act as cofactor for specific enzymes of intermediary metabolism

Vitamin D (Chapter 40), K (Chapter 31), folic acid and vitamin B_{12} (Chapter 30) have already been discussed.

FAT SOLUBLE VITAMINS

Vitamin A

It exists in nature in two forms:

- Retinol (vitamin A_1) is unsaturated alcohol. It is present in marine fish (cod, shark, and halibut) liver oils, egg yolk, milk and butter.
- Dehydroretinol (vitamin A_2) is present in fresh water fish, carrot, turnip, and spinach.

In plants, it is present as carotenoids (β carotene). Retinyl palmitate is the chief retinyl ester in diet. In intestine, it is hydrolysed to retinol which is absorbed by carrier transport and re-esterified. Retinol ester is stored in liver cells from where it is released and transported to the target cells after combining with retinol binding protein. Small amount is conjugated with glucuronic acid and undergoes enterohepatic circulation. Its water soluble metabolites are excreted in urine and faeces.

Retinal is generated by reversible oxidation of retinol. Retinal is a component of light sensitive pigment Rhodopsin which is synthesized by rods during dark adaptation. In case of prolonged vitamin A deficiency, permanent night blindness occurs. Vitamin A plays an important role in the maintenance of epithelia all over, spermatogenesis and fetal development. It is required for bone growth and improves resistance to infection. Manifestations of vitamin A deficiency are:

- Dryness (xerosis) of eye, 'Bitots spots', keratomalacia (softening of cornea), corneal opacities, night blindness and finally total blindness
- Increased susceptibility to infection due to keratinization of bronchopulmonary epithelium
- Diarrhoea due to unhealthy gastrointestinal mucosa
- Dry and rough skin
- Growth retardation
- Sterility due to faulty spermatogenesis
- Abortions and fetal abnormalities

Therapeutic Uses

- To prevent vitamin deficiency during pregnancy, lactation, infancy, hepatobiliary diseases and steatorrhoea 3000–5000 IU are administered per day.
- To treat vitamin A deficiency 50000–100,000 IU of vitamin A i.m. or orally are administered for 1–3 days followed by intermittent supplemental doses.
- Systemic retinoids (analogues of vitamin A) have antiproliferative and differentiating effects on human squamous epithelial cells. So they have been used in the treatment of leukoplakia in dental practice.

  Hypervitaminosis A occurs due to regular ingestion of excess of retinol (100,000 IU daily) for months. It is characterized by nausea, vomiting, itching, erythema, dermatitis, exfoliation, hair loss, bone and joint pains, loss of appetite, irritability, bleeding, increased intracranial tension and chronic liver disease.

Treatment
- Stop further ingestion of vitamin A
- Vitamin E is given to promote storage of retinol in tissues
- Supportive measures

Vitamin—Analogues

- β-carotene: It is derived from carrot and cabbage. It is a precursor of vitamin A and is converted to vitamin A in the wall of intestine prior to its absorption. It is then oxidized to retinoic acid and retinol. It is mainly used as oxidant in doses of 30–300 µg/day (1 µg of retinol = 6 µg of β-carotene).
- Retinoic acid has vitamin A activity in epithelial tissues and promotes growth. However, it is inactive in eye and reproductive organs. It has been applied topically in the treatment of leukoplakia in dental practice.
- Tretinoin (All-*trans* retinoic acid) is similar in actions as that of retinoic acid. It is used topically for acne vulgaris and to reverse the signs of photoaging.
- Isotretinoin (13-*cis* retinoic acid) is given orally for treatment of nodulocystic acne vulgaris and prevention of skin cancer. It is absolutely contraindicated in pregnancy. Its adult dose is 500 µg/kg daily in two divided doses for 3–4 months.
- Eteritinate is used orally for refractory psoriasis. It is also contraindicated in pregnancy.
- Tazarotene and bexarotene are used as gels for topical application in patients of psoriasis and acne. It is contraindicated in pregnancy. Contraception during child bearing age is necessary on its clinical use.

Vitamin E

Vitamin E activity is present in a number of tocopherols, particularly in α-tocopherol. The d-isomer is more potent than l-isomer. It is present in wheat, germ oil, cereals, nuts, spinach and egg yolk. The daily requirement of vitamin E is 10 mg. Vitamin E is absorbed from intestine through lymph with the help of bile. It circulates in plasma in association with β-lipoprotein. It is stored in tissues. It is excreted slowly in bile and urine as metabolites.

Vitamin E acts as antioxidant. It protects unsaturated lipids in cell membrane, coenzyme Q, etc. from oxidation damage due to free radicals. Thus it stops generation of toxic per oxidation products.

Clinical vitamin E deficiency may lead to:

- Certain neuromuscular diseases in children
- Neurological manifestations in adults with hepatobiliary disease
- Increased oxidative fragility of erythrocytes
- Haemolytic anaemia in premature infants and in patients of acanthocytosis due to genetic absence of β-lipoprotein
- Malabsorption syndrome

Therapeutic Uses

It is used:

- To avoid vitamin E deficiency; supplement doses (10–30 mg) may be given to patients at risk.
- To increase survival time of erythrocytes in patients with glucose-6-phosphate dehydrogenase deficiency (100 mg/day for long period).
- To normalize oxidatives fragility of erythrocytes in patients of acanthocytosis (100 mg/week i.m.).
- To enhance absorption and storage of vitamin A
- To afford symptomatic improvement in intermittent claudication, fibrocystic breast disease and nocturnal muscle cramps (400 mg/day).

WATER SOLUBLE VITAMINS

The Vitamin B Complex Group

The vitamins of this group are considered together because they are present in same foods. This group includes thiamine (B_1), riboflavin (B_2), nicotinic acid (B_3), pyridoxine (B_6) and cynocobalamine (B_{12}).

Thiamine (B₁)

It is mainly obtained from pork, beef, liver, whole or enriched grains and legumes, green vegetables, yeast, eggs. It is mainly absorbed by active transport from gut. However, some passive diffusion also occurs when large oral doses are given. It is stored in tissues in limited amount. About 1 mg is metabolized in the body. Excess amount of vitamin is rapidly excreted in urine.

Thiamine acts as a coenzyme in the carbohydrate metabolism after conversion into thiamine pyrophosphate in the body. It may also play some role in neuromuscular transmission. Pyrithiamine and oxythiamine are synthetic thiamine antagonists. A thiamine antagonist is also present in tea.

Deficiency of thiamine leads to beriberi (loss of peripheral nerve function) which is seen in dry (with prominent neurological symptoms) and wet (with prominent cardiovascular system involvement) forms. Neuritis due to B_1 deficiency is also observed in alcoholics and in pregnancy. The daily requirement is about 1 mg. In state of deficiency, it is given up to 30 mg per day.

Therapeutic Uses

- Beriberi
- Chronic alcoholics
- Prophylactically (2–10 mg) in infants, pregnant women, chronic diarrheas, patients on parenteral alimentation

Riboflavin (B₂)

It is found in milk, eggs, liver, green leafy vegetables and cereals. It is phosphorylated in the intestine and absorbed by active transport. It is not stored significantly in the body. Large doses are excreted unchanged in urine. It acts as coenzyme for flavoproteins which are involved in many oxidation-reduction reactions. Its deficiency leads to poor wound healing process, glossitis, eye irritation, photophobia and dermatitis. Daily requirement is about 0.6 mg/100 calories/day. In deficiency states, it is administered in a dose of 5–10 mg orally along with other B-complex vitamins.

Nicotinic Acid (Nicotinamide, Niacin, Vitamin B₃)

Dietary source of vitamin B_3 is meat, liver, fish, peanuts, and enriched grains. It is completely absorbed from gut and physiological amounts are metabolized in the body. However, large doses are excreted unchanged in urine. Only modest amounts are stored in liver.

Nicotinamide acts as a coenzyme in several protein utilization processes and in tissue respiration.

Its deficiency leads to pellagra in man and black tongue in dogs. Cardinal manifestations of pellagra are:

- Dermatitis
- Diarrhoea
- Dementia

In addition to these manifestations anaemia, intestinal haemorrhage, hypoproteinemia, anorexia, lassitude, weakness, inability to digest and assimilate food may occur. Daily requirement is 14–19 mg.

Therapeutic Uses

- **Pellagra:** 200–500 mg/day in divided doses orally or parenterally. Nicotinamide is preferred because it does not cause flushing and other side effects.
- Hartnup's disease in which tryptophan transport is impaired.
- Carcinoid tumours which use tryptophan for manufacturing 5-HT.
- Peripheral vascular disease
- Hypolipoproteinemia
- Prophylactically (20–50 mg/day oral) in people at risk

Pyridoxine (Vitamin B₆)

Dietary sources of this vitamin are wheat, corn, meat and liver. It is well absorbed from gut and oxidized in the body. It is excreted as pyridoxic acid. Little is stored in the body. It is used as a coenzyme in the form of pyridoxal phosphate in the amino acid metabolism.

Deficiency state leads to epileptiform convulsions which are due to lack of GABA whose formation is dependent on B_6. There also occurs dermatitis, skin lesions, peripheral neuritis and anaemia. Daily requirement of pyridoxine is 2 mg. Its dose in deficiency state varies from 5–500 mg per day. Several drug interactions of B_6 are reported such as with oral contraceptive, levodopa and hydralazine.

Therapeutic Uses

- Used to treat and prevent isoniazid, hydralazine and cycloserine induced neurological disturbances.
- Used to treat mental symptoms on oral contraceptives.
- Convulsions in infants and children.
- Prophylactically in infants with deficiency of other B vitamins.

Cynocobalamine (Vitamin B₁₂)

The main use of vitamin B_{12} and folic acid is in megaloblastic anaemia. So they have been described in chapter of haematinics. Biotin (100–300 µg), choline (500–900 mg), pantothenic acid (5–10 mg) are usually included in the B-complex vitamins. They all act as coenzymes in vital body metabolic pathways.

Vitamin C (Ascorbic Acid)

It is a potent reducing agent and its L-isoform is biologically active. It is freely soluble in water and readily destroyed by exposure to air and heat. The main source of vitamin C is fresh fruits and vegetables. It is completely absorbed from gut and widely distributed extra- and intracellularly. It is partly metabolized to active (dehydroascorbic acid) and inactive (oxalic acid) metabolites.

Its important physiological actins are:

- Ascorbic acid is essential for the maintenance of cellular structure and for the synthesis of collagen.

- It plays a role in wound healing and bone matrix formation.
- It is involved in the synthesis of adrenal steroids.

Its deficiency in man leads to scurvy. The characteristic features of scurvy are pathological lesions of teeth, gums, skin and blood vessels. Daily requirement of vitamin C is about 30–60 mg. It increases in disease, pregnancy, peptic ulcer, stress and surgery. Scurvy is usually treated with 1–2 gm per day of vitamin C where as in other conditions it is given in doses of 200–500 mg per day.

Therapeutic Uses

It is used:
- In scurvy
- Postoperatively and in post-injury periods where requirement of ascorbic acid is increased.
- In anaemia because ascorbic acid enhances absorption of iron.
- To acidify urine (1 gm three times or four times a day) in urinary tract infections.
- To prevent ascorbic acid deficiency in individuals at risk.
- In large doses (2–6 gm per day) as a prophylactic in common cold, viral infection, allergies, aging and cancer. But there is no established evidence on its value in above conditions.

TO REMEMBER

1. Vitamins are chemical substances. They are essential dietary factors. These are required in small quantities for various metabolic processes.
2. Vitamins are classified as fat soluble (A, D, E, K) and water soluble (B, C) compounds.
3. Vitamin A is essential for the structural integrity of epithelial cells and the production of photosensitive pigment of the retina.
4. Vitamin A deficiency leads to night blindness, keratinization of the epithelia of cornea, conjunctiva, broncho- respiratory tract, genitourinary tract and gastrointestinal tract.
5. Vitamin E is α-tocopherol. It is an anti-oxidant. Its exact role in man is not known.
6. Vitamin B-complex is made up of different substances that tend to occur together in foods.
7. Thiamine (vitamin B_1) acts as a coenzyme in the carbohydrate metabolism. Its deficiency leads to beriberi (dry, and wet).
8. Riboflavin (vitamin B_2) acts as a coenzyme for flavoproteins which are involved in many oxidation-reduction reactions. Its deficiency leads to poor wound healing process, glossitis, eye irritation, photophobia and dermatitis.
9. Nicotinamide acts as a coenzyme in several protein utilization processes and in tissue respiration. Its deficiency leads to pellagra in man.
10. Pyridoxine (vitamin B_6) acts as a co-enzyme in the amino acid metabolism. Its deficiency leads to epileptiform convulsions, dermatitis, skin lesions, peripheral neuritis and anaemia.
11. Vitamin C is a potent reducing agent. Its deficiency leads to scurvy.

Chapter 80

Antioxidants in Health

Oxygen is required to sustain aerobic organisms. However, it also poisons them through reactive intermediates produced during respiration. These reactive intermediates are powerful oxidants and are called 'free radicals', e.g.

- Superoxide anions
- Hydroxyl radicals
- Nitric oxide
- Transition metal ions such as iron and copper

Hydrogen peroxide, hypochlorous acid and singlet oxygen are not free radicals. They are called reactive oxygen species. They react much faster with biological molecules than normal oxygen. So they are powerful oxidizing agents. Singlet oxygen has been implicated in causation of photosensitization reactions.

Orbitals are spaces in an atom. These spaces are occupied by electrons. Each orbital can hold a maximum of two electrons spinning in opposite directions. Most biological molecules belong to this group. Such molecules can be termed as non-radicals.

Free radicals may independently exist with one or more unpaired electrons. The unpaired electrons are highly energetic. They seek out other electrons to pair from another molecule, which is damaged and changed to reactive second molecule. This reactive second molecule damages the third molecule and thus the process goes on. The activity of the free radical can only be terminated when a free radical pairs up with another free radical. So free radicals are unguided missiles. They bounce round and attack healthy cells. They tear the cell membrane and spill its cytoplasm. Thus they subject the cells to:

- Infection
- Genetic damage
- Mutations

They react with serum lipoprotein (LDL) and cause formation of atheromatous plaques.

They may react with cell membrane lipid and cause peroxidation of polyunsaturated fatty acids and induce generation of further free radicals. Free radicals have been implicated in the following disorders:

- Alzheimer's disease
- Arthritis
- Hemorrhoids
- Parkinsonism
- Rheumatism
- Heart attack
- AIDS
- Cataract
- Stroke
- Cancer
- Stress
- Jet lag
- Senility
- Varicose veins
- Phlebitis
- Immune system disorders

- Long list of degenerative disorders including aging

Free radicals are not entirely bad. The macrophages and neutrophils use them to destroy bacteria and other foreign invaders. However, they become harmful when their production is too much or occurs at a wrong place. This is why the body needs antioxidant compounds.

Antioxidants are also called free radical scavengers. They absorb a free radical. For this, they 'trap' (de-energize or stabilize) the lone free radical electron and make it stable enough to be transported to an enzyme. In turn, enzyme combines two stabilized free radicals together to neutralize.

Antioxidants are needed in the different compartments of the body like the cell membranes, inside the cells, the circulating system and across the "blood–brain" barrier to the brain and the central nervous system. So a variety of different types of antioxidants are needed to combat the damaging effects of free radicals in the body. Important antioxidants are:

1. **Natural (enzyme antioxidants and metal carrier proteins in the body):**
   - *Tocopherol (vitamin E):* It is a fat soluble vitamin. It neutralizes free radicals which are responsible to cause damage to the membranes of cells and to low density lipoproteins.
   - *Vitamin C:* It is soluble in water and is also powerful antioxidant because it is distributed to all parts of the body.
   - Cysteine ⎫ They act either by
   - Glutethione ⎪ preventing free
   - D-penicillamine ⎬ radical production
   - Transferrin ⎪ or by mopping them
   - Ceruloplasmin ⎭ up

2. **Selenium:** It is a trace mineral. It enhances the properties of vitamin E. It is also involved in the synthesis of the enzyme glutathione peroxidase in the body. It also helps the immune system by increasing the antibody response to infection.

3. **Scavenging or chain breaking antioxidant:** These are vitamin A and beta carotene. Beta carotene is a precursor to vitamin A (retinol). It is present in carrots, egg yolk, milk, butter, liver, spinach, tomato, peaches and fortified grain products.

4. **Melatonin** is a hormone and an important antioxidant. It permeates into any cell with in the body. It is an efficient direct and indirect antioxidant. Its important functions are:
   - It detoxifies the highly reactive hydroxyl radicals.
   - It neutralizes single oxygen, hydrogen peroxide, nitric oxide and peroxynitrite anion.
   - It stimulates several antioxidative enzymes.

5. **The building blocks nutrients** are the minerals manganese, zinc and copper. They are required for making superoxide dismutase, glutathione peroxidase, glutethione reductase, catalase and other metalloenzymes. These are called repair enzymes that can regenerate some anti-oxidants. Superoxide dismutase converts superoxide free radicals to the less reactive hydrogen peroxide, which is immediately broken down by catalase into water and oxygen. Glutathione peroxidase is another natural antioxidant enzyme which also reduces hydrogen peroxide to harmless water.

6. **Lycopene:** It is an antioxidant. It is found in tomatoes. Cooking of tomatoes makes it even easier for the body to use their lycopene. As lycopene level in the blood goes up, the levels of oxidized lipoprotein, protein and DNA compounds come down. It reduces risk of prostate cancer, heart attack. Low lycopene concentrations are

found to be associated with early atherosclerosis.

7. Other antioxidants used by the body are:
   • Lipoic acid
   • Albumin
   • Billirubin
   • Coenzyme-Q10
   • Flavonoids
   • Thiols
   • Uric acid

8. Other antioxidants which have been suggested as preventive against heart disease and cancer are:
   • Garlic
   • Resveratrol from grapes
   • Soy isoflavones
   • Turmic

No doubt free radicals are implicated in many diseases. However, it is not impossible that those free radicals are not the cause but the consequences of the disease at least in some situations. Further, it is not possible to give targeted therapy of antioxidants at the site of injury. No doubt for good health antioxidants are necessary but recently we are becoming aware of their toxicities also. Under a range of circumstances, many oxidants can act as pro-oxidants. It is also possible that antioxidants may cause unforeseen metabolic disturbances after chronic use of highly bioavailable pure compounds. However, when antioxidants are procured from natural food, such effects may not be seen. So to supplement antioxidants, natural sources should be used.

Chapter 81

Treatment of Heavy Metal Poisoning

Heavy metals such as mercury, lead, arsenic, iron and gold may lead to poisoning due to:

- Occupational reasons (e.g. in persons working in mines, paint industry, glass industry, pesticide industry and petroleum industry)
- Their use as salts in some medicines of alternative therapy
- Their use as ashes in many Ayurvedic industry

Heavy metals produce their toxic effects by combining with and inactivating the functional groups ($-SH$; $-S-S-$; $-NH_2$; $-OH$; $-PO_3$) of vital enzymes. Due to this they interfere with the normal physiological functions of these enzymes in the body and lead to toxic effects. These groups are called as "ligands". Metal poisoning is treated by using chelating agents (Greek word, *chele* = claw). A chelating agent also consists of polar groups such as $-SH$, $-OH$, $-NH_2$, $-COOH$. These groups can bind a metal ion in a similar way as endogenous ligands bind to metal ions. So chelating agents compete with body ligands (for heavy metal binding) to form stable, non-toxic, water soluble complexes, which are then easily excreted from the body.

Toxicity of Heavy Metals

Mercury

- Inhalation of inorganic elemental mercury usually causes acute poisoning characteri-

zed by severe tremors, chest pain, and shortness of breath, gastroenteritis, nausea, vomiting, kidney inflammation and central nervous system damage.
- Inorganic mercury ($HgCl_2$) also leads to acute poisoning on oral administration. It is characterized by severe haemorrhagic gastroenteritis followed by renal failure.
- Chronic mercury poisoning may result after slow but prolonged exposure of mercury (mercuric chloride or methyl mercury). It is characterized by central nervous system and neurological effects along with behavioural changes (erethism; irritability, memory loss, personality derangement, depression).

Lead

Acute inorganic lead poisoning is less common. It may occur from industrial exposure. Chronic lead poisoning is more common. It occurs through diet or occupational exposure to lead in mine workers, smelter and lead acid battery workers. The characteristic features of lead poisoning are anaemia, and urinary porphyrins. Other features are abdominal colic, reversible or irreversible tubular damage, neuropathies and encephalopathy. In children, there occurs growth retardation, neuro-cognitive deficits and loss in IQ.

Organic lead poisoning results due to tetra-ethyl lead in gasoline and is characterized by hallucinations, convulsions and coma.

Arsenic

It is an environmental as well as occupational hazard. It is an established carcinogen which can cause cancer of lungs and skin. Acute arsenic poisoning causes gastroenteritis, laryngitis, dehydration and shock. A sweet garlicky odour in breath and of stool is indicative of arsenic poisoning. Chronic arsenic poisoning is characterized by skin irritation and colour change, hair loss, nausea, gastrointestinal tract disturbances, bone marrow depression and anaemia.

Arsenic causes massive haemoglobulinuria, and acute renal failure.

Iron

- Chronic toxicity is due to genetic disposition. Due to this, the individual absorbs excessive amount of iron taken orally. So there occurs accumulation of haemosiderin in liver, spleen with haemochromatosis.
- Acute toxicity is characterized by vomiting, diarrhoea, acidosis, shock, convulsions, cardiovascular collapse and coma ensues.

Chelating Agents in the Management of Heavy Metal Poisoning

Chelators spare endogenous ligands, i.e. vital enzymes and proteins. Further they facilitate excretion of toxic metal as chelator-metal complex. Selective chelating agent is needed for treating specific metal ions. Clinically useful chelating agents are as under:

Dimercaprol (BAL—British anti-Lewisite): It is available in peanut oil vehicle. It is used for the treatment of mercury and arsenic poisoning. It is contraindicated in iron poisoning because BAL-Fe complex, formed, is itself toxic. The dose schedule is 5 mg/kg i.m. stat followed by 2–3 mg/kg 8 hourly for two days and then once a day for 10 days.

In a prescribed protocol with edetate calcium disodium, BAL is also used for the treatment of lead poisoning. In case of mercury poisoning, keep the urine alkaline to avoid dissociation of BAL-mercury complex and subsequent reabsorption of metal.

Pain at the site of injection, tachycardia, mild increase in blood pressure, vomiting, tingling, and burning sensation in extremities, sweating, cramps and headache may appear as side effects.

Succimer: It is a structural analogue of dimercaprol (2, 3-dimercaptosuccinic acid). It is orally effective, less toxic and more water soluble. It is more specific for lead chelation and needs no combination with edetate calcium disodium. It is given orally in doses of 10 mg/kg every 8 hours for 5 days followed by 10 mg/kg every 12 hours for 14 days.

It is equally effective in the treatment of acute mercury poisoning. It prevents distribution of orally given mercury into brain and also reduces mercury contents of kidney. Common adverse effects are anorexia, vomiting and diarrhoea. Occasionally, rashes and elevation of liver aminotransferase - enzyme may also occur.

Unithiol: It is also a structural analogue of dimercaprol (dimercaptopropane sulfonic acid—DMPS). It is soluble in water. It can be administered orally as well as i.v. It is used for the treatment of severe acute inorganic mercury and arsenic poisoning. For this purpose, it is administered in doses of 3–5 mg/kg every 4 hours by i.v. infusion over 20 minutes. When the condition of the patient is stabilized, switch over to oral administration in doses of 4–8 mg/kg every 6 to 8 hours. It is also effective in the treatment of lead poisoning.

It may cause self-limited urticaria. On rapid i.v. infusion, it may cause vasodilatation and hypotension.

Edentate calcium disodium (ethylene diamine tetra-acetic acid, EDTA disodium salt): Editate calcium disodium complex chelates with many divalent (Pb, Zn, Cd, Mn and Hg) as well as trivalent (Fe) metals. This salt is used to avoid EDTA induced life-threatening hypocalcaemia as a side effect. It is highly polar compound. So it is not absorbed from gut and poorly crosses cell membranes. It does not cross blood brain–barrier. Hence it is given parenterally. It is usually given by slow i.v. route because i.m. injection is very painful. It is rapidly eliminated through glomerular filtration.

It is primarily used in lead poisoning in combination with dimercaprol as EDTA disodium salt has only poor penetration in the tissues. It forms edetate-lead complex which is water soluble. The treatment protocol includes 50–75 mg/kg/day of EDTA disodium salt by slow i.v. injection 6 hourly and dimercaprol 4 mg/kg i.m. every 4 hours for 3 to 5 days. Adverse effects include nephrotoxicity (can be prevented by maintaining adequate urine flow), myalgia, lacrimation, hypotension and congestion.

Structural analogues of EDTA are still under investigation. These are:

- *Diethylenetriamine penta-acetic acid (DTPA) calcium disodium:* It is less toxic, more effective but has a very poor tissue distribution. It has been found useful in removing radioactive uranium and plutonium.

- *Dicobalt edentate:* It has been used to treat cyanide poisoning. It forms cobalt-cyanide complex which is stable, water soluble and non-toxic.

D-penicillamine (dimethylcystein or 3-mercapto-D-valine): It is a water soluble degradation product of penicillamine. It is readily absorbed from the gut and is resistant to metabolic degradation. It is highly effective chelator of copper. It can also be used to treat lead or mercury poisoning but succimer is more preferred. To treat copper poisoning, it is given in doses of 500 mg twice a day, 2 hours after meals to avoid chelation of other dietary metals. Its other uses are:

- It is also a drug of choice in the management of Wilson's disease heptolenticular dege-neration due to accumulation of copper in brain, kidney, liver, and cornea). It results due to genetic deficiency of ceruloplasmin whose physiological role is to eliminate excess copper, if absorbed from food.

- Used to treat cystinuria (cystine stones) because it complexes with cystine and prevents precipitation in the urinary tract.

- Occasionally used for the treatment of rheumatoid arthritis but its use has declined.

- Used to treat scleroderma patients because it increases the solubility of collagen.

Adverse effects include hypersensitivity (not alarming) and proteinuria (rare), leucopenia and aplastic anaemia.

Trientine (triethylene teramine-dehydro-chloride): It is another acceptable alternative to penicillamine. It is given in doses of 1 gm twice a day on empty stomach. It causes iron deficiency as side effect. Hence to overcome this problem, short courses of iron therapy are given during and after therapy.

Deferoxamine: It is ferrioxamine derivative which is devoid of iron. Ferrioxamine is an iron chelate. It is obtained from *Streptomyces pilosus* and degraded chemically to obtain iron-free ligand deferoxamine. Its unique property is that it can remove iron from ferritin, haemosiderin and to some extent from transferrin, but not from haemoglobin or cytochrome. Since it is poorly absorbed from gut, it is administered parenterally. Its dose schedules are:

- For serious iron toxicity, it is given by i.v. infusion (10–15 mg/kg/hr).

- In moderate iron toxicity, it is administered i.m. (50 mg/kg).

- For chronic iron intoxication (e.g. thalassemia), an i.m. dose of 0.5–1.0 gm per day or oral dose of 500 mg twice a day is recommended.

It is also used to treat aluminium toxicity along with haemodialysis in renal failure. Its adverse effects are diarrhoea, hypotension (if i.v. infusion is rapid), flushing and acute respiratory distress syndrome (rare and with high dose).

Deferiprone: It is an orally effective iron chelator which is used to treat iron overload in patients of thalassemia major. However, prolonged use may lead to Zn depletion. Anorexia, altered taste, joint pain and reversible neutropenia are other minor side effects.

Appendix

QUESTION BANK

1. Discuss biotransformation of drugs in the body.
2. Write the factors which modify the effect of drugs. Give examples for each.
3. Describe briefly:
   - Adverse drug reactions
   - Drug interactions
   - Prescription writing
   - Methods of prolonging the duration of action of drugs
   - Drug addiction
4. Write the general principles of mechanism of action of a drug.
5. What are the different routes of administration of drugs? Discuss their merits and demerits.
6. Discuss combination of drugs.
7. Describe in brief:
   - Sources of drugs
   - Development of bacterial resistance to drugs
   - Factors modifying the absorption of drugs
   - Xylocaine
   - Types of local anaesthetic administration
8. List local anaesthetic agents. Write the mechanism of action, side effects and their management.
9. Describe hypersensitivity reactions to drugs. How will you manage a case of anaphylactic shock due to injection of penicillin?
10. Write short notes on:
    - Preanaesthetic medication
    - Nitrous oxide (N_2O) as gas general anaesthetic agent.
    - Therapeutic uses of morphine
    - Benzodiazepines
11. Write the basis for the use of:
    - Atropine as preanaesthetic agent
    - Dopamine in cardiogenic shock
    - Adrenaline in anaphylactic shock
    - Atropine in pesticide poisoning
12. Give reasons for the use of:
    - Adrenaline with local anaesthetics
    - Combination therapy in tuberculosis
13. Give therapeutic uses of:
    - Atropine
    - Propranolol
    - Morphine
    - Plasma expanders
14. Describe toxicity of:
    - Morphine
    - Phenytoin
    - Barbiturates
    - Alcohol
    - Aspirin
    - Ether
    - Chloroform
15. Describe antiepileptic agents in brief.

16. Name the benzodiazepines used as hypnotic/sedative. Give reasons why they are now preferred over barbiturates for inducing sleep.
17. Classify opioid analgesics. Give the pharmacological actions, therapeutic uses and adverse effects of morphine.
18. Give some points of distinction among morphine, codeine and pethidine.
19. Describe the pharmacological actions, therapeutic uses and toxicity of phenobarbitone.
20. What are sedatives and hypnotics? Classify hypnotics. Describe the pharmacology of important hypnotics.
21. Classify non-narcotic analgesics. Give the pharmacological actions, therapeutic uses and adverse effects of acetyl salicylic acid.
22. List the non-narcotic anti-inflammatory drugs. Write the mechanism of action, side effects and therapeutic uses of aspirin.
23. Describe toxicity of:
    • Atropine
    • Adrenaline
    • Chloramphenicol
    • Chloroquin
    • Sulphonamides
    • Streptomycin
    • Digitalis
    • Corticoids
    • Tetracycline
24. Describe the pharmacological actions, adverse effects and therapeutic use of atropine.
25. Enumerate antiemetics. Give the mechanism of action and therapeutic uses of metochlopramide.
26. Enumerate tetracyclines antibiotics. Describe their therapeutic uses and adverse effects.
27. Enumerate vasopressor agents. Give the management of shock.
28. Describe the mechanism of action of heparin and adverse effects associated with its use.
29. Write therapeutic uses and adverse effects of:
    • Magnesium sulphate
    • Phenytoin
30. Write short notes on:
    • Tolbutamide
    • Cotrimoxazole
    • Oral prophylactic agents
    • Vitamin C
    • Vitamin D
    • Castor oil as purgative
    • Chelating agents
31. Describe briefly:
    • Chloramphenicol
    • Potassium sparing diuretics
    • Insulin of long duration
    • Antihypertensive agents
    • Heparin
    • General principles of antimicrobial therapy
    • Haemostatics and styptics
    • Antiarrhythmic agents
    • Volatile anaesthetic agents
32. Write short notes on:
    • Astringents
    • Bleeching agents
    • Caustics
    • Dentifrices
    • Obtundents
    • Mouth washes
    • Mummifying agents
33. Describe local anti-infective agents in detail.
34. Describe the drug therapy of dental caries.
35. Describe in brief drugs used in the management of dentoalveolar abscess.
36. Describe briefly the drug treatment of:
    • Oral candidiasis
    • Recurrent ulcerative stomatitis.

INDEX